Image-guided Focused Ultrasound Therapy

Ultrasound has been widely used in diagnostic imaging for a long time. In the past 10 years, image-guided focused ultrasound therapy has seen rapid growth in biomedical science and engineering and in clinical medicine. The purpose of this book is to bring internationally renowned authorities and experts in this field together to provide up-to-date and comprehensive reviews of basic physics, biomedical engineering, and clinical applications of focused ultrasound therapy in a widely accessible fashion.

Focusing on applications in cancer treatment, this book covers basic principles, practical aspects, and clinical applications of focused ultrasound therapy. It reviews the medical physics and bio-effects of focused ultrasound beams on living tissues, dosimetric methods and measurements, transducer engineering, image guidance and monitoring (including magnetic resonance imaging (MRI) and ultrasound), treatment delivery systems, and clinical applications. The book also gives practical guidelines on patient setup, target localisation, treatment planning, and image-guided procedures for treatment in various sites, including the prostate, liver, pancreas, breast, kidney, uterus, bone, and brain.

The book discusses major challenges for the use of focused ultrasound energy on living tissues and explores the cellular and physiological responses that can be employed in the fight against cancer from biological, physics, and engineering perspectives. It also highlights recent advances, including the treatment of solid tumours using image-guided drug delivery, and the exploitation of microbubbles, nanoparticles, and other cutting-edge techniques. Readers who are interested in learning more about the technique and the clinical applications described in each chapter can find more information in the comprehensive bibliographies provided.

This book is suitable for anyone involved in, or looking to become involved in, the research and clinical applications of focused ultrasound therapy, including medical professionals, physicists, biomedical engineers, graduate students, and others working in this multidisciplinary field. It offers a balanced and critical assessment of state-of-the-art technologies, major challenges, and an outlook on the future of focused ultrasound therapy. It presents a thorough introduction for those new to the field while providing helpful, up-to-date information and guidelines for readers already using this therapy in clinical and pre-clinical settings.

Key Features:

- Brings together a wide range of world-leading experts in this new field, presenting the latest clinical outcomes of using focused ultrasound for the treatment of benign and malignant diseases.
- Covers the fundamental physics of focused ultrasound therapy and ultrasound-mediated drug delivery, including chapters on the mechanism of sonoporation, microbubble and ultrasound interaction, and their potential clinical applications.
- Introduces clinical guidelines for focused ultrasound therapy, including indications and contraindications, treatment goals, the selection of patients, clinical observation during treatment procedure and follow-up, and characteristics of image changes after treatment.

Series in Medical Physics and Biomedical Engineering

Series Editors: Kwan-Hoong Ng, E. Russell Ritenour, and Slavik Tabakov

Recent books in the series:

Clinical Nuclear Medicine Physics with MATLAB: A Problem Solving Approach
Maria Lyra Georgosopoulou (Ed)

Handbook of Nuclear Medicine and Molecular Imaging for Physicists – Three Volume Set
Volume I: Instrumentation and Imaging Procedures
Michael Ljungberg (Ed)

Practical Biomedical Signal Analysis Using MATLAB®
Katarzyna J. Blinowska, Jaroslaw Zygierewicz

Handbook of Nuclear Medicine and Molecular Imaging for Physicists – Three Volume Set
Volume II: Modelling, Dosimetry and Radiation Protection
Michael Ljungberg (Ed)

Handbook of Nuclear Medicine and Molecular Imaging for Physicists – Three Volume Set
Volume III: Radiopharmaceuticals and Clinical Applications
Michael Ljungberg (Ed)

Electrical Impedance Tomography: Methods, History and Applications, Second Edition
David Holder and Andy Adler (Eds)

Introduction to Medical Physics
Cornelius Lewis, Stephen Keevil, Anthony Greener, Slavik Tabakov, Renato Padovani

Calculating X-ray Tube Spectra: Analytical and Monte Carlo Approaches
Gavin Poludniowski, Artur Omar, Pedro Andreo

Problems and Solutions in Medical Physics: Radiotherapy Physics
Kwan-Hoong Ng, Ngie Min Ung, Robin Hill

Biomedical Photonics for Diabetes Research
Andrey Dunaev and Valery Tuchin (Eds)

Spectral Multi-detector Computed Tomography (sMDCT): Data Acquisition, Image Formation, Quality Assessment and Contrast Enhancement
Xiangyang Tang

Monte Carlo in Heavy Charged Particle Therapy: New Challenges in Ion Therapy
Pablo Cirrone and Giada Petringa

Radiotheranostics – A Primer for Medical Physicists I: Physics, Chemistry, Biology and Clinical Applications
Cari Borrás and Michael Stabin

Image-guided Focused Ultrasound Therapy: Physics and Clinical Applications
Feng Wu, Gail ter Haar, and Ian Rivens

Clinical Insights for Image-Guidance Radiation Therapy: Prostate
Mike Kirby and Kerrie-Anne Calder

For more information about this series, please visit: www.routledge.com/Series-in-Medical-Physics-and-Biomedical-Engineering/book-series/CHMEPHBIOENG

Image-guided Focused Ultrasound Therapy

Physics and Clinical Applications

Edited by Feng Wu, Gail ter Haar, and Ian Rivens

CRC Press
Taylor & Francis Group
Boca Raton London New York

CRC Press is an imprint of the
Taylor & Francis Group, an **informa** business

Front cover image: John Civale (Institute of Cancer Research)

First edition published 2024
by CRC Press
2385 NW Executive Center Drive, Suite 320, Boca Raton FL 33431

and by CRC Press
4 Park Square, Milton Park, Abingdon, Oxon, OX14 4RN

CRC Press is an imprint of Taylor & Francis Group, LLC

Library of Congress Cataloging-in-Publication Data
Names: Haar, G. ter (Gail), editor. | Rivens, Ian, editor. | Wu, Feng, 1962 September 24– editor.
Title: Image-guided focused ultrasound therapy : physics and clinical applications / edited by Feng Wu, Gail ter Haar, and Ian Rivens.
Other titles: Series in medical physics and biomedical engineering.
Description: First edition. | Boca Raton, FL : CRC Press, 2024. | Series: Series in medical physics and biomedical engineering | Includes bibliographical references and index.
Identifiers: LCCN 2023055205 | ISBN 9781498711357 (hardback) | ISBN 9781032756639 (paperback) | ISBN 9780429162671 (ebook)
Subjects: MESH: Ultrasonic Therapy—methods | Magnetic Resonance Imaging—methods | Neoplasms—therapy | Drug Delivery Systems
Classification: LCC RC78.7.U4 | NLM WB 515 | DDC 616.07/543—dc23/eng/20240405
LC record available at https://lccn.loc.gov/2023055205

ISBN: 978-1-498-71135-7 (hbk)
ISBN: 978-1-032-75663-9 (pbk)
ISBN: 978-0-429-16267-1 (ebk)

DOI: 10.1201/9780429162671

Typeset in Minion
by Apex CoVantage, LLC

Contents

About the Series

The *Series in Medical Physics and Biomedical Engineering* describes the applications of physical sciences, engineering, and mathematics in medicine and clinical research.

The series seeks (but is not restricted to) publications in the following topics:

- Artificial organs
- Assistive technology
- Bioinformatics
- Bioinstrumentation
- Biomaterials
- Biomechanics
- Biomedical engineering
- Clinical engineering
- Imaging
- Implants
- Medical computing and mathematics
- Medical/surgical devices
- Patient monitoring
- Physiological measurement
- Prosthetics
- Radiation protection, health physics, and dosimetry
- Regulatory issues
- Rehabilitation engineering
- Sports medicine
- Systems physiology
- Telemedicine
- Tissue engineering
- Treatment

The *Series in Medical Physics and Biomedical Engineering* is an international series that meets the need for up-to-date texts in this rapidly developing field. Books in the series range in level from introductory graduate textbooks and practical handbooks to more advanced expositions of current research.

The Series in Medical Physics and Biomedical Engineering is the official book series of the International Organization for Medical Physics.

The International Organization for Medical Physics

The International Organization for Medical Physics (IOMP) represents over 18,000 medical physicists worldwide and has a membership of 80 national and 6 regional organizations, together with a number of corporate members. Individual medical physicists of all national member organisations are also automatically members.

The mission of IOMP is to advance medical physics practice worldwide by disseminating scientific and technical information, fostering the educational and professional development of medical physics, and promoting the highest-quality medical physics services for patients.

A World Congress on Medical Physics and Biomedical Engineering is held every three years in cooperation with the International Federation for Medical and Biological Engineering (IFMBE) and International Union for Physics and Engineering Sciences in Medicine (IUPESM). A regionally based international conference, the International Congress of Medical Physics (ICMP) is held between world congresses. IOMP also sponsors international conferences, workshops, and courses.

The IOMP has several programmes to assist medical physicists in developing countries. The joint IOMP Library Programme supports 75 active libraries in 43 developing countries, and the Used Equipment Programme coordinates equipment donations. The Travel Assistance Programme provides a limited number of grants to enable physicists to attend the world congresses.

IOMP co-sponsors the *Journal of Applied Clinical Medical Physics*. The IOMP publishes an electronic bulletin twice a year: *Medical Physics World*. IOMP also publishes e-Zine, an electronic newsletter, about six times a year. IOMP has an agreement with Taylor & Francis for the publication of the *Medical Physics and Biomedical Engineering* series of textbooks. IOMP members receive a discount.

IOMP collaborates with international organizations, such as the World Health Organization (WHO), the International Atomic Energy Agency (IAEA), and other international professional bodies such as the International Radiation Protection Association (IRPA) and the International Commission on Radiological Protection (ICRP), to promote the development of medical physics and the safe use of radiation and medical devices.

Guidance on education, training, and professional development of medical physicists is issued by IOMP, which is collaborating with other professional organisations in development of a professional certification system for medical physicists that can be implemented on a global basis.

The IOMP website (www.iomp.org) contains information on all the activities of the IOMP, policy statements 1 and 2, and the "IOMP: Review and Way Forward", which outlines all the activities of IOMP and plans for the future.

About the Editors

Professor Gail ter Haar, DSc, is a renowned expert who works at the intersection of focused ultrasound and physics and leads the therapeutic ultrasound team at The Institute for Cancer Research (ICR), UK. Gail is founding president of the International Society for Therapeutic Ultrasound (ISTU).

Dr Ian Rivens, PhD, is a staff scientist at The Institute for Cancer Research (ICR), UK, with a background in biomedical physics and 35 years of experience of developing equipment and techniques in the laboratory and translating them to bedside research via clinical trials in oncology and fetal medicine He is a founding member of ISTU with extensive experience supervising PhD and MD students.

Professor Feng Wu, MD, PhD, is a world-leading HIFU surgeon who works in clinical applications of focused ultrasound therapy. Feng is currently working as HIFU consultant at Oxford University Hospitals and also serving as senior clinical scientist at Nuffield Department of Surgical Sciences, University of Oxford, UK. He is a co-founder and the first secretary of the International Society for Therapeutic Ultrasound (ISTU).

Contributors

Rodi Abdalkader
Ritsumeikan Global Innovation Research Organization (R-GIRO)
Ritsumeikan University
Shiga, Japan

M. Ahmed
Breast Unit
Royal Free Hospital
London, UK

Giulia Alfieri
Radiological, Oncological and Pathological Sciences
Sapienza University of Rome
Rome, Italy

David Aum
Department of Neurosurgery, Brigham and Women's Hospital, Harvard Medical School
Boston, Massachusetts

David Brenin
University of Virginia Medical Center
Charlottesville, Virginia

Matthew R.D. Brown
The Magnetic Resonance Imaging Unit and Cancer Research UK Imaging Centre
The Institute of Cancer Research
Sutton, Surrey, UK
Pain Medicine Department
The Royal Marsden Hospital
London, UK

Charles A. Cain
Department of Biomedical Engineering
University of Michigan,
Ann Arbor, Michigan

Robert Carlisle
Institute of Biomedical Engineering
University of Oxford
Oxford, UK

Carlo Catalano
Department of Diagnostic Radiology
Sapienza University of Rome
Rome, Italy

Tan To Cheung
Chief, Hepatobiliary and Pancreatic Surgery
Queen Mary Hospital
Clinical Associate Professor
Department of Surgery
University of Hong Kong
Hong Kong

Daniel Y.F. Chung
Academic Clinical Fellow
Oxford Thermal Ablation Service
Churchill Hospital
Oxford, UK

John Civale
Therapy Ultrasound, Physics Department
Division of Radiotherapy & Imaging
The Institute of Cancer Research
London, UK

Constantin C. Coussios
Institute of Biomedical Engineering
University of Oxford
Oxford, UK

David Cranston
Clinical Director
Oxford HIFU Unit
Associate Professor
Nuffield Department of Surgical Sciences
University of Oxford
Oxford, UK

Alessandro De Maio
Department of Radiological, Oncological and Pathological Sciences
Policlinico Umberto I
Sapienza University of Rome
Rome, Italy

Nandita M. deSouza
The Magnetic Resonance Imaging Unit and Cancer Research UK Imaging Centre
The Institute of Cancer Research
Sutton, Surrey, UK

Luisa Di Mare
Dept of Radiology
Azienda Ospedaliera Bolognini
Seriate, Italy

M. Douek
Nuffield Department of Surgical Sciences
University of Oxford
Oxford, UK

Paul Farquhar-Smith
Pain Medicine Department
The Royal Marsden Hospital
London, UK

Stecia-Marie Fletcher
Department of Radiology
Focused Ultrasound Laboratory
Brigham and Women's Hospital
Harvard Medical School
Boston, Massachusetts

Wladyslaw M. Gedroyc
Department of Radiology
St Mary's Hospital
Imperial College London
London, UK

Gail ter Haar
Therapy Ultrasound, Physics Department
The Institute of Cancer Research
Sutton, Surrey, UK

Timothy L. Hall
Department of Biomedical Engineering
University of Michigan
Ann Arbor, Michigan

Maya Harary
Department of Neurosurgery
Brigham and Women's Hospital
Harvard Medical School
Boston, Massachusetts

Mitsuru Hashida
Kyoto University
Institute for Integrated Cell-Material Science (iCeMS)
Kyoto, Japan

Yuexi Huang
Physical Sciences Platform
Sunnybrook Research Institute
Toronto, Ontario, Canada

Kullervo Hynynen
Physical Sciences Platform
Sunnybrook Research Institute
Toronto, Ontario, Canada
Department of Medical Biophysics
Institute of Biomedical Engineering
University of Toronto
Toronto, Ontario, Canada

Jordi Isern-Quitllet
Head of the Department of Gynecology and Obstetrics
Hospital de Figueres
Fundació Salut Empordà
Girona, Spain
Clinique Ambroise Paré
Toulouse, France

Ryan M. Jones
Physical Sciences Platform
Sunnybrook Research Institute
Toronto, Ontario, Canada

Thiele Kobus
Erasmus MC Cancer Institute
Department of Radiotherapy
University Medical Center Rotterdam
Rotterdam, Netherlands

Nicholas Kotewall
Queen Mary Hospital, Department of Surgery
The University of Hong Kong
Hong Kong

Fa-Qi Li
State Key Laboratory of Ultrasound in Medicine and Engineering
Chongqing Medical University
Chongqing, China

Paul Lyon
Department of Radiology
Oxford University Hospitals NHS Foundation Trust
Churchill Hospital
Oxford, UK
Institute of Biomedical Engineering
University of Oxford
Oxford, UK
Nuffield Department of Surgical Sciences
Oxford, UK

Monica Mattone
Department of Radiological, Oncological and Pathological Sciences
Policlinico Umberto I
Sapienza University of Rome
Rome, Italy

Nathan J. McDannold
Department of Radiology, Focused Ultrasound Laboratory
Brigham and Women's Hospital
Harvard Medical School
Boston, Massachusetts

Alessandro Napoli
Department of Radiological, Oncological & Pathological Sciences
Sapienza University of Rome
Rome, Italy

Mirjam C.L. Peek
Research Oncology Division of Cancer Studies
King's College London
London, UK

Stephen Derek Quinn
Department of Obstetrics and Gynecology
St. Mary's Hospital
Imperial College London
London, UK

Natalya Rapoport
Professor Emerita, Department of Bio-engineering
University of Utah
Salt Lake City, Utah

Ian Rivens
Therapy Ultrasound, Physics Department
The Institute of Cancer Research
Sutton, Surrey, UK

Shaun H. Scott
Consultant Anaesthetist
Nuffield Department of Anaesthetics
Oxford University Hospitals
Oxford, UK

David Sinden
Fraunhofer Institute for Digital Medicine MEVIS
Bremen, Germany

Jonathan Sutton
Senior Scientist, Philips Ultrasound Research
Boston, Massachusetts

Amy K. Swinson
Consultant Anaesthetist
Nuffield Department of Anaesthetics
Oxford University Hospitals
Oxford, UK

Travis S. Tierney
Department of Neurosurgery
Brigham and Women's Hospital
Harvard Medical School
Boston, Massachusetts

Joan Vidal-Jové
Director, Comprehensive Tumour Center
Institute Khuab for Interventional Oncology
Barcelona, Spain

Feng Wu
Nuffield Department of Surgical Sciences
University of Oxford
Oxford, UK
State Key Laboratory of Ultrasound in Medicine and Engineering
Chongqing Medical University
Chongqing, China

Junru Wu
Formerly Department of Physics, University of Vermont
Burlington, Vermont

Zhen Xu
Department of Biomedical Engineering
University of Michigan
Ann Arbor, Michigan

Foreword

It gives us great pleasure to have worked with so many expert contributors on this book. Our aim is to provide a "one-stop shop" for those with a clinical or scientific interest in focused ultrasound therapy. We review the fundamentals that are necessary for all keen biologists, chemists, engineers, and physicists working in the area to have an appreciation of. The chapters have been written in such a way that the information is accessible to the many, at the cost of omitting the extreme details that would interest the few. Of course, these can be found in the many important and informative references that we cite. Many of the most exciting and well-established clinical applications are reviewed, but we recognise that we fall short of a truly comprehensive review of all topics, particularly as this is a very fast evolving field. We hope that this volume will inspire the interested reader to push forward the clinical and scientific frontiers of this exciting non-invasive treatment tool.

When focused ultrasound therapy is guided by real-time ultrasound imaging, it can be thought of as a dynamic "seek and destroy" technique. Ultrasound imaging techniques allow targets to be visualised, and the ability to focus an ultrasound beam allows their selective targeting. An advantage of using ultrasound for both imaging and therapy is that a similar beam path is involved for both. However, there are many applications for which target visualisation and treatment monitoring are better achieved using magnetic resonance imaging (MRI), especially where bone lies in the beam path, as in brain applications, and where temperature mapping is considered essential. Thus, the term image-guided focused ultrasound, used in the title of this volume, refers to a technique that can be guided and monitored by either ultrasound or MRI.

At first sight, focused ultrasound therapy seems to have huge advantages over many other therapeutic techniques. It is a non-invasive modality that is capable of highly selective tissue modification using thermal or mechanical means. This volume reflects many of the potential applications for this versatile technique, with the brain, liver, prostate, uterus, breast, thyroid, bone, soft tissues, kidney, and pancreas being included in organs targeted, and thermal ablation, tissue emulsification, and enhanced drug delivery and immune response being discussed as sought-after effects.

The clinical take-up of focused ultrasound therapies has been disappointingly slow, despite its exciting pre-clinical promise. There may be a number of reasons for this, including the lack of available commercial devices. This has meant that many of the early clinical trials have been conducted using "home-made" systems. In addition, the need to occupy an MRI system for extended periods of time may prove challenging and costly for busy departments. Perhaps therapeutic ultrasound has suffered from its own state of infancy as the development of therapeutic devices such as phased array transducers with many thousands of elements has demonstrated a potential that is difficult to implement in the clinic for reasons of cost and complexity. In addition, the essential fields of calibration and quality assurance (QA) have needed to be developed hand-in-hand with clinical implementation, whereas many better-accepted therapies such as radiotherapy have a long history of well-established and widely used processes and procedures. Finally, as the therapeutic potential of focused ultrasound has been realised in a greater breadth of clinical applications and over an increasing width of deployment modalities (from high-intensity focused ultrasound [HIFU] and histotripsy to blood-brain barrier opening and sonoporation for delivery of systemically delivered therapeutics), there has been rapid development of imaging techniques for both guidance and monitoring. In many ways, focused ultrasound therapy was developed ahead of its time, but recent technological advances have meant that clinical realisation of the use of multimodality, multi-element arrays is now possible at reasonable cost. This will reduce treatment times and allow previously "difficult to treat" applications. The treatment of essential tremor through the skull is an early example of this.

Chapter 22 covers the field of sonoporation and was contributed by our esteemed colleague, Professor Junru Wu. Sadly, Professor Wu passed away during the preparation of this volume, but we feel enormously privileged that he was able to finish this chapter, and thus to give us the benefit of his considerable knowledge in this area. We are very grateful to his family, who have given permission to include this chapter here.

Gail ter Haar, Ian Rivens, Feng Wu
November 2023

1

Image-Guided Focused Ultrasound Therapy: Past, Current and Future

Gail ter Haar

1.1 Early History

There are two ways in which the history of therapy ultrasound might logically be traced: by mechanism of action for producing the desired biological effects (thermal ablation, hyperthermia, cavitation, etc.) or by consideration of its applications. In what follows it has been decided to follow the latter approach, as this reflects the structure of this book.

1.1.1 The Brain

The first paper to describe detailed preclinical studies of high-power ultrasound in the brain was published in 1942 by Lynn et al., who were based in Columbia University departments of Neurology and Anatomy in New York, and at the Piezoelectric Research Laboratories in New Jersey.[1] Their paper, published in *The Journal of General Physiology* and entitled 'A new method for the generation and use of focused ultrasound in experimental biology', described their initial investigations into the design, build and output of a focused ultrasound transducer using studies in paraffin blocks and excised beef livers. After achieving good ablation in slabs of fresh liver, they exposed the brains of 3 cats and 2 dogs. As predicted from their preliminary experiments, the main effect they saw was damage to the scalp, with any sign of effects in the brain being seen only at the highest powers used. Subsequent studies by this and other groups involved removal of a bone flap to create a window to facilitate ultrasound exposure of the brain parenchyma without absorption in the overlying skull. The Fry brothers working in Illinois were pioneers of studies in the brain, building a confocal 4-transducer system to study the effects of localised ultrasound exposures in the brains of large animals.[2, 3]

One of the earliest clinical applications was described in 1954 by Lindström et al. This Swedish group removed two bone 'buttons' to allow pre-frontal ultrasound exposure in 25 patients who they treated for carcinomatosis and cancer-related pain.[4] Autopsy in 14/15 patients who subsequently died of cancer, showed successful lobotomy with minimal brain tissue damage outside the target volume. 10/17 patients who were reported as being in 'excruciating pain' were reported as having 'practically complete' relief during the 2-week to 11-month follow-up observation period. Lindström worked with Leksell to develop a system for treating psychiatric disorders using high-intensity frequency ultrasound (HIFU).[5] The necessity for a craniotomy led Leksell to abandon ultrasound and to develop frame-based stereotactic radiosurgery (and later the Gamma knife). Around the same time, Ballantine and colleagues at Massachusetts General Hospital (MGH) were investigating the use of a device referred to as the 'Cosman machine' (a HIFU system mounted on a milling machine) to treat a number of conditions, including psychiatric disorders, and the Fry team targeted a number of brain disorders, including Parkinson's disease, with their system.[6–10]

Despite early promise, HIFU did not become widespread. Two major challenges confronted HIFU's protagonists. The first was the need to create an acoustic window in the skull, and the second was the inability to visualise targets within the brain. Targeting became much easier with the introduction of magnetic

DOI: 10.1201/9780429162671-1

resonance (MR) imaging guidance for HIFU exposures of the brain.[11, 12] This allowed both imaging of the brain and thermometry based on MR imaging parameters.[13] MR-guided treatments were initially performed through a craniotomy, but the introduction of hemispherical phased array transducers allowed transcranial exposures. Fry and Goss had shown that it was possible to focus ultrasound fields through the skull, but that the phase aberrations introduced by the non-uniformity of the skull caused the focus to distort and shift position.[14] If a hydrophone was implanted into the brain, these phase aberrations could be corrected by altering the drive (phase and amplitude) to the various transducer array elements. The need for the implanted hydrophone is obviated by simulations of the acoustic pathway through the skull based on a pre-operative computed tomography (CT) scan that allows the skull thickness to be mapped. This was originally implemented by groups in North America and France.[15–19]

While early clinical trials revolved mainly around the ablative treatment of brain cancer and Parkinson's disease, it was not until the introduction of large phased arrays and phase aberration correction techniques that the range of brain applications could be expanded considerably, with treatment of essential tremor being one of the most exciting.[20–23]

The ability of relatively low ultrasound energy to open the blood-brain barrier (BBB) was first mentioned by Bakay and colleagues, who observed localised uptake of trypan blue, with no damage to surrounding tissue, on exposure of cat brain to pulsed ultrasound.[24] In more recent years renewed interest in this, spawned by a seminal publication by Hynynen et al. in 2001 that demonstrated BBB opening, has led to substantial interest in using this technique for enhanced delivery of a variety of agents to the brain for conditions such as cancer and Alzheimer's disease.[25–34]

1.1.2 Cancer Outside the Brain

The first published mention of the possibility of using ultrasound to treat cancer was not encouraging. Szent-Gyorgi, in a letter to *Nature* on 'The chemical and biological effects of ultra-sonic radiation', refers to the work of a colleague, saying 'The effect of this radiation on Ehrlich's carcinoma has been studied by B Gŏzsi and found to have no specific effect on this tumour'.[35]

The main early focus of ultrasound clinical trials in oncology were in urology. Guy Vallancien in Paris ran a clinical trial on the treatment of patients with bladder cancer using an extracorporeal HIFU system (the Pyrotherm).[36, 37] He reported on 20 patients of whom 75% showed normal cytology at 1 month, 67% had had no recurrence after 1 year, and 33% had recurrence of their disease. At around the same time devices that allowed HIFU to be delivered to the prostate via a trans-rectal route were being developed. These were the Ablatherm (from Edap Technomed, France) and the Sonablate (from Focus Surgery, USA). They were first trialled on benign prostatic hyperplasia (BPH) with some success,[38–41] but their potential for treating prostate cancer was also soon explored.[38–40, 42–45] These urological applications were all guided using diagnostic ultrasound imaging. More recently MR-guided systems have been introduced.[46–49]

The introduction of devices that could combine either ultrasound (US) or MR guidance with HIFU led to the investigation of the treatment of other tumour sites within the body. The Chongqing HAIFU company (China) led the way with their JC system that allowed ablation of tumours in the abdomen and of bone cancers under ultrasound guidance.[50–54] Insightec (Israel) developed their Exablate system that allowed MR-guided ablation of abdominal and bone targets, although initially predominantly uterine fibroids.[55–62] Philips also produced an MR-guided system for extra-corporeal treatments. This system (the Sonalleve, now developed by Profound) has been used for cancer treatments, the treatment of benign tumours such as uterine fibroids and osteoid osteomas and for alleviation of pain.[63–70]

1.1.3 Other Applications

One area that was investigated in the early days of therapy US, and is now enjoying more interest, is the ability to stop blood flow using thermal ablation.[71–73] This has been used to produce haemostasis as a solution for battlefield injuries, to treat varicose veins and, most recently, to treat twin-twin transfusion syndrome.[74–78]

Therapy US at lower output levels has experienced a considerable renaissance in interest. It has found application in physiotherapy, bone fracture repair, neuromodulation and pain relief.[67, 69, 70, 79–86]

1.2 Current Status of Therapy Ultrasound

A number of clinical trials have now been undertaken to explore the role of US thermal ablation in the treatment of conditions as diverse as the symptoms arising from uterine fibroids, benign and malignant prostate disease, the pain induced by secondary bone tumours, primary and secondary tumours of the abdomen, osteoid osteomas, the region of the brain responsible for essential tremor, and fetal medicine. Despite these, the weight of clinical evidence is still insufficient for widespread uptake of the HIFU technique. There may be a number of reasons for this. It is in part, a case of the chicken and the egg – which comes first? Broader availability of clinical HIFU devices will lead to more patient treatments, but in the absence of convincing clinical evidence of efficacy, centres are unlikely to invest in such systems, especially where there is the need to combine them with busy MR scanners.

Although progress is slow, HIFU is becoming more widely used, and treatment protocols are becoming more rigorous. Figure 1.1 shows a timeline for HIFU uptake in the clinic. Figure 1.2 shows the number of patients treated for each indication. Both the cumulative number (to 2022) and the numbers in 2022 are shown. While HIFU treatments are perceived as being slow to deliver, they do have the advantage, when properly executed, of being single treatments, with the target tissue being thermally ablated in a single session.

While not yet widely available clinically, the technique known as histotripsy, in which the action of ultrasonically driven bubbles is used to cause disintegration of tissue, is starting to gain traction. This method uses high-amplitude, short pulses either to draw gas out of solution (intrinsic cavitation histotripsy) or to induce shock waves, which lead to a local temperature rise, and activate the bubbles produced by boiling (boiling histotripsy). The shear stresses induced by the driven bubbles in both cases lead to rapid breakdown of neighbouring cells (see Chapter 3). This mechanical form of tissue ablation has the advantage that while the spatial and temporal peak pressures required are high, the time-averaged intensities are relatively low, thus reducing the risk of skin burn and other thermally associated side effects. In addition, as histotripsy involves the action of bubbles, this activity can be readily visualised on a diagnostic US scan.

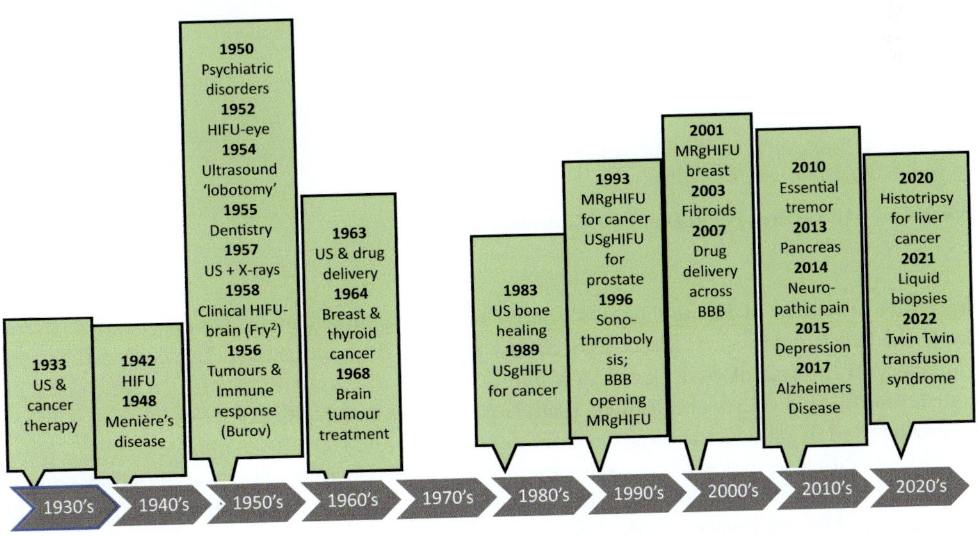

FIGURE 1.1 Timeline showing the date on which various indications were first described in the literature.

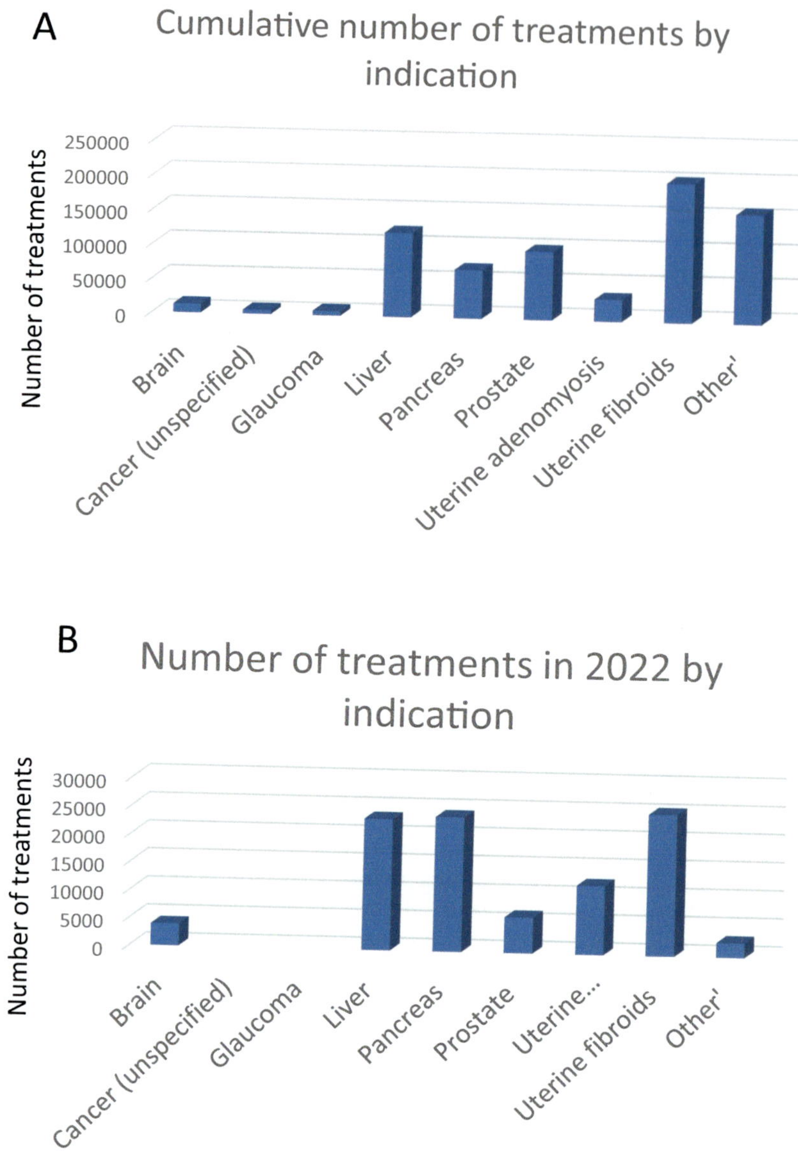

FIGURE 1.2 A. Cumulative numbers of patients treated with HIFU for different applications. B. Numbers of patients treated with HIFU for various indications in 2022.

(Source: Focused Ultrasound Foundation; www.fusfoundation.org.)

Alternative methods of harnessing US energy for therapeutic benefit are now under discussion. Probably the most widely researched, and closest to clinical application, is the potential to enhance drug delivery. If the transit of drug across a blood vessel wall can be improved (in terms of either its concentration or the distance it can travel from the vessel, or both), efficacy may be increased, or lower doses may be used to achieve the required cellular response, and side effects may be reduced. Using US, this is achieved either by exposing the target vasculature (whether in benign or malignant tissue) simultaneously to both the drug of interest and cavitation (promoted in a number of ways, see Chapter 3) or by selectively heating regions while drugs encapsulated in thermally sensitive carriers (commonly liposomes) pass through them. An advantage of these types of approaches is that the lower intensity required is lower than for ablation, and so tight focusing of the US beam is not essential. The field of neuromodulation is growing fast, with recent trials reporting the use of very low US energies to treat depression, obsessive-compulsive disorder (OCD) and other brain-related conditions, echoing the early work of Leksell and Ballantine.[7, 8]

Associated with these lower-intensity applications of US is the field of US-mediated hyperthermia for cancer therapy. In this, the aim is to raise the tissue temperature of a target volume by 6–9°C (to temperatures in the range of 43–46°C) for times of the order of 10–60 minutes, with the shorter times being associated with the higher temperatures. For comparison, it should be noted that thermal ablation is considered to have been achieved at the equivalent temperature/time combination of 43°C for 240 minutes. At these lower raised temperatures, the aim is not to cause tissue damage from the heat alone, but to potentiate the effects of systemically or locally introduced chemotherapeutic agents or of ionising radiation therapy.

While thermal and mechanical ablation, and enhancement of drug delivery, remain the main clinical thrust of therapy US usage, longer-standing applications of this versatile energy form remain in use. Physiotherapists still use US, mainly to address soft tissue injuries, and it is still used, at very low intensities, to stimulate fracture repair.

1.3 Place of Therapeutic Ultrasound amongst Other Minimally Invasive Therapies

It is often claimed that a major, and unique, feature of HIFU and other therapy US applications is that they can be delivered completely non-invasively. At first this may seem to be a self-evident advantage. However, given that surgeons are not averse to intervention, it is instructive to analyse the need for non-invasiveness over alternative minimally invasive approaches.

Table 1.1 shows the relative advantages and disadvantages of non-invasive and minimally invasive techniques. HIFU is a competitor to other thermal ablation techniques such as deep brain stimulation (DBS), radiofrequency ablation (RFA), microwave ablation (MWA), laser ablation and cryosurgery. It should, of course, be remembered that interstitial US probes are also under serious consideration.

RFA uses heat generated in target tissues by 350–500 kHz alternating current.[87–89] Since nerves and cardiac muscle are not stimulated by the RF signal, ablation can be carried out under local anaesthetic or conscious sedation. Usually guided by X-ray, CT or ultrasound, it can be delivered via catheter or needle electrodes. RFA is used for treatment of cancers of the lung, liver, kidney, bone and pancreas. It is also used for management of pain, treatment of hypertension by renal denervation and cardiac arrhythmias.

MWA uses frictional heating generated by 300 MHz–300 GHz electromagnetic waves. MWA can generate larger heated volumes than RFA, using single or multiple antennae. The most common application is ablation of lung or liver cancer using 915 MHz.[88, 90]

Cryoablation uses low temperatures (~–75°C) to create intracellular ice crystals, which disrupt cells. This can be performed as an open technique, laparoscopically, but more commonly, is delivered

TABLE 1.1

Advantages and Disadvantages of Minimally and Non-invasive Approaches

	Advantages	Disadvantages
Minimally invasive	Exact targeting Faster Tissue movement irrelevant	Skin is breached Anaesthesia may be needed
Non-invasive	Skin not breached Reduction in infection Trackless Anaesthesia unlikely to be needed	Targeting more difficult Slow Tissue movement may be important

percutaneously. Cryoablation is largely used for treating cancers of the kidney and prostate, but also for those of lung, liver and breast.[91] It is also used for treatment of cardiac arrythmias.

DBS is used by neurosurgeons to treat movement and neuropsychiatric disorders. Electrical impulses delivered using a neuro-stimulating electrode interfere with neural activity.[92–94]

1.4 Future/Summary

It is hard to predict the future of the different therapeutic US applications. It seems likely that the wide range of potential treatments will continue to be explored, both as a method of ablating selected regions and as a method of improving uptake of therapeutic agents, capitalising, for example, on the ability to temporarily open the BBB. It seems likely that thermal ablation (HIFU) devices will become more available, and it may be that this will be accelerated by the advent of smaller, application-specific systems. This process may be made easier by the incorporation of dedicated imaging to provide targeting and treatment monitoring. At present, this would favour diagnostic US-based guidance.

US treatments have, to some extent, come full circle. HIFU was first proposed in the 1940s and 1950s for selective ablation in the brain. The brain is again the target organ attracting the most activity, with thermal ablation and neuromodulatory techniques exciting considerable interest. Therapeutic US underwent a resurgence in interest with the growth of hyperthermia in the 1970s and 1980s. There is now renewed interest in combining US with chemo- and/or radiotherapy, using either thermal or cavitational effects to improve these treatments. This 'rediscovery' of therapy US is due, in part, to improvements in imaging (both US and MR) and to more sophisticated US energy sources, usually involving phased arrays.

REFERENCES

1. Lynn JG, Zwemer RL, Chick AJ, Miller AE. A new method for the generation and use of focused ultrasound in experimental biology. The Journal of General Physiology. 1942;26(2):179.
2. Fry W, Wulff V, Tucker D, Fry F. Physical factors involved in ultrasonically induced changes in living systems: I. Identification of non-temperature effects. The Journal of the Acoustical Society of America. 1950;22(6):867–76.
3. Fry WJ. Intense ultrasound in investigations of the central nervous system. Advances in Biological and Medical Physics. 6. Elsevier; 1959. p. 281–348.
4. Lindstrom PA. Prefrontal ultrasonic irradiation – a substitute for lobotomy. AMA Archives of Neurology & Psychiatry. 1954;72(4):399–425.
5. Nelson E, Lindstrom PA, Haymaker W. Pathological effects of ultrasound on the human brain: A study of 25 cases in which ultrasonic irradiation was used as a lobotomy procedure. Journal of Neuropathology & Experimental Neurology. 1959;18(4):489–508.
6. Åström K, Bell E, Ballantine Jr H, Heidensleben E. An experimental neuropathological study of the effects of high-frequency focused ultrasound on the brain of the cat. Journal of Neuropathology & Experimental Neurology. 1961;20(4):484–520.
7. Ballantine H, Bell E, Manlapaz J. Progress and problems in the neurological applications of focused ultrasound. Journal of neurosurgery. 1960;17(5):858–76.
8. Ballantine Jr H, Cotter W, Hueter T. On brain lesions by focused ultrasound. The Journal of the Acoustical Society of America. 1956;28(6):1292–3.
9. Fry F, Johnson L. Tumor irradiation with intense ultrasound. Ultrasound in Medicine & Biology. 1978;4(4):337–41.
10. Heimburger R, Fry F, Franklin T, Eggleton R, editors. Ultrasound potentiation of chemotherapy for brain malignancy. Ultrasound in Medicine: Volume 1 Proceedings of the 19th Annual Meeting of the American Institute of Ultrasound in Medicine. Springer; 1975.
11. Cline HE, Schenck JF, Hynynen K, Watkins RD, Souza SP, Jolesz FA. MR-guided focused ultrasound surgery. Journal of Computer Assisted Tomography. 1992;16(6):956–65.

12. Jolesz FA, Hynynen K. Magnetic resonance image-guided focused ultrasound surgery. Cancer Journal (Sudbury, Mass). 2002;8:S100–12.
13. Cline HE, Hynynen K, Hardy CJ, Watkins RD, Schenck JF, Jolesz FA. MR temperature mapping of focused ultrasound surgery. Magnetic Resonance in Medicine. 1994;31(6):628–36.
14. Fry FJ, Goss SA, Patrick JT. Transkull focal lesions in cat brain produced by ultrasound. Journal of Neurosurgery. 1981;54(5):659–63.
15. Hynynen K, Clement GT, McDannold N, Vykhodtseva N, King R, White PJ, et al. 500-element ultrasound phased array system for noninvasive focal surgery of the brain: A preliminary rabbit study with ex vivo human skulls. Magnetic Resonance in Medicine: An Official Journal of the International Society for Magnetic Resonance in Medicine. 2004;52(1):100–7.
16. Lipsman N, Schwartz ML, Huang Y, Lee L, Sankar T, Chapman M, et al. MR-guided focused ultrasound thalamotomy for essential tremor: A proof-of-concept study. The Lancet Neurology. 2013;12(5):462–8.
17. McDannold N, Clement GT, Black P, Jolesz F, Hynynen K. Transcranial magnetic resonance imaging–guided focused ultrasound surgery of brain tumors: Initial findings in 3 patients. Neurosurgery. 2010;66(2):323–32.
18. Sun J, Hynynen K. Focusing of therapeutic ultrasound through a human skull: A numerical study. The Journal of the Acoustical Society of America. 1998;104(3):1705–15.
19. Pernot M, Aubry J-F, Tanter M, Boch A-L, Marquet F, Kujas M, et al. In vivo transcranial brain surgery with an ultrasonic time reversal mirror. Journal of Neurosurgery. 2007;106(6):1061–6.
20. Weintraub D, Elias WJ. The emerging role of transcranial magnetic resonance imaging–guided focused ultrasound in functional neurosurgery. Movement Disorders. 2017;32(1):20–7.
21. Elias WJ, Huss D, Voss T, Loomba J, Khaled M, Zadicario E, et al. A pilot study of focused ultrasound thalamotomy for essential tremor. New England Journal of Medicine. 2013;369(7):640–8.
22. Dobrakowski PP, Machowska-Majchrzak AK, Łabuz-Roszak B, Majchrzak KG, Kluczewska E, Pierzchała KB. MR-guided focused ultrasound: A new generation treatment of Parkinson's disease, essential tremor and neuropathic pain. Interventional Neuroradiology. 2014;20(3):275–82.
23. Elias WJ, Lipsman N, Ondo WG, Ghanouni P, Kim YG, Lee W, et al. A randomized trial of focused ultrasound thalamotomy for essential tremor. New England Journal of Medicine. 2016;375(8):730–9.
24. Bakay L, Hueter T, Ballantine H, Sosa D. Ultrasonically produced changes in the blood-brain barrier. AMA Archives of Neurology & Psychiatry. 1956;76(5):457–67.
25. Hynynen K, McDannold N, Vykhodtseva N, Jolesz FA. Noninvasive MR imaging–guided focal opening of the blood-brain barrier in rabbits. Radiology. 2001;220(3):640–6.
26. Aryal M, Arvanitis CD, Alexander PM, McDannold N. Ultrasound-mediated blood–brain barrier disruption for targeted drug delivery in the central nervous system. Advanced Drug Delivery Reviews. 2014;72:94–109.
27. Choi JJ, Pernot M, Small SA, Konofagou EE. Noninvasive, transcranial and localized opening of the blood-brain barrier using focused ultrasound in mice. Ultrasound in Medicine & Biology. 2007;33(1):95–104.
28. Deng CX. Targeted drug delivery across the blood–brain barrier using ultrasound technique. Therapeutic Delivery. 2010;1(6):819–48.
29. Kinoshita M, McDannold N, Jolesz FA, Hynynen K. Noninvasive localized delivery of Herceptin to the mouse brain by MRI-guided focused ultrasound-induced blood–brain barrier disruption. Proceedings of the National Academy of Sciences. 2006;103(31):11719–23.
30. Lipsman N, Meng Y, Bethune AJ, Huang Y, Lam B, Masellis M, et al. Blood–brain barrier opening in Alzheimer's disease using MR-guided focused ultrasound. Nature Communications. 2018;9(1):2336.
31. Mainprize T, Lipsman N, Huang Y, Meng Y, Bethune A, Ironside S, et al. Blood-brain barrier opening in primary brain tumors with non-invasive MR-guided focused ultrasound: A clinical safety and feasibility study. Scientific Reports. 2019;9(1):321.
32. McDannold N, Vykhodtseva N, Raymond S, Jolesz FA, Hynynen K. MRI-guided targeted blood-brain barrier disruption with focused ultrasound: Histological findings in rabbits. Ultrasound in Medicine & Biology. 2005;31(11):1527–37.
33. Treat LH, McDannold N, Zhang Y, Vykhodtseva N, Hynynen K. Improved anti-tumor effect of liposomal doxorubicin after targeted blood-brain barrier disruption by MRI-guided focused ultrasound in rat glioma. Ultrasound in Medicine & Biology. 2012;38(10):1716–25.

34. Vykhodtseva N, McDannold N, Hynynen K. Progress and problems in the application of focused ultrasound for blood–brain barrier disruption. Ultrasonics. 2008;48(4):279–96.
35. Szent-Györgyi A. Chemical and biological effects of ultra-sonic radiation. Nature. 1933;131(3304):278.
36. Vallancien G, Chartier-Kastler E, Chopin D, Veillon B, Brisset J, Andre-Bougaran J. Focussed extracorporeal pyrotherapy: Experimental results. European Urology. 1991;20(3):211–9.
37. Vallancien G, Harouni M, Veillon B, Mombet A, Prapotnich D, Brisset J, et al. Focused extracorporeal pyrotherapy: Feasibility study in man. Journal of Endourology. 1992;6(2):173–81.
38. Chapelon J-Y, Rouvière O, Crouzet S, Gelet A. Prostate focused ultrasound therapy. Therapeutic Ultrasound. 2016:21–41.
39. Beerlage H, Thüroff S, Debruyne F, Chaussy C, de la Rosette J. Transrectal high-intensity focused ultrasound using the Ablatherm device in the treatment of localized prostate carcinoma. Urology. 1999;54(2):273–7.
40. Chaussy CG, Thüroff S. High-intensity focused ultrasound for the treatment of prostate cancer: A review. Journal of Endourology. 2017;31(S1):S-30-S-7.
41. Sanghvi N, Foster R, Bihrle R, Casey R, Uchida T, Phillips M, et al. Noninvasive surgery of prostate tissue by high intensity focused ultrasound: An updated report. European Journal of Ultrasound. 1999;9(1):19–29.
42. Bakavicius A, Marra G, Macek P, Robertson C, Abreu AL, George AK, et al. Available evidence on HIFU for focal treatment of prostate cancer: A systematic review. International Brazilian Journal of Urology. 2022;48:263–74.
43. Madersbacher S, Pedevilla M, Vingers L, Susani M, Marberger M. Effect of high-intensity focused ultrasound on human prostate cancer in vivo. Cancer Research. 1995;55(15):3346–51.
44. Poissonnier L, Murata F, Chapelon J, Gelet A, editors. Indications, Techniques and Outcomes of High-intensity Focused Ultrasound (HIFU) for the Treatment of Localized Prostate Cancer. Annales D'urologie; 2007.
45. Rebillard X, Gelet A, Davin JL, Soulie M, Prapotnich D, Cathelineau X, et al. Transrectal high-intensity focused ultrasound in the treatment of localized prostate cancer. Journal of Endourology. 2005;19(6):693–701.
46. Anttinen M, Mäkelä P, Suomi V, Kiviniemi A, Saunavaara J, Sainio T, et al. Feasibility of MRI-guided transurethral ultrasound for lesion-targeted ablation of prostate cancer. Scandinavian Journal of Urology. 2019;53(5):295–302.
47. Dora C, Clarke GM, Frey G, Sella D. Magnetic resonance imaging-guided transurethral ultrasound ablation of prostate cancer: A systematic review. Journal of Endourology. 2022;36(6):841–54.
48. Galgano SJ, Planz VB, Arora S, Rais-Bahrami S. MR-Guided High-Intensity directional ultrasound ablation of prostate cancer. Current Urology Reports. 2021;22:1–6.
49. Lumiani A, Samun D, Sroka R, Muschter R, editors. Single Center Retrospective Analysis of Fifty-two Prostate Cancer Patients with Customized MR-guided Transurethral Ultrasound Ablation (TULSA). Urologic Oncology: Seminars and Original Investigations. Elsevier; 2021.
50. Wu F, Chen W-Z, Bai J, Zou J-Z, Wang Z-L, Zhu H, et al. Pathological changes in human malignant carcinoma treated with high-intensity focused ultrasound. Ultrasound in Medicine & Biology. 2001;27(8):1099–106.
51. Wu F, Chen W-Z, Bai J, Zou J-Z, Wang Z-L, Zhu H, et al. Tumor vessel destruction resulting from high-intensity focused ultrasound in patients with solid malignancies. Ultrasound in Medicine & Biology. 2002;28(4):535–42.
52. Wu F, Wang Z-B, Cao Y-D, Chen W, Bai J, Zou J, et al. A randomised clinical trial of high-intensity focused ultrasound ablation for the treatment of patients with localised breast cancer. British Journal of Cancer. 2003;89(12):2227–33.
53. Wu F, Wang Z-B, Chen W-Z, Bai J, Zhu H, Qiao T-Y. Preliminary experience using high intensity focused ultrasound for the treatment of patients with advanced stage renal malignancy. The Journal of Urology. 2003;170(6):2237–40.
54. Wu F, Wang Z-B, Chen W-Z, Wang W, Gui Y, Zhang M, et al. Extracorporeal high intensity focused ultrasound ablation in the treatment of 1038 patients with solid carcinomas in China: An overview. Ultrasonics Sonochemistry. 2004;11(3–4):149–54.

55. Chapman A, ter Haar G. Thermal ablation of uterine fibroids using MR-guided focused ultrasound-a truly non-invasive treatment modality. European Radiology. 2007;17:2505–11.
56. Hesley GK, Gorny KR, Henrichsen TL, Woodrum DA, Brown DL. A clinical review of focused ultrasound ablation with magnetic resonance guidance: An option for treating uterine fibroids. Ultrasound Quarterly. 2008;24(2):131–9.
57. Verpalen IM, Anneveldt KJ, Nijholt IM, Schutte JM, Dijkstra JR, Franx A, et al. Magnetic resonance-high intensity focused ultrasound (MR-HIFU) therapy of symptomatic uterine fibroids with unrestrictive treatment protocols: A systematic review and meta-analysis. European Journal of Radiology. 2019;120:108700.
58. Alfieri G, Mattone M, Manganaro L, Pecorini F, Catalano C, Napoli A. High-Intensity Focused Ultrasound Surgery of Uterine Myomas. Diagnostic and Interventional Radiology in Gynecological and Obstetric Diseases. Springer; 2023. p. 153–61.
59. Bazzocchi A, Napoli A, Sacconi B, Battista G, Guglielmi G, Catalano C, et al. MRI-guided focused ultrasound surgery in musculoskeletal diseases: The hot topics. The British Journal of Radiology. 2016;89(1057):20150358.
60. Napoli A, Alfieri G, Andrani F, Scipione R, Manganaro L, Pecorini F, et al., editors. Uterine myomas: Focused ultrasound surgery. Seminars in Ultrasound, CT and MRI. Elsevier; 2021.
61. Pediconi F, Marzocca F, Cavallo Marincola B, Napoli A. MRI-guided treatment in the breast. Journal of Magnetic Resonance Imaging. 2018;48(6):1479–88.
62. Peek M, Ahmed M, Napoli A, ten Haken B, McWilliams S, Usiskin S, et al. Systematic review of high-intensity focused ultrasound ablation in the treatment of breast cancer. Journal of British Surgery. 2015;102(8):873–82.
63. Dorenberg EJ, Courivaud F, Ring E, Hald K, Jakobsen JÅ, Fosse E, et al. Volumetric ablation of uterine fibroids using Sonalleve high-intensity focused ultrasound in a 3 Tesla scanner–first clinical assessment. Minimally Invasive Therapy & Allied Technologies. 2013;22(2):73–9.
64. Jeong J-H, Hong GP, Kim Y-R, Ha J-E, Lee K-S. Clinical consideration of treatment to ablate uterine fibroids with magnetic resonance imaging-guided high intensity focused ultrasound (MRgFUS): Sonalleve. Journal of Menopausal Medicine. 2016;22(2):94–107.
65. Thiburce AC, Frulio N, Hocquelet A, Maire F, Salut C, Balageas P, et al. Magnetic resonance-guided high-intensity focused ultrasound for uterine fibroids: Mid-term outcomes of 36 patients treated with the Sonalleve system. International Journal of Hyperthermia. 2015;31(7):764–70.
66. Giles SL, Imseeh G, Rivens I, ter Haar GR, Taylor A, Desouza NM. MR guided high intensity focused ultrasound (MRgHIFU) for treating recurrent gynaecological tumours: A pilot feasibility study. The British Journal of Radiology. 2019;92(1098):20181037.
67. Harding D, Giles S, Brown M, ter Haar G, van den Bosch M, Bartels L, et al. Evaluation of quality of life outcomes following palliative treatment of bone metastases with magnetic resonance-guided high intensity focused ultrasound: An international multicentre study. Clinical Oncology. 2018;30(4):233–42.
68. Imseeh G, Giles SL, Taylor A, Brown MR, Rivens I, Gordon-Williams R, et al. Feasibility of palliating recurrent gynecological tumors with MRGHIFU: Comparison of symptom, quality-of-life, and imaging response in intra and extra-pelvic disease. International Journal of Hyperthermia. 2021;38(1):623–32.
69. Huisman M, Lam MK, Bartels LW, Nijenhuis RJ, Moonen CT, Knuttel FM, et al. Feasibility of volumetric MRI-guided high intensity focused ultrasound (MR-HIFU) for painful bone metastases. Journal of Therapeutic Ultrasound. 2014;2(1):1–10.
70. Huisman M, ter Haar G, Napoli A, Hananel A, Ghanouni P, Lövey G, et al. International consensus on use of focused ultrasound for painful bone metastases: Current status and future directions. International Journal of Hyperthermia. 2015;31(3):251–9.
71. Denbow M, Rivens I, Rowland I, Leach M, Fisk N, ter Haar G. Preclinical development of noninvasive vascular occlusion with focused ultrasonic surgery for fetal therapy. American Journal of Obstetrics and Gynecology. 2000;182(2):387–92.
72. Rivens I, Rowland I, Denbow M, Fisk N, ter Haar G, Leach M. Vascular occlusion using focused ultrasound surgery for use in fetal medicine. European Journal of Ultrasound. 1999;9(1):89–97.
73. Hynynen K, Colucci V, Chung A, Jolesz F. Noninvasive arterial occlusion using MRI-guided focused ultrasound. Ultrasound in Medicine & Biology. 1996;22(8):1071–7.

74. Shaw C, ter Haar G, Rivens I, Giussani D, Lees C. Pathophysiological mechanisms of high-intensity focused ultrasound-mediated vascular occlusion and relevance to non-invasive fetal surgery. Journal of the Royal Society Interface. 2014;11(95):20140029.
75. Shaw CJ. Developing a non-invasive treatment for twin-twin transfusion syndrome using high intensity focused ultrasound in an animal model. PhD thesis, University of Cambridge; 2017.
76. Shaw CJ, Civale J, Botting KJ, Niu Y, ter Haar G, Rivens I, et al. Noninvasive high-intensity focused ultrasound treatment of twin-twin transfusion syndrome: A preliminary in vivo study. Science Translational Medicine. 2016;8(347):347ra95-ra95.
77. Okai T, Ichizuka K, Hasegawa J, Matsuoka R, Nakamura M, Shimodaira K, et al. First successful case of non-invasive in-utero treatment of twin reversed arterial perfusion sequence by high-intensity focused ultrasound. Ultrasound in Obstetrics & Gynecology. 2013;42(1):112–4.
78. Seo K, Ichizuka K, Okai T, Dohi S, Nakamura M, Hasegawa J, et al. Treatment of twin-reversed arterial perfusion sequence using high-intensity focused ultrasound. Ultrasound in Obstetrics & Gynecology. 2019;54(1):128–34.
79. Bertrand A-S, Iannessi A, Natale R, Beaumont H, Patriti S, Xiong-Ying J, et al. Focused ultrasound for the treatment of bone metastases: Effectiveness and feasibility. Journal of Therapeutic Ultrasound. 2018;6(1):1–9.
80. Catane R, Beck A, Inbar Y, Rabin T, Shabshin N, Hengst S, et al. MR-guided focused ultrasound surgery (MRgFUS) for the palliation of pain in patients with bone metastases – preliminary clinical experience. Annals of Oncology. 2007;18(1):163–7.
81. Gianfelice D, Gupta C, Kucharczyk W, Bret P, Havill D, Clemons M. Palliative treatment of painful bone metastases with MR imaging–guided focused ultrasound. Radiology. 2008;249(1):355–63.
82. Li C, Zhang W, Fan W, Huang J, Zhang F, Wu P. Noninvasive treatment of malignant bone tumors using high-intensity focused ultrasound. Cancer. 2010;116(16):3934–42.
83. Napoli A, Anzidei M, Marincola BC, Brachetti G, Noce V, Boni F, et al. MR imaging–guided focused ultrasound for treatment of bone metastasis. Radiographics. 2013;33(6):1555–68.
84. Baek H, Pahk KJ, Kim H. A review of low-intensity focused ultrasound for neuromodulation. Biomedical Engineering Letters. 2017;7:135–42.
85. Blackmore J, Shrivastava S, Sallet J, Butler CR, Cleveland RO. Ultrasound neuromodulation: A review of results, mechanisms and safety. Ultrasound in Medicine & Biology. 2019;45(7):1509–36.
86. Bowary P, Greenberg BD. Noninvasive focused ultrasound for neuromodulation: A review. Psychiatric Clinics. 2018;41(3):505–14.
87. Curley SA. Radiofrequency ablation of malignant liver tumors. Annals of Surgical Oncology. 2003;10:338–47.
88. Izzo F, Granata V, Grassi R, Fusco R, Palaia R, Delrio P, et al. Radiofrequency ablation and microwave ablation in liver tumors: An update. The Oncologist. 2019;24(10):e990-e1005.
89. Ni Y, Mulier S, Miao Y, Michel L, Marchal G. A review of the general aspects of radiofrequency ablation. Abdominal Imaging. 2005;30:381–400.
90. Liang P, Wang Y. Microwave ablation of hepatocellular carcinoma. Oncology. 2007;72(Supplement 1):124–31.
91. Hu K-Q. Advances in clinical application of cryoablation therapy for hepatocellular carcinoma and metastatic liver tumor. Journal of Clinical Gastroenterology. 2014;48(10):830–6.
92. Dostrovsky JO, Lozano AM. Mechanisms of deep brain stimulation. Movement Disorders: Official journal of the Movement Disorder Society. 2002;17(S3):S63–S8.
93. Montgomery Jr EB, Gale JT. Mechanisms of action of deep brain stimulation (DBS). Neuroscience & Biobehavioral Reviews. 2008;32(3):388–407.
94. Perlmutter JS, Mink JW. Deep brain stimulation. Annual Review of Neuroscience. 2006;29:229–57.

2

Physical Principles of Focused Ultrasound Therapy

Gail ter Haar

2.1 An Introduction to the Physics of Ultrasound Wave Propagation

Ultrasound travels through tissue in the form of a pressure wave. Medical ultrasound fields are most usually generated using the phenomenon of piezo-electricity. A piezo-electric crystal has the property that it can expand and contract in response to a varying applied voltage across its faces. This has the effect of changing the pressure in whatever medium the crystal is in contact with. Here, for simplicity, we will take that medium to be soft tissue. An applied sinusoidally varying voltage, for example, will lead to a pressure wave in tissue that has a sinusoidal profile. Ultrasound travels through tissue as a longitudinal wave, with regions of compression (high pressure) and rarefaction (low pressure).

The time taken for a point in tissue to experience the cycle of peak high pressure, down through low pressure and back to the peak high pressure (one cycle) is known as the 'period' (τ), with the number of periods occurring in 1 second being the 'frequency' (f). The unit in which frequency is quoted is the Hertz (1 cycle/second [Hz]), with ultrasound frequencies in the low MegaHertz (MHz) range being used for diagnostic and therapy ultrasound (1MHz = 10^6 Hz). The distance between adjacent regions of tissue that are undergoing the same motion is known as the 'wavelength' (λ), and the speed at which the peak pressure 'crest' moves is the speed (c). These concepts are illustrated in Figure 2.1.

A wave can thus be described in terms of its wavelength (λ), frequency (f), period (τ) and speed (c), with these parameters being related by the following equations:

$$f = 1/\tau \qquad \text{eqn 2.1}$$

$$c = \lambda/\tau \qquad \text{eqn 2.2}$$

$$c = f\lambda \qquad \text{eqn 2.3}$$

The energy carried by an ultrasound wave can be characterised in terms either of pressure (commonly used units in therapy ultrasound are MegaPascals MPa) or intensity (units used W cm^{-2}). Pressure (P) and intensity (I) are related in a plane wave by the equation:

$$I = P^2/2\rho c \qquad \text{eqn 2.4}$$

where ρ is the medium density. Intensity is the energy crossing unit area per unit time (energy flux). Strictly, consistent units should be those of W m^{-2}, but for clinical applications, the square meter is inappropriately large, and so intensity is quoted in W cm^{-2}, where 1 W m^{-2} = 10^4 W cm^{-2}. This energy may be delivered in continuous or pulsed mode.

As a rule of thumb, intensity is the most relevant parameter for describing an ultrasound field for thermal treatments, whereas where mechanical effects, such as those arising from acoustic cavitation, are sought, it is usually more appropriate to cite pressure values.

An ultrasound beam may be both spatially and temporally variant. The acoustic pressure varies both along and transverse to, the beam axis, regardless of whether the beam is focused or not. The most commonly quoted pressure parameter is the peak pressure amplitude. This may be the peak to peak (P-P),

DOI: 10.1201/9780429162671-2

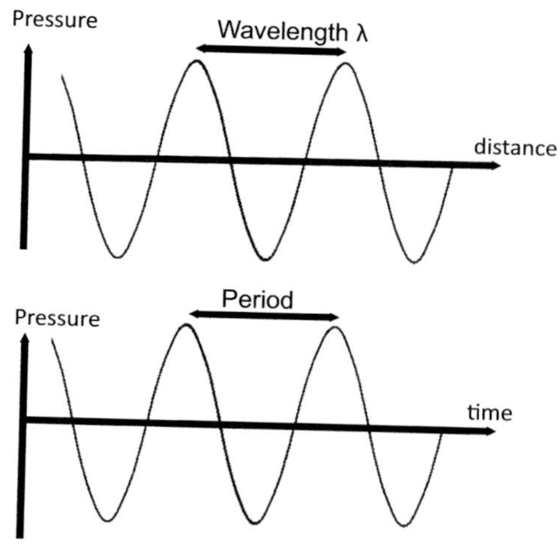

FIGURE 2.1 Diagram showing a sinusoidal pressure wave, plotted as a function of time and of distance. The wavelength is shown. This is the distance between two points on the wave undergoing the same behaviour.

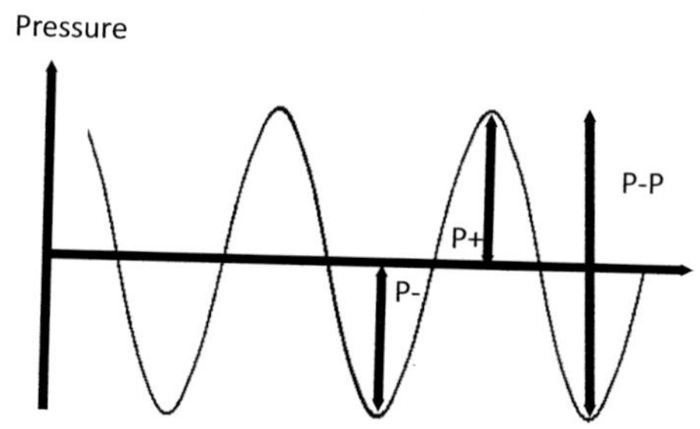

FIGURE 2.2 Graph showing pressure as a function of distance. The peak positive, peak negative and peak-to-peak amplitudes are shown.

peak negative (P–) or peak positive (P+) value. When the output is pulsed, it is essential also to describe the pulsing regime in terms of both pulse length and pulse repetition frequency.

When intensity is the quoted parameter, it is important, when it has been averaged, to describe over what area (I_{SA}) this has been carried out. For focused ultrasound therapies, the focal peak intensity (or pressure) is most usually given ($I_{focal\ peak}$), but here it is also important to describe the focal dimensions. For pulsed fields, it is necessary to state whether the quoted intensity is for a single pulse (I_{pulse}) or is time averaged over a pulse train (I_{TA}). Clearly these temporal and spatial averages can be combined to give, for example, a spatial and temporal average (I_{SATA}). These concepts are demonstrated in Figure 2.3.

It should be remembered that ultrasound fields are usually characterised in large water baths under 'free field' conditions. In order to know the energy incident on a target volume, the intensity (or pressure) must be reduced (derated) to take into account the attenuation that takes place in the overlying tissues. This requires a knowledge of the acoustic properties of these tissue layers (see §2.4). It is important, when describing treatments, or in pre-clinical research, to describe the ultrasound exposure delivered as fully as possible.[1, 2]

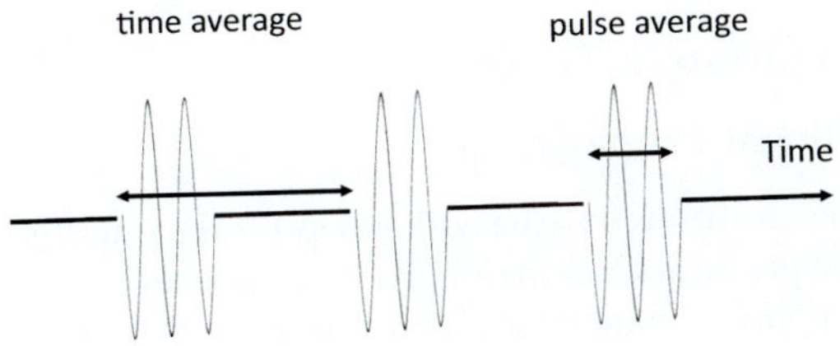

FIGURE 2.3A Diagram illustrating the concepts of time and pulse average for pulsed beams.

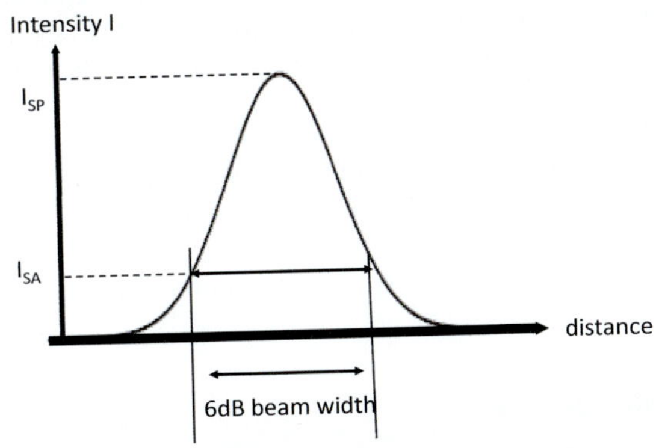

FIGURE 2.3B Diagram showing a Gaussian intensity beam profile. The spatial peak and spatial average levels are shown, as is the 6dB beam width.

TABLE 2.1

Acoustic properties for a range of tissue types. These are representative values as there is considerable variation in published values, depending on the temperature and status of the tissue, and the measurement technique.[6–8]

Tissue Type	Speed of Sound C (ms^{-1})	Amplitude Attenuation Coefficient at 1 MHz μ ($dB\ cm^{-1}/Np\ cm^{-1}$)	Frequency Dependence of Attenuation n	Acoustic Impedance Z ($kg\ m^{-2}s^{-1}$)
Non-fatty tissue	1575	0.6/0.07	1.2	$1.66\ 10^6$
Fat	1465	1.0/0.12	1.0	$1.44\ 10^6$
Bone	3635	20/0.23		$6.98\ 10^6$
Blood	1584	0.15/0.02	1.2	$1.68\ 10^6$
Water	1530	0.004/0.0004	2.0	$1.53\ 10^6$
Air				$0.0004\ 10^6$

The acoustic impedance (Z) of a tissue is used to describe how much resistance an ultrasound beam meets as it passes through tissue and is given by the equation:

$$Z = pc \quad \text{eqn 2.5}$$

where ρ is the medium's density. The SI units for impedance are Rayls (kg/m^2s). Table 2.1 shows impedance values for different tissues.

2.2 Ultrasound Propagation in Tissue

2.2.1 Linear and Non-linear Propagation

An ultrasound wave that passes through tissue with low-pressure amplitude is referred to as propagating linearly. In this case, the pressure train maintains its sinusoidal form, with little loss of amplitude. However, as the pressure amplitude is increased, non-linear effects kick in. Particles in the ultrasound field (taken to be tiny volumes in the propagation medium, whether water or tissue) will move faster in the regions of compression than those in the regions of rarefaction. This means that the peak positive pressure 'crest' moves faster than the peak negative 'trough', thus distorting the wave form away from its pure sinusoidal form. This distortion increases with distance from the source. A pure sine wave can be represented by a single frequency (known as the fundamental) in the frequency domain, but as the wave distorts, more and more frequencies are seen in its spectrum, all of which are integer multiples of the fundamental. The wave can distort until a shock front is formed. At this point the wave form resembles an N shape as shown in Figure 2.4.

Since the attenuation coefficient increases with rising frequency (see §2.4), as the wave becomes more distorted, the energy in the beam is reduced more than it would be if the propagation were linear. The higher-frequency components are attenuated most rapidly, and thus the wave distortion reduces with distance.

For therapy ultrasound, the increased absorption due to non-linearity can be used to advantage to enhance local heating.

2.2.2 Reflection and Refraction

When an ultrasound wave meets an interface, some of its energy is reflected back into the medium it has just passed through, and some is transmitted across the interface. This interface may, for instance, be composed of water and skin, fat and muscle, or muscle and bone. The amount of energy that is transmitted depends on the difference in impedance between the media involved. A line drawn at right angles to the interface is known as the 'normal'. The Law of Reflection states that the angle between the incident wave and the normal is always equal to the angle between the reflected wave and the normal. For B-mode imaging, it is the reflected component of the beam at an interface that gives rise to the echoes whose amplitudes are converted into grey-scale levels to produce the image.

If the ultrasound beam hits the interface at an angle to the normal, it may undergo refraction. If the second medium has a lower sound speed than the first, the beam axis will bend towards the normal direction. If the angle of the incident beam to the normal is θ_1 and the sound speed is c_1 in the first medium and c_2 in the second, then the beam direction in this second medium (θ_2) is given by Snell's Law:

$$\mathrm{Sin}\left(\frac{\sin\theta_1}{\sin\theta_2}\right) = \frac{c_1}{c_2} \qquad \text{eqn 2.6}$$

In France this is referred to as the 'Loi de Descartes' or 'Loi de Snell-Descartes'.

The ratio of the incident pressure to the reflected pressure (P_r/P_i) is known as the reflection coefficient, R, and is determined by the acoustic impedances of the two media (Z_1 and Z_2). R is given by:

$$R = \frac{Z_2 - Z_1}{Z_2 + Z_1} \qquad \text{eqn 2.7}$$

for normal incidence. The transmission coefficient, T, is given by:

$$T = 1 - R \qquad \text{eqn 2.8}$$

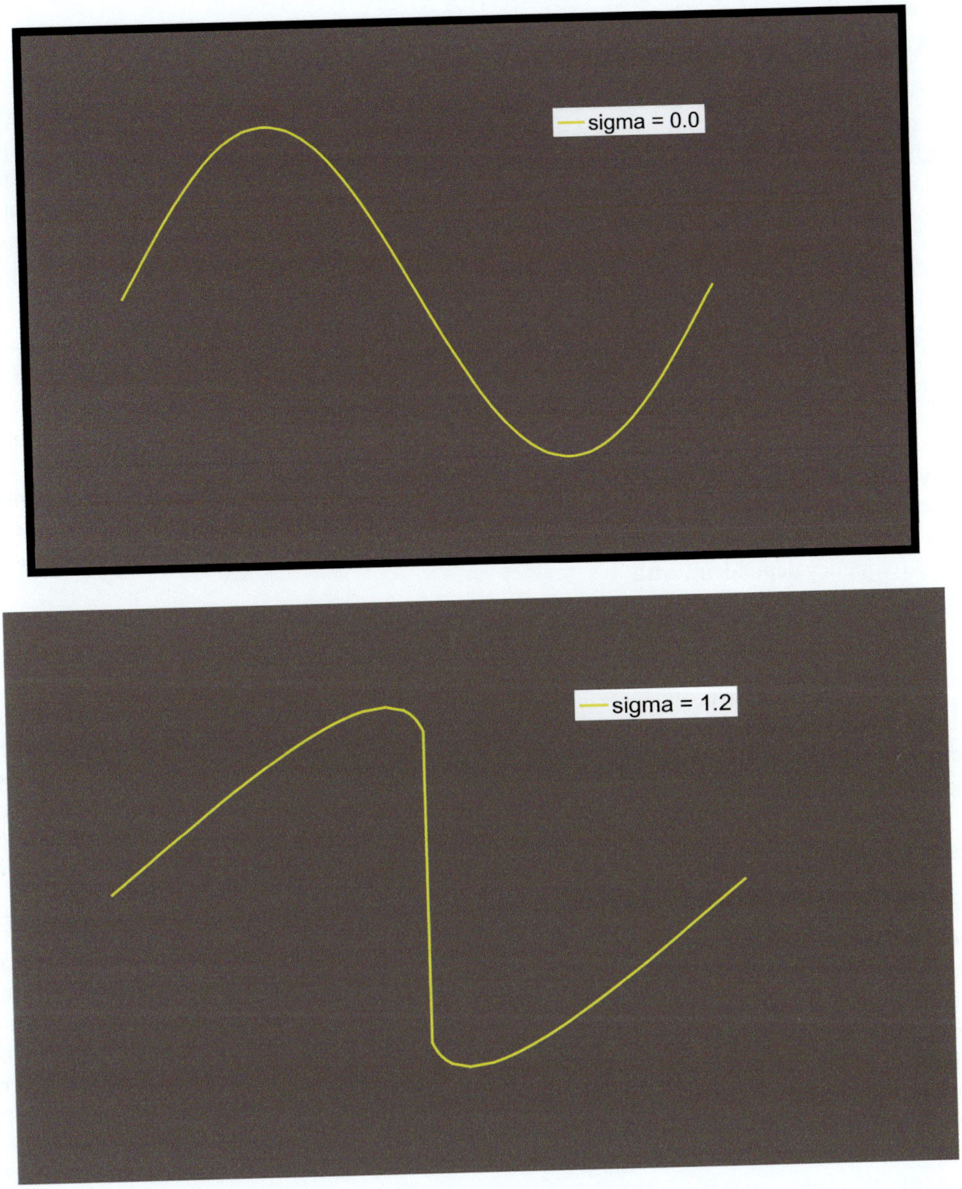

FIGURE 2.4 Diagram showing a linear waveform (top) and a highly non-linear (N wave) waveform (bottom). Sigma (σ) is a dimensionless distance. σ <<1 non-linearity is negligible; σ <1 non-linearity becomes significant; σ >1 shocks form.

Where the beam hits the interface at an angle and the beam is refracted, these relationships become:

$$R = \frac{Z_2 cos\theta_1 - Z_1 cos\theta_2}{Z_2 cos\theta_1 + Z_1 Cos\theta_2} \qquad \text{eqn 2.9}$$

and

$$T = \frac{2Z_2 cos\theta_I}{Z_2 cos\theta_I + Z_1 cos\theta} \qquad \text{eqn 2.10}$$

2.3 Acoustic Properties of Tissue

As ultrasound passes through tissue it loses energy; that is, it is attenuated. The energy is lost due to a combination of reflection, refraction, scatter, and absorption. The mechanisms for absorption are complex and beyond the scope of this chapter, but have been reviewed extensively elsewhere.[3–5] The reduction in pressure amplitude is characterised by the amplitude attenuation coefficient α where $\alpha = \alpha_a + \alpha_s$, α_a representing loss by absorption and α_s that by scattering. The intensity, after the beam has travelled a distance *x*, is given by

$$P = P_0 e^{-\alpha x} \quad \text{eqn 2.11}$$

where P_0 is the starting pressure. It follows that the intensity loss is described by the equation:

$$I = I_0 e^{-\mu x} \quad \text{eqn 2.12}$$

where $\mu = 2\alpha$, and I_0 is the initial pressure. α is the amplitude attenuation coefficient, and μ is the intensity attenuation coefficient. The units of the attenuation coefficient most commonly quoted are dB/cm/MHz, but nepers/cm/MHz are often used as well, where 1 Np/cm = 8.68 dB/cm. The attenuation coefficient is frequency dependent, with

$$\alpha = \alpha_0 f^n \quad \text{eqn 2.13}$$

Table 2.1 shows attenuation coefficients for a number of different tissues. It can be seen that bone has the highest attenuation and impedance values of all the tissues in the body, and so it is to be expected that there is very significant reflection from a bone/soft tissue interface, with very rapid attenuation of any energy entering the bone itself.

2.4 Thermal Properties of Tissue

The loss of energy as an ultrasound wave travels through tissue and its conversion into heat is a partial expression of the first law of thermodynamics: 'in all processes occurring in an isolated system, the energy of the system remains constant'. The concepts of heat and temperature are differentiated in physics. The temperature achieved with a given amount of thermal energy (heat) will depend on the volume in which it is dissipated, with larger volumes having a lower temperature. Thermodynamic temperature is an absolute measure of the average total internal energy of an object or objects – namely its kinetic energy (energy of motion) plus contributions from other factors. Its base unit is the kelvin. Lord Kelvin introduced a linear scale of temperature which started at absolute zero (0 K). The Celsius scale is subdivided into the same intervals as the Kelvin scale, but absolute zero is now at –273.5 C. It is divided into 100 intervals between the condensing point of steam (100°C = 371.315 K) and the melting point of ice (0°C = 273.15 K). For reference, the Fahrenheit scale gives 0°C as 32°F and 100°C as 212°F (i.e. 1°C = 1.8°F). The unit used to describe the quantity of heat is the joule (J).

The most useful parameter to judge tissue's ability to heat up is its heat capacity, C. This is defined as the amount of heat required to raise the temperature by 1°C and has units of $J\ °C^{-1}$. Most commonly, this is expressed as the heat required to raise the temperature of 1 g of the substance, the specific heat capacity, with units of $J\ g^{-1}\ °C^{-1}$. For water, this is 4.185 $J\ g^{-1}\ °C^{-1}$, whereas for air it is ~1.01 $J\ g^{-1}\ °C^{-1}$, which indicates that far less energy is needed to heat air than water. The specific heats of various representative tissues are shown in Table 2.2. It follows that the amount of thermal energy required to raise the temperature of a mass *m* by ΔT, Q, is:

$$Q = mC\,\Delta T = \rho V C \Delta T \quad \text{eqn 2.14}$$

where ρ is the density.

TABLE 2.2

Representative literature values for specific heats and thermal conductivity of tissues.[6, 8, 9] The value depends to some extent on the tissue state when measured, and the temperature of measurement. Those cited are primarily for body temperature. The ability of a material to conduct heat across its volume is described by its thermal conductivity coefficient (κ), with units of W cm^{-1}°C^{-1}.

Tissue Type	Specific Heat Capacity J g^{-1}°C^{-1}	Thermal Conductivity W cm^{-1} °C^{-1}
Skin	3.39–3.77	0.2–0.6 10^{-3}
Muscle	3.5–3.8	0.38–0.46 10^{-3}
Fat	2.2–2.4	0.20–0.23 10^{-3}
Liver	3.59	0.57 10^{-3}
Brain	3.59	0.16–0.57 10^{-3}
Bone	1.59	0.68 10^{-3}

It can be seen from equation 2.10 that the energy lost across a unit area in travelling a distance, dx, by an ultrasound wave, dI/dx, is μI. If we assume that all this energy loss goes to heating the tissue, then the rate of heat deposition Q is given by

$$\dot{Q} = \mu I \qquad \text{eqn 2.15}$$

From equation 2.12 we know that Q can also be written as

$$\dot{Q} = \rho C \frac{dT}{dt} \qquad \text{eqn 2.16}$$

where $\frac{dT}{dt}$ is the rate of temperature rise. This gives, for example, a temperature rise of ~14.4°C s^{-1} for a tissue exposed to 100 Wcm^{-2} at 1 MHz for which μ is 0.6 Np/cm and density is 1 g cm^{-3}.

In reality, while ultrasound can heat tissue, physiological cooling mechanisms exist that will carry some of the heat away, reducing the final temperature. The temperature rise can be calculated using the Pennes bio-heat equation, which takes into account both the heat source and any cooling mechanisms.[10–14] The temperature rise is given by:

$$\rho C \frac{\partial T}{\partial t} = \kappa \nabla^2 T - A(x, y, z, t) + \dot{Q} \qquad \text{eqn 2.17}$$

where $A(x,y,z,t)$ is the cooling term that depends on thermal conductivity and blood flow to the region. If the cooling is considered to be primarily due to vascular perfusion, then

$$A(x, y, z, t) = W_b C_b (T - T_b) \qquad \text{eqn 2.18}$$

where W_b, C_b and T_b are the perfusion, specific heat and temperature of the blood, respectively. This assumes that blood enters the volume at body core temperature and leaves at the temperature of the volume being heated.

The Pennes bio-heat equation is the basis for most simulations used in planning thermal treatments, with the most common solvers being based on finite element or finite difference methods (see Chapter 6 for a more complete description of the simulation methods used).

The temperature distribution achieved depends on the geometry of the ultrasound source (the transducer) as well as the target tissue. Plane waves, weakly, and strongly, focused beams, can be achieved. These are discussed in more detail in Chapter 4.

An important aspect for ensuring the safety and efficacy of any therapy is dosimetry. In radiotherapy, for example, a distinction is made between exposure and dose, with dose being described in terms of the gray (Gy) which describes the absorption of 1 joule of energy in 1 kg of tissue. No such distinction is made in ultrasound therapy, and in fact no universal 'dose' unit exists. However, heat-based therapies can be quantified in terms of the thermal dose, with units of cumulative minutes at 43°C (CEM_{43}). This concept was first proposed by Sapareto and Dewey in 1984,[15] and is discussed further in Chapter 3.

2.5 Summary

A knowledge of the nature of ultrasonic propagation through tissue is essential for a proper understanding of therapy ultrasound and for its most efficient application for a wide range of indications. Acoustic and thermal parameters are available in the literature, but almost inevitably these are limited in their accuracy by the inability to be measured in perfused tissues in vivo. The vast majority of the data are acquired using freshly excised tissues and are measured at room, rather than body, temperature. Nevertheless the Pennes bio-heat equation can be used to predict the temperature distribution with sufficient accuracy to allow treatment planning.

REFERENCES

1. Padilla F, ter Haar G. Recommendations for reporting therapeutic ultrasound treatment parameters. Ultrasound in Medicine & Biology. 2022;48(7):1299–308.
2. Shaw A, ter Haar G, Haller J, Wilkens V. Towards a dosimetric framework for therapeutic ultrasound. International Journal of Hyperthermia. 2015;31(2):182–92.
3. Bamber JC. Ultrasonic properties of tissues. Ultrasound in Medicine. CRC Press; 2020. p. 57–88.
4. Pauly H, Schwan H. Mechanism of absorption of ultrasound in liver tissue. The Journal of the Acoustical Society of America. 1971;50(2B):692–9.
5. Ziskin MC. Fundamental physics of ultrasound and its propagation in tissue. Radiographics. 1993;13(3):705–9.
6. Duck FA. Acoustic properties of tissue at ultrasonic frequencies. Physical Properties of Tissues. 1990:73–135.
7. Fairhead AC. ICRU report 61: Providing reference data for tissue properties. The Journal of the Acoustical Society of America. 1999;105(2_Supplement):1324.
8. Giering K, Minet O, Lamprecht I, Müller G. Review of Thermal Properties of Biological Tissues. SPIE Optical Engineering Press; 1995.
9. Feldmann AN, Wili P, Maquer GB, Zysset P. The thermal conductivity of cortical and cancellous bone. European Cells & Materials eCM. 2018;35:25–33.
10. Pennes HH. Analysis of tissue and arterial blood temperatures in the resting human forearm. Journal of Applied Physiology. 1948;1(2):93–122.
11. Attar MM, Haghpanahi M, Amanpour S, Mohaqeq M. Analysis of bioheat transfer equation for hyperthermia cancer treatment. Journal of Mechanical Science and Technology. 2014;28:763–71.
12. Vanne A, Hynynen K. MRI feedback temperature control for focused ultrasound surgery. Physics in Medicine & Biology. 2002;48(1):31.
13. Xuan Y, Roetzel W. Bioheat equation of the human thermal system. Chemical Engineering & Technology: Industrial Chemistry-Plant Equipment-Process Engineering-Biotechnology. 1997;20(4):268–76.
14. Wissler EH. Pennes' 1948 paper revisited. Journal of Applied Physiology. 1998;85(1):35–41.
15. Sapareto SA, Dewey WC. Thermal dose determination in cancer therapy. International Journal of Radiation Oncology* Biology* Physics. 1984;10(6):787–800.

3

Mechanisms for Induction of Bio-effects of Focused Ultrasound in Tissue

Gail ter Haar

3.1 Heating

The varying pressures in an ultrasound wave alternately compress and decompress the medium through which it passes. Since soft tissues are composed of cells surrounded by an extracellular matrix, they can be pushed and pulled at the frequency of the ultrasound wave. When this motion is sufficiently rapid and the amplitude of motion is sufficiently high, some parts of the tissue move at slightly different rates than their surroundings. This results in frictional forces that will convert some of the kinetic energy into heat in a process known as viscous heating.[1] Focused beams allow the ultrasonic energy to be concentrated into a specific volume, creating localised regions of elevated temperatures, with the surroundings remaining unheated.

Cells can respond to elevated temperatures in a number of ways. Ultrasound exposures that result in temperature rises of ~1–2°C are used to stimulate wound healing[2–4] and muscle regeneration[5–7] and are thus used in physiotherapy.[8, 9] The exact mechanisms by which these effects are achieved are still poorly understood.

Temperature rises of 5–15°C maintained for several minutes are capable of permanently damaging (or killing) cells. The mechanism for this type of cell killing is reproductive death, meaning the cells are unable to divide successfully. This type of heating is used in hyperthermia treatments in which tumours are heated to 43–45°C for many minutes, in conjunction with chemo- or radiotherapy.

In contrast, high-intensity focused ultrasound (HIFU) is a technique in which cells are heated very rapidly, to temperatures in excess of 56°C for a few seconds, resulting in instantaneous cell death through a process of thermal necrosis. HIFU treatments are based on this type of heating regime, inducing thermal ablation, which is so rapid that tissues undergo the process of coagulative necrosis. Whereas hyperthermic temperatures cause cells to undergo programmed cell death over longer time periods, or sensitise cells to other insults, ablation causes immediate denaturation of proteins and coagulation.

A dosimetric quantity, known as the *thermal dose*, has been devised. This is mainly used to describe ablative treatments. It relates temperature rises in tissue to their biological effect, depending on the time for which cells are at an elevated temperature, and is an attempt to normalise ‘time at temperature’ data in order to allow comparison between different heating regimes.

Arrhenius measured reaction rates (k_1 and k_2) at different temperatures (T_1 and T_2) and found that their temperature dependence could be fitted with an exponential dependence of temperature difference[10–12]:

$$\frac{k_2(T_2)}{k_1(T_1)} = exp\left\{\frac{\mu(T_2 - T_1)}{2T_2T_1}\right\} \qquad \text{eqn 3.1}$$

This relationship has been used to generate Arrhenius plots in which the reciprocal of some measure of effect – in cancer biology, usually the dose required to generate a given level of cell killing – is plotted against the reciprocal of temperature at which this point was generated. These plots are usually biphasic

DOI: 10.1201/9780429162671-3

with a break point that lies at about 43°C. This break point varies a little between different species and cell lines, as does the gradient of the two lines involved, R.[13, 14]

The general expression for thermal dose, usually quoted in cumulative equivalent minutes at 43°C (CEM_{43}) is given by equation 3.2:

$$CEM_{43} = tR^{(43-T)} \quad \text{eqn 3.2}$$

where t is a time interval in minutes, and from above, R is the number of minutes needed to compensate for a 1°C temperature change. R is taken as 0.5 above the break point and 0.25 below it.[15, 16]

However, the temperature-time curve during a thermal treatment does not have a 'top hat' shape, but rather has heating up, steady-state and cooling phases, all of which contribute to the thermal dose and need to be summed, giving:

$$CEM_{43} = \sum_{t=t_{initial}}^{t=t_{final}} R^{43-T} \Delta t \quad \text{eqn 3.3}$$

where T is the temperature of tissues over a given time interval Δt. Although there is a slight dependence on tissue type, a CEM_{43} value of 240 minutes is generally accepted as the threshold for denaturation of proteins in mammalian cells.[16, 17] The thermal dose relationship roughly halves this time for each 1°C increase in temperature from this level. Thus, in order to cause rapid cell death in 1–2 seconds, as is required in HIFU, the temperature required is 56°C.[18]

While thermal dose is a useful comparator of different heating regimes designed to achieve the same clinical ends, it is not completely accurate. Its derivation comes from cell experiments carried out at temperatures around 43°C, and it is less clear that the relationship holds good for temperatures above 44–45°C. The experimental evidence for these temperatures, and indeed for a range of different tissues in vivo, is very sparse. A value of 240 minutes for ablation was somewhat arbitrarily chosen and may not be the correct value for all tissue types. Moreover, it has been shown that the cellular heating history has an impact on the response to thermal insult, with 'slow' heating resulting in lower cell survival than 'rapid heating'.[19, 20]

3.2 Acoustic Cavitation

Cavitation has many different definitions. These range from 'the formation of one or more pockets of gas (or cavities) in a liquid'[21] to 'the activities, simple or complex, of bubbles or cavities containing gas or vapour, in liquids or any media with liquid content'.[22] A much broader definition is that of Neppiras, namely 'whenever a new surface is created in the body of a liquid'.[23] This definition includes boiling and effervescence. Cavitation in an ultrasound field is known as acoustic cavitation. While the positive pressure components of the ultrasound pressure wave compress tissue, the negative-going portion (rarefaction) pulls the tissue apart. A sufficiently great negative pressure can draw dissolved gas in the tissue out of solution, leading to bubble formation. Acoustic cavitation has been defined in a number of ways, but the most commonly used definition is the 'behaviour, growth and subsequent motion' of these bubbles.[18] Bubble activity under the action of an ultrasound wave in water or in tissue is an enormously complex topic and cannot be covered comprehensively here. The reader is directed towards the many more detailed texts that are available for a deeper treatment of this topic.[24–29]

Bubbles oscillate in response to the incident ultrasound field. Two types of bubble activity are distinguished: *inertial* (formerly referred to as collapse or transient) and *non-inertial* (formerly referred to as stable) *cavitation*. Inertial cavitation occurs when a gas-filled cavity expands during a part of the pressure cycle and then collapses very rapidly to a volume that is a small fraction of its original volume. The name derives from the fact that the behaviour is controlled by the bubble's inertia.[30, 31] High temperatures and pressures are generated at the point of collapse.

At lower-pressure amplitudes, bubbles can oscillate stably, in phase with the ultrasonic field. Gas can diffuse in and out of a bubble as it expands and contracts. Since the surface area is greater on expansion than on contraction, more gas is pulled into the bubble during rarefaction than can diffuse back out during compression, and so the bubble will gradually grow. This process is known as rectified diffusion. The behaviour of stably oscillating bubbles leads to streaming of fluids surrounding the bubble. For example, when a bubble oscillates within an extracellular space, the fluid surrounding it begins to move. This is known as microstreaming. Stable cavitation bubbles exert forces on their surroundings, due directly to their oscillation or to this microstreaming flow. If cavitation occurs close to the wall of a blood vessel, the force may be enough to stretch the vessel wall, making it more permeable to therapeutic agents. Similarly, forces on nearby membranes may increase their permeability, allowing drugs to enter cells for a number of therapeutic applications.[32–34] This is discussed in more detail later.

Cavitation is a threshold phenomenon. The different regimes kick in at defined negative pressures. These thresholds are frequency and temperature dependent. Considerable effort is put into measuring these thresholds, but there is a strong dependence on tissue type and tissue status. Thresholds are usually expressed in terms of the pressure needed to induce cavitation in a given percentage of exposures, with that percentage usually being 50% or 75%.

Cavitation occurring in tissue is usually identified by monitoring the characteristic acoustic emissions that accompany inertial and non-inertial bubble behaviour. Cavitating bubbles themselves act as sources of sound. These can be picked up using a sensitive hydrophone operating in the required frequency range.

Oscillating bubbles emit sound at the half-order subharmonic ($f_0/2$). Several mechanisms for this have been postulated, but it is still not fully understood.[25] Explanations have included the surface vibrations on the bubble,[35] the behaviour of bubbles that are larger than the resonant size at the drive frequency, f_0[36], and chaos theory.[37] At high pressures (above the inertial cavitation threshold) the subharmonic signal amplitude rises. This may come from bubbles taking two pressure cycles to collapse.[38] In non-inertial cavitation fields, the second harmonic, $2f_0$, is also prominent, and the $(2n+1)\ f_0/2$ harmonics are also seen. As the acoustic pressure increases and cavitation activity builds up, so does the level of white noise, detected as broadband emissions.

The cavitation phenomenon is harnessed for therapies that use very high powers, such as HIFU, lithotripsy[39, 40] and histotripsy.[41–43] In particular, lithotripsy and histotripsy rely on significant amounts of inertial cavitation, using large populations of violently collapsing bubbles to break up tissues or calcifications. Cavitation bubbles may be advantageous in HIFU treatments since they enhance absorption locally, increasing the thermal effects achieved.[44] It is important to know whether cavitation is occurring for any given therapeutic ultrasound exposure regime, as its effects may be detrimental as well as beneficial. Bubbles may scatter the sound beam in an unpredictable way, diverting the ultrasonic energy away from the desired target.[45] In many cases, cavitation is not specifically monitored during clinical treatments, although the ability to do this during HIFU can help to determine whether a treatment is being delivered in the optimum way.[24, 46, 47]

Stably oscillating cavitation bubbles can also have a therapeutic effect. As they oscillate within extracellular spaces, for example, the fluids surrounding them begin to move in a fashion known as microstreaming. This has been of particular interest in the brain, where it has been shown that ultrasound exposures in the presence of microbubbles can temporarily open the blood-brain barrier (BBB).[34, 48–54] This topic is addressed in Chapters 25 and 26.

3.3 Radiation Force and Acoustic Streaming

There is another class of phenomena that may give rise to biological effects in tissue, and that are non-thermal and non-cavitational in origin. These are radiation pressure and streaming (including microstreaming).

An ultrasound pressure wave exerts a force on any boundary or inhomogeneity that lies in its path. The force has two components, a time varying component that has the frequency of the ultrasound beam and which time-averages to zero, and a steady component which has a non-zero time average. This steady component is known as the *radiation force* and arises from non-linearities in the sound field.[55–57]

For a perfectly reflecting target with area A, the radiation force F_{RP} can be expressed as:

$$F_{RP} = \frac{2IA}{c} \quad \text{eqn 3.4}$$

where I is the intensity and c is the speed of sound. For an absorbing target, this force is halved.

The biological consequences of this force are generally subtle. An early paper reported the transient blanching of rabbit eye choroid during the treatment of retinal tears with HIFU.[58] It has been known for a while that ultrasound can stimulate sensory receptors, with temperature receptors having been studied,[59–61] as have pain receptors on the skin.[62] More recently the neuromodulatory effects seen to result from ultrasound exposures are thought to be in part due to radiation pressure.[63–68]

The passage of an ultrasound beam through a fluid results in a radiation force which sets up unidirectional fluid motion in the fluids contained in cells and extracellular spaces. This is known as *acoustic streaming*. Streaming can increase heat transfer, accelerate rate processes and strip cell surfaces. The velocity gradients set up in the fluid are due to the spatially non-uniform nature of streaming, and these lead to shear stresses on objects within the field. These are highest against boundaries (for example, a blood vessel wall) because a non-slip condition dictates that the velocity is zero at a boundary, and they may be sufficient to cause changes – either beneficial or damaging, depending on their magnitude and the application. The region in which the velocity varies from zero to the bulk velocity of fluid is known as the boundary layer and is determined by the sound field frequency, the density, ρ, and viscosity, η, of the fluid by the relationship[69]:

$$\beta^{-1} = \sqrt{\frac{2\eta}{2\pi f \rho}} \quad \text{eqn 3.5}$$

At 1 MHz this boundary layer is ~0.56 μm. Acoustic streaming sets up a steady time invariant velocity gradient. The variations in acoustic pressure caused by the ultrasound beam also lead to oscillatory velocity gradients at the boundaries. It can be calculated that the steady stress is an order of magnitude lower than the oscillatory stress, but since it acts for longer, it may be more significant in causing biological effects.[70, 71]

Acoustic microstreaming is the term used to describe the eddying motions that are set up around an oscillating bubble in a sound field. These may have complex patterns, depending on the location of the bubble.[72] For example, vortices may develop around a bubble sitting on a surface. A schematic of this is shown in Figure 3.1. This streaming is small scale, and high-velocity gradients which lead to significant shear stresses developing. The shearing forces that may act on cells in the microstreaming fields around these oscillating bubbles can cause detrimental biological effects such as haemolysis or endothelial cell damage,[73–75] but can also be used to enhance drug delivery.[34, 50, 52–54]

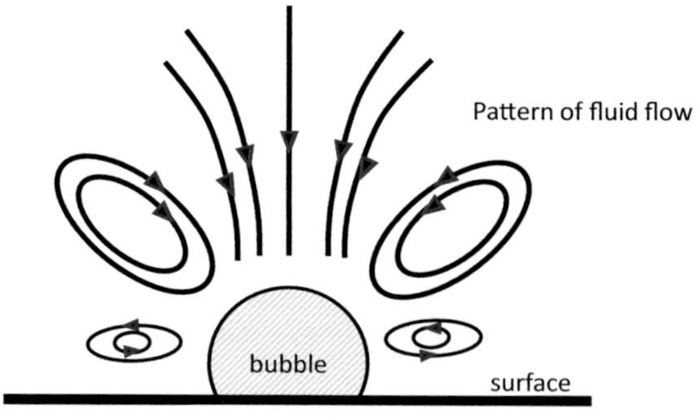

FIGURE 3.1 Schematic of an acoustic streaming regimen when a bubble is sitting on a surface.

Source: Adapted from[35].

The threshold pressures that are required to draw gas out of solution in tissue are still poorly quantified, but it is known that the negative pressure required to draw gas out of solution when using microsecond pulses (intrinsic histotripsy) is ~ 25 MPa, and when shock scattering is used to induce highly localised heating with millisecond pulses resulting in boiling (boiling or cavitation cloud histotripsy), this reduces to ~17 MPa.[41–43, 76–78] These are high pressures that can be difficult to achieve safely at depth in tissue, however, when drug delivery is the aim, the required exposures can be reduced by introducing stabilised microbubbles, such as are commonly used as diagnostic ultrasound contrast agents.[79, 80] These can be driven to produce the same microstreaming patterns as seen with naturally occurring bubbles. The most actively explored exploitation of these at present is their ability to temporarily open the BBB.[48, 81–84] These are discussed in more detail in Chapters 25 and 26.[ibid] Ultrasound thrombolysis (sonothrombolysis) also depends on bubble activity for its action.[85, 86]

3.4 Summary

MHz ultrasonic energy is remarkably versatile in nature. The combination of the pressure variations and its millimetric wavelengths in tissue means that exposures can be designed to result in purely thermal or purely mechanical (including cavitation) effects in tissue. There are occasions when a combination of these effects may be beneficial, for example in cancer therapy. An example of this might be the use of thermally ablative exposures to destroy the hypoxic centre of a tumour combined with hyperthermia-enhanced radiotherapy in its better oxygenated outer regions. There is no doubt that the full potential of the different mechanisms by which ultrasound can produce effects in tissue has not as yet been fully realised.

REFERENCES

1. Hill C, Bamber J, ter Haar G. Attenuation and absorption. Physical Principles of Medical Ultrasonics. Wiley; 1986. p. 495.
2. Byl NN, McKenzie AL, West JM, Whitney JD, Hunt TK, Scheuenstuhl HA. Low-dose ultrasound effects on wound healing: A controlled study with Yucatan pigs. Archives of Physical Medicine and Rehabilitation. 1992;73(7):656–64.
3. Ennis WJ, Lee C, Gellada K, Corbiere TF, Koh TJ. Advanced technologies to improve wound healing: Electrical stimulation, vibration therapy, and ultrasound – what is the evidence? Plastic and Reconstructive Surgery. 2016;138(3S):94S-104S.
4. Yadollahpour A, Mostafa J, Samaneh R, Zohreh R. Ultrasound therapy for wound healing: A review of current techniques and mechanisms of action. Journal of Pure and Applied Microbiology. 2014;8(5):4071–85.
5. Nagata K, Nakamura T, Fujihara S, Tanaka E. Ultrasound modulates the inflammatory response and promotes muscle regeneration in injured muscles. Annals of Biomedical Engineering. 2013;41:1095–105.
6. Rantanen J, Thorsson O, Wollmer P, Hurme T, Kalimo H. Effects of therapeutic ultrasound on the regeneration of skeletal myofibers after experimental muscle injury. The American Journal of Sports Medicine. 1999;27(1):54–9.
7. Wilkin L, Merrick M, Kirby TE, Devor ST. Influence of therapeutic ultrasound on skeletal muscle regeneration following blunt contusion. International Journal of Sports Medicine. 2004;25(01):73–7.
8. Warden SJ, McMeeken JM. Ultrasound usage and dosage in sports physiotherapy. Ultrasound in Medicine & Biology. 2002;28(8):1075–80.
9. Watson T. Ultrasound in contemporary physiotherapy practice. Ultrasonics. 2008;48(4):321–9.
10. Arrhenius S. Über die Reaktionsgeschwindigkeit bei der Inversion von Rohrzucker durch Säuren. Zeitschrift für physikalische Chemie. 1889;4(1):226–48.
11. Dewey WC. Arrhenius relationships from the molecule and cell to the clinic. International Journal of Hyperthermia. 2009;25(1):3–20.
12. Laidler KJ. The development of the Arrhenius equation. Journal of Chemical Education. 1984;61(6):494.
13. Hall EJ, Roizin-Towle L. Biological effects of heat. Cancer Research. 1984;44(10_Supplement):4708s–13s.
14. Roizin-Towle L, Pirro JP. The response of human and rodent cells to hyperthermia. International Journal of Radiation Oncology* Biology* Physics. 1991;20(4):751–6.

15. Sapareto SA. Practical concepts of thermal dose. Thermal Effects on Cells and Tissues. CRC Press; 2023. p. 201–12.
16. Sapareto SA, Dewey WC. Thermal dose determination in cancer therapy. International Journal of Radiation Oncology* Biology* Physics. 1984;10(6):787–800.
17. Damianou C, Hynynen K. The effect of various physical parameters on the size and shape of necrosed tissue volume during ultrasound surgery. The Journal of the Acoustical Society of America. 1994;95(3):1641–9.
18. ter Haar G. Therapeutic and Surgical Applications-physical Principles of Medical Ultrasonics. Ellis Horwood Ltd; 1986.
19. Mouratidis P, ter Haar G. An investigation of thermal dose as a parameter to model the thermal effects of high intensity focused ultrasound in cancer therapy. Cancer Research. 2015;75(15_Supplement):3611.
20. Mouratidis PX, Rivens I, Civale J, Symonds-Tayler R, ter Haar G. Relationship between thermal dose and cell death for "rapid" ablative and "slow" hyperthermic heating. International Journal of Hyperthermia. 2019;36:229–43.
21. Apfel R. Methods of Experimental Physics: Ultrasonics. Academic Press; 1981.
22. Coakley W, Nyborg W. Ultrasound: Its Applications in Medicine and Biology. Part I. F.J. Fry (ed.). Elsevier Scientific Publishing; 1978. p. 77–159.
23. Neppiras EA. Acoustic cavitation. Physics Reports. 1980;61(3):159–251.
24. Coussios C, Farny C, ter Haar G, Roy R. Role of acoustic cavitation in the delivery and monitoring of cancer treatment by high-intensity focused ultrasound (HIFU). International Journal of Hyperthermia. 2007;23(2):105–20.
25. Leighton T. The Acoustic Bubble. Academic Press; 2012.
26. Stride E, Coussios C. Nucleation, mapping and control of cavitation for drug delivery. Nature Reviews Physics. 2019;1(8):495–509.
27. Lajoinie G, De Cock I, Coussios CC, Lentacker I, Le Gac S, Stride E, et al. In vitro methods to study bubble-cell interactions: Fundamentals and therapeutic applications. Biomicrofluidics. 2016;10(1).
28. Stride E, Coussios C. Cavitation and contrast: The use of bubbles in ultrasound imaging and therapy. Proceedings of the Institution of Mechanical Engineers, Part H: Journal of Engineering in Medicine. 2010;224(2):171–91.
29. Kooiman K, Roovers S, Langeveld SA, Kleven RT, Dewitte H, O'Reilly MA, et al. Ultrasound-responsive cavitation nuclei for therapy and drug delivery. Ultrasound in Medicine & Biology. 2020;46(6):1296–325.
30. Flynn H. Physics of acoustic cavitation in liquids. Physical Acoustics. 1964;1(Part B):57–172.
31. Flynn HG. Physics of acoustic cavitation. The Journal of the Acoustical Society of America. 1959;31(11_Supplement):1582.
32. Costley D, Mc Ewan C, Fowley C, McHale AP, Atchison J, Nomikou N, et al. Treating cancer with sonodynamic therapy: A review. International Journal of Hyperthermia. 2015;31(2):107–17.
33. McHale AP, Callan JF, Nomikou N, Fowley C, Callan B. Sonodynamic therapy: Concept, mechanism and application to cancer treatment. Therapeutic Ultrasound. 2016:429–50.
34. Rosenthal I, Sostaric JZ, Riesz P. Sonodynamic therapy-a review of the synergistic effects of drugs and ultrasound. Ultrasonics Sonochemistry. 2004;11(6):349–63.
35. Esche R. Untersuchung der schwingungskavitation in flüssigkeiten. Acta Acustica united with Acustica. 1952;2(6):208–18.
36. Eller A, Flynn H. Generation of subharmonics of order one-half by bubbles in a sound field. The Journal of the Acoustical Society of America. 1969;46(3B):722–7.
37. Lauterborn W, Parlitz U. Methods of chaos physics and their application to acoustics. The Journal of the Acoustical Society of America. 1988;84(6):1975–93.
38. Parlitz U, Englisch V, Scheffczyk C, Lauterborn W. Bifurcation structure of bubble oscillators. The Journal of the Acoustical Society of America. 1990;88(2):1061–77.
39. Cleveland RO, McAteer JA. Physics of shock-wave lithotripsy. Smith's Textbook of Endourology. 2012:527–58.
40. Lingeman JE, McAteer JA, Gnessin E, Evan AP. Shock wave lithotripsy: Advances in technology and technique. Nature Reviews Urology. 2009;6(12):660–70.
41. Bader KB, Vlaisavljevich E, Maxwell AD. For whom the bubble grows: Physical principles of bubble nucleation and dynamics in histotripsy ultrasound therapy. Ultrasound in Medicine & Biology. 2019;45(5):1056–80.

42. Khokhlova VA, Fowlkes JB, Roberts WW, Schade GR, Xu Z, Khokhlova TD, et al. Histotripsy methods in mechanical disintegration of tissue: Towards clinical applications. International Journal of Hyperthermia. 2015;31(2):145–62.
43. Xu Z, Hall TL, Vlaisavljevich E, Lee Jr FT. Histotripsy: The first noninvasive, non-ionizing, non-thermal ablation technique based on ultrasound. International Journal of Hyperthermia. 2021;38(1):561–75.
44. Farny CH, Holt RG, Roy RA. The correlation between bubble-enhanced HIFU heating and cavitation power. IEEE Transactions on Biomedical Engineering. 2009;57(1):175–84.
45. Bailey MR, Couret LN, Sapozhnikov OA, Khokhlova VA, ter Haar G, Vaezy S, et al. Use of overpressure to assess the role of bubbles in focused ultrasound lesion shape in vitro. Ultrasound in Medicine & Biology. 2001;27(5):695–708.
46. Gyongy M, Arora M, Noble JA, Coussios C-C, editors. Use of passive arrays for characterization and mapping of cavitation activity during HIFU exposure. 2008 IEEE Ultrasonics Symposium. IEEE; 2008.
47. Rabkin BA, Zderic V, Vaezy S. Hyperecho in ultrasound images of HIFU therapy: Involvement of cavitation. Ultrasound in Medicine & Biology. 2005;31(7):947–56.
48. Aryal M, Arvanitis CD, Alexander PM, McDannold N. Ultrasound-mediated blood–brain barrier disruption for targeted drug delivery in the central nervous system. Advanced Drug Delivery Reviews. 2014;72:94–109.
49. Deng CX. Targeted drug delivery across the blood–brain barrier using ultrasound technique. Therapeutic Delivery. 2010;1(6):819–48.
50. Ferrara KW. Driving delivery vehicles with ultrasound. Advanced Drug Delivery Reviews. 2008;60(10):1097–102.
51. Lyon PC, Gray MD, Mannaris C, Folkes LK, Stratford M, Campo L, et al. Safety and feasibility of ultrasound-triggered targeted drug delivery of doxorubicin from thermosensitive liposomes in liver tumours (TARDOX): A single-centre, open-label, phase 1 trial. The Lancet Oncology. 2018;19(8):1027–39.
52. Mitragotri S. Healing sound: The use of ultrasound in drug delivery and other therapeutic applications. Nature Reviews Drug Discovery. 2005;4(3):255–60.
53. Mo S, Coussios C-C, Seymour L, Carlisle R. Ultrasound-enhanced drug delivery for cancer. Expert Opinion on Drug Delivery. 2012;9(12):1525–38.
54. Mørch Ý, Hansen R, Berg S, Åslund AK, Glomm WR, Eggen S, et al. Nanoparticle-stabilized microbubbles for multimodal imaging and drug delivery. Contrast Media & Molecular Imaging. 2015;10(5):356–66.
55. Hasegawa T, Yosioka K. Acoustic-radiation force on a solid elastic sphere. The Journal of the Acoustical Society of America. 1969;46(5B):1139–43.
56. Sarvazyan AP, Rudenko OV, Nyborg WL. Biomedical applications of radiation force of ultrasound: Historical roots and physical basis. Ultrasound in Medicine & Biology. 2010;36(9):1379–94.
57. Torr G. The acoustic radiation force. American Journal of Physics. 1984;52(5):402–8.
58. Lizzi F, Coleman D, Driller J, Franzen L, Leopold M. Effects of pulsed ultrasound on ocular tissue. Ultrasound in Medicine & Biology. 1981;7(3):245–52.
59. Gavrilov L, Tsirulnikov E, Davies IA. Application of focused ultrasound for the stimulation of neural structures. Ultrasound in Medicine & Biology. 1996;22(2):179–92.
60. Gavrilov LR. Use of focused ultrasound for stimulation of nerve structures. Ultrasonics. 1984;22(3):132–8.
61. Gavrilov LR. The possibility of generating focal regions of complex configurations in application to the problems of stimulation of human receptor structures by focused ultrasound. Acoustical Physics. 2008;54:269–78.
62. Dalecki D, Child SZ, Raeman CH, Carstensen EL. Tactile perception of ultrasound. The Journal of the Acoustical Society of America. 1995;97(5):3165–70.
63. Baek H, Pahk KJ, Kim H. A review of low-intensity focused ultrasound for neuromodulation. Biomedical Engineering Letters. 2017;7:135–42.
64. Blackmore J, Shrivastava S, Sallet J, Butler CR, Cleveland RO. Ultrasound neuromodulation: A review of results, mechanisms and safety. Ultrasound in Medicine & Biology. 2019;45(7):1509–36.
65. Bowary P, Greenberg BD. Noninvasive focused ultrasound for neuromodulation: A review. Psychiatric Clinics. 2018;41(3):505–14.
66. Darmani G, Bergmann T, Pauly KB, Caskey C, De Lecea L, Fomenko A, et al. Non-invasive transcranial ultrasound stimulation for neuromodulation. Clinical Neurophysiology. 2022;135:51–73.

67. Darrow DP. Focused ultrasound for neuromodulation. Neurotherapeutics. 2019;16(1):88–99.
68. Di Biase L, Falato E, Di Lazzaro V. Transcranial focused ultrasound (tFUS) and transcranial unfocused ultrasound (tUS) neuromodulation: From theoretical principles to stimulation practices. Frontiers in Neurology. 2019;10:549.
69. Nyborg WLM. Physical Mechanisms for Biological Effects of Ultrasound. US Department of Health, Education, and Welfare, Public Health Service, Food . . .; 1978.
70. Rooney JA. Shear as a mechanism for sonically induced biological effects. The Journal of the Acoustical Society of America. 1972;52(6B):1718–24.
71. Wu J. Shear stress in cells generated by ultrasound. Progress in Biophysics and Molecular Biology. 2007;93(1–3):363–73.
72. Elder SA. Cavitation microstreaming. The Journal of the Acoustical Society of America. 1959;31(1):54–64.
73. Daniels S, Kodama T, Price D. Damage to red blood cells induced by acoustic cavitation. Ultrasound in Medicine & Biology. 1995;21(1):105–11.
74. Wong Y, Watmough D. Haemolysis of red blood cells in vitro and in vivo induced by ultrasound at 0.75 MHz and at therapeutic intensity levels. Ultrasound Interactions in Biology and Medicine. Springer; 1983. p. 179–84.
75. Saad A, Bahakim H, Helmi A, Bashandi A, Lim L. Therapeutic ultrasound and the liver in vivo: Action and possible mechanisms. Ultrasound in Medicine & Biology. 1986;12(11):855–63.
76. Pahk KJ, Lee S, Gélat P, de Andrade MO, Saffari N. The interaction of shockwaves with a vapour bubble in boiling histotripsy: The shock scattering effect. Ultrasonics Sonochemistry. 2021;70:105312.
77. Vlaisavljevich E, Gerhardson T, Hall T, Xu Z. Effects of f-number on the histotripsy intrinsic threshold and cavitation bubble cloud behavior. Physics in Medicine & Biology. 2017;62(4):1269.
78. Vlaisavljevich E, Xu Z, Maxwell AD, Mancia L, Zhang X, Lin K-W, et al. Effects of temperature on the histotripsy intrinsic threshold for cavitation. IEEE Transactions on Ultrasonics, Ferroelectrics, and Frequency Control. 2016;63(8):1064–77.
79. Cosgrove D. Ultrasound contrast agents: An overview. European Journal of Radiology. 2006; 60(3):324–30.
80. Frinking P, Segers T, Luan Y, Tranquart F. Three decades of ultrasound contrast agents: A review of the past, present and future improvements. Ultrasound in Medicine & Biology. 2020;46(4):892–908.
81. Alkins R, Burgess A, Ganguly M, Francia G, Kerbel R, Wels WS, et al. Focused ultrasound delivers targeted immune cells to metastatic brain tumors. Cancer Research. 2013;73(6):1892–9.
82. Alonso A. Ultrasound-induced blood-brain barrier opening for drug delivery. Translational Neurosonology. 2015;36:106–15.
83. Hynynen K. Ultrasound for drug and gene delivery to the brain. Advanced Drug Delivery reviews. 2008;60(10):1209–17.
84. McDannold N, Vykhodtseva N, Hynynen K. Effects of acoustic parameters and ultrasound contrast agent dose on focused-ultrasound induced blood-brain barrier disruption. Ultrasound in Medicine & Biology. 2008;34(6):930–7.
85. Datta S, Coussios C-C, McAdory LE, Tan J, Porter T, De Courten-Myers G, et al. Correlation of cavitation with ultrasound enhancement of thrombolysis. Ultrasound in Medicine & Biology. 2006;32(8):1257–67.
86. Francis CW. Ultrasound-enhanced thrombolysis. Echocardiography. 2001;18(3):239–46.

4

Imaged-Guided Focused Ultrasound Therapy: Physics and Clinical Applications

Ian Rivens and John Civale

4.1 Introduction: Physics of Ultrasound Generation

This chapter outlines methods of generating ultrasound fields for therapeutic medical use, from the simplest earliest systems that used naturally occurring materials, to the most complex modern manufactured devices consisting of thousands of miniature sources driven by highly complex electronics to achieve impressive feats such as dynamic steering of the focal position for volumetric treatment, aberration correction for treatment of the brain through the highly attenuating skull, and the simultaneous creation of multiple focal peaks to create homogeneous heating in a region much larger than the geometric focus.

The fields of diagnostic and therapeutic ultrasound exist thanks to the discovery in 1880 by Pierre Curie and his brother Jacques of a phenomenon known as piezoelectricity.[1] They found that some materials, such as Rochelle salt (sodium potassium tartrate tetrahydrate), produced a voltage when compressed. The inverse piezoelectric behaviour of creating a mechanical stress in response to a voltage difference was mathematically deduced from thermodynamic principles[2] by physicist Gabriel Lippman in 1881, was experimentally verified by the Curie brothers, and provides us with the ability to generate ultrasound.

By applying an alternating voltage using electrodes attached to opposing surfaces of a piezoelectric material, it can be set into oscillation, thus producing a continuously varying thickness change in the direction between 2 electrodes. Simplistically, the resonant frequency of the device depends on the thickness of the material, with a 5-mm-thick manufactured piezoelectric having a fundamental resonance around 1 MHz. Higher ultrasound frequencies can be generated with thinner disks or by using odd-integer harmonic resonances of the fundamental. When such a device is loaded by an elastic medium such as water, MegaHertz (MHz) frequency ultrasound (pressure) waves can be produced and propagated. The ability to transduce energy from electricity into ultrasound has spawned a wide range of applications from non-destructive testing of structural materials (e.g. railway tracks) to medical applications, including the imaging of fetuses, and therapy that exploits either the ultrasound absorption that leads to heating (hyperthermia or ablation) and/or pressure-induced acoustic cavitation (bubble formation) to break kidney stones or gallstones, emulsify diseased soft tissue, or alter tissue permeability or functionality. The life-improving range of medical applications of ultrasound only became possible following intensive work on sound navigation and ranging (sonar), developed initially after the sinking of the *Titanic* to detect icebergs, and subsequently during World War I for detecting submarines.

The resonant frequency of a piezoelectric crystal is related to twice its thickness since waves reflected from the internal surfaces interfere coherently under this condition. Transducer design[3] is therefore fundamentally relatively simple. For broadband (wide frequency) operation, such as used in diagnostic ultrasound imaging, matching the rear surface of the device with a material of similar acoustic impedance (defined as the product of density and sound speed in the material) to that of the transducer is

DOI: 10.1201/9780429162671-4

beneficial, whereas for high-power applications, the rear transducer surface is usually air backed. The low acoustic impedance of air strongly reflects energy at this rear interface and maximises the coherent interference of the sound waves within the crystal, thus maximising the energy output from the front surface in a narrow band around the crystal's natural resonance frequency.

Because piezoelectric materials generally have a much higher acoustic impedance than human soft tissues, the transducer's front surface is typically matched to the load material (often water or skin) using a quarter wavelength thick layer with an acoustic impedance between that of the transducer and the load. Since the speed of sound in a piezoelectric is fixed and the output frequency is determined by reflections from the surface material, the material's thickness dictates the fundamental resonant frequency (this frequency increases as thickness decreases). Additionally, a transducer's natural resonance (internal reflection coherence) at all odd integer multiples of the fundamental frequency may be exploited, commonly by driving devices at their 3rd (or higher order) harmonic to obtain higher frequency output without the need to use thinner, less robust transducer elements, but at the cost of a reduction in transduction efficiency.

Transducers are driven using a signal generator (or arbitrary waveform generator) set to the required voltage amplitude and frequency. If the voltage output is insufficient for the therapy application under investigation, an additional power amplifier may be used. Best practice involves measurement of the electrical power delivered to the transducer. For this, either a forward and reflected power meter may be inserted into the drive circuit, or the drive voltage and current may be measured. Finally, before the 50-Ω electrical impedance drive chain is connected to the transducer, there is usually an electrical matching network[4] designed to minimise the difference between the electrical impedance of the transducer and the drive components. This is electrically analogous to the use of matching layers on the transducer surface to optimise acoustic power output by minimising energy reflection, with the aim of transduction efficiency maximisation.

For the treatment of tissue targets at depth in the human body, the attenuation of ultrasound in the tissue overlying the target (due to scattering and local absorption) has to be overcome in order to provide sufficient intensity to heat the target (focal) region or induce sufficiently high-pressure fields to produce acoustic cavitation, both of which can be used to damage tissue in a therapeutic way. This is achieved remarkably simply by focusing the ultrasound beam. To ensure effective and safe treatment delivery, the beam should avoid any regions of high acoustic impedance change (usually bone or air interfaces), and the device used should be of sufficient area to reduce the energy density on the skin which, as the body's waterproof covering, has a particularly high ultrasound attenuation and absorption, rendering it more highly susceptible to unintended damage, a situation which is drastically worsened if air is trapped on the skin during coupling for therapeutic ultrasound treatments.

4.2 Ultrasound Transducer Materials

Some piezoelectric materials are naturally occurring (such as certain types of quartz), while others are manmade. While natural materials may be machined to provide, for example, focusing, artificial materials may be readily moulded to required shapes. This is true of both piezoceramics and of the more highly engineered piezocomposites, which are described in more detail later.

For medical purposes, and therapy in particular, transducers need to have the following characteristics:

Electromechanical coupling (transducer efficiency) as close to 100% as possible.

Specific acoustic impedance should be well matched to the intended propagation medium to minimise reflected energy at the transducer/medium interface.

Dielectric constant and *electrical and mechanical losses* in the transducer should be minimised.

Thermal stability and *structural strength* are important for the longevity of devices. Strength may be problematic at high frequencies, where thinner materials provide the required resonant frequency.

Shaping of the transducer material is important if geometrically focused devices are required.

4.2.1 Piezoceramic Transducers

The first major advance in transducer technology came after World War II when lead zirconium titanate (PZT) piezoceramic[5] was developed at the Tokyo Institute of Technology (~1952). PZT offers better electromechanical coupling (better power output or detection sensitivity) and higher operating temperatures (up to ~ 250°C) than its predecessor, barium titanate, whilst remaining physical strong, chemically inert, and relatively low cost to manufacture. For these reasons, PZT remains the most commonly used piezoelectric ceramic. Different formulations are preferred for different applications, and for high-intensity frequency ultrasound (HIFU), high-power options, such as PZT4 (Navy Type I) and PZT8 (Navy Type III), are generally chosen.[6] PZT8 was named to indicate that it is roughly twice as good as PZT4 in terms of producing high-power output. The only significant drawback with PZT is its high acoustic impedance compared to water and soft tissue. However, by using "matching layers", as described earlier, it is possible to greatly improve the acoustic coupling.

Whilst any planar piezoelectric material can be focused using lenses or reflectors, artificial materials can be moulded or shaped more easily than those occurring naturally (see Figure 4.1). In 1942, Lynn et al. published details of a system[7] for which quartz crystal had to be ground to provide focusing, and the diameter of the devices was limited by the size of available natural crystals. This explains why the pioneering clinical work of the Fry brothers in the 1950s into brain disorders required 4 planar quartz crystals, each of which was lens focused and then aligned so that their focal regions overlapped in order to obtain sufficient power concentration for therapeutic effect.[8, 9] These crystals were small compared to modern artificial ones, which can also easily be shaped into spherical bowls to provide inherent focusing.

4.2.2 Piezocomposite Transducers

The development of piezocomposite materials, an important advance following the creation of artificial piezoceramics, was largely pioneered by R. Newnham at the Materials Research Laboratory of Pennsylvania State University.[10–12] With piezocomposites, a mixture of polymer material and piezoceramic is used to modify specific features of the ceramic.[13] Currently the "1–3" type piezocomposite is preferred for ultrasonic transducers.[14] Here parallel piezoceramic rods are embedded in a polymer matrix, usually by dicing the ceramic into rectangular rods before filling the gaps with epoxy polymer. The ceramic plate is typically cut to ~80% of its thickness, with the pitch of the cuts being small

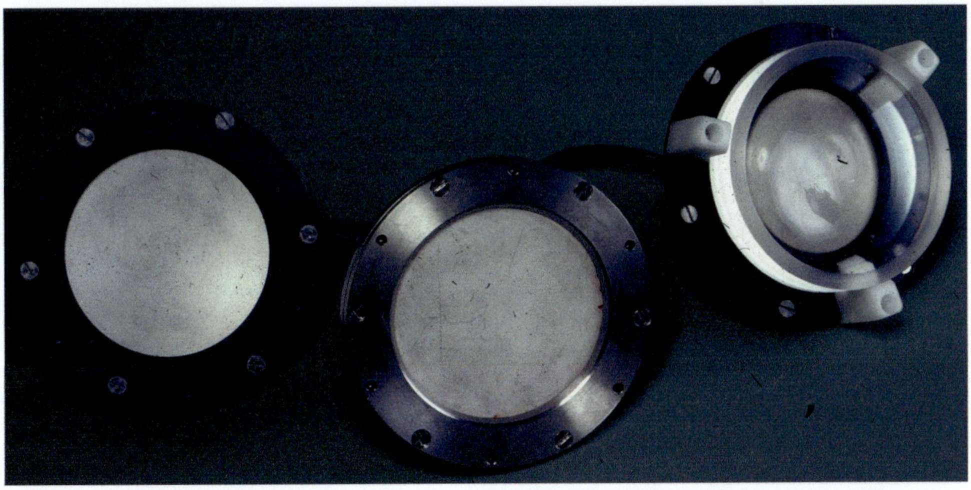

FIGURE 4.1 PZT transducers, from left to right, a spherical focused bowl, a planar transducer, and a planar transducer with Perspex lens. *Image courtesy of the Institute of Cancer Research.*

compared to the wavelength (e.g. <0.1 mm at 5 MHz) to avoid the formation of ultrasound radial modes and grating lobes (see Chapter 5 *ibid*). The notches are filled with epoxy or other polymers. Once cured, the uncut ceramic is ground smooth before each surface is plated with electrodes and the material polarised using high magnetic fields and heat to give the required piezoelectric properties. This method makes it possible to fabricate relatively large piezocomposite plates, which can be used to produce one large or multiple smaller transducers. Polymers have more tissue-like acoustic impedance than PZT, but worse electromechanical coupling and dielectric properties. Piezocomposites may have superior (greater) electromechanical coupling, specific acoustic impedance (lower), and dielectric and mechanical losses (lower). The manufacture of optimal piezocomposites is a highly skilled process that is dependent on efficient modelling of these complex multi-layered devices for success. Combining piezoceramic with polymers means that unlike conventional piezoceramic, piezocomposites can be tailored to specific needs. For example, the thickness coupling factor can be modified to control the acoustic impedance without significant coupling losses. Varying ceramic volume fraction, and selection of the best PZT material, allows adjustment of the dielectric constant to yield the optimum pulse form and amplitude. Polymer choice (hard or flexible epoxy) allows control of the acoustic and mechanical performance of the piezocomposite transducer, including the internal attenuation of the transducer and the reduction of planar coupling, and hence suppression of radial modes. The use of flexible epoxy also allows the piezocomposite to be formed into a spherical shape to produce a focused transducer. One example is shown in Figure 4.2. In summary, piezocomposite offers superior mechanical flexibility, electroacoustic efficiency, and beneficially reduced planar coupling and acoustic impedance. Unfortunately, the cost is reduced mechanical strength and lower tolerance to heating (particularly if the focus is inadvertently reflected back onto the transducer surface). The use of both piezoceramic (Figures 4.1 and 4.4) and piezocomposite (Figures 4.2, 4.3, and 4.8) transducers in therapeutic ultrasound is widespread.

4.2.3 CMUT Transducers

A more recent, and still developing, alternative transducer technology, is the capacitive micromachined ultrasonic transducer (CMUT) in which ultrasound is generated by a change in capacitance rather than by the piezoelectric effect. Here the transducer consists of a back plate beneath a cavity over which a thin metal electrode is mounted. The stretching and displacement of the electrode relative to the back plate by an applied voltage produces the ultrasound waves. These devices are micro electromechanical systems (MEMS)-based structures that can transmit (and receive) ultrasonic signals. They have enabled novel ultrasound technology to be used in diverse industries including inkjet printing. Compared to conventional transducers, CMUTs naturally have a wide frequency bandwidth and are easy to fabricate

FIGURE 4.2 An example of an asymmetric, curved piezocomposite endorectal transducer (black region) designed for the treatment of the prostate under MR guidance. *Image courtesy of the Institute of Cancer Research.*

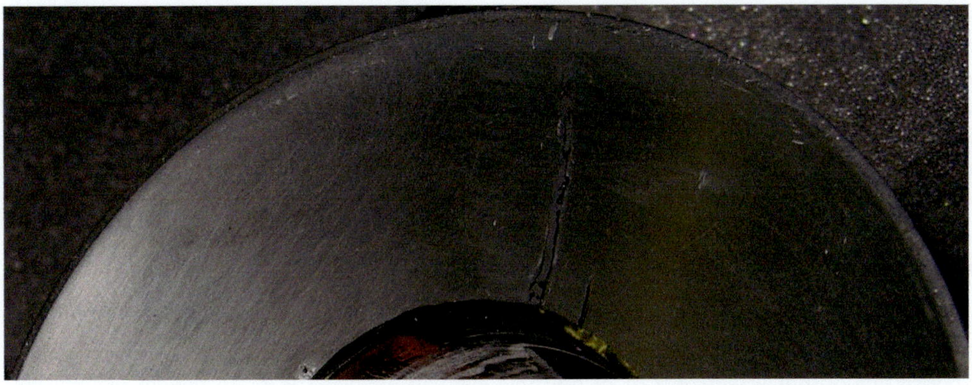

FIGURE 4.3 Mechanical damage (after repair) to the surface of a piezoceramic transducer's matching layer due to insertion into the central aperture of an ill-fitting imaging probe. *Image courtesy of the Institute of Cancer Research.*

as large arrays of very small elements, with simple integration of drive electronics via CMUT-on-CMOS (complementary metal-oxide semiconductors, currently the mostly widely used technology for integrated circuits). CMUT technology offers design freedom, high volume transducer manufacture, and high levels of integration at a lower cost. CMUTs can operate from –40° to 200°C at pressures up to 10 bar and can easily be made resistant to abrasion and chemical damage. But their biggest advantage is the simplicity with which array transducers with high numbers of elements can be fabricated. The advantages of such devices are described in Section 4.4.

The feasibility of producing HIFU using CMUTs was first reported in 2008 when magnetic resonance (MR) temperature mapping with a single-element, unfocused, 2.5-MHz CMUT was demonstrated in a hydrogel. The CMUT tested produced a relatively modest peak-to-peak output pressure of 1.4 MPa (16.3 Wcm^{-2}).[15] Following this, a concentric annular CMUT array[16] with axial steering capability was fabricated to produce a high intensity focus. These reports demonstrated the feasibility of using CMUTs for HIFU, but lateral steering and beam shaping were not possible with these early devices. In 2016, the fabrication of a 5-MHz 8 × 8-mm^2, 32 × 32-element 2-D CMUT array for HIFU was reported. To reduce system complexity the 1024 CMUT transducer elements were grouped into eight HIFU channels (based on the phase delay from the CMUT element to the targeted focal point 8 mm away). The measured peak-to-peak focal pressure was 8.5 MPa, which was expected to generate a lesion in 60 seconds according to the temperature simulations. Ex vivo tissue experiments successfully demonstrated this capability in both bovine muscle and liver tissue.[17] By 2018, Bawiec et al. had demonstrated a planar 64-element annular CMUT design with central imaging aperture capable of dynamically focusing a 3-MHz ultrasound beam at axial distances ranging from 32 to 72 mm, producing lesions comparable in size and shape to those obtained with a clinical transrectal prostate device.[18] The acoustic intensity from a single CMUT ring-element was measured to be over 6 Wcm^{-2}, which was shown in simulations to be sufficient for the generation of thermal lesions when using all 1024 elements, suggesting the feasibility of dynamic HIFU focusing with planar CMUT probes for the treatment of prostate tissue using an endo-cavitary approach. A comprehensive introduction to CMUT technology, with a detailed review of the literature including HIFU and dual-mode HIFU and ultrasound imaging applications was published in 2022.[19]

4.2.4 Transducer Preservation

Transducers are susceptible to damage from several sources. Heating of the piezoelectric can cause depoling of the magnetic field and destroy the device's piezoelectric capabilities. Typical Curie temperatures of piezoceramics mean that the temperature has to exceed several hundred °C for this to happen,[20] but piezocomposites can be particularly susceptible to thermal damage, affecting their structure. Most matching layers on the front of therapy ultrasound transducers will melt at lower temperatures, affecting device performance. Of particular concern is the unintended reflection of the focused beam back onto the transducer surface, which can result in damaged regions. As with any ceramic object, mechanical impact can shatter it, so dropping the device or driving it into solid objects using a gantry or robotic arm should be avoided. Transducer housings with purpose-built imaging apertures can also be susceptible to damage from insertion of wrong sized or excessively tight-fitting imaging probes. Transducer matching layers may not be suitable for use in highly alkaline or acidic environments, so cleaning materials should be carefully chosen, in accordance with manufacturer's recommendations.

4.3 Ultrasound Transducer Design: Single Elements

Ultrasound transducers consist of either single elements (where the entire device is driven in phase to produce one output wavefront) or of multiple element arrays. The main benefit of focused ultrasound therapy is that tissue damage only occurs within and around the focal region, where the acoustic pressure (intensity) is significantly higher than anywhere else in the beam. This specificity allows the delivery of both effective and safe treatment by maximising the power in one volume and minimising it everywhere else. For single element spherical bowl transducers (or plane transducers used with lenses), the approximately ellipsoidal focal region's size may be predicted[21] from the speed of sound (c), frequency (f), and transducer geometry (where the f-number (F#) is given by the focal length (radius of curvature) divided by the effective diameter of the ultrasound source), with the length usually being approximately 10 times the width.[22] More specifically, the full-width half-maximum (FWHM) pressure (P) dimensions for the lateral (L) and axial (A) focal directions are roughly:

$$FWHMP_L = 1.4\frac{c}{f}F\#$$

$$FWHMP_A = 7.2\frac{c}{f}(F\#)^2$$

4.3.1 Advantages of Single Elements

Single-element transducers are the simplest to set up, drive, and use safely because:

- only one drive channel needs to be monitored to ensure operation is within expected limits
- fault finding involves the minimum number of components as there is only one drive channel
- replacement of faulty transducers is simple, device performance should always be measured as it cannot be assumed that a nominally similar device will operate in the same way as the one it replaces
- the fixed geometry means that the focal region is always in the same position relative to the device, which means that:
  - it is possible to design pointers that are able to provide a physical indication of the position of the focus
  - the focal position is likely to only vary by a few millimetres at most. Variations are due to temperature changes and other factors affecting sound speed in the propagation medium, and to the effects of attenuation which may shift the focal point in tissue slightly towards the source

Single-element devices may be planar with low-cost focusing achieved using a lens,[23–26] but lenses may also be designed for single-element devices that are already focused.[27] In either case, different (relatively cheap) lenses may be used to achieve different focal distances (treatment depths), focal sizes, and peak pressures or intensities, using one (relatively expensive) ultrasound source. Recent developments in lens design mean that complex patterns, such as multiple foci, can be formed, allowing the delivery of larger volume uniform heating for hyperthermia.[27] Focusing may also be achieved using geometrical shaping of the transducer (e.g. into a spherical bowl) to give a fixed focal geometry (position, size, and shape). Scope for further flexibility derives from devices that are electrical-impedance matched at more than one frequency. For a fixed geometry, higher ultrasound frequencies will produce smaller focal regions and, due to the enhanced focusing, higher focal peak pressures/intensities unless this is offset by a reduction in transduction efficiency and pre-focal tissue absorption.

4.3.2 Practical Devices

Single element transducers have been used in many laboratory studies, some of which have spawned clinical devices for extracorporeal,[28, 29] endocavitary,[30, 31] or interstitial[32, 33] treatments. A single element transducer requires one drive channel and therefore electrical safety monitoring of that channel is simple and relatively inexpensive to achieve. Additionally, the simplicity means there are fewer drive components that can malfunction. The cost of these benefits may include the need to move devices with high accuracy when extended volumes need to be exposed, usually to many treatment positions, using an automated gantry or robotic arm. This introduces new patient safety concerns. Such systems are often best suited to one, or a small number of, applications that target similar depths within the body since the device and focal geometry are fixed. A number of commercial systems which incorporate a single-element focused ultrasound transducer are available for pre-clinical laboratory use in ex vivo or in vivo studies e.g. Alpinion's VIFU[34–37] and Sonic Concepts' HIFUplex.[38, 39] Additionally there are a number of commercially available clinical systems such as Chongqing HAIFU's JC200[29] (see Figure 4.4) or the Echopulse from Theraclion.[40]

4.4 Ultrasound Transducer Design: Phased Arrays

Focused ultrasound phased arrays have provided game-changing capability, ranging from finally achieving the holy grail of focusing ultrasound through the intact skull into pre-selected regions of the brain, to providing the potential to perform interleaved therapy and imaging guidance and monitoring with a single transducer probe. An investment in expensive and complex equipment can provide researchers with an incredibly flexible tool. Understandably, early array designs incorporated a small number of relatively large transducer elements, but as engineering and an understanding of their potential has improved, the trend has been towards larger numbers of smaller elements which provide more flexible beam modulation.[41]

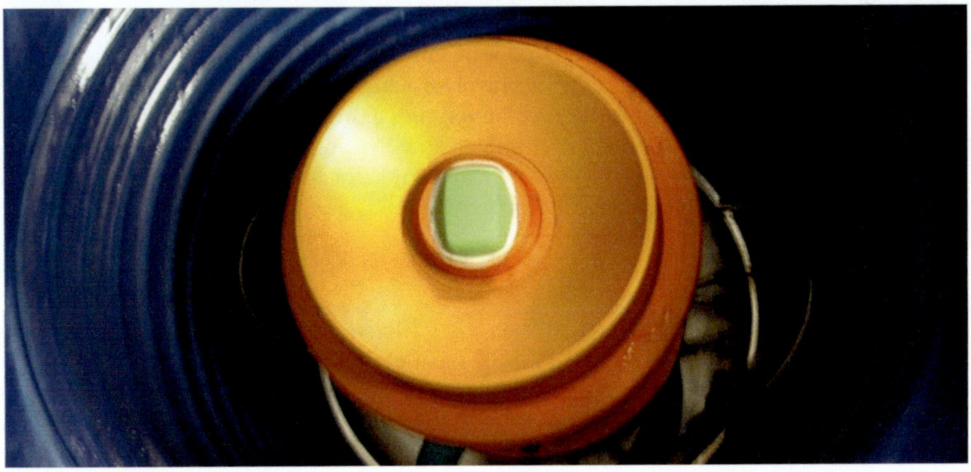

FIGURE 4.4 Therapy transducer with centrally mounted ultrasound imaging transducer from an early model Chongqing HAIFU system installed in the John Radcliffe Hospital, Oxford, UK. *Image courtesy of the Institute of Cancer Research.*

4.4.1 Reasons for Choosing an Array

Array transducers consisting of multiple transducer elements have the advantage that they can be used electronically to:

- steer the position of the focus (without the need to move the treatment head, reducing the risk of mechanical injury to patients or operators, and loss of coupling)
- alter the size and/or shape (in addition to the position) of the focus
- change the number (and size/shape/position) of foci
- compensate for tissue heterogeneity

Each of these is possible as long as individual elements, or subsets of elements, can be driven independently, but the efficacy with which this can be achieved depends on both the layout and number of elements. Typically the phase (essentially the time at which a voltage is applied to the elements and therefore the time at which each element begins to contribute to the wavefront) is changed to achieve the desired field shape at the intended treatment position.

Annular arrangements of elements,[42–44] also known as concentric rings,[45–47] allow the position of the focus to be adjusted towards, or away from, the source along the beam axis. This requires relatively few elements (e.g. from 4 to 20) to provide a few centimetres of adjustment either side of a geometric focus. Strip elements can allow lateral steering or treatment through the rib cage, again with a relatively small number of elements (e.g. 10) by aligning elements to lie along ribs.[48] Sector-based arrays are those in which the transducer surface is segmented radially into wedges. This is another deployment in which only a small number of elements are required to allow some widening of focal regions and hence the potential for more rapid volume ablation.[49–52] Combining sector and annular (ring) arrays is another option. Transducer arrays in which the surface is populated with high numbers of elements (see Figure 4.6 for example), generally either rectangular or circular in cross-section, can provide the functionality of the simpler arrays with greater potential for defocusing or spreading energy into larger volumes by producing multiple foci.[53–56] For the ultimate "fully steerable" arrays (that can theoretically steer over up to 2 π steradians of solid angle i.e. an entire hemisphere in front of them), the requirement is to have each element emit a spherical wave. This in turn requires elements that are $\leq \lambda/2$ (half a wavelength) in width. The wavelength in room temperature water at 1 MHz is approximately 1.5 mm, while at 3 MHz this drops to 0.5 mm.

The simplest beam forming option for an array is to move a single focal region in space. This can be useful for covering a target volume more rapidly than by mechanical means.[57–59] But one of the main clinical drivers for transducer array development was the overcoming of tissue heterogeneity, and specifically of beam aberrations caused by the skull in order to be able to deliver HIFU to the brain non-invasively.[60, 61] This achievement was later adapted to allow treatments through the rib cage[62–64] (see Figure 4.5). Transducer arrays are ideal for bespoke beamforming, such as creating ring-shaped foci for more uniform volumetric heating.[65] Usually this involves achieving a field with multiple foci[56, 58, 66, 67] or even anti-foci[68] which may be used to spare specific volumes or organs at risk. Generally, an array drive configuration may be designed to produce multiple, accurately controlled in shape or size focal regions. The accuracy with which these foci can be produced, and any associated unwanted features in the acoustic field away from the focus can be avoided ultimately depends on the size, number, and configuration of the available elements.

4.4.2 Design Challenges

While 2D transducer arrays have been used for diagnostic ultrasound imaging for many years, their therapeutic deployment has been restrained by technical issues related to manufacturing high power, densely populated, large footprint arrays. So called 1D arrays,[55, 69–72] a term which can either describe the device shape or its ability to provide one-dimensional beam modification, include concentric ring (annular) arrays that only allow steering in depth and linear arrays (strips) of elements that allow steering to a focal position that may be "moved" along the long direction of the array, lateral to the wave propagation. Improvements in 1D arrays have seen 1.25D, 1.5D, and 1.75D devices investigated.[73–75]

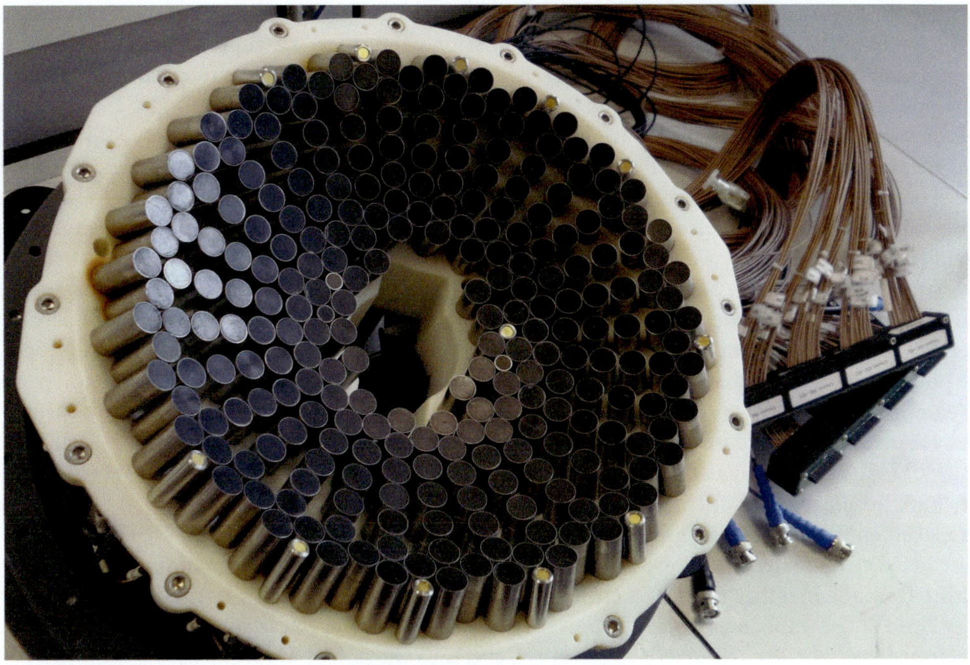

FIGURE 4.5 A 254-element, sparse, aperiodic array consisting of individual piezoceramic transducers mounted in a 3D printed shell with a spherical curvature, designed for the transcostal exposure of liver tumours. *Courtesy of the Institute of Cancer Research.*

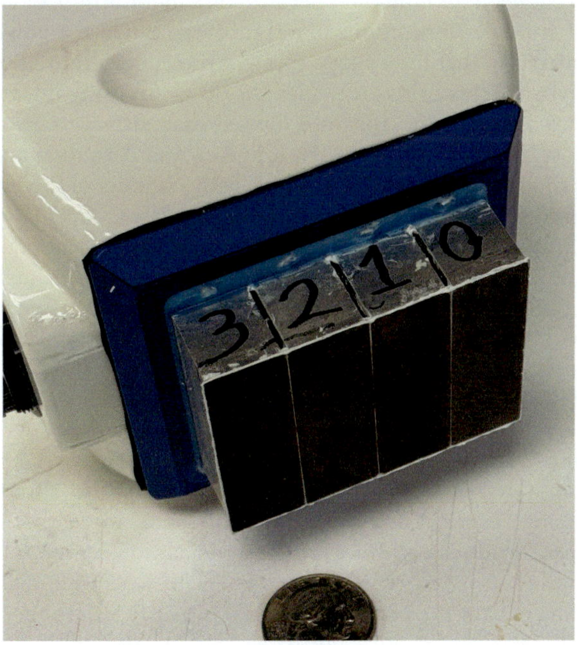

FIGURE 4.6 An example of a fully sampled, high power, high density therapeutic ultrasound array. Four modules, each composed of 1152 individual transducers (4608 elements in total), are mounted in a handheld device. For scale the "quarter" coin is 2.4 cm in diameter. *Photograph courtesy of Acoustiic, Inc, Washington, USA.*

To have "full" 2D steering capability with a planar device, the spacing of element centres needs to be ≤ $\lambda/2$ which means that the wavelength in the transmission medium puts an upper limit on element size. If this condition is not met, constructive interference at positions away from the focus forms so called grating (or side) lobes which waste energy and risk tissue damage in unintended locations. Thus, for steering and beam shaping, smaller elements are beneficial. Higher acoustic power output is required for ultrasound therapy than for imaging in order to create the focal pressures/intensities necessary to damage tissue at depth within the human body. Large elements are typically more robust and have a higher transduction efficiency and lower electrical impedance than smaller ones. The higher impedance of smaller elements causes more energy wastage (heating and energy reflection), requiring greater electrical energy delivery to achieve the same acoustic output. Thus the requirements of full steering and therapeutic use are in direct conflict with each other. By using a higher number of elements (high element density), the power handling requirement of each element may be reduced, but each therapy element usually requires more power than that used for US imaging. If a device is curved to provide a natural geometric focus, the element size that allows full steering can be increased beyond $\lambda/2$. This was exploited in early studies of array transducers to circumvent the manufacturing challenge of producing high-density high-power arrays.[46, 47, 53, 65] Various ways of achieving clinically usable transducer arrays with larger than ideal elements have been proposed, including sparse (or random) arrays. Simulations are used to optimise element placement by minimising grating lobes and/or maximising steering range.[76–78] The main problem with reduced element density arrays is the loss of total power (which limits maximum treatment depth) resulting from the inability to use the entire available surface. A secondary, but related, issue is that the energy close to the transducer will be less evenly spread than if the whole surface were used, increasing the energy density in any skin overlying a target, and thus the potential for burns.

Studies have shown that phased array connection and drive circuitry simplification can successfully reduce the number of drive circuits required. By using isolation transformers (switches) to connect elements with the closest phase requirements,[26] as few as 4 separate driving circuits could be used to drive a 64-element array.[79] This was in part possible due to the phase resolution requirements not being particularly high (digital quantisation as low as 4-bit being acceptable) for effective focusing.[80] For maximum flexibility, each transducer element needs to be connected to its own drive circuit, resulting in the need for many electrical connections (and their performance monitoring), often within a relatively tight space. The advantage of multiple connections to a transducer is that the power handling of each may be greatly reduced compared to that for a single-element transducer, thus allowing miniaturisation of drive components and wiring. This brings into play the option of using integrated circuits for driving arrays[81] as is the standard approach for (the lower power) diagnostic ultrasound imaging. Whilst this keeps manufacturing cost relatively low, the high initial cost of designing and testing chips makes it better suited to a mass production market. Unfortunately the number of therapy array systems in use is currently orders of magnitude fewer than that of imaging arrays.

Solutions to the problem of smaller array elements having higher electrical impedance are limited. One successful technique is to place the electrodes on the sides of each element instead of on the front and rear surfaces.[82, 83] The ability to control electrical impedance by adjusting the distance between electrodes in this way without affecting the resonant frequency of the device has been demonstrated in 1D[4] and 2D[84] therapy arrays.

Performance measurement with arrays is significantly more challenging than for single-element sources. By driving an array transducer to produce a single focal peak, a device's performance may be assessed in the same way as a single element device (see Chapter 5). However, an array presents the additional challenge of knowing that each element is working correctly. While relative performance may be adequately monitored using electrical drive power, an ultrasonic method of measuring absolute performance is also desirable. Rather than taking the time-consuming approach of obtaining hydrophone beam plots across the entire surface of a device, it is possible to measure at high resolution closer to the focus and to use modelling to back project the beam onto the surface of the array to verify and quantify the functionality of each element.[85–88] Such measurements are also critically important for allowing the relative phase and efficiency of all elements to be assessed so that starting phase and drive voltage conditions that will allow each element to be driven in phase with the same acoustic power output can be identified.

4.4.3 Design Realisation

Goss et al. published the first paper to describe a sparse therapy ultrasound array, based on communication antenna design from the 1960s in 1996.[78] They built an array with hexagonal element packing and randomly selected a subset (64/108) of elements to drive and demonstrated, both theoretically and experimentally, the benefit in terms of the reduction of grating lobes.

The first clinical use of a HIFU phased array was in the early 2000s, for the treatment of uterine fibroids using magnetic resonance for imaging guidance (MRg),[89, 90] and 2 decades later there are several commercial imaging-guided focused ultrasound phased array systems available,[91, 92] with two MR-guided systems having been proven to provide effective treatment of uterine fibroids.[89, 91] The system with clinical feasibility results published in 2003 was built by InSightec, Inc. (Israel). A 12-cm-diameter, fully populated (208 element), hybrid sector-vortex and concentric ring phased array allows focal steering, mostly in depth, but with a limited lateral capability (see Figure 4.7). The array, which operates between 0.96 and 1.14 MHz, can be mechanically positioned in 3 linear and 2 angular directions to allow targeting while avoiding organs or other structures at risk of unwanted damage. Initial, low power, exposures verify the focal targeting, followed by additional sonications at therapeutic power levels to achieve adequate heating, monitored using MR thermometry. The updated 2013 version of the system allows spatially interleaved exposures, to deliver more sonications in a given treatment time.[92] The other clinical system (2009) was built by Philips Healthcare, Inc. (Finland). This system is now being further developed by Profound Medical Corp. (USA). It uses a 12–14-cm-diameter spherically curved, randomised 256-element piezocomposite sparse array (see Figure 4.7), driven at either 1.2 or 1.45 MHz. It can be mechanically translated in 3 linear and 2 rotational directions for initial targeting. Exposures can either be for fixed times determined by the chosen exposure volume or can be for durations controlled using MR thermometry feedback. The array begins by sonicating at the geometrical focus, then scans the focal volume around a 4-mm diameter circle centred on this beam axis (a 4-mm treatment cell) electronically. Larger, 8-, 12-, or 16-mm (diameter) treatment cells can also be chosen, which, in addition to the 4-mm cell, treat concentric rings at each diameter up to the largest selected by the user.

These MRg FUS systems have also been used to treat bone pain from secondary tumours. The Israeli MRg system previously used for fibroids was successfully tested in 2007,[93] with additional publications following in 2014 from both the systems detailed earlier.[94, 95]

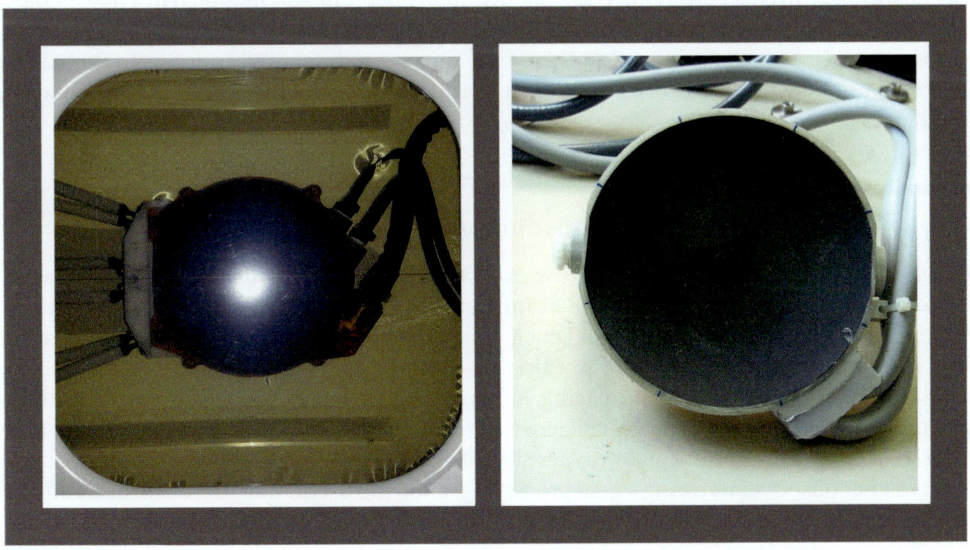

FIGURE 4.7 Left: Sonalleve piezocomposite array transducer used for treating bone pain from metastatic cancer and gynaecological recurrent cancer at the Royal Marsden Hospital, Sutton, UK (system initially supplied by Philips N.V. and later by Profound Medical Corp.). Right: Insightec Exablate array transducer used for uterine fibroid treatment at St. Mary's Hospital, London, UK. Both are MRg FUS devices.

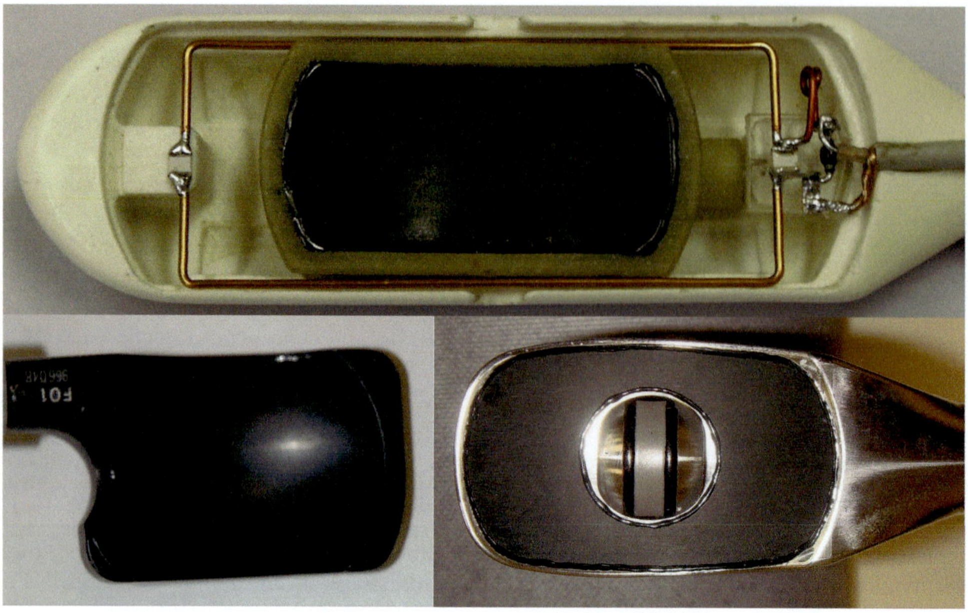

FIGURE 4.8 Transrectal HIFU transducers designed for the treatment of prostate cancer. Top: MR-guided experimental device developed at the Institute of Cancer Research, Sutton, UK. Bottom: Two piezocomposite transducers used in the EDAP Ablatherm system. Left: An earlier single-element transducer with slot to allow an imaging probe to be inserted in front of it for planning. Right: A phased array device with centrally mounted imaging. *Photographs courtesy of Institute of Cancer Research.*

Two phased array focused ultrasound systems have been developed for transrectal prostate cancer treatment. The first came from EDAP TMS (France) and was an US imaging guided, 3 MHz, 5.6 cm long device consisting of 16 concentric ring elements. The imaging probe was mounted in a hole in the centre of the therapy device[96] (see Figure 4.8). The more recent MR imaging guided array from Insightec Inc. (Israel) is a 2-MHz, 990-element array.[97] There have also been unfocused transurethral planar arrays (Tulsa Pro, Profound Medical Corp.) developed that have been used to ablate prostate tissue under MR guidance.[98]

4.5 Hybrid Imaging/Therapy Transducers

In 2006, Ebbini et al. presented the ex vivo use of a 1.1 MHz, 64 element dual-mode (therapy and imaging) piezocomposite ultrasound array with its inherent registration for therapy guidance and monitoring.[99] They simulated both the narrow band, high power therapeutic and the synthetic aperture imaging performance, and demonstrated that despite the low-contrast, high-speckle images, optimisation of the array was possible using ~2λ element spacing, although this produced higher than ideal grating lobes. Despite the need for therapeutic power efficiency restricting the imaging bandwidth to less than 40% at 1.1 MHz, the strong non-linear signals (hyperechoes) produced during thermal lesion formation could be detected after post-beamforming signal processing, allowing useful imaging during and after lesioning. Experimental results showed that therapy beams that ablated ex vivo porcine liver with submillimetre targeting precision were formed and that the lateral (1 mm) and axial (2.6 mm) imaging resolution was governed by the fractional bandwidth and imaging frequency. In their full synthetic aperture image reconstruction, they used array gain compensation to provide uniform contrast resolution within the image, accounted for element directivity to reduce grating lobes and increase dynamic range, and compensated for element performance heterogeneity to correct side lobe non-uniformity. In addition, they used a single transmit focus with an interrogation time of 200 μs which allowed short interruptions of the therapy exposure to be used to acquire images. This facilitated detection of non-linear bubble activity during lesioning. The ability to obtain dual-mode array images in real time,[100] coupled with development of closed loop control of lesion formation[101] led to the in vivo use of a dual-mode array in 2014. It was deployed for precise ablation of fine neurovascular structures (carotid bodies) in rodents as a treatment for hypertension. High frame-rate imaging provided closed-loop control over lesion formation via intensity and exposure duration modulation to avoid over-exposure (indicated by hyperechoes caused by tissue boiling)[102] and demonstrated sufficient efficacy to advance to large animal testing prior to clinical trials.

Bouchoux et al. (2008) also used piezocomposite technology to obtain high-quality imaging and effective focused ultrasound ablation within the same transducer array.[103] Air backing the low-loss material, which had stable output over a wide range of temperature, provided maximal power output. Endoscopic prototypes were designed and built for treating cholangiocarcinomas in the biliary ducts. The 2.5 by 7.5 mm transducer was cylindrically focused at 10 mm and was operated at 11 MHz. Measured transducer efficiency was 71%, with an axial imaging resolution of 0.2 mm.[103] Device performance was evaluated in ex vivo tissue[104] and in vivo.[105]

More recently, dual-mode transducers have been used for focused ultrasound blood-brain barrier opening via efficacy monitoring using passive acoustic mapping (see Chapter 7) to identify regions of therapy ultrasound induced bubble activity[106, 107] and for correcting for propagation path aberration when exposing the brain through the intact skull.[108–110]

4.6 Application-Specific Transducers

The following sections describe transducers that have been specifically designed and deployed for applications in the brain (such as essential tremor), for benign and malignant disease of the prostate, for the treatment of conditions in the eye including glaucoma, treatment of benign and malignant liver disease, and for transoesophageal treatment of cancer or for cardiac ablations.

4.6.1 Transducers for Brain Applications

The first clinical treatments in the brain were carried out by the Fry brothers at the University of Illinois in the late 1950s and early 1960s. X-ray guidance[9] was used due to the lack of our modern ultrasound and magnetic resonance imaging techniques. A main challenge was the focusing of ultrasound through the highly attenuating and spatially variant skull bone. This was avoided by removing a skull flap and exposing through the intact dura. Despite this easier access, treatment typically took 12–14 hours.[111] They used 1 MHz ultrasound with intensities in the range of 50–1000 Wcm^{-2}.[8]

Focusing ultrasound through the intact skull has been one of the most sought-after capabilities of therapy ultrasound since the 1950s. The earliest papers by Fry and Goss in the early 1980s achieved results by judicious choice of exposure parameters, including reducing the frequency to 500 kHz.[112, 113] The advent of multi-element phased arrays offered the potential for aberration correction, the challenge being to work out the phase and amplitude correction needed to focus successfully through the non-uniformly thick skull. Two teams suggested effective solutions around the same time in the mid-1990s. In Paris, Fink et al worked on "time reversal" techniques[61, 114] and at Harvard, Hynynen et al. worked on aberration correction using forward modelling based on CT scans.[60, 115] The work in the United States evolved into a 1024-element array that was commercialised by Insightec as a clinical MR-guided system (the Exablate Neuro) that is Food and Drug Administration (FDA) approved for use in tremor-dominated Parkinson's dyskinesia and essential tremor.

4.6.2 Transducers for Prostate Applications

Asymmetrical trans-rectal devices for prostate ablation were originally developed into clinical systems in the early 1990s in Europe and the United States (see Figure 4.8). They are generally longer than they are wide to facilitate transrectal application and use frequencies between 2 and 4 MHz as the target distance from the transducer is relatively short compared to most extracorporeal applications. Early clinical devices were single-element HIFU transducers either with apertures for US imaging guidance or with US imaging probes that were advanced in front of the therapy device for treatment planning and then withdrawn during exposures. The preference for single elements was understandable for cost and simplicity reasons, even though earlier work had looked at the feasibility of using transducer arrays for the induction of non-ablative hyperthermia.[71] The earliest publication of clinical results used a 4.00 ± 0.02 MHz device with 3- or 3.5-cm focal length but no details of the transducer size were provided.[116] The first Ablatherm (EDAP Technomed) system[117] worked at between 2.25 and 3 MHz, with a 3.5-cm-diameter transducer with 3.5-cm focal length, while the system used in the United States (Focal Surgery, Inc.) used a 4-MHz transrectal probe with a 30 by 22 mm transducer.[118] MR imaging guided systems developed rather differently, potentially due to the higher cost of the imaging systems. Here array transducers were developed fairly early on[119] with a recent development seeing a 1000-element device in a commercial system available from Exablate.[120, 121] Although the details are not always published, it is most likely the early devices were piezoceramic, while the modern clinical devices, especially those manufactured in Europe, are more likely to be piezocomposite.

US imaging guided transurethral transducers for prostate treatment have been in development since the mid-1990s.[72, 122–124] Their use has been far less widespread than transrectal devices, due in part to the challenge of making smaller probes. MR-guided transurethral devices first developed around 2010[33] have progressed through pre-clinical studies[125] and into clinical trials.[126, 127]

4.6.3 Ophthalmic Transducers

The treatment of ophthalmic conditions was one of the earliest clinical applications for HIFU, being introduced between the 1960s and 1980s. A variety of transducers were used in different studies, but typically a focused, robust (thick, low-frequency PZT4 ceramic) single-element transducer (resonant around 1.4 MHz and driven at its 7th harmonic) was used to produce 9.8 MHz ultrasound. Fixed geometry transducers directly coupled to the eye using a saline bath could be used to expose the retina, choroid, sclera, or ciliary processes.[128] With the advent of clinical lasers, this application lost popularity as lasers were easier to target into the eye and provided more rapid treatments. However, modern advances have resulted in a new clinical offering. The 21-MHz HIFU device (Eye Tech Care) is 30 mm in diameter with 6 rectangular transducers spaced around the device, each of which targets a separate region of the ciliary processes as a treatment for glaucoma. Treatment takes around 5 minutes and can be readily repeated if required.[129]

4.6.4 Transducers for Liver Applications

Early investigations into the treatment of the liver, mainly in cancer applications, used simple single-element transducers. Beyond having an appropriately long focal length, such transducers were not really optimised for the complexity of liver applications. In 1988, Frizzell et al. repurposed a transducer that had previously been used in brain studies[130] for studies in cat liver. It consisted of a 1-MHz fundamental quartz disc coupled to a stepped plastic lens. The transducer aperture was 10 cm and the focal length was 13.7 cm, resulting in FWHM power focal dimensions of 0.95 mm transverse to the axis and 5.8 mm along the axis when driven at 3 MHz.[131] The thermal damage threshold in (highly perfused) liver was found to be more than twice that in brain (for exposure durations of 0.1–10 s), approximately following the relation $It^{0.5} = 460\ Wcm^{-2}.\ s^{0.5}$ where I is spatial peak intensity and t the exposure duration in seconds. ter Haar et al. performed preliminary ex vivo and in vivo experiments using a 1.7-MHz, 10-cm diameter planar piezoceramic (PZT4) transducer focused using a biconcave Perspex lens in the late 1980s. A gap between the transducer and lens allowed fluid circulation for cooling. The focal length was 14 cm and the ellipsoidal focal region was about 21 mm long by 2.1 mm wide (full-width, half-pressure maximum).[132–135] Varying the electrical input to the transducer from 57 to 154 W resulted in spatial peak pressures in the range of 6.4–10.24 MPa (peak focal intensities 1.4–3.5 $kWcm^{-2}$). Exposure of 15–5 s produced lesions in rat liver in vivo. At intensities between 67 W cm^{-2} and 425 W cm^{-2},[7, 53] with an exposure duration of 2–20 s, a marked difference was found between the lesion dimensions obtained with normal and reduced blood flow. Yang et al. (1991) also used a lens-focused single-element transducer for liver studies in mice, but at 4-MHz.[136] In 1993, Sibille presented work with a 1.1-MHz spherical bowl transducer[137] that was later used in studies of perfused isolated porcine liver. The ultrasound source was a 150-mm diameter air-backed piezocomposite annular array, with a geometric focal length of 150 mm that was driven at its fundamental resonance.[138] The Biomedical Ultrasound Laboratory, Shanghai Jiaotong University (in 1997) developed a 1.1-MHz transducer with an array of 16 pistons distributed on a 14-cm-diameter concave spherical surface with a focal distance of 11 cm that produced an acoustic beam with half-intensity axial and lateral dimensions of 10 mm and 8 mm, respectively.[139] In 1999, Daum et al. reported the first use of a transducer array designed for clinical liver treatments. A 256-element 1.1-MHz array was built in-house from a 1 to 3 piezocomposite shell with a 10 cm radius of curvature and 12 cm diameter. The array elements were etched onto the surface of the curved bowl to form a grid of 6.5 by 6.5 mm squares. Although the piezoelectric material's electroacoustic efficiency was measured as 64%, ~50% electrical loss in the array cable reduced the overall efficiency to just 27%. They demonstrated ex vivo and in vivo liver ablation using single and multiple foci (in a variety of different configurations) that allowed faster volume ablation.[140]

The earliest clinical treatments of liver tumours were extracorporeal and carried out in the UK and China. The UK study treated a variety of solid soft tissue tumours using a 1.7-MHz, 12-cm focal length, 8.4-cm-diameter, single-element piezoceramic transducer.[28] Chongqing Medical University in collaboration with the Institute of Acoustics of Nanjing University reported liver exposures, but device details were only cross referenced.[141] A later paper provided details of the JC type device, which was probably used in the earlier studies too, as a 0.8-MHz transducer with a focal distance of 135 mm yielding a mean focal diameter of 1.1 mm and length of 9.8 mm (whether this was pressure or intensity and full width or FWHM was not specified).[142]

As the field developed, innovative methods of overcoming one of the most significant challenges, namely the lack of energy propagation through the overlying rib cage, were investigated. Quesson et al. used a commercial MRgHIFU system to identify which elements of an array transducer should be deactivated since the underlying liver was obscured by the ribs. The 256-element piezocomposite pseudo-random array on a spherical bowl with a 12-cm focal length and 13-cm-diameter aperture was used to demonstrate a simple, rapid and effective method of transcostal ablation in ex vivo tissue[64] and in vivo.[143]

Another significant problem is respiratory motion of the liver which sits just beneath the diaphragm and moves several centimetres during each breathing cycle. Whilst breath holding can be effective for exposures shorter than 20 s in duration,[28] it requires outcome-critical cooperation from the patient that would be better avoided. Respiratory gating and respiratory motion modelling have been investigated to overcome these issues,[144] with the potential to used phased array transducers to dynamically steer to the target position.

One of the most recent and innovative transducer developments (in 2023) from Switzerland is a liver-specific MRgHIFU 0.65-MHz piezocomposite transducer composed of 256 elements distributed across 5 emitters, but with complex emitter geometry and arrangement. In effect, a solid transducer has been broken into concentric emitters, with the outer emitters being stepped backward, away from the patient as shown in Figure 4.9. The stepped device allows a wide aperture without reducing the practical focal depth due to the proximity of the device to the patient. The innermost section has a central aperture which can house an US imaging probe. The next emitters out are located to either side of the central one but stepped backwards along the sound axis, away from the focus. The next 2 are more lateral and recessed yet further. The overall appearance is of a stepped series of truncated annuli. The concentric segments have specific radii of 100, 111, or 125 mm increasing towards the centre of the device. Since it is a phased array, the elements can be driven as if they were located on a continuous spherical surface. The focal region at the geometric focus was measured to have -6dB profiles approximately 8 mm axially, by 4 mm and 1 mm laterally, with the largest dimension of the ultrasound source giving the tightest lateral focal dimension.[145]

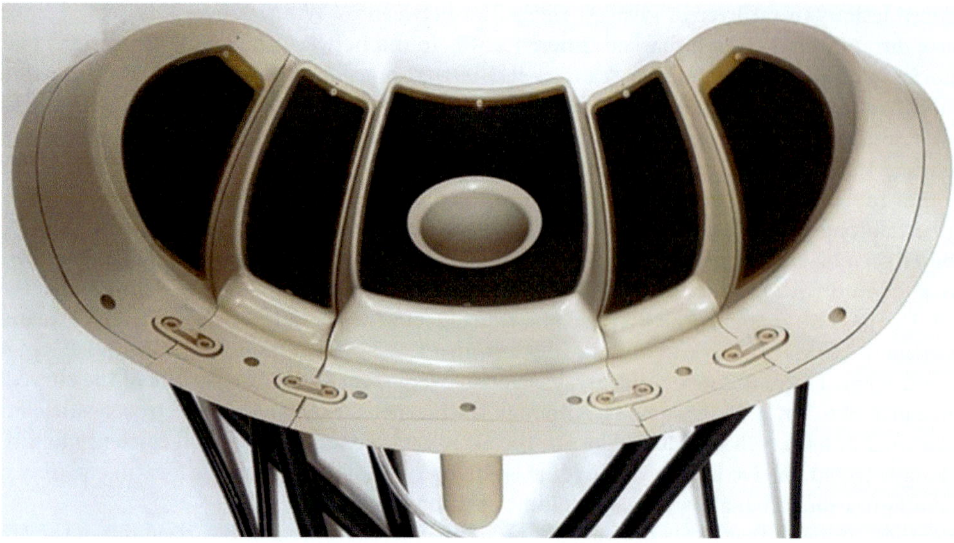

FIGURE 4.9 Novel design of an MR compatible transducer dedicated to liver ablation. The transducer is an assembly of 5 concentric parts of spheres of different radii (100, 111, and 125 mm) providing a wide contact surface with the patient skin while keeping the natural focal point 100 mm deep. The central aperture allows US imaging of the focal area. *Photograph curtesy of Mrs Orane Lorton, MS, Image Guided Interventions Laboratory, University of Geneva.*

In France, Melodelima et al. developed a novel toroidal HIFU transducer to provide a larger ablative region than the ellipsoidal focus created by an equivalent spherical bowl. The first prototype was demonstrated to be safe and effective in excised tissue[146] and pre-clinical studies.[147] The 3-MHz piezocomposite HIFU transducer's toroidal emitting surface geometry (diameter and radius of curvature of 70 mm) produces a conical focal zone. The surface is divided radially into 8 (sector) emitters, each of which is subdivided into concentric rings to create a 32-element phased array with elements of surface area 0.13 mm^2. An ultrasound imaging probe is mounted in a central aperture for guidance and monitoring. Therapeutic exposures are performed using an acoustic power of 60 W for 5 s per emitter with each activated alternately and consecutively to give a total exposure time for a single lesion of 40 s. In cross-section at the focal plane, the conical focal zone is a ring. The −6 dB length of the focus is 28.8 mm and the outer diameters in orthogonal directions at the focal plane are 19.5 and 18.0 mm.[147] In collaboration with EDAP Technomed, they produced a clinical prototype which, after evaluation for colorectal liver metastases treatment, they showed could be used intraoperatively for reducing blood loss during hepatic surgery.[148] By combining control of the volume of coupling liquid and electronic steering in depth the focal zone to be placed anywhere up to 9 cm below the surface of the liver.

Outside oncological applications, a 3.3-MHz HIFU transducer developed to stop bleeding after traumatic liver injury had an aperture of 6.34 cm^2 and was spherically curved to produce a focus at 4 cm.[149] It produced an acoustic power of 65 W when a 300-V peak-to-peak voltage was applied to the transducer matching network. The half-maximum beam width and length were 1 mm and 10 mm (pressure or intensity not specified), respectively. The spatial peak intensity at the focus (acoustic power divided by the cross-sectional area of the focal spot) was approximately 3000 Wcm^{-2}. This device evolved into an intraoperative 5.47 MHz, 3.7 cm aperture, 6.4 cm focal length transducer equipped with a solid titanium conical coupler to allow direct tissue coupling. Drive powers of 80 and 100 W produced acoustic intensities of 2264 and 2829 Wcm^{-2}, respectively. Using funding from the U.S. Army and NASA, they went on to develop devices for haemorrhagic control of visible wounds and internal injuries[150] beyond applications in the liver. A spin-out company clinically trialled a 3.2-MHz, f-number of 1 transducer for speeding up arterial coagulation after catheter based medical interventions, which although successful in over 160 patients, was not a commercially successful. Acoustic haemostasis was ultimately developed into a Deep Bleeder Acoustic Coagulation device (DBAC) as a cuff[151, 152] to be strapped to the patient's limb to provide control of deep bleeding. This array technology, likened to that of Dr McCoy in *Star Trek*, consisted of multiple imaging and therapy transducer array tiles. A therapy array which resulted from this project, and the subject of new commercialisation from Acoustiic Inc., is shown in Figure 4.6.

4.6.5 Transoesophageal Transducers

Transoesophageal transducers have been developed for 2 main purposes, the first being the ablation of oesophageal tumours and the second being ablation of cardiac tissue. The first US imaging guided therapy ultrasound transducer (1998) for treating oesophageal tumours was unfocused.[153] The first focused device (2002) was a sector-based phased array that was a 10.6-mm diameter cylindrical 4.55 MHz transducer comprising 16 plane elements 0.45 mm wide, 15 mm long, and 390 μm thick, separated by 70 μm.[154] This was superseded by a very similar 64-element array.[155]

Devices for cardiac ablation began appearing around the mid-2000s, with non-invasive transoesophageal cardiac thermal ablation using focused ultrasound first being demonstrated around 2008 in China, using an electronically steered 2280-element planar phased array (1 MHz, 60 by 10 mm, 0.525-mm element centre spacing).[156] Subsequently, in the United States, a 1.6-MHz sparse phased array prototype, designed based on ultrasound field simulations, was made from a rectangular ceramic PZT-8 diced into 195 (15 by 13) elements. Rather than having a randomised distribution of elements, they used a uniform distribution but obtained a partially periodic arrangement by activating only a subset of 64. The transducer, which was mounted in a 19-mm-diameter by 53-mm-long cylindrical housing, was shown to ablate cardiac tissue ex vivo and subsequently in vivo.[157, 158]

Another US imaging guided device that has been developed and tested is an a 3-MHz spherical truncated (30 by 14 mm) piezocomposite HIFU transducer divided into 8 ring elements, with a 40 mm radius of curvature (developed around 2013)[159] deployed in an 18-mm-diameter and 50-mm-long housing. This transducer is shown in Figure 4.10. Electronic focusing provided treatment depths of 15–55 mm and maximum acoustic intensity at the transducer surface of 9 and 12 Wcm^{-2} depending on whether it was in a rigid or flexible housing, respectively.[160, 161]

A more recent entry into the cardiac ablation field (2019) is a 3.8-MHz focused ultrasonic array consisting of 6 (4.5 by 4.5 mm) elements with a focal length of 17 mm built into a 30F transoesophageal catheter[162] and used to modify the stellate ganglion as a treatment for arrhythmia, with positive outcomes in preclinical testing. Although technological developments in the cardiac ablation arena are rife, major obstacles to successful clinical deployment include identification of the location of the electrical pathway that needs to be ablated, and safe targeting of that position in the beating heart.

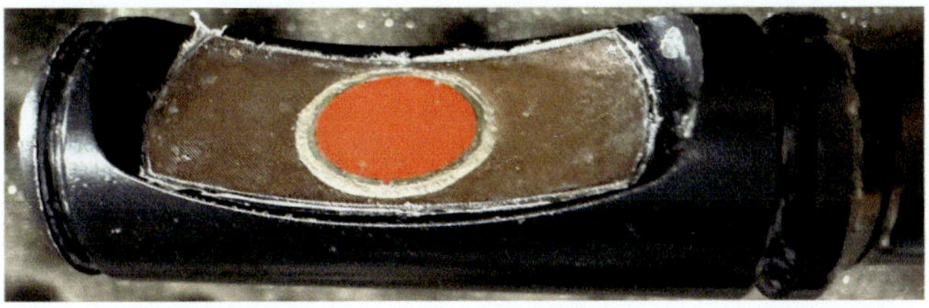

FIGURE 4.10 Example of a transoesophageal probe. The 3-MHz, 8-element piezocomposite annular array has a centrally mounted 5-MHz US imaging probe and a radius of curvature of 40 mm. *Photograph courtesy of LabTAU, INSERM, Lyon and Vermon S.A., Tours, France.*

4.7 Summary

Pivotal moments in history which have facilitated focused ultrasound transducer technology's reach to where it is today include the discovery of the (inverse) piezoelectric effect, curiosity about whether underwater detection sonar could be adapted for medical use, the invention of artificial PZT, and the application of communications antenna technology to ultrasound phased arrays. However, it has taken pioneers from around the world to produce medical devices that include FUS transducers, that are MR or US imaging guided and that can focus on targets in the brain or liver, after overcoming field aberration caused by the skull or rib cage, or which can dynamically steer a focal region in such a way as to produce thermal damage and avoid the confounding effects of acoustic cavitation. Yet a relatively simple single element spherical bowl can still be used in the laboratory to investigate whether therapy ultrasound can promote drug uptake beyond the blood-brain barrier or to stimulate the innate immune system to destroy cancer cells. The evolution and fundamental importance of FUS or HIFU transducers in their many guises have been described in detail in this chapter.

REFERENCES

1. Duck F. 'The Electrical Expansion of Quartz' by Jacques and Pierre Curie. Ultrasound. 2009;17(4):197–203.
2. Lippman G. Principe de la conservation de l'électricité. Annales de Chimie et Physique. 1881;5(24):145–78.
3. Gooberman GL. Ultrasonics: Theory and Application. London: English Universities Press; 1968.
4. Song J, Lucht B, Hynynen K. Large improvement of the electrical impedance of imaging and high-intensity focused ultrasound (HIFU) phased arrays using multilayer piezoelectric ceramics coupled in lateral mode. IEEE Transactions on Ultrasonics, Ferroelectrics, and Frequency Control. 2012;59(7):1584–95.
5. Shirane G, Takeda A. Phase transitions in solid solutions of PbZrO3 and PbTiO3 (I) small concentrations of PbTiO3. Journal of the Physical Society of Japan. 1952;7(1):5–11.
6. DeAngelis DA, Schulze GW. Performance of PZT8 versus PZT4 piezoceramic materials in ultrasonic transducers. 44th Annual Symposium of the Ultrasonic Industry Association (UIA 44th Symposium) and 45th Annual Symposium of the Ultrasonic Industry Association (UIA 45th Symposium). 2016;87:85–92.
7. Lynn JG, Zwemer RL, Chick AJ, Miller AE. A new method for the generation and use of focused ultrasound in experimental biology. Journal of General Physiology. 1942;26(2):179–93.
8. Fry WJ, Mosberg W, Barnard J, Fry F. Production of focal destructive lesions in the central nervous system with ultrasound. Journal of Neurosurgery. 1954;11(5):471–8.
9. Meyers R, Fry FJ, Fry WJ, Eggleton RC, Schultz DF. Determination of topologic human brain representations and modifications of signs and symptoms of some neurologic disorders by the use of high level ultrasound. Neurology. 1960;10(3):271–7.
10. Newnham RE, Bowen LJ, Klicker KA, Cross LE. Composite piezoelectric transducers. Materials & Design. 1980;2(2):93–106.
11. Newnham RE, Markley DC, Meyer RJ, Hughes WJ, Hladky-Hennion AC, Cochran JK. Multimode underwater transducers. Ceramic Transactions. 2003;150:427–43.
12. Hladky-Hennion AC, Uzgur AE, Newnham RE. Monolithic class IV type flextensional transducers. Journal of Electroceramics. 2008;20:139–144.
13. Fleury G, de Lima DM, Hynynen K, Berriet R, Le Baron O, Huguenin B, editors. New piezocomposite transducers for therapeutic ultrasound. In: Thermal Treatment of Tissue. Energy Delivery and Assessment II: SPIE – The International Society for Optical Engineering (Washington, USA); 2003.
14. Smith WA, Shaulov AA. Composite piezoelectrics: Basic research to a practical device. Ferroelectrics. 1988;87(1):309–20.
15. Wong SH, Watkins RD, Kupnik M, Pauly KB, Khuri-Yakub BT. Feasibility of MR-temperature mapping of ultrasonic heating from a CMUT. IEEE Transactions on Ultrasonics, Ferroelectrics, and Frequency Control. 2008;55(4):811–8.
16. Wong SH, Kupnik M, Watkins RD, Butts-Pauly K, Khuri-Yakub BT. Capacitive micromachined ultrasonic transducers for therapeutic ultrasound applications. IEEE Transactions on Biology Medicine and Engineering. 2010;57(1):114–23.

17. Yoon HS, Chang C, Jang JH, Bhuyan A, Choe JW, Nikoozadeh A, et al. Ex vivo HIFU experiments using a 32 times 32 -element CMUT array. IEEE Transactions on Ultrasonics, Ferroelectrics, and Frequency Control. 2016;63(12):2150–8.
18. Bawiec CR, N'Djin WA, Bouchoux G, Sénégond N, Guillen N, Chapelon JY. Preliminary investigation of a 64-element capacitive micromachined ultrasound transducer (CMUT) annular array designed for high intensity focused ultrasound (HIFU). Innovation and Research in BioMedical Engineering. 2018;39(5):295–306.
19. Joseph J, Ma B, Khuri-Yakub BT. Applications of capacitive micromachined ultrasonic transducers: A comprehensive review. IEEE Transactions on Ultrasonics, Ferroelectrics, and Frequency Control. 2022;69(2):456–67.
20. Hiruma Y, Nagata H, Takenaka T. Thermal depoling process and piezoelectric properties of bismuth sodium titanate ceramics. Journal of Applied Physics. 2009;105(8).
21. Cobbold RSC. Foundations of Biomedical Ultrasound. Oxford: Oxford University Press; 2007.
22. Fry WJ, Dunn F. In: Nastuk WL, editor. Physical Techniques in Biological Research. 4. New York, NY: Academic Press; 1962. p. 322.
23. Hynynen K. The construction and assessment of lenses for local treatment of malignant tumours by ultrasound. Ultrasound in Medicine and Biology. 1983;9(1):33–8.
24. Londe RJ, Worthington A, Hunt JW. Field conjugate acoustic lenses for ultrasound hyperthermia. IEEE Transactions on Ultrasonics, Ferroelectrics, and Frequency Control. 1993;40(5):592–602.
25. Fjield T, Sorrentino V, Cline H, Hynynen K. Design and experimental verification of thin acoustic lenses for the coagulation of large tissue volumes. Physics in Medicine and Biology. 1997;42:2341–54.
26. Fjield T, Silcox CE, Hynynen K. Low-profile lenses for ultrasound surgery. Physics in Medicine and Biology. 1999;44(7):1803–13.
27. Andrés D, Rivens I, Mouratidis P, Jiménez N, Camarena F, ter Haar G. Holographic focused ultrasound hyperthermia system for uniform simultaneous thermal exposure of multiple tumor spheroids. Cancers. 2023;15(9).
28. Visioli AG, Rivens IH, ter Haar GR, Horwich A, Huddart RA, Moskovic E, et al. Preliminary results of a phase I dose escalation clinical trial using focused ultrasound in the treatment of localised tumours. European Journal of Ultrasound. 1999;9(1):11–8.
29. Wu F, Chen WZ, Bai J, Zou JZ, Wang ZL, Zhu H, et al. Pathological changes in human malignant carcinoma treated with high-intensity focused ultrasound. Ultrasound in Medicine and Biology. 2001;27(8):1099–106.
30. Gelet A, Chapelon JY. Effects of high-intensity focused ultrasound on the human prostate. Journal of Urology (Paris). 1993;99(6):350.
31. Bihrle R, Foster RS, Sanghvi NT, Donohue JP, Hood PJ. High intensity focused ultrasound for the treatment of benign prostatic hyperplasia: Early United States clinical experience. Journal of Urology. 1994;151(5):1271–5.
32. Prakash P, Salgaonkar VA, Clif Burdette E, Diederich CJ. Multiple applicator hepatic ablation with interstitial ultrasound devices: Theoretical and experimental investigation. Medical Physics. 2012;39(12):7338–49.
33. Siddiqui K, Chopra R, Vedula S, Sugar L, Haider M, Boyes A, et al. MRI-guided transurethral ultrasound therapy of the prostate gland using real-time thermal mapping: Initial studies. Urology. 2010;76(6):1506–11.
34. Li T, Wang YN, Khokhlova TD, D'Andrea S, Starr F, Chen H, et al. Pulsed high-intensity focused ultrasound enhances delivery of doxorubicin in a preclinical model of pancreatic cancer. Cancer Research. 2015;75(18):3738–46.
35. Burks SR, Nguyen BA, Tebebi PA, Kim SJ, Bresler MN, Ziadloo A, et al. Pulsed focused ultrasound pretreatment improves mesenchymal stromal cell efficacy in preventing and rescuing established acute kidney injury in mice. Stem Cells. 2015;33(4):1241–53.
36. Mouratidis PXE, Costa M, Rivens I, Repasky EE, ter Haar G. Pulsed focused ultrasound can improve the anti-cancer effects of immune checkpoint inhibitors in murine pancreatic cancer. Journal of the Royal Society Interface. 2021;18(180).
37. Li T, Chen H, Khokhlova T, Wang YN, Kreider W, He X, et al. Passive cavitation detection during pulsed HIFU exposures of ex vivo tissues and in vivo mouse pancreatic tumors. Ultrasound in Medicine and Biology. 2014;40(7):1523–34.

38. Basavarajappa L, Rijal G, Hoyt K. Multifocused ultrasound therapy for controlled microvascular permeabilization and improved drug delivery. IEEE Transactions on Ultrasonics, Ferroelectrics, and Frequency Control. 2021;68(4):961–8.
39. Margolis R, Basavarajappa L, Li J, Obaid G, Hoyt K. Image-guided focused ultrasound-mediated molecular delivery to breast cancer in an animal model. Physics in Medicine and Biology. 2023;68(15):155012.
40. Peek MC, Ahmed M, Douek M. High-intensity focused ultrasound for the treatment of fibroadenomata (HIFU-F) study. Journal of Therapeutic Ultrasound. 2015;3:6. https://jtultrasound.biomedcentral.com/articles/10.1186/s40349-015-0027-6
41. Hynynen K, Jones RM. Image-guided ultrasound phased arrays are a disruptive technology for non-invasive therapy. Physics in Medicine and Biology. 2016;61(17):R206–R48.
42. Held RT, Zderic V, Nguyen TN, Vaezy S. Annular phased-array high-intensity focused ultrasound device for image-guided therapy of uterine fibroids. IEEE Transactions on Ultrasonics, Ferroelectrics, and Frequency Control. 2006;53(2):335–48.
43. Christopher T. HIFU focusing efficiency and a twin annular array source for prostate treatment. IEEE Transactions on Ultrasonics, Ferroelectrics, and Frequency Control. 2005;52(9):1523–33.
44. Dupenloup F, Chapelon JY, Cathignol DJ, Sapozhnikov OA. Reduction of the grating lobes of annular arrays used in focused ultrasound surgery. IEEE Transactions on Ultrasonics, Ferroelectrics, and Frequency Control. 1996;43(6):991–8.
45. Jeong J. Dual concentric-sectored HIFU transducer with phase-shifted ultrasound excitation for expanded necrotic region: A simulation study. IEEE Transactions on Ultrasonics, Ferroelectrics, and Frequency Control. 2013;60(5):924–31.
46. Fjield T, Fan X, Hynynen K. A parametric study of the concentric-ring transducer design for MRI guided ultrasound surgery. The Journal of the Acoustical Society of America. 1996;100(2):1220–30.
47. Ibbini MS, Cain CA. The concentric-ring array for ultrasound hyperthermia: Combined mechanical and electrical scanning. International Journal of Hyperthermia. 1990;6(2):401–19.
48. Civale J, Clarke R, Rivens I, ter Haar G. The use of a segmented transducer for rib sparing in HIFU treatments. Ultrasound in Medicine and Biology. 2006;32(11):1753–61.
49. Liu HL, Chen HW, Ju KC, Shih TC, Chen WS. Heating efficiency improvement by using a spherically-concaved sectored array in focused ultrasound thermal therapy. 2006 28th Annual International Conference of the IEEE Engineering in Medicine and Biology Society, Vols 1–15. IEEE; 2006. p. 754–7. https://ieeexplore.ieee.org/document/4462629
50. Melodelima D, Lafon C, Prat F, Theillere Y, Arefiev A, Cathignol D. Transoesophageal ultrasound applicator for sector-based thermal ablation: First in vivo experiments. Ultrasound in Medicine and Biology. 2003;29(2):285–91.
51. Umemura SI, Holmes KR, Frizzell LA, Cain CA. Insonation of fixed porcine kidney by a prototype sector-vortex-phased array applicator. International Journal of Hyperthermia. 1992;8(6):831–42.
52. Umemura SI, Cain CA. Analysis of temperature responses to diffused ultrasound focal fields produced by a sector-vortex phased array. International Journal of Hyperthermia. 1990;6(3):641–54.
53. Ebbini ES. A spherical-section ultrasound phased array applicator for deep localized hyperthermia. IEEE Transactions on Biomedical Engineering. 1991;38(7):634–43.
54. McGough RJ, Ebbini ES, Cain CA. Direct computation of ultrasound phased-array driving signals from a specified temperature distribution for hyperthermia. IEEE Transactions on Biomedical Engineering. 1992;39(8):825–35.
55. Buchanan MT, Hynynen K. Design and experimental evaluation of an intracavitary ultrasound phased array system for hyperthermia. IEEE Transactions on Biomedical Engineering. 1994 41(12):1178–87.
56. Fan X, Hynynen K. Control of the necrosed tissue volume during noninvasive ultrasound surgery using a 16-element phased array. Medical Physics. 1995;22(3):297–306.
57. Moros EG, Roemer RB, Hynynen K. Simulations of scanned focused ultrasound hyperthermia – the effects of scanning speed and pattern on the temperature-fluctuations at the focal depth. IEEE Transactions on Ultrasonics, Ferroelectrics, and Frequency Control. 1988;35(5):552–60.
58. Wan H, VanBaren P, Ebbini ES, Cain CA. Ultrasound surgery: Comparison of strategies using phased array systems. IEEE Transactions on Ultrasonics, Ferroelectrics, and Frequency Control. 1996;43(6):1085–98.
59. Rieke V, Instrella R, Rosenberg J, Grissom W, Werner B, Martin E, et al. Comparison of temperature processing methods for monitoring focused ultrasound ablation in the brain. Journal of Magnetic Resonance Imaging. 2013;38(6):1462–71.

60. Hynynen K, Jolesz FA. Demonstration of potential noninvasive ultrasound brain therapy through an intact skull. Ultrasound in Medicine and Biology. 1998;24(2):275–83.
61. Thomas JL, Fink MA. Ultrasonic beam focusing through tissue inhomogeneities with a time reversal mirror: Application to transskull therapy. IEEE Transactions on Ultrasonics, Ferroelectrics, and Frequency Control. 1996;43(6):1122–9.
62. Botros YY, Ebbini ES, Volakis JL. Two-step hybrid virtual array ray (VAR) technique for focusing through the rib cage. IEEE Transactions on Ultrasonics, Ferroelectrics, and Frequency Control. 1998;45(4):989–1000.
63. Aubry JF, Pernot M, Marquet F, Tanter M, Fink M. Transcostal high-intensity-focused ultrasound: Ex vivo adaptive focusing feasibility study. Physics in Medicine and Biology. 2008;53(11):2937–51.
64. Quesson B, Merle M, Kohler MO, Mougenot C, Roujol S, de Senneville BD, et al. A method for MRI guidance of intercostal high intensity focused ultrasound ablation in the liver. Medical Physics. 2010;37(6):2533–40.
65. Cain CA, Umemura S. Concentric-ring and sector-vortex phased-array applicators for ultrasound hyperthermia. IEEE Transactions on Microwave Theory and Techniques. 1986;34(5):542–51.
66. Ebbini ES, Cain CA. Optimization of the intensity gain of multiple-focus phased-array heating patterns. International Journal of Hyperthermia. 1991;7(6):953–73.
67. McGough RJ, Wang H, Ebbini ES, Cain CA. Mode scanning: Heating pattern synthesis with ultrasound phased arrays. International Journal of Hyperthermia. 1994;10(3):433–42.
68. Seo J, Lee J. Anti-foci for focused ultrasound. International Journal of Hyperthermia. 2009;25(7):566–80.
69. Kuen-Cheng J, Yung-Yaw C, Win-Li L, Te-Son K. One-dimensional phased array with mechanical motion for conformal ultrasound hyperthermia. Physics in Medicine and Biology. 2003;48(2):167.
70. Hao-Li L, Yung-Yaw C, Jia-Yush Y, Win-Li L. Treatment time reduction for large thermal lesions by using a multiple 1D ultrasound phased array system. Physics in Medicine and Biology. 2003;48(9):1173.
71. Gavrilov LR, Hand JW. Development and investigation of ultrasound linear phased arrays for transrectal treatment of prostate. Ultrasonics Sonochemistry. 1997;4(2):173–4.
72. Diederich CJ, Burdette EC. Transurethral ultrasound array for prostate thermal therapy: Initial studies. IEEE Transactions on Ultrasonics, Ferroelectrics, and Frequency Control. 1996;43(6):1011–22.
73. Curiel L, Chavrier F, Souchon R, Birer A, Chapelon JY. 1.5-D high intensity focused ultrasound array for non-invasive prostate cancer surgery. IEEE Transactions on Ultrasonics, Ferroelectrics, and Frequency Control. 2002;49(2):231–42.
74. Saleh KY, Smith NB. A 63 element 1.75 dimensional ultrasound phased array for the treatment of benign prostatic hyperplasia. Biomedical Engineering Online. 2005;4:39. https://biomedical-engineering-online.biomedcentral.com/articles/10.1186/1475-925X-4-39
75. Wildes DG, Chiao RY, Daft CMW, Rigby KW, Smith LS, Thomenius KE. Elevation performance of 1.25D and 1.5D transducer arrays. IEEE Transactions on Ultrasonics, Ferroelectrics, and Frequency Control. 1997;44(5):1027–37.
76. Nikolov SI, Jensen JA. Application of different spatial sampling patterns for sparse array transducer design. Ultrasonics. 2000;37(10):667–71.
77. Hutchinson EB, Buchanan MT, Hynynen K. Design and optimisation of an aperiodic ultrasound phased array for intracavity prostate thermal therapies. Medical Physics. 1996 23:767–78.
78. Goss SA, Frizzell LA, Kouzmanoff JT, Barich JM, Yang JM. Sparse random ultrasound phased array for focal surgery. IEEE Transactions on Ultrasonics, Ferroelectrics, and Frequency Control. 1996;43(6):1111–21.
79. Caulfield R, Yin X, Juste J, Hynynen K. A novel phase assignment protocol and driving system for a high-density focused ultrasound array. IEEE Transactions on Ultrasonics, Ferroelectrics and Frequency Control. 2007;54(4):793–801.
80. Wang H, Ebbini E, Cain CA. Effect of phase errors on field patterns generated by an ultrasound phased-array hyperthermia applicator. IEEE Transactions on Ultrasonics, Ferroelectrics, and Frequency Control. 1991;38(5):521–31.
81. Gougheri HS, Kiani M. A high-voltage ASIC for ultrasound neuromodulation with a piezoelectric transducer. IEEE International Symposium on Circuits and Systems (ISCAS 22). 2022:951–5.
82. Song J, Hynynen K. Feasibility of using lateral mode coupling method for a large scale ultrasound phased array for noninvasive transcranial therapy. IEEE Transactions on Biomedical Engineering. 2010;57(1):124–33.

83. Hynynen K, Yin JH. Lateral mode coupling to reduce the electrical impedance of small elements required for high power ultrasound therapy phased arrays. IEEE Transactions on Ultrasonics, Ferroelectrics, and Frequency Control. 2009;56(3):557–64.
84. Ellens NP, Lucht BB, Gunaseelan ST, Hudson JM, Hynynen KH. A novel, flat, electronically-steered phased array transducer for tissue ablation: Preliminary results. Physics in Medicine and Biology. 2015;60(6):2195–215.
85. Schafer ME, Lewin PA. Transducer characterization using the angular spectrum method. Journal of the Acoustical Society of America. 1989;85(5):2202–14.
86. Clement GT, Hynynen K. Field characterization of therapeutic ultrasound phased arrays through forward and backward planar projection. The Journal of the Acoustical Society of America. 2000;108(1):441–6.
87. Kreider W, Yuldashev PV, Sapozhnikov OA, Farr N, Partanen A, Bailey MR, et al. Characterization of a multi-element clinical HIFU system using acoustic holography and nonlinear modeling. IEEE Transactions on Ultrasonics, Ferroelectrics, and Frequency Control. 2013;60(8):1683–98.
88. Sapozhnikov OA, Tsysar SA, Khokhlova VA, Kreider W. Acoustic holography as a metrological tool for characterizing medical ultrasound sources and fields. Journal of the Acoustical Society of America. 2015;138(3):1515–32.
89. Tempany CMC, Stewart EA, McDannold N, Quade BJ, Jolesz FA, Hynynen K. MR Imaging-guided focused ultrasound surgery of uterine leiomyomas: A feasibility study. Radiology. 2003;226(3):897–905.
90. Stewart EA, Gedroyc WMW, Tempany CMC, Quade BJ, Inbar Y, Ehrenstein T, et al. Focused ultrasound treatment of uterine fibroid tumors: Safety and feasibility of a noninvasive thermoablative technique. American Journal of Obstetrics and Gynecology. 2003;189(1):48–54.
91. Kohler MO, Mougenot C, Quesson B, Enholm J, Le Bail B, Laurent C, et al. Volumetric HIFU ablation under 3D guidance of rapid MRI thermometry. Medical Physics. 2009;36(8):3521–35.
92. Fennessy FM, Tempany CM. An update on magnetic resonance guided focused ultrasound surgery (MRgFUS) of uterine fibroids. Current Radiology Reports. 2013;1(2):136–46.
93. Catane R, Beck A, Inbar Y, Rabin T, Shabshin N, Hengst S, et al. MR-guided focused ultrasound surgery (MRgFUS) for the palliation of pain in patients with bone metastases-preliminary clinical experience. Annals of Oncology. 2007;18(1):163–7.
94. Hurwitz MD, Ghanouni P, Kanaev SV, Iozeffi D, Gianfelice D, Fennessy FM, et al. Magnetic resonance-guided focused ultrasound for patients with painful bone metastases: Phase III trial results. Journal of the National Cancer Institute. 2014;106(5).
95. Huisman M, Lam MK, Bartels LW, Nijenhuis RJ, Moonen CT, Knuttel FM, et al. Feasibility of volumetric MRI-guided high intensity focused ultrasound (MR-HIFU) for painful bone metastases. Journal of Therapeutic Ultrasound. 2014;2:16.
96. Petrusca L, Ngo J, Brasset L, Blanc E, Murillo A, Auboiroux V, et al. Experimental investigation of MRgHIFU sonication with interleaved electronic and mechanical displacement of the focal point for transrectal prostate application. Physics in Medicine and Biology. 2012;57(15):4805–25.
97. Napoli A, Anzidei M, De Nunzio C, Cartocci G, Panebianco V, De Dominicis C, et al. Real-time magnetic resonance-guided high-intensity focused ultrasound focal therapy for localised prostate cancer: Preliminary experience. European Urology. 2013;63(2):395–8.
98. Muschter R, Steinmeister L, Lumiani A. A retrospective clinical service evaluation of lesion-targeted mri-guided transurethral ultrasound ablation (tulsa) for the treatment of localized prostate cancer. Journal of Urology. 2023;209:E1038.
99. Ebbini ES, Yao H, Shrestha A. Dual-mode ultrasound phased arrays for image-guided surgery. Ultrasonic Imaging. 2006;28(2):65–82.
100. Casper AJ, Liu D, Ballard JR, Ebbini ES. Real-time implementation of a dual-mode ultrasound array system: In vivo results. IEEE Transactions on Biomedical Engineering. 2013;60(10):2751–9.
101. Liu DL, Haritonova A, Ebbini E. Close-loop lesion formation control using multiple-focus dual mode ultrasound array. IEEE International Ultrasonics Symposium (IUS). 2014:1634–7.
102. Almekkawy M, Casper A, Ballard J, Ebbini E. Non-linear modeling of pulsed and CW HIFU beams for dual-mode ultrasound arrays. 11th International Symposium on Therapeutic Ultrasound. 2012;1481:3–8.
103. Bouchoux G, Lafon C, Berriet R, Chapelon JY, Fleury G, Cathignol D. Dual-mode ultrasound transducer for image-guided interstitial thermal therapy. Ultrasound in Medicine and Biology. 2008;34(4):607–16.

104. Owen NR, Bouchoux G, Murillo A, Merouche S, Birer A, Chapelon JY, et al. In vitro evaluation of an oscillating dual-mode ultrasound probe for sector imaging and directive therapy. Conference Proceedings of the IEEE Engineering in Medicine and Biology Society. IEEE; 2008. p. 3669–72. https://ieeexplore.ieee.org/document/4650003
105. Owen NR, Bouchoux G, Seket B, Murillo-Rincon A, Merouche S, Birer A, et al. In vivo evaluation of a mechanically oscillating dual-mode applicator for ultrasound imaging and thermal ablation. IEEE Transactions on Biomedical Engineering. 2010;57(1):80–92.
106. Hoang TN, Lin HC, Tsai CH, Jan CK, Liu HL. Passive cavitation enhancement mapping via an ultrasound dual-mode phased array to monitor blood-brain barrier opening. Journal of Medical and Biological Engineering. 2022;42(6):757–66.
107. Crake C, Brinker ST, Coviello CM, Livingstone MS, McDannold NJ. A dual-mode hemispherical sparse array for 3D passive acoustic mapping and skull localization within a clinical MRI guided focused ultrasound device. Physics in Medicine and Biology. 2018;63(6).
108. Lin HC, Yeh CK, Liu HL. Strategy in passively reconstructing and correcting transcranial focal beam via dual-mode ultrasound phased array. IEEE International Ultrasonics Symposium (IUS). 2021:1–4
109. Aldiabat H, O'Brian P, Liu DL, Ebbini ES. Wideband image-based transskull refocusing using dual-mode ultrasound arrays. IEEE International Ultrasonics Symposium (IUS). 2018:1–4.
110. Haritonova A, Liu DL, Bayat M, Ebbini ES. Transcranial focusing and HIFU beam localization with dual-mode ultrasound arrays. IEEE International Ultrasonics Symposium (IUS). 2014:1638–41.
111. Meyers R, Fry WJ, Fry FJ, Dreyer LL, Schultz DF, Noyes RF. Early experiences with ultrasonic irradiation of the pallidofugal and nigral complexes in hyperkinetic and hypertonic disorders. Journal of Neurosurgery. 1959;16(1):32–54.
112. Fry FJ, Goss SA, Patrick JT. Transkull focal lesions in cat brain produced by ultrasound. Journal of Neurosurgery. 1981;54(5):659–63.
113. Fry FJ, Goss SA. Further studies of the transkull transmission of an intense focused ultrasonic beam: Lesion production at 500 kHz. Ultrasound in Medicine and Biology. 1980;6(1):33–8.
114. Aubry JF, Tanter M, Pernot M, Thomas JL, Fink M. Experimental demonstration of noninvasive transskull adaptive focusing based on prior computed tomography scans. Journal of the Acoustical Society of America. 2003;113(1):84–93.
115. McDannold N, King RL, Jolesz FA, Hynynen K. The use of quantitative temperature images to predict the optimal power for focused ultrasound surgery: In vivo verification in rabbit muscle and brain. Medical Physics. 2002;29(3):356–65.
116. Madersbacher S, Kratzik C, Susani M, Marberger M. Tissue ablation in benign prostatic hyperplasia with high intensity focused ultrasound. Journal of Urology. 1994;152(6 Pt 1):1956–60; discussion 1960–1.
117. Gelet A, Chapelon JY, Margonari J, Theillere Y, Gorry F, Cathignol D, et al. Prostatic tissue destruction by high-intensity focused ultrasound: Experimentation on canine prostate. Journal of Endourology. 1993;7(3):249–53.
118. Sanghvi NT, Hynynen K, Lizzi FL. New developments in therapeutic ultrasound. IEEE Engineering in Medicine and Biology Magazine. 1996 15(6):83–92.
119. Hutchinson EB, Hynynen K. Intracavitary ultrasound phased arrays for prostate thermal therapies: MRI compatibility and testing. Medical Physics. 1998;25(12):2392–9.
120. Ozhinsky E, Salgaonkar VA, Diederich CJ, Rieke V. MR thermometry-guided ultrasound hyperthermia of user-defined regions using the ExAblate prostate ablation array. Journal of Therapeutic Ultrasound. 2018;6.
121. Perlis N, Hlasny E, Kucharczyk W, Haider M, Finelli A, Zlotta A, et al. Safety and feasibility of real-time mri-guided focused ultrasound for focal therapy of localized prostate cancer using the exablate 2100 device: Phase 1 study. Journal of Urology. 2017;197(4):E941–E.
122. Schatzl G, Madersbacher S, Djavan B, Lang T, Marberger M. Two-year results of transurethral resection of the prostate versus four 'less invasive' treatment options. European Urology. 2000;37(6):695–701.
123. Lafon C, Koszek L, Chesnais S, Theillere Y, Cathignol D. Feasibility of a transurethral ultrasound applicator for coagulation in prostate. Ultrasound in Medicine and Biology. 2004;30(1):113–22.
124. Ross AB, Diederich CJ, Nau WH, Rieke V, Butts RK, Sommer G, et al. Curvilinear transurethral ultrasound applicator for selective prostate thermal therapy. Medical Physics. 2005;32(6Part1):1555–65.

125. Burtnyk M, Hill T, Cadieux-Pitre H, Welch I. Magnetic resonance image guided transurethral ultrasound prostate ablation: A preclinical safety and feasibility study with 28-day followup. Journal of Urology. 2015;193(5):1669–75.
126. Klotz L, Penson D, Chin J, Pavlovich C, Relle J, Koch M, et al. MRI-guided transurethral ultrasound ablation (TULSA) in patients with localized prostate cancer: Preliminary results of tact pivotal study. Journal of Urology. 2018;199(4):E1077–E8.
127. Miura M, Takahashi S, Fukumoto M, Higashiyama H. Initial experience of transurethral ultrasound ablation (TULSA) of the prostate in Asia. International Journal of Urology. 2022;29:54.
128. Coleman DJ, Lizzi FL, Jakobiec FA. Therapeutic ultrasound in the production of ocular lesions. American Journal of Ophthalmology. 1978;86(2):185–92.
129. Aptel F, Begle A, Razavi A, Romano F, Charrel T, Chapelon JY, et al. Short- and long-term effects on the ciliary body and the aqueous outflow pathways of high-intensity focused ultrasound cyclocoagulation. Ultrasound in Medicine and Biology. 2014;40(9):2096–106.
130. Dunn F. Frequency dependence of threshold ultrasonic dosages for irreversible structural changes in mammalian brain. Journal of the Acoustical Society of America. 1975;58:512–4.
131. Frizzell LA. Threshold dosages for damage to mammalian liver by high intensity focused ultrasound. IEEE Transactions on Ultrasonics, Ferroelectrics, and Frequency Control. 1988;35(5):578–81.
132. ter Haar G, Sinnett D, Rivens I. High intensity focused ultrasound-a surgical technique for the treatment of discrete liver tumours. Physics in Medicine and Biology. 1989;34(11):1743–50.
133. Chen L, Rivens I, ter Haar G, Riddler S, Hill CR, Bensted JP. Histological changes in rat liver tumours treated with high-intensity focused ultrasound. Ultrasound in Medicine and Biology. 1993;19(1):67–74.
134. Chen L, ter Haar G, Hill CR, Dworkin M, Carnochan P, Young H, et al. Effect of blood perfusion on the ablation of liver parenchyma with high-intensity focused ultrasound. Physics in Medicine and Biology. 1993;38(11):1661–73.
135. Chen LL, ter Haar G, Hill CR, Eccles SA, Box G. Treatment of implanted liver tumors with focused ultrasound. Ultrasound in Medicine and Biology. 1998;24(9):1475–88.
136. Yang R, Reilly CR, Rescorla FJ, Faught PR, Sanghvi NT, Fry FJ, et al. High-intensity focused ultrasound in the treatment of experimental liver cancer. Archives of Surgery. 1991;126(8):1002–9; discussion 9–10.
137. Sibille A, Prat F, Chapelon JY, abou el Fadil F, Henry L, Theilliere Y, et al. Characterization of extracorporeal ablation of normal and tumor-bearing liver tissue by high intensity focused ultrasound. Ultrasound in Medicine and Biology. 1993;19(9):803–13.
138. Arefiev A, Prat F, Chapelon JY, Tavakkoli J, Cathignol D. Ultrasound-induced tissue ablation: Studies on isolated, perfused porcine liver. Ultrasound in Medicine and Biology. 1998;24(7):1033–43.
139. Cheng SQ, Zhou XD, Tang ZY, Yu Y, Bao SS, Qian DC. Ultrastructural observation of liver tissue ablation induced by high-intensity focused ultrasound. World Journal of Gastroenterology. 1997;3(3):134–6.
140. Daum DR, Smith NB, King R, Hynynen K. In vivo demonstration of noninvasive thermal surgery of the liver and kidney using an ultrasonic phased array. Ultrasound in Medicine & Biology. 1999;27(7):1087–98.
141. Wang ZB, Wu F, Wang ZL, Zhang Z, Zou JZ, Liu C, et al. Targeted damage effects of high intensity focused ultrasound (HIFU) on liver tissues of Guizhou Province miniswine. Ultrasonic Sonochemistry. 1997;4(2):181–2.
142. Li CX, Xu GL, Jiang ZY, Li JJ, Luo GY, Shan HB, et al. Analysis of clinical effect of high-intensity focused ultrasound on liver cancer. World Journal of Gastroenterology. 2004;10(15):2201–4.
143. Quesson B, Laurent C, Maclair G, de Senneville BD, Mougenot C, Ries M, et al. Real-time volumetric MRI thermometry of focused ultrasound ablation in vivo: A feasibility study in pig liver and kidney. NMR in Biomedicine. 2011;24(2):145–53.
144. Rijkhorst EJ, Rivens I, Haar G, Hawkes D, Barratt D. Effects of respiratory liver motion on heating for gated and model-based motion-compensated high-intensity focused ultrasound ablation. Medical Image Computing and Computer Assisted Interventions. 2011;14(Pt 1):605–12.
145. Lorton O, Guillemin PC, M'Rad Y, Peloso A, Boudabbous S, Charbonnier C, et al. A novel concept of a phased-array HIFU transducer optimized for MR-guided hepatic ablation: Embodiment and first studies. Frontiers in Oncology. 2022;12:1-12
146. Melodelima D, N'Djin WA, Parmentier H, Chesnais S, Rivoire M, Chapelon J-Y. Ultrasound surgery with a toric transducer allows the treatment of large volumes over short periods of time. Applied Physics Letters. 2007;91(19):193901.

147. Chenot J, Melodelima D, N'Djin W A, Souchon R, Rivoire M, Chapelon JY. Intra-operative ultrasound hand-held strain imaging for the visualization of ablations produced in the liver with a toroidal HIFU transducer: First in vivo results. Physics in Medicine and Biology. 2010;55(11):3131–44.
148. Dupre A, Perol D, Blanc E, Peyrat P, Basso V, Chen Y, et al. Efficacy of high-intensity focused ultrasound-assisted hepatic resection (HIFU-AR) on blood loss reduction in patients with liver metastases requiring hepatectomy: Study protocol for a randomized controlled trial. Trials. 2017;18(1):57.
149. Vaezy S, Martin R, Schmiedl U, Caps M, Taylor S, Beach K, et al. Liver hemostasis using high-intensity focused ultrasound. Ultrasound in Medicine and Biology. 1997;23(9):1413–20.
150. Vaezy S, Zderic V. Hemorrhage control using high intensity focused ultrasound. International Journal of Hyperthermia. 2007;23(2):203–11.
151. Sekins KM, Barnes SR, Fan L, Hopple JD, Hsu SJ, Kook J, et al. Deep bleeder acoustic coagulation (DBAC)-Part I: Development and in vitro testing of a research prototype cuff system. Journal of Therapeutic Ultrasound. 2015;3:16.
152. Sekins KM, Barnes SR, Fan L, Hopple JD, Hsu SJ, Kook J, et al. Deep Bleeder Acoustic Coagulation (DBAC)-part II: In vivo testing of a research prototype system. Journal of Therapeutic Ultrasound. 2015;3:17.
153. Lafon C, Chapelon JY, Prat F, Gorry F, Theillere Y, Cathignol D. Design and in vitro results of a high intensity ultrasound interstitial applicator. Ultrasonics. 1998;36(1–5):683–7.
154. Melodelima D, Lafon C, Prat F, Birer A, Cathignol D. Ultrasound cylindrical phased array for transoesophageal thermal therapy: Initial studies. Physics in Medicine and Biology. 2002;47(23):4191–203.
155. Melodelima D, Salomir R, Mougenot C, Moonen C, Cathignol D. 64-element intraluminal ultrasound cylindrical phased array for transesophageal thermal ablation under fast MR temperature mapping: An ex vivo study. Medical Physics. 2006;33(8):2926–34.
156. Yu R, Ma C, Dong J, Liu X, Kang J. Transesophageal high intensity focused ultrasound ablation of left atrium posterior wall: New method for treating atrial fibrillation. Medical Hypotheses. 2008;70(3):654–6.
157. Lee H, Francischelli D, Smith NB. Design of focused ultrasound array for non-invasive transesophageal cardiac ablation. The Open Medical Devices Journal. 2010;2(1).
158. Werner J, Park EJ, Lee H, Francischelli D, Smith NB. Feasibility of in vivo transesophageal cardiac ablation using a phased ultrasound array. Ultrasound in Medicine and Biology. 2010;36(5):752–60.
159. Constanciel E, N'Djin WA, Bessiere F, Chavrier F, Grinberg D, Vignot A, et al. Design and evaluation of a transesophageal HIFU probe for ultrasound-guided cardiac ablation: Simulation of a HIFU minimaze procedure and preliminary ex vivo trials. IEEE Transactions on Ultrasonics, Ferroelectrics, and Frequency Control. 2013;60(9):1868–83.
160. Bessiere F, N'Djin W A, Colas EC, Chavrier F, Greillier P, Chapelon JY, et al. Ultrasound-guided transesophageal high-intensity focused ultrasound cardiac ablation in a beating heart: A pilot feasibility study in pigs. Ultrasound in Medicine & Biology. 2016;42(8):1848–61.
161. Greillier P, Ankou B, Bour P, Zorgani A, Abell E, Lacoste R, et al. Myocardial thermal ablation with a transesophageal high-intensity focused ultrasound probe: Experiments on beating heart models. Ultrasound in Medicine and Biology. 2018;44(12):2625–36.
162. Yao Y, Qian J, Rong S, Huang Y, Xiong B, Yang G, et al. Cardiac denervation for arrhythmia treatment with transesophageal ultrasonic strategy in canine models. Ultrasound in Medicine and Biology. 2019;45(2):490–9.

5

Calibration and Quality Assurance for High Intensity Focused Ultrasound Fields

Ian Rivens and John Civale

5.1 Introduction

Calibration of high-intensity frequency ultrasound (HIFU) devices is becoming increasingly important as the number of studies increases, especially those with ethical implications i.e. clinical trials on humans and pre-clinical in vivo studies. In clinical studies the absolute quantification of ultrasound field parameters (calibration) may be less frequently performed than in the laboratory, with quality assurance (QA) measurements ideally being made prior to each treatment in order to confirm that the system is working within the manufacturer's recommended tolerances. For example, with MR-guided systems the QA measurement may be to confirm a maximum (MR thermometry measured) temperature rise and expected spatial extent of heating in a specially designed QA phantom by using a prescribed therapy ultrasound exposure level and exposure duration. Increasingly, there is also development of lower intensity applications of focused ultrasound, for which most calibration devices and techniques reviewed here are applicable.

QA may also be used to ensure that nominally identical devices (clinical systems or laboratory setups) are similar within manufacturing tolerance and are operating consistently over time. This allows patient treatments to be carried out consistently, safely, and effectively; ensures that research studies are well controlled; and enables data obtained with different devices by different groups in different locations to be compared properly. This is particularly important because whilst HIFU drive electronics (e.g. waveform generators, power amplifiers and electrical impedance matching circuits) can be manufactured with variations in performance of a few percent, piezoelectric crystals are prone to much greater variation in transduction efficiency, both within a single crystal's surface area and between different batches of piezoceramics. Additional variation may occur due to further processing of the ceramic, such as its incorporation into a piezocomposite transducer, or to the addition of a quarter wavelength matching layer designed to maximise ultrasound output. Although electrical impedance matching optimises the electrical power delivered to the transducer, it is not typically used to ensure output uniformity between devices. As a result, the production of multiple systems with similar performance can be challenging and costly. In addition to the variation between devices, calibration or QA measurement should allow changes due to device deterioration, whether it be rapid (a malfunction) or slow (ceramic ageing), to be identified or accounted for.

Focused ultrasound calibration is particularly challenging compared, for example, to radiotherapy, because the field covers an ever-increasing number of ultrasound mediated or enhanced therapies. Some applications use a few ultrasonic cycles, either at low pressure (<1 MPa) e.g. with microbubbles or nanodroplets injected into the blood stream to disrupt the blood-brain barrier[1] or at extremely high pressures designed to induce intrinsic histotripsy (~30 MPa peak negative pressure).[2] Other applications use many millions of cycles in continuous or tone-burst exposures. The intention here may be to induce mild heating (e.g. ~43°C) for many minutes (known as hyperthermia)[3] or it could be to raise the temperature rapidly above 55°C, in some cases as high as the boiling point of water, to thermally ablate tissue.[4, 5]

DOI: 10.1201/9780429162671-5

For most applications, the focal region (and wider beam) shape, size, and position are important. Which other calibration parameters are the most useful often depends on the anticipated mechanism of ultrasound interaction with tissue, be it thermal or non-thermal. For heating, the ultrasonic intensity, and more specifically the spatial-peak temporal-average intensity (I_{SPTA}) is likely to be the most appropriate parameter. For lower power applications, such as wound or fracture healing, I_{SATA} (spatial averaged temporal averaged intensity) may be required. For ultrasonic cavitation mediated applications, the peak pressure amplitudes negative (and positive) provide the most useful measure of exposure level. Peak negative pressures are associated with the likelihood of bubble formation, and peak positive pressures affect the likelihood of highly energetic bubble collapse due to restoring forces within the bubble being overcome.

There are a range of commercially available ultrasound calibration and QA devices, some developed originally for imaging applications, others specifically designed to tolerate HIFU fields. Although the choice may be a compromise between science and economics, the measurement device should be the most appropriate for the parameters of most interest, the energy levels involved, and the available budget. The higher the energy to be measured, the greater the risk of damaging an expensive measurement device. Whichever devices are chosen and used, the best approach is to deploy standardised methods for making measurements and data analysis (including accounting for both type I and type II uncertainties) and publication of comprehensive, statistically rigorous data.

5.2 Transducer Geometry Challenges

HIFU transducers can have a variety of application dependent geometries (characterised by outer dimensions, radius of curvature, and dimensions of any central aperture) and drive frequencies. With the resurgence of interest in trans-skull brain treatment, and the development of histotripsy expanding the exploitation of cavitation, the use of frequencies below 1 MHz is increasingly popular. Current clinical HIFU applications generally lie within the range of 0.3 to 4.0 MHz, with the highest frequencies being used where the target is closest to the transducer e.g. for the transrectal treatment of prostate cancer.

Single-element devices generally have an ellipsoidal focus around 1–2 mm wide and 8–15 mm long (smaller at higher frequencies and lower F-numbers). Around 80% of the total ultrasonic energy is contained within the focus, the rest being distributed into rings surrounding it (side lobes).[6, 7] Whilst side lobes are often ignored clinically, they can be responsible for significant energy deposition during steering or during the placement of multiple adjacent exposures, and so should be accounted for in any calibration process. The relatively small size of the focus compared to the overall ultrasound beam volume yields the ability to ablate target (focal) tissue and spare that overlying and surrounding the target. The energy density at the transducer surface (area of ~cm^2) is orders of magnitude lower than in the focal peak (area of mm^2), where, for ablation, it is generally >1000 W/cm^2.

Generally, an F-number (ratio of the focal length to diameter) around 1 is favoured. For deeper targets, a larger radius of curvature (focal length) is required and potentially a wider device, as this has a greater surface area over which to generate energy. This may also be coupled with the use of lower frequencies to reduce the energy loss (attenuation) in tissue overlying the focus, although this will also reduce absorption in the focal region. Transducers will often be circularly symmetric, but minimally invasive devices such as those used for the trans-rectal treatment of prostate cancer,[8, 9] may benefit from being asymmetric. Alternatively, a rectangular central aperture may be favoured to incorporate a linear or curvilinear array diagnostic ultrasound probe.

As clinical applications have become more challenging, there has been a shift towards multi-element phased arrays, and away from single-element bowls.[6, 10] Phased arrays offer the potential to steer the position of the focus to a range of locations (without the need for mechanical transducer movement) to shape the volume of influence of the ultrasound beam, often by simultaneously creating multiple foci (which can also be achieved using bespoke lenses, such as those designed holographically[11] or to treat larger volumes by sweeping the focus in a prescribed trajectory (such as in concentric circles[12]) during exposures. Such versatility complicates formulating a standard calibration or QA process and renders reporting of just the most basic exposure conditions e.g. electrical or acoustical power rather inadequate. Whilst the reporting of positional variations in field parameters is generally preferred for phase arrays, its usefulness may be somewhat limited.

5.3 Imaging Guidance Challenges

Where the calibration of image-guided systems is required, the imaging guidance may play a confounding role if the HIFU cannot be easily decoupled from it. The two main methods of providing imaging guidance are magnetic resonance (MR) and ultrasound (US) imaging.

MR-guided HIFU (MRgHIFU) is often built into MR scanners in a way that makes it difficult to remove e.g. by being built into the bed.[13, 14] Since most HIFU calibration devices are not specifically designed to be MR compatible, calibration can be particularly challenging in these cases. Even if the HIFU module can be decoupled from the MR system, non-clinical control software may be required in order to avoid any reliance on images for transducer positioning. Finally, devices designed for brain treatments, via direct coupling to the human head, may make coupling to field measurement devices a particular challenge.

Generally, ultrasound guided devices (USgHIFU) tend to have imaging probes mounted within them, often centrally.[15] Calibration difficulties relating to the length of the imaging cable restricting positioning of the HIFU transducer may sometimes be overcome as easily as unplugging the imaging probe from the scanner. Challenges relating to the imaging probe either increasing the size of the treatment head or preventing submersion in water may be less trivial to deal with.

5.4 Tissue Considerations

A HIFU beam consists of many pressure peaks and troughs, which increase in amplitude in all directions as the focal peak is approached. During a clinical treatment, there may be key positions (organs or structures at risk) at which it is particularly useful to know the incident beam parameters. The most common organ in which unwanted damage needs to be avoided is the skin, where adjacent beam positions produce the most energy overlap. Within the body, there may be other particularly important organs or nerves where avoidance of over-exposure is vitally important.

Therefore, understanding the interaction of the beam with biological tissue can be very important. Ultrasound absorption is used in the focal region to obtain sufficient tissue heating to lead to necrosis, but elsewhere in the body, heating is normally unwanted. Some tissues, such as bone and soft tissues containing gas e.g. the intestines or bowel, have significantly elevated levels of ultrasound absorption and/or reflection, leading to significant disturbance of the beam, potentially causing adverse heating and damage at tissue interfaces.[16, 17] Tissue overlying the target volume reduces the energy in a HIFU beam by scattering, in addition to absorption and reflection (at interfaces). This may be an important factor when assessing the impact of calibration measurements made in water. The effects of tissue on ultrasound propagation can be complex, resulting in de-focusing of the beam, usually asymmetrically, and shifting the position of the focal peak, usually towards the transducer. Additionally, differences in sound speed between tissues can affect focal shape and position. On top of this, tissue sound speed, absorption, and scattering are usually temperature dependent, so their effects may change during the delivery of thermal treatments.[18] During non-thermal exposures, microbubbles are usually formed and/or forced into oscillation. These can have a highly significant effect on local tissue properties including scatter and absorption. It can be difficult to account for all these potential changes (which are also discussed in chapter 3) when trying to translate the relevance of water-based calibration measurements into clinical or experimental tissues or phantoms.

5.5 Ultrasound Characterisation Standards and Guidelines

The International Electrotechnical Commission (IEC) standards provide guidance on characterisation of acoustic fields. IEC 62555 relates to HIFU power measurement,[19] IEC 62556 to acoustic field measurements,[20] IEC 61161 gives guidance for the use of acoustic radiation force balances for measuring power,[21] and IEC 62127–1 advises on the use of hydrophones for beam plotting.[22] In addition, it is highly recommended that careful consideration be given to published guidance on reporting ultrasound exposure conditions.[23]

5.6 Hydrophone Measurements

A direct method of quantifying (absolute) HIFU field values is to use a (calibrated) hydrophone to provide a localised measure of acoustic pressure. Measurements are usually performed under 'free-field' conditions in which the ultrasound propagates through non-attenuating water, in the absence of reflecting or absorbing structures in its path. Ideally, the water should be filtered to remove scatterers ≥5 or 10 μm in diameter, deionised to reduce its electrical conductivity (particularly important for some membrane or co-planar devices with exposed electrodes), and, most importantly for high-power devices, degassed to minimise the risk of forming acoustic cavitation bubbles, which may cause measurement artefacts and irreversible hydrophone damage.[24] This relatively simple calibration technique requires a water tank sufficiently large to minimise or avoid, the impact of signals being reflected back to the hydrophone and interfering with the signal of interest. If continuous exposures need to be characterised, reflections may be reduced by lining the tank with ultrasound absorbing material, ideally placed so that any reflections do not travel directly back to the hydrophone, although the use of a rubber which is closely impedance matched to water will minimise any reflection. Sheets of absorbing material are commercially available from companies providing calibration devices or complete systems. Water tanks are normally made of transparent plastic to allow functionality such as visual alignment of the transducer and hydrophone. One method of achieving this rapidly is to build a pointer that can physically indicate the approximate 3D location of the focal peak. This may be inserted into a central aperture of a transducer or mounted on to the ultrasound source in another way. Gross localisation of the hydrophone to within a millimetre or so of the focal peak can greatly reduce the time required for focal alignment. After this, finer localisation can usually be achieved rapidly by manual movement in 3D while visually maximising the hydrophone detected waveform e.g. on the screen of an oscilloscope (or secondary monitor mounted above the beam plotting tank), or by performing small scale automated linear beamplots.

While manual beam plotting, for example using a micrometer actuated gantry, is possible, the use of a precise, automated positioning system can be an expensive, but hugely time saving, investment. Typically, localising precision of better than 100 μm is achievable. Scans that take several hours when performed manually can be obtained in minutes. Automated gantries can be programmed to move rapidly between measurement positions, but it can be beneficial to allow a dwell time before each measurement, especially if using wide surface area hydrophones (membranes) that displace a large volume of water when moved axially, as this can result in axial oscillatory motion after such repositioning. Lateral movement is much less prone to this issue.

Although, manual reading of the hydrophone signal is possible, computerised data recording from a digital oscilloscope is faster and less prone to inaccuracies. In practice, it is beneficial to average over a number of waveforms (e.g. between 20 and 100) to increase reading accuracy and reduce artefacts caused by noise sources such as electronic jitter. Most modern oscilloscopes are easily connected to a control and/or read-out computer via standard communication cables and protocols (e.g. RS232, USB or Ethernet). It is preferable to record whole waveforms rather than just maxima or minima values since these peaks are more prone to noise fluctuations. While the laboratory QA environment may be purpose built, the same may not be true for clinical installations of commercially available therapy ultrasound devices. In particular, the MR guidance of HIFU presents considerable challenges since MR compatibility of acoustic field characterisation equipment is rarely part of their manufacturing design criteria. Similarly, the spatial resolution at which a clinical transducer may be repositioned, may not be optimal for beam plotting. Furthermore, the standard range of clinical exposure conditions may not be well suited to hydrophone measurements, and it may be beneficial to be able to control HIFU transducer output outside the clinical software environment, although without support from the device manufacturer this may be challenging. It is particularly useful to be able to control the number of cycles the transducer produces. Too few cycles and the device may still be ramping up to its maximum steady state output level, too many and multiple ultrasound reflections can cause interference (or in the case of continuous excitation, standing waves) that artificially elevate peak measured values. In addition, hydrophones exhibit different sensitivities to electromagnetic signals, so exciting the HIFU transducer at the same time as making a hydrophone measurement (i.e. by using too long a pulse) can result in an artefactually high signal being measured due to radio frequency (RF) pickup. Since the speed of sound at room temperature in water is roughly 1500 m/s, this is sufficiently different to the speed of light (electrical signals) that even for transducer-hydrophone separations as short as 2–3 cm, pulses of around 30–40 cycles can be enough to avoid this artefact. These are usually sufficiently long for the transducer to reach its peak output level, but this can be checked by making measurements further away from the source.

Hydrophones are available commercially from manufacturers such as Precision Acoustics Ltd. based in Europe and Onda Corp. based in the United States. These have often been designed for the characterisation of both diagnostic and therapeutic ultrasound fields in the 'standard' 1–20 MHz range. As ultrasound applications diversify, with HIFU being used more frequently at 0.1–1 MHz, particularly for brain applications, and with pre-clinical imaging and microscopy applications using frequencies from 20 to 100 MHz and above, systems may be less well suited to calibration using existing devices. For low amplitude sensitivity, it may be necessary to couple a hydrophone to a pre-amplifier, often providing an additional 20 dB of low noise amplification. Hydrophones will normally be supplied with a manufacturer provided calibration – sensitivity values in mV/MPa at a set of frequencies within the user's range of interest). Such calibrations are essential, and if greater traceability is required it may be necessary to make an additional investment in a 3rd-party calibration, often by a national standards institute such as the Food and Drug Administration (FDA) in the United States, National Physical Laboratory (NPL) in the UK, or Physikalisch-Technische Bundesanstalt (PTB) in the European Union. Manufacturer-supplied calibrations may be for the sensor and pre-amplifier separately, in which case the user has to combine the data, or it may be provided as a combined sensitivity, but the user must always be careful to use the correct combination of devices. Broadly, there are three categories of hydrophones: membrane, probe (or needle), and fibre-optic. Membrane and probe/needle hydrophones are piezoelectric sensors, relying on the same technology and phenomena as for ultrasound beam generation. They commonly employ a polyvinylidene fluoride (PVdF) polymer as the sensor. Fibre-optic hydrophones measure changes in light reflection at the tip of an optical fibre caused by pressure induced changes either in the fibre's refractive index[25] or in a Fabry-Perot interferometer design.[26] A summary of typical hydrophone specifications is shown in Table 5.1, and photographs of a range of hydrophone types are shown in Figure 5.1.

Choosing the best hydrophone to characterise HIFU fields should take into account:

i. how high an intensity or pressure needs to be measured (device robustness);
ii. the required spatial resolution (sensor size);
iii. the frequency range of interest (frequency response flatness);
iv. noise level (pressure resolution);
v. temporal stability;
vi. response time of the device;
vii. temperature range over which it can operate;
viii. suitability to the measurement environment (e.g. for the magnetic fields necessary for MRgHIFU);
ix. the size and shape best suited to the measurement environment

For applications involving HIFU ablation, via heating or histotripsy, large peak negative pressures are likely, increasing the risk of inertial cavitation destroying the sensor or altering its response (sensitivity). The quality of the degassing and removal of potential cavitation nuclei (by filtering) from the water in the measurement tank becomes of paramount importance. Assuming this can be optimised, membrane hydrophones are relatively robust and can measure peak negative pressures of several MPa at frequencies above 1 MHz. Traditionally, needle-type sensors are much more susceptible to cavitation damage,[27]

TABLE 5.1

Summary of Hydrophone Capability Ranges

	FOPH 2000	HFO-690	Onda Membrane	Onda Capsule	Onda Needle	PA Needle	PA Membrane	PA Fibre Optic
Spatial resolution/sensor size (µm)	100	100	200 or 500	85 to 400	200 or 400	40 to 4000	200 or 400	10
Sensitivity (mV/MPa)	2	6	~0.1 to 0.6	1.3 to 2.8	1.3 to 5.0	~0.6 to 8000	35	250
Acoustic pressure range (MPa)	-60 to +400	Up to 500	7 to 53 (p-p)	n/a	n/a	0.2 kPa to 2.33 MPa	14 kPa to 20 MPa	16 kPa to 8 MPa
Bandwidth (MHz)	DC to 150	0.003 to 150	0.5 to 45 (3dB)	0.25 to 40 (3 dB)	1 to 20 (6 dB)	1 to 30 (4 dB)/0.08 to 8	1 to 40	0.25 to 40
Temperature range (°C)	5 to 95	5 to 95	Up to 40	Up to 50	Up to 50	5 to 50	5 to 50	5 to 50
Accuracy (%)	5%					9–18%	8–15%	8–15%
Device dimension	20 m fibre	2 m fibre	~100 mm dia.	~12 mm dia.	2.4 mm dia.	40 mm long	~100 mm dia.	125 µm dia.
Optimum application	Histotripsy	Histotripsy	Thermal/histotripsy	Thermal	Thermal	Thermal	Thermal	Thermal

Note that the stated ranges may be applicable across a range of devices (e.g. needle hydrophones) rather than being specific to one device. Manufacturer's advice should be sought on the best device for specific needs. Abbreviations: DC – direct current, PA – precision acoustics, dia – diameter.

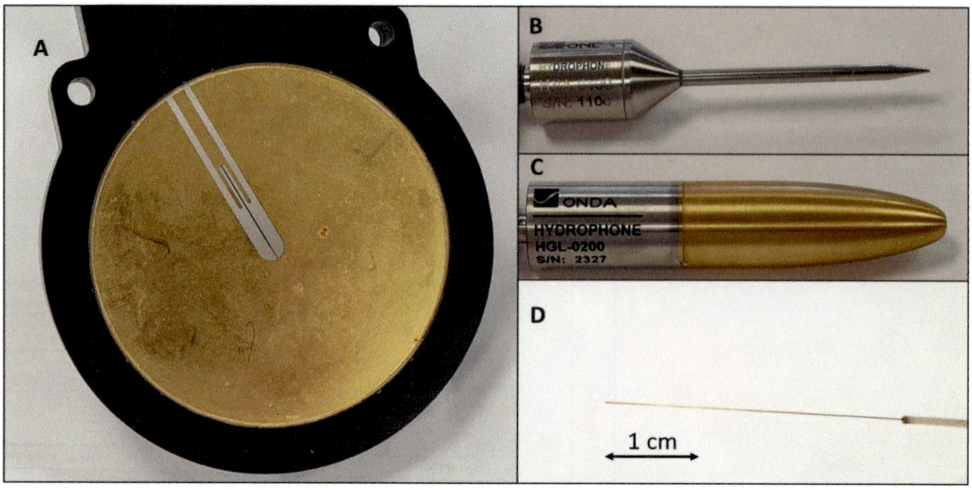

FIGURE 5.1 Examples of hydrophones which may be used to characterise HIFU acoustic fields: A) 0.4-mm membrane (Precision Acoustics); B) 'rugged' 0.4-mm needle (Onda Corp); C) 0.2-mm capsule ('lipstick' type (Onda Corp); and D) a Fabry-Perot fibre-optic hydrophone (Precision Acoustics).

but some needle-like probes have been specifically developed to be more robust. These include the HNA and HGL series of hydrophones (Onda Corp., Sunnyvale, CA). Finally, specialist, very high pressure, fibre-optic hydrophones have been developed recently which can measure pressure amplitudes from −60 MPa to +400 MPa with a precision of up to +−0.7 MPa (FOPH 2000, RP-Acoustics, Lautenbach, Germany) or pressures up to 500 MPa with a sensitivity of 6 mV/MPa (HFO-690 Onda Corp, USA).[25, 28] Although such devices are not immune to damage, the tip of the fibre can be cut-off by the user once damaged to restore performance.

Hydrophone sensor size is particularly important for accurate pressure measurements at the focal peak of a highly focused beam because of the spatial averaging that occurs across its surface area. To minimise such errors, the smallest available sensor should be deployed. IEC standards[20, 22] recommend a sensor radius no larger than a quarter of the acoustic wavelength, although larger sensors may be acceptable for far field measurements where pressure fluctuations are less rapid. A smaller sensor will also have a lower variation in angular response, making it more suitable for measurements away from the focal peak where the angle between the sensor and the sound propagation axis may be up to 45 degrees. Figure 5.3 shows an example of one hydrophone's angular response at two frequencies. Since piezoelectric sensor size correlates with sensitivity, the advantages of a small sensor have to be weighed against its relatively low sensitivity, a more significant problem for low pressure applications than for HIFU. As a result, PVDF hydrophones are more effective in the focal region than farther from it, where the signal-to-noise ratio reduces. For pressures below ~0.1 MPa, hydrophone sensitivity may be the dominant device selection criterion; see Table 5.1 and Figure 5.2.

A flat frequency response over the range of 1–20 MHz, or better still 0.1–40 MHz, is ideal for HIFU measurements, since the detected voltage waveform will closely resemble that of the acoustic pressure. Membrane hydrophones typically offer the flattest frequency response and are therefore best suited to measuring acoustic signals which contain multiple harmonics of the drive frequency. Such harmonics are often generated by non-linear wave propagation, resulting from high pressures or intensities. The less frequency dependent a hydrophone's sensitivity, the lower the error that would be introduced if only the drive frequency sensitivity is used to convert measured voltage into acoustic pressure.[29] Needle or fibre-optic hydrophones, due to their shape and construction, often have a more variable frequency response with resonances and phase distortions.[26, 29, 30] For this reason, it is more important that the frequency dependent sensitivity is used.[22] Regardless of hydrophone type, this more rigorous approach improves calibration reliability provided accurate characterisation of the hydrophone magnitude and

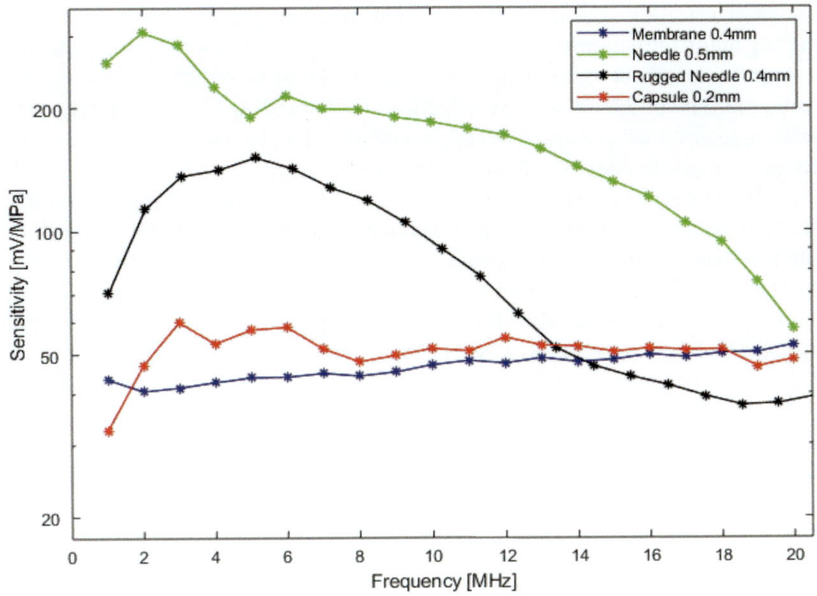

FIGURE 5.2 Examples of sensitivity frequency dependence for a range of hydrophones.

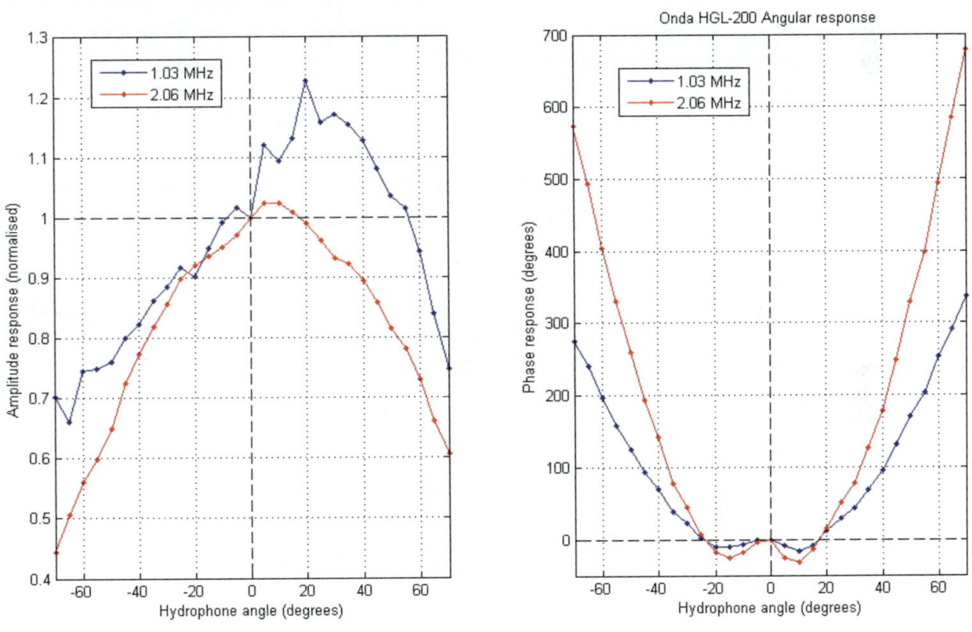

FIGURE 5.3 An example of hydrophone angular sensitivity and phase response.

phase response is available. Further practical considerations influencing hydrophone choice include how easily the device can be mounted into a measurement system (see Figure 5.1), which device size and shape is best suited to the application or environment (for example, needle-type devices are better than membranes for measuring close to bowl shaped devices or within apertures or restricted spaces) and the relative cost of different options.[31] However, needle and fibre-optic devices, which are essentially narrow cylinders, can be susceptible to pressure-pulse distortion which may be complex to correct.[32]

HIFU field characterisation should ideally be performed using a tone-burst excitation. This is best suited for avoiding many measurement problems and minimises the risk of hydrophone damage. Pulsed exposure measurements can be made while the drive is signal is 'off' thus avoiding electromagnetic pickup, and can eliminate problems such as reflections (and standing waves) that may occur under continuous sonication. In addition, pulsing reduces the risk of thermal or cavitation damage. Typically, fewer than 20 cycles are enough to allow the transducer to ramp up to a steady output level. However, if the hydrophone is to be used many centimetres from the focal peak, the time-of-flight variation to it from all points across the transducer surface to the hydrophone needs to be taken into account. Usually, 40–50 cycles are sufficient in such cases. For data processing, it is best to analyse a smaller number of cycles e.g. 5–10 close to the centre of the burst, chosen to be where the pressure amplitude is the most stable.

Conversion of hydrophone measured voltage to acoustic pressure requires knowledge of the sensitivity of both the hydrophone and any associated pre-amplifier. Calibration data is usually provided in units of mV/MPa or μV/Pa, with an indication of measurement uncertainty, often at integer MHz intervals above 1 MHz, and/or 0.05 or 0.1 MHz increments below this. The simplest conversion is to use the quoted sensitivity closest to the transducer's working frequency. A slight improvement on this would be to assume a linear variation between the two closest data points and linearly interpolate to obtain a sensitivity value for the transducer drive frequency. If multiple harmonics are present at the sensor, and the hydrophone response is not flat, a frequency-dependent deconvolution will perform better. A fast Fourier transform (FFT) of the measured waveform can be used to identify the drive frequency harmonics present in the frequency spectrum. After converting the amplitude of each to pressure using the appropriate sensitivity value at each frequency, an inverse FFT can be used to yield a more accurate estimate of the ultrasonic waveform. A full deconvolution with hydrophone sensitivity and phase response can provide better quantification of the positive and negative acoustic pressure peaks. Whilst the advantage of this is that drive harmonics, usually created by non-linear propagation, are taken into account, the power distribution across harmonics may only be relevant for the medium in which the measurement was made. Usually water is used for 'free-field' measurements, which has a coefficient of non-linearity (B/A)[33] of around 5,. However predicting in situ pressures (i.e. attenuation corrected values) in tissues is not straightforward as they may have very different acoustic properties from water in terms of attenuation and B/A coefficient. A simple but not particularly satisfactory approach is to calculate derated pressures/intensities from the free-field water measurements. In this approach tissue attenuation is modelled assuming a linear relationship between attenuation coefficient and frequency, essentially ignoring effects due to the development of higher harmonic components. Another limitation is that it is much more complex to determine calculation uncertainty when numerous sensitivity values are used. Measurement uncertainties are high for HIFU calibration, compared to those for radiotherapy. A hydrophone calibration measurement from NPL, for example, has a quoted measurement uncertainty on site of ±7%. When the device is used under less ideal circumstances in a HIFU laboratory this probably increases to at least ±10%, which results in the best possible accuracy being e.g. 5 ± 0.5 MPa or 2000 ± 400 Wcm^{-2} (the percentage error doubling for intensity which depends on pressure squared).

Usually, the pressure values of most interest are the peak negative and positive pressures, indicators of potential cavitation activity. Typically, these differ in terms of their location, magnitude and focal width, due to non-linear propagation and diffraction of the focused beam. The root-mean-square (RMS) pressure is useful because it does not suffer from the kind of distortions that affect the negative and positive pressure amplitudes. This value, which averages the positive and negative measurements, is inherently less noisy and can be used to estimate intensity. Assuming transducer performance is comparable during continuous wave and low duty cycle tone-burst exposures (i.e. that the ceramic does not heat significantly during use), the RMS pressure can be used to determine temporal-average intensity (I_{ta}):

$$I_{ta} = (P_{RMS})^2/\rho\, c$$

where ρ is the density and c the sound speed in water. Although the expression is strictly only valid for plane waves, where the pressure and velocity are in phase, it is a reasonable approximation at the focal or spatial peak. I_{SPTA} is thus useful for practical purposes such as comparisons between different transducers, or modelling tissue heating.

The spectral content of the pressure waveform may be analysed using FFTs to identify the total pressure (intensity) distribution amongst the harmonics, each of which will have a different (frequency dependent) absorption and scatter in tissue. Ensuring the FFT window is an exact number of cycles of the fundamental frequency guarantees that the FFT frequency bins are exactly centred on the harmonic frequencies, and that the power spectrum is correctly calculated with the intensity being distributed at the harmonics only, minimising frequency leakage effects. Such analysis allows more comprehensive comparison of different transducers and may be of use for treatment planning, taking into account nonlinear propagation. In HIFU treatments, the effects of frequency-dependent attenuation and the non-linear properties (B/A) of tissue are likely to have a significantly different impact on the waveform shape, and frequency content at the focus than that observed in water.

Hydrophones may be used to obtain spatial beam plots in a number of ways. Linear (1D) scans through the focal peak can be used to determine focal size, for example by quantifying the full-width half-pressure maximum (6 dB) or full-width half-intensity maximum (3 dB) beam widths. This is often done along the sound axis (axially) and in two orthogonal trans-axial (lateral) directions. Such dimensions are often used to indicate the extent of a 'typical' single HIFU lesion, although in practice, lesion size is affected by the exposure time (via thermal conduction). It is important that lateral measurements are made in orthogonal axes as radial symmetry should not be assumed, especially for asymmetric transducers such as those used for prostate exposures. Linear scans are quick to obtain, generally taking minutes, even for submillimetric resolution scans over several centimetres. Planar (2D) scans are useful for visualising the HIFU beam shape, highlighting any asymmetry and identifying regions of highest intensity outside the focus. In addition to plots centred around the focal peak, 2D plots in the pre-focal field can be used to back-project data onto the transducer surface and examine field homogeneity at the source.[34] This is particularly useful for phased (multi-element) arrays as it allows identification of malfunctioning elements. It is also possible to use 2D pre-focal scans to predict the pressure in the focal plane using a non-linear forward projection,[20] allowing estimation of focal pressures likely to be too high to be measured with a hydrophone. Pre-focal scans could also be obtained over a curved grid just in front of a transducer's surface for the same purpose. Obtaining 2D plots with reasonable, but lower spatial resolution than linear plots, in both directions, usually takes several hours. As a result 2D plots generally have lower resolution than linear plots, providing less accurate quantitative data. Volume or orthogonal-planar (3D) scans are possible; but rapidly become prohibitive in terms of scan times, bearing in mind that it is not good practice to leave hydrophones immersed in water for periods >12 hours. Whilst it is possible to perform scans at variable spatial resolution these are relatively complex to setup, and usually require the user to control automated beamplotting systems with their own software rather than commercially available software. However, such flexibility would also allow beam plotting over arbitrary orthogonal axes rather than having to carefully align the transducer's sound axis with the gantry. The use of hydrophones in all biomedical applications of ultrasound has recently been thoroughly reviewed by Harris et al.[35]

5.7 Electrical Power Measurement

Although measuring the electrical drive to a HIFU transducer yields no information about the acoustic field, it is a fundamental characteristic of the drive system that should remain relatively stable. Measuring electric power is relatively cheap and simple. In-line RF power meters, usually measuring forward and/or reflected power, are commercially available or can be purchased as a component of a HIFU drive system. As a result, even in the absence of HIFU calibration equipment, it may be possible to quantify and monitor this useful parameter. Given knowledge of the transducer efficiency (often in the range of 50–70%), which may be provided by the manufacturer, it is possible to estimate acoustic power from total electrical power. Knowing the electrical drive power as well as the ultrasonic properties of a system can be advantageous, as it allows verification of the transducer efficiency either as part of acceptance testing or for routine monitoring of system performance stability. As an alternative to monitoring power it is also possible to monitor drive voltage (using a potential divider or bridge) and current (using an inductor placed around an unshielded drive cable). Power may then be calculated from voltage and current, ideally with relative phase taken into account. Electrical power monitoring will alert system users to changes in either the performance of the transducer or any electrical matching network, both of which can lead to acoustic power not being the expected value.

5.8 Acoustic Power Measurement

Measurement of acoustic power provides a simple quantitative description of a transducer's output, at one, or a series of, drive levels. This is preferable to only measuring electrical power. Repeated monitoring of acoustic power over days, months, and years demonstrates a system's stability over the short or long term. While piezoceramics are known to lose efficiency over a time scale of years, a sudden decrease in acoustic power is likely to indicate a problem with a HIFU transducer, its electrical impedance matcher or another component of its drive system. Compared to beam characterisation with a hydrophone, power measurement is simpler and faster.

There are two approaches to measuring ultrasonic power. One exploits radiation force, and the other calorimetry. The radiation force technique makes use of the fact that propagating ultrasound carries momentum. Absorption or reflection of this momentum will result in a net force being applied on a target.[19, 21, 36–38] Calorimetric methods require the complete absorption of the beam's ultrasound energy and its conversion to heat.[39, 40] Calorimetry can be challenging due to the difficulties of accurately measuring volumetric heating and of limiting thermal losses from the measurement environment. A relatively recently developed buoyancy approach[41] combines both radiation force and calorimetry methods in one device.

5.8.1 Radiation Force Methods

Although the radiation force generated by ultrasound is relatively small (equivalent to 0.67 mN/W for an absorbing target[42]), this method is the primary standard for measuring acoustic power. Under standardised measurement conditions, it is possible to measure acoustic powers down to ~1 mW using a precision balance.[43] As a result, this technique is widely used for both imaging and therapy devices, with commercially available measurement systems (PA www.acoustics.co.uk/product/radiation-force-bala nce/, ONDA www.ondacorp.com/radiation-force/).

Radiation force (at a propagation medium/air interface) was used as early as 1956 during the scientific development of HIFU for treating cancer. By measuring the height of the fountain of water at an air interface it was possible to perform rudimentary QA on a transducer to ensure its continued functionality.[44]

Measured radiation force can be converted to acoustic power by multiplying by sound speed in the propagation medium. The only complications are the type of target (absorbing or reflecting), its alignment with the ultrasonic beam, and the need for geometrical correction factors for beam convergence or diffraction.[19] For reflecting targets, it is important to direct the reflected beam away from the transducer, to avoid interference and potential standing waves that may result from the continuous or long tone-burst exposures that are usually used for these measurements. Typically, conical[45] or otherwise angled reflecting[46] targets are used. There is however the potential for significant error in position, and alignment for correct interception of the acoustic beam using these kinds of targets with highly focused transducers.[47] For absorbing targets,[48] ideally none of the incident ultrasound power is reflected and so alignment and target geometry are less critical, providing the target intercepts the entire width of the beam and the HIFU axis is aligned normally to the balance. The main problem with absorbing targets is their potential to heat. This can lead to thermal expansion, changes in the target's properties, or target damage, all of which can produce unstable or unreliable results. A brush-type absorber which avoids many such problems has been proposed[49] with promising results when used with pulsed HIFU exposures. A commercially available radiation force balance system with multiple target options that can be mounted above a balance is shown in more detail in Figure 5.4. The tank must be filled with degassed water and bubble-free coupling of the transducer under test must be ensured.

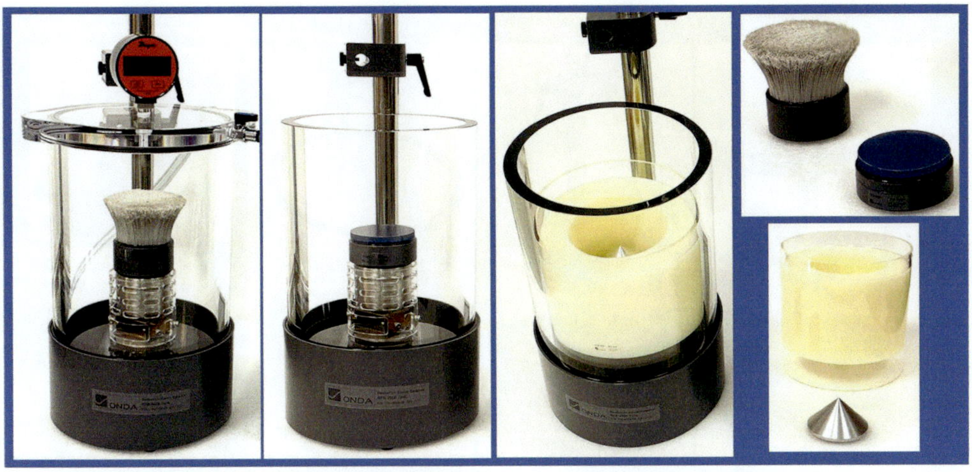

FIGURE 5.4 One example of a commercially available radiation force balance system with 3 target options: brush for powers up to 100 W, cone for powers up to 20 W and absorber (blue) for 1 mW–2 W. Photographs courtesy of Sam Howard, Onda Corporation, Inc.

A method that neatly combines radiation force and calorimetry (Figure 5.5) uses an absorbing target made from a large (>8 cm diameter, >15 cm long) cylinder filled with castor oil.[19, 41, 50] The cylinder is submerged in a tank of degassed water and is suspended below a precision balance using thin wires. The cylinder has an acoustically transparent membrane (window) through which the HIFU beam propagates into the oil. The flexible membrane allows expansion and contraction of the heated castor oil. Beam alignment is not critical as long as the whole beam enters the castor oil, and no correction due to the focused nature of the beam is necessary. When the HIFU is switched on (and off) the absorbing target experiences a change in applied force, which is measured by the balance. A second effect is expansion of the castor oil as it continuously heats during exposure (typically 10–20 s), resulting in a change in buoyancy which is also detected by the balance (Figure 5.6). Because castor oil has a relatively high attenuation coefficient, the ultrasonic energy is absorbed and the thermal energy distributed through much of the available volume. Radiation force promotes acoustic streaming in the oil, which also helps redistribute the heat. This avoids excessive heating and effects such as acoustic cavitation. For ideal measurements, the heat from the phantom during each exposure should be negligible. Heat travels relatively slowly (mm/s), and the Perspex cylinder is relatively large and thermally insulating. Although the buoyancy effect is small compared to the radiation force (0.35 mg/J sensitivity[41]) it is easily measurable provided exposures are at high enough power and/or of long enough duration to build up ~5 J of heat.[50] Thermal losses may need to be considered at frequencies above 3 MHz,[50] but provided the target is thermally large, (which is necessary to enclose the entire beam of typical HIFU transducers), the time scale over which heat is lost to the surrounding fluid will be longer than the measurement duration. The castor oil buoyancy system is suitable for power measurements up to hundreds of watts.

Acoustic power can be used to estimate spatial peak intensity providing the relevant acoustic pressure or intensity distributions are known. Even if this is only possible at lower power settings, focal peak intensities may then be extrapolated for higher power settings. Hill et al. used this approach with radiation force data and hydrophone focal width (6 dB) measurements at lower power to derive estimates of spatial-peak temporal-average intensity.[46] This approach can be useful where the focal pressures or intensities cannot safely be measured using an existing hydrophone; however, care must be taken since this relies on a set of assumptions regarding the HIFU transducer and how the intensity is distributed within the beam. For the case where the transducer geometry is not a simple spherical bowl, such as transducers with a central aperture or asymmetric insertable probes, it may be possible to determine appropriate corrections to improve the accuracy of spatial-peak-temporal-average intensity estimated by considering transducer geometry alone or by performing hydrophone measurements in the focal plane.[51]

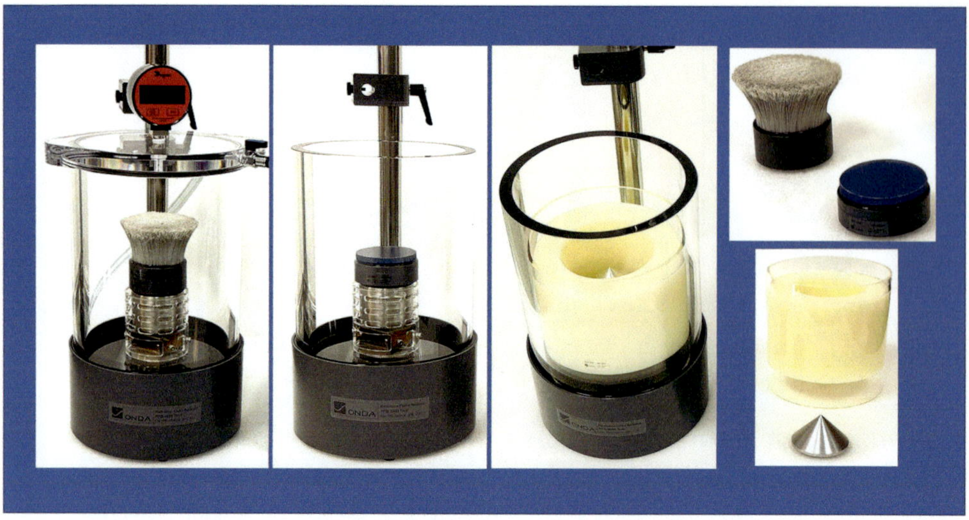

FIGURE 5.5 Buoyancy calibration system. Left: A castor oil filled phantom is suspended from the under pan weighing mechanism of a high accuracy balance using nylon fishing twine. Middle: Liquid crystal thermochromic strips allow monitoring of the castor oil temperature to avoid significant heating during high power/long duration exposures. A HIFU transducer can be seen submerged in the degassed water within the tank such that the focal region is at depth in the castor oil phantom. Right: The HIFU transducer must be placed so that the entire beam enters the phantom via an acoustically transparent membrane which is flexible to allow for thermal expansion of the oil during heating. Precise alignment is not required.

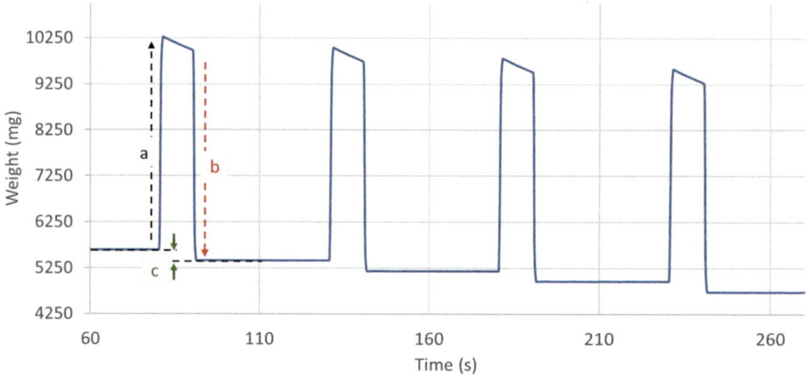

FIGURE 5.6 Example of acoustic power measurement (at ~70 W) using a radiation force/buoyancy system showing the weight measured by a precision balance (Sartorius LA230S) for a set of 4 repeat 10-s sonications. The radiation force at onset (a), and offset (b) are indicated, together with the shift in baseline weight (c) due to the change in the buoyancy force acting on the target.

5.9 Phantom and Test Devices

Comprehensive calibration, or QA, requires a means of assessing both the HIFU and of any targeting/guidance capability, since correct placement of the focus during clinical treatment is of critical importance. Here, phantoms or test objects can perform a vital role in checking the alignment of a HIFU focal region with respect to its positioning and/or imaging system, and, ideally, by providing a means of quantifying the acoustic or thermal effects induced in a reference material.

For ultrasound-guided systems (USgHIFU), a phantom or test object which includes an embedded reflector (such as a small ball or end of a rod) or acoustic or thermal sensor can be used. By independently localising the HIFU and imaging beam on the target, it is possible to estimate the extent of any misalignment between the two in 3D. Acoustic reflectors may be used to locate the HIFU beam using pulse echo techniques, provided there is access to the transducer's drive voltage, and to targeting verification using standard B-mode imaging. An implanted hydrophone may be localised using a short HIFU burst as described earlier, and the tips of needle-like devices should be visible on B-mode images. An embedded thermocouple may be used for HIFU localisation, albeit being a rather more time-consuming process than acoustic pressure localisation. This method needs additional thermal monitoring hardware and software. Another disadvantage of this technique is the difficultly in imaging the thermal junction accurately, especially if a fine wire thermocouple (<100 μm) is used. A Fabry-Perot fibre-optic hydrophone[26] offers the opportunity for the use of an embedded or implantable probe to monitor both acoustic pressure and temperature change simultaneously. The tip of such a probe can usually be imaged using ultrasound, or localisation using a pulsed-Doppler gate is an option.

In an MR guided system, a purely thermal test phantom is likely to be the simplest approach as MR thermometry is the standard method for HIFU monitoring. A homogeneous material that provides a strong MR signal with minimal artefacts (from its bulk or its housing), has tissue-like ultrasound properties (absorption, attenuation, sound speed, B/A parameter) and that remains stable over time is ideal. The MRI system can be used to verify both the extent and location of the heating for a standard QA exposure regime. Whilst any hydrogel may be suitable for such an application, some equipment manufacturers provide a polyacrylamide-based phantom for routine QA.

Although quantification of absolute values for parameters is essential for comparing both clinical and laboratory HIFU data, there is a valuable contribution to be made by qualitative or semi-quantitative techniques, particularly for the visualisation of acoustic or thermal distributions for QA purposes. A relatively simple technique is to use thermochromic dyes. As an example, these have been in the form of a film attached to a 3D printed bone mimic, to demonstrate the ability to avoid rib heating using a 10 strip-element transducer[52] or a highly absorbing rubber sheet.[53] The thermochromic effect is reversible unless the film is damaged through over-heating or cavitation. More recently, a blue dye within a translucent phantom which loses its colour above a threshold temperature of 50 ± 3°C has been reported.[54] Similar, but irreversible, results have been obtained in PVA doped with thermochromic dye[55] and in translucent polyacrylamide gels containing either bovine serum albumin[56] or egg white,[57, 58] where heat denaturated protein has increased opacity. Polyacrylamide gels mixed with corn syrup and a non-ionic surface-active agent (NiSAA), polyoxyethylene alkyl ether series, provide a temperature-dependent clouding point.[59] Although the clouding is mainly reversible, some hysteresis has been reported. The clouding temperatures investigated were in the range of 66–80°C.

Another method for thermal beam visualisation exploits ultrasound absorption at an air interface, using a 0.2-mm-thick sheet. For this, infra-red (IR) imaging was used to obtain a series of 2D thermal images through a HIFU beam (with 0.044 mm and 0.05°C resolution) to assess the potential to construct a 3D image in real time.[60] This technique can cover wider temperature ranges than thermochromic dyes or NiSAAs and is independent of the starting temperature. As clinical interest in HIFU has burgeoned, the desire for more rapid methods of performing QA measurements has increased. IR has been used with HIFU arrays,[6, 61] and shown to correlate well with hydrophone scans[62] for focused and unfocused beams, and the use of an MR compatible system has also been demonstrated.[63] A similar idea, but using an acoustically absorbing, thermochromic dye impregnated tile developed for rapid visualisation of time-averaged intensity profiles, has been tested, but only at relatively low power for physiotherapy ultrasound equipment.[64, 65] Direct comparison of hydrophone plots between IR thermography in an absorbing phantom and thermochromic film embedded in a phantom[66] showed the potential benefits and limitations of each technique for qualitative or quantitative assessment.

An optical approach to HIFU beam visualisation, Schlieren imaging,[67, 68] takes advantage of pressure-induced changes in refractive index of the propagation medium. This relatively simple technique is good for rapid visualisation of a beam, but does not readily provide quantitative information. Other visualisation options include holography of the ultrasound beam[34, 69, 70] and vibrometry of the transducer surface.[71, 72] These methods may also be used in conjunction with a suitable model to predict the acoustic field in the focal region. Holography methods are based on characterising the amplitude and phase of the acoustic field over a 2D plane normal to the direction of beam propagation, usually at a location between the transducer and the focus. This characterisation requires a relatively large scan with fine resolution ($\leq\lambda/2$), usually performed with a hydrophone. The recorded information may then be used to back-project the acoustic field on to the transducer surface, giving a 2D image of amplitude and phase at the transducer, or forward-project to determine the acoustic field in the focal region. In practice the latter is rarely performed, as projection methods rely on linear acoustics calculations, such as the use of the Rayleigh integral or angular spectrum methods, which do not readily incorporate non-linear propagation effects. One advantage of characterising the acoustic field with a hydrophone at a pre-focal location is that the pressure amplitudes will be lower, reducing the risk of hydrophone damage in particular due to acoustic cavitation. A drawback is the need for a relatively large scan typically requiring a few thousand measurements, which can be time consuming. The long time required for the scan also poses the problem of potential errors due to changes in sound speed in the propagation medium due to drift in water temperature. Back-projection of the acoustic field on to the transducer surface can be invaluable from a QA perspective, as it can readily identify transducer defects. For example, on simple bowl transducers it may help identify 'dead' areas, or apodisation, and on multi-element arrays it may help identify individual elements that have either failed or are not working effectively. The Rayleigh integral is most often used for the back-projection, as it lends itself easily to calculation along the typically curved surface of HIFU transducers. A characterisation of the acoustic output at the transducer, via holography or other methods, may then be used as input to a more sophisticated model, for example, one that incorporates non-linear propagation effects, to predict the properties of the acoustic beam up to and beyond the focal region.

5.10 Measurement Reporting

As the clinical applications of HIFU/FUS expand, the science and technology associated with the accurate and rigorous characterisation of device output become increasingly important. Calibration of ultrasound transducers and their drive electronics is essential. In summary, relatively simple radiation force (with or without buoyancy) measurements can provide accurate measurements of total acoustic power which can be used to estimate I_{SPTA}. Hydrophones can be used to measure focal peak pressure, from which intensity may be calculated, and the spatial distribution of pressure in 1, 2, or 3D. Focal peak and focal dimension values are essential for characterising exposures.

Simple quantification of acoustic power output (ideally as a function of drive conditions over a commonly used range) is useful for reporting clinical and laboratory work. Additionally, or alternatively, calculation of the focal (spatial) peak intensity (often the temporal average) is important. Beam profiling in 1, 2, or 3D, describing the size of the focal regions either in terms of pressure (6 dB) or intensity (3 dB) iso-contours, adds important information. High fidelity and accurate quality assurance enables valid comparisons between studies across different sites around the world, using different clinical or laboratory systems in different exposure regimes, whether they be pulsed or continuous. While the high powers (pressure/intensity) involved in HIFU present significant challenges, a number of solutions exist for measuring output parameters. In addition, recommended methods and available measurement device types are detailed in IEC standards.[19–22] It is advisable to consider methods of quantifying ultrasound exposures and to make baseline measurements of system performance carefully before clinical trials, pre-clinical experiments or laboratory studies commence.[73] The aim should always be to measure and report the parameters (pressure amplitudes, intensity, acoustic frequency, acoustic power, duty cycles, beam width, etc.) used in the study[23] so that others may replicate the work or move forward from a solid scientific foundation. Measurements performed under free-field conditions are the easiest to perform, are widely published and provide an acceptable option. Where de-rating factors are used to determine in situ values, these must be fully explained and quantified. Wide uptake of the recommendations for a more rigorous approach to reporting of exposure conditions and standardised use of measurement techniques will encourage regular quality assurance on clinical systems and ultimately lead towards more widely accepted safety and quality assurance protocols which will give further credence to HIFU as a therapeutic modality in the clinic.[74]

REFERENCES

1. Morse SV, Pouliopoulos AN, Chan TG, Copping MJ, Lin JL, Long NJ, et al. Rapid short-pulse ultrasound delivers drugs uniformly across the murine blood-brain barrier with negligible disruption. Radiology. 2019;291(2):458–65.
2. Vlaisavljevich E, Xu Z, Maxwell A, Mancia L, Zhang X, Lin KW, et al. Effects of temperature on the histotripsy intrinsic threshold for cavitation. IEEE Transactions on Ultrasonics, Ferroelectrics, and Frequency Control. 2016;63(8):1064–77.
3. Marmor JB, Pounds D, Hahn GM. Clinical studies with ultrasound-induced hyperthermia. National Cancer Institute of Monographs. 1982;61:333–7.
4. Fry WJ, Mosberg W, Barnard J, Fry F. Production of focal destructive lesions in the central nervous system with ultrasound. Journal of Neurosurgery. 1954;11(5):471–8.
5. Lynn JG, Zwemer RL, Chick AJ, Miller AE. A new method for the generation and use of focused ultrasound in experimental biology. Journal of General Physiology. 1942;26(2):179–93.
6. Bobkova S, Gavrilov L, Khokhlova V, Shaw A, Hand J. Focusing of high-intensity ultrasound through the rib cage using a therapeutic random phased array. Ultrasound in Medicine and Biology. 2010;36(6):888–906.
7. O'Neil HT. Theory of focusing radiators. The Journal of the Acoustical Society of America. 2005;21(5):516–26.
8. Foster RS, Bihrle R, Sanghvi N, Fry F, Kopecky K, Regan J, et al. Production of prostatic lesions in canines using transrectally administered high-intensity focused ultrasound. European Urology. 1993;23(2):330–6.
9. Gelet A, Chapelon JY, Margonari J, Theillere Y, Gorry F, Cathignol D, et al. Prostatic tissue destruction by high-intensity focused ultrasound: Experimentation on canine prostate. Journal of Endourology. 1993;7(3):249–53.
10. Hynynen K, Jones RM. Image-guided ultrasound phased arrays are a disruptive technology for non-invasive therapy. Physics in Medicine and Biology. 2016;61(17):R206-R48.
11. Andrés D, Rivens I, Mouratidis P, Jiménez N, Camarena F, ter Haar G. Holographic focused ultrasound hyperthermia system for uniform simultaneous thermal exposure of multiple tumor spheroids. Cancers. 2023;15(9).
12. Mougenot C, Kohler MO, Enholm J, Quesson B, Moonen C. Quantification of near-field heating during volumetric MR-HIFU ablation. Medical Physics. 2011;38(1):272–82.
13. Voogt MJ, Trillaud H, Kim YS, Mali WP, Barkhausen J, Bartels LW, et al. Volumetric feedback ablation of uterine fibroids using magnetic resonance-guided high intensity focused ultrasound therapy. European Radiology. 2012;22(2):411–7.
14. Illing RO, Kennedy JE, Wu F, ter Haar GR, Protheroe AS, Friend PJ, et al. The safety and feasibility of extracorporeal high-intensity focused ultrasound (HIFU) for the treatment of liver and kidney tumours in a Western population. British Journal of Cancer. 2005;93(8):890–5.
15. Wu F, Wang ZB, Chen WZ, Zhu H, Bai J, Zou JZ, et al. Extracorporeal high intensity focused ultrasound ablation in the treatment of patients with large hepatocellular carcinoma. Annals of Surgical Oncology. 2004;11(12):1061–9.
16. Kennedy JE, Wu F, ter Haar GR, Gleeson FV, Phillips RR, Middleton MR, et al. High-intensity focused ultrasound for the treatment of liver tumours. Ultrasonics. 2004;42(1–9):931–5.
17. Li JJ, Gu MF, Luo GY, Liu LZ, Zhang R, Xu GL. Complications of high intensity focused ultrasound for patients with hepatocellular carcinoma. Technology in Cancer Research and Treatment. 2009;8(3):217–24.
18. Bamber JC, Hill CR. Ultrasonic attenuation and propagation speed in mammalian tissues as a function of temperature. Ultrasound in Medicine and Biology. 1979;5:149–57.
19. I.E.C. Ultrasonics – Power measurement – High intensity therapeutic ultrasound (HITU) transducers and systems. IEC 62555. Geneva: International Electrotechnical Commission; 2014.
20. I.E.C. Ultrasonics – Surgical systems – Specification and measurement of field parameters for High Intensity Therapeutic Ultrasound (HITU) transducers and systems. IEC/TS 62556. Geneva: International Electrotechnical Commission; 2014.
21. I.E.C. Ultrasonics – Power measurement – Radiation force balances and performance requirements. IEC 61161. Geneva: International Electrotechnical Commission; 2013.

22. I.E.C. Ultrasonics – Hydrophones – Part 1: Measurement and characterization of medical ultrasonic fields up to 40 MHz. IEC 62127-1. Geneva: International Electrotechnical Commission; 2007.
23. ter Haar G, Shaw A, Pye S, Ward B, Bottomley F, Nolan R, et al. Guidance on reporting ultrasound exposure conditions for bio-effects studies. Ultrasound in Medicine and Biology. 2011;37(2):177–83.
24. Zanelli CI, Howard SM. A robust hydrophone for HIFU metrology. AIP Conference Proceedings. 2006;829(1):618–22.
25. Staudenraus J, Eisenmenger W. Fibre-optic probe hydrophone for ultrasonic and shock-wave measurements in water. Ultrasonics. 1993;31(4):267–73.
26. Morris P, Hurrell A, Shaw A, Zhang E, Beard P. A Fabry-Perot fiber-optic ultrasonic hydrophone for the simultaneous measurement of temperature and acoustic pressure. The Journal of the Acoustical Society of America. 2009;125(6):3611–22.
27. Haller J, Jenderka KV, Durando G, Shaw A. A comparative evaluation of three hydrophones and a numerical model in high intensity focused ultrasound fields. The Journal of the Acoustical Society of America. 2012;131(2):1121–30.
28. Canney MS, Khokhlova VA, Bessonova OV, Bailey MR, Crum LA. Shock-induced heating and millisecond boiling in gels and tissue due to high intensity focused ultrasound. Ultrasound in Medicine and Biology. 2010;36(2):250–67.
29. Wear KA, Gammell PM, Maruvada S, Liu Y, Harris GR. Improved measurement of acoustic output using complex deconvolution of hydrophone sensitivity. IEEE Transactions on Ultrasonics, Ferroelectrics, and Frequency Control. 2014;61(1):62–75.
30. Haller J, Wilkens V, Jenderka KV, Koch C. Characterization of a fiber-optic displacement sensor for measurements in high-intensity focused ultrasound fields. The Journal of the Acoustical Society of America. 2011;129(6):3676–81.
31. Liu YB, Wear KA, Harris GR. Variation of high-intensity therapeutic ultrasound (hitu) pressure field characterization: Effects of hydrophone choice, nonlinearity, spatial averaging and complex deconvolution. Ultrasound in Medicine and Biology. 2017;43(10):2329–42.
32. Wear KA, Liu YB, Harris GR. Pressure pulse distortion by needle and fiber-optic hydrophones due to nonuniform sensitivity. IEEE Transactions on Ultrasonics, Ferroelectrics, and Frequency Control. 2018;65(2):137–48.
33. Dong F, Madsen EL, MacDonald MC, Zagzebski JA. Nonlinearity parameter for tissue-mimicking materials. Ultrasound in Medicine & Biology. 1999;25(5):831–8.
34. Kreider W, Yuldashev PV, Sapozhnikov OA, Farr N, Partanen A, Bailey MR, et al. Characterization of a multi-element clinical HIFU system using acoustic holography and non-linear modeling. IEEE Transactions on Ultrasonics, Ferroelectrics, and Frequency Control. 2013;60(8):1683–98.
35. Harris GR, Howard SM, Hurrell AM, Lewin PA, Schafer ME, Wear KA, et al. Hydrophone measurements for biomedical ultrasound applications: A review. IEEE Transactions on Ultrasonics, Ferroelectrics, and Frequency Control. 2023;70(2):85–100.
36. Torr GR. The acoustic radiation force. American Journal of Physics. 1984;52(5):402–8.
37. Beissner K. Minimum radiation force target size for power measurements in focused ultrasonic fields with circular symmetry. The Journal of the Acoustical Society of America. 2010;128(6):3355–62.
38. Davidson F. Ultrasonic power balances. In: Preston RC, editor. Output measurements for medical ultrasound. London: Springer Verlag; 1991. p. 75–89.
39. Delchar TA, Melvin RJ. A calorimeter for ultrasound total power measurements. Measurement Science and Technology. 1994;5(12):1533.
40. Herman B, Stewart HF. An ultrasonic radiation calorimeter. The Journal of the Acoustical Society of America. 2005;53(1_Supplement):341.
41. Shaw A. A buoyancy method for the measurement of total ultrasound power generated by HIFU transducers. Ultrasound in Medicine and Biology. 2008;34(8):1327–42.
42. Civale J, Rivens I, ter Haar G. Quality assurance for clinical high intensity focused ultrasound fields. International Journal of Hyperthermia. 2015;31(2):193–202.
43. Hekkenberg RT, Beissner K, Zeqiri B, Bezemer RA, Hodnett M. Validated ultrasonic power measurements up to 20 w. Ultrasound in Medicine & Biology. 2001;27(3):427–38.
44. Burov AK. High-intensity ultrasonic vibrations for action on animal and human malignant tumours. Dokl Akad Nauk SSSR. 1956;106:239–41.

45. Shotton KC. A tethered float radiometer for measuring the output power from ultrasonic therapy equipment. Ultrasound in Medicine & Biology. 1980;6(2):131–3.
46. Hill CR, Rivens I, Vaughan MG, ter Haar GR. Lesion development in focused ultrasound surgery: A general model. Ultrasound in Medicine & Biology. 1994;20(3):259–69.
47. Shaw A, Hodnett M. Calibration and measurement issues for therapeutic ultrasound. Ultrasonics. 2008;48(4):234–52.
48. Sutton Y, Shaw A, Zeqiri B. Measurement of ultrasonic power using an acoustically absorbing well. Ultrasound in Medicine & Biology. 2003;29(10):1507–13.
49. Maruvada S, Harris GR, Herman BA, King RL. Acoustic power calibration of high-intensity focused ultrasound transducers using a radiation force technique. The Journal of the Acoustical Society of America. 2007;121(3):1434–9.
50. Rajagopal S, Shaw A. The buoyancy method – a potential new primary ultrasound power standard. Metrologia. 2012;49(3):327.
51. Civale J, Rivens I, Shaw A, ter Haar G. Focused ultrasound transducer spatial peak intensity estimation: A comparison of methods. Physics in Medicine & Biology. 2018;63(5):055015.
52. Civale J, Clarke R, Rivens I, ter Haar G. The use of a segmented transducer for rib sparing in HIFU treatments. Ultrasound in Medicine and Biology. 2006;32(11):1753–61.
53. Eames M, Larrabee Z, Hananel A, Padilla F, Aubry JF. Low-cost thermochromic quality assurance phantom for therapeutic ultrasound devices: A proof of concept. Ultrasound in Medicine and Biology. 2023;49(1):269–77.
54. Dabbagh A, Abdullah BJ, Abu Kasim NH, Ramasindarum C. Reusable heat-sensitive phantom for precise estimation of thermal profile in hyperthermia application. International Journal of Hyperthermia. 2014;30(1):66–74.
55. Ambrogio S, Baêsso RD, Gomis A, Rivens I, ter Haar G, Zeqiri B, et al. A polyvinyl alcohol-based thermochromic material for ultrasound therapy phantoms. Ultrasound in Medicine and Biology. 2020;46(11):3135–44.
56. Lafon C, Zderic V, Noble ML, Yuen JC, Kaczkowski PJ, Sapozhnikov OA, et al. Gel phantom for use in high-intensity focused ultrasound dosimetry. Ultrasound in Medicine and Biology. 2005;31(10):1383–9.
57. Divkovic GW, Liebler M, Braun K, Dreyer T, Huber PE, Jenne JW. Thermal properties and changes of acoustic parameters in an egg white phantom during heating and coagulation by high intensity focused ultrasound. Ultrasound in Medicine and Biology. 2007;33(6):981–6.
58. Takegami K, Kaneko Y, Watanabe T, Maruyama T, Matsumoto Y, Nagawa H. Polyacrylamide gel containing egg white as new model for irradiation experiments using focused ultrasound. Ultrasound in Medicine and Biology. 2004;30(10):1419–22.
59. Park SK, Guntur SR, Lee KI, Paeng DG, Choi MJ. Reusable ultrasonic tissue mimicking hydrogels containing nonionic surface-active agents for visualizing thermal lesions. IEEE Transactions on Biomedical Engineering. 2010;57(1):194–202.
60. Shaw A, Nunn J. The feasibility of an infrared system for real-time visualization and mapping of ultrasound fields. Physics in Medicine and Biology. 2010;55(11):N321–7.
61. Hand JW, Shaw A, Sadhoo N, Rajagopal S, Dickinson RJ, Gavrilov LR. A random phased array device for delivery of high intensity focused ultrasound. Physics in Medicine and Biology. 2009;54(19):5675–93.
62. Khokhlova VA, Shmeleva SM, Gavrilov LR, Martin E, Sadhoo N, Shaw A. Infrared mapping of ultrasound fields generated by medical transducers: Feasibility of determining absolute intensity levels. The Journal of the Acoustical Society of America. 2013;134(2):1586–97.
63. Miloro P, Civale J, Rivens I, Shaw A. The feasibility of thermal imaging as a future portal imaging device for therapeutic ultrasound. Ultrasound in Medicine and Biology. 2016;42(8):2033–8.
64. Martin K, Fernandez R. A thermal beam-shape phantom for ultrasound physiotherapy transducers. Ultrasound in Medicine & Biology. 1997;23(8):1267–74.
65. Butterworth I, Barrie J, Zeqiri B, Zauhar G, Parisot B. Exploiting thermochromic materials for the rapid quality assurance of physiotherapy ultrasound treatment heads. Ultrasound in Medicine and Biology. 2012;38(5):767–76.
66. Gutierrez MI, Leija L, Vera A, editors. Therapy ultrasound equipment characterization: Comparison of three techniques. 2008 30th Annual International Conference of the IEEE Engineering in Medicine and Biology Society; 2008 20–25 Aug. 2008.

67. Johns LD, Demchak TJ, Straub SJ, Howard SM. The role of quantitative Schlieren assessment of physiotherapy ultrasound fields in describing variations between tissue heating rates of different transducers. Ultrasound in Medicine and Biology. 2007;33(12):1911–7.
68. Kudo N, Ouchi H, Yamamoto K, Sekimizu H. A simple Schlieren system for visualizing a sound field of pulsed ultrasound. Journal of Physics: Conference Series. 2004;1:146–9.
69. Sapozhnikov OA, Tsysar SA, Khokhlova VA, Kreider W. Acoustic holography as a metrological tool for characterizing medical ultrasound sources and fields. The Journal of the Acoustical Society of America. 2015;138(3):1515–32.
70. Maynard JD, Williams EG, Lee Y. Nearfield acoustic holography: I. Theory of generalized holography and the development of NAH. The Journal of the Acoustical Society of America. 1985;78(4):1395–413.
71. Wang Y, Tyrer J, Zhihong P, Shiquan W. Measurement of focused ultrasonic fields using a scanning laser vibrometer. The Journal of the Acoustical Society of America. 2007;121(5):2621–7.
72. Song J, Hynynen K. Feasibility of using lateral mode coupling method for a large scale ultrasound phased array for noninvasive transcranial therapy. IEEE Transactions on Biomedical Engineering. 2010;57(1):124–33.
73. Shaw A, ter Haar GR. Telling it like it is. Journal of Therapeutic Ultrasound. 2013;1(1):4.
74. Padilla F, ter Haar G. Recommendations for reporting therapeutic ultrasound treatment parameters. Ultrasound in Medicine and Biology. 2022;48(7):1299–308.

6

Numerical Modelling for Simulation and Planning of Focused Ultrasound Treatments

David Sinden

6.1 Introduction

Treatment planning is an optimisation problem which can be approached in one of two ways: as a forward problem, or as an inverse problem:

- For a *forward problem*, given a set of specified initial conditions such as the position of the transducer, phase, amplitude and duty cycle, the fields are simulated. Based on the outcome from these simulations, the operator may decide to proceed with a treatment. This is applicable in cases for which there are no significant organs at risk during the treatment.
- In more complicated cases, treatment planning may take the form of an *inverse problem*. In this case, an intended outcome which delivers the dose at the planned treatment volume while sparing healthy surrounding tissue is defined, and an algorithm will seek to discover the initial set of conditions, such as phase, amplitude duty cycle and exposure duration, which produce a solution very close to the desired outcome. Inverse problems can be solved either directly or indirectly through an iterative process.

For both forward and inverse planning, as stated earlier, the principal challenge is the simulation of the desired field. In many applications, this requires the computation of acoustic, thermal and (intended) dose models. However, for some, such as those in which the propagation of the acoustic field is nonlinear, solving the inverse problem directly may be intractable. In this case, treatment planning may require an iterative method, involving the repeated computation of a large number of solutions until convergence close to the desired solution is reached. This places further computational demands on treatment planning.

Thus, the computational cost of performing simulations is important. However, as will be described in this chapter, the implementation of the most appropriate numerical method to model the acoustic, thermal or intended dose field is highly dependent on the application.

Motion compensation,[1] segmentation and registration algorithms,[2] propagation through bubbly media[3] and the numerical modelling of cavitation or drug delivery[4] are beyond the scope of this chapter, and the reader is referred to the more detailed texts referenced. Instead, this chapter will describe the various models which may be used to model the acoustic, thermal and dose fields, outlining the assumptions employed and how appropriate the assumptions are in differing clinical contexts.

In the absence of temperature-dependent changes in material properties,[5] or boiling bubbles (which lead to enhanced local absorption),[6,7] the acoustic field is independent of any thermal effects. Thus, once the acoustic field has been computed, the thermal field can be computed without a need to update the acoustic field. This reduces the computational demands significantly. However, even allowing for such assumptions, the acoustic field is more computationally demanding than the thermal field, which in turn is more computationally demanding than the 'dose' field, such as that described by the cumulative equivalent minutes formulation (see later).[8] The thermal simulations are less computationally demanding

DOI: 10.1201/9780429162671-6

than the acoustic simulations because the spatial resolution required to compute the thermal field accurately is far lower than that for the acoustic field. The dose field is often simply post-processed from the thermal field. That is, quantities which have been computed from differential equations are simply computed using a simple algorithm which does not require any spatial or temporal information. This chapter will therefore primarily focus on methods for solving acoustic equations which are appropriate for a number of different clinical applications. The governing equations for acoustic, thermal and dose formulations are presented and the limitations discussed, as well as consequent clinical implications. The range of numerical implementations for linear and nonlinear equations are then outlined and their limitations presented in the context of specific clinical implementations.

6.2 Current State of the Art and Challenges

The pipeline for treatment planning and delivery for external beam therapies can be summarised as follows:

1. Preclinical image acquisition: This may involve magnetic resonance imaging (MRI) or X-ray computed tomography (CT). Markers that allow the patient position to be registered in space with the images on which treatment planning is performed during treatment ensure that the target can be registered to the planning image in order to deliver the treatment to the intended location.
2. Target motion is acquired: This is on a different time scale from the planning images, so that the full detail of the motion can be captured. For example, if images are acquired in slices in the transverse plane on the same time scale as the respiratory cycle, it may be the case that the images simply track the displacements of an object.
3. Image segmentation[9]: Here the preoperative images are partitioned into segments so that organs and objects of interest (e.g. tumours) can be identified. At its most basic level, segmentation can be performed by thresholding data and then associating each region with a tissue type based on a table of values.
4. Identification of planned treatment volume, gross tumour margin and organs at risk, such as the spinal column, significant vascular, nerve or lymphatic structures, healthy tissue to be spared, etc.
5. Treatment planning: The outputs here are the positions and drive settings of the therapy head (source), such as the phase and amplitude for all elements, This ensures that the intended dose is delivered to the planned treatment volume, while sparing the organs at risk.
6. Registration of target to therapy head to ensure correct positioning for treatment delivery following the treatment plan.
7. Treatment delivery and monitoring: It is necessary that any intra-operative imaging system clearly delineates the target region, identifies any objects within the beam path which may adversely affect delivery (such as bowel gas) and associates the focal region with the target region.

There have been many clinical studies into a number of applications of image-guided therapeutic ultrasound. However, in all reported cases, treatment[11–13] planning consists of using an imaging system to locate the focus through a series of targeting shots used to ascertain its correct position (Figure 6.1).[14, 15] For ultrasound-guided systems the therapeutic transducer has a central aperture in which a diagnostic probe is placed confocally. The position of the focus can then be overlaid on top of the ultrasound images. For MR-guidance, T_2-weighted fast spin echo images are used to locate the focus. In one study Pulkkinen[16] states that the location of the focus was determined using low power sonications, and the sonications were then repeated with increasing power until the desired temperature was reached. This is currently the most commonly used targeting procedure. After locating an initial focal region and deciding on the treatment volume, planning software may determine a set of sonication locations to cover this region. This process is

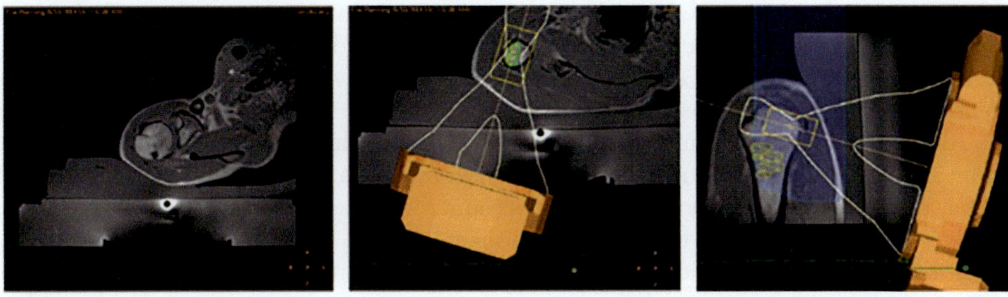

FIGURE 6.1 Targeting of periosteal nerves for pain palliation using MR-guided therapy.[10]

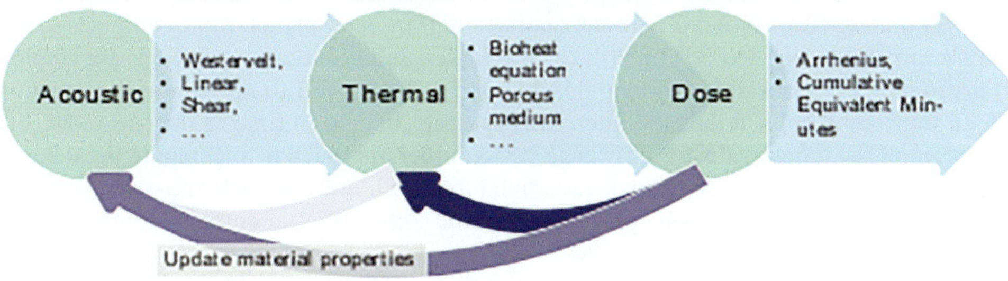

FIGURE 6.2 Schematic of simulation pipeline.

described by Scherrer et al.[17, 18], who formulated the optimisation problem as two sub-problems: the ideal location of the transducer and the location of the individual focal volumes.

The treatment of an entire volume requires an optimisation routine to ensure complete coverage. If it assumed that each dose volume delivered is spherical or ellipsoidal in shape, there are many algorithms that can ensure complete coverage.[19] Rather than assuming that the focal volume will always be ellipsoidal, Fedewa et al.[20] precomputed a number of typical focal volumes, described as a lesion library, at various powers, obtained from exposure through inhomogeneous tissue for use in treatment planning in prostate therapy.

A factor that influences the size of the lesion is the sequencing of the lesion placement. In order to ensure a uniform dose and avoid distortions in the focal volume due to changes in material properties in the beam path, treatment is usually performed from the furthermost plane to the nearest.[21]

The selection of a scanning path that treats the tumour volume as fast as possible, while minimising temperature rise in healthy tissue, would increase the efficiency of ultrasound surgery. Malinen et al.[22] developed a computationally efficient method, based on optimal control theory, which optimised sequencing using quadratic cost criteria to obtain the desired thermal dose in the target region. The authors showed that both treatment times and the total applied energy can be decreased from 16% to 43%, compared to standard sonication sequences.

As mentioned, although treatment planning for therapeutic ultrasound shares many similarities with that for other external beam therapies, the physical mechanisms that come into play in dose delivery, such as thermal and mechanical mechanisms, are different from those due to ionising radiation, and lead to different challenges. The following sections describe some of the challenges, how they affect treatment planning and the techniques which have been proposed to overcome them (Figure 6.2).

6.2.1 Motion Management

One characteristic feature of therapeutic ultrasound that differs from external beam radiotherapy is that the relative size of a single focal volume of the dose delivered under clinically relevant conditions is far smaller than the gross tumour volume. The precise size and shape of the focal region is determined by a number of factors, such as the transducer geometry and phasing configuration, depth of treatment, tissue properties, power and frequency. Typically, for a clinical transducer at low MegaHertz frequencies, ablated regions may be the size of a grain of rice.[23, 24] Thus, an advantage of therapeutic ultrasound is the potential to selectively target pathogenic tissue precisely. However, where the target volume undergoes large displacements, such as in transcostal applications[25] in which maximum displacements due to respiration are of the order of 10 mm,[26] the ratio between the size of the lesion and the amplitude of the motion may be small. Thus, failure to adequately account for motion in treatment delivery may lead to entire lesions being placed outside the planned treatment volume.

An additional challenge is to predict the motion of the target from preoperative images. For example, the motion of the liver can be predicted, due to periodic forcing from the diaphragm. However, the exact motion of the diaphragm, the coupling between the diaphragm and the liver, and the constraints due to the ribs and skin are difficult to establish precisely.

For simple cases, motion can be managed based on the assumption of incompressibility, in which organs simply undergo translation in coronal, sagittal and transverse planes. More complicated deformable models can also be applied.[27, 28] In such cases complex finite element simulations are employed to predict organ motion. Naturally, such methods do not capture the full complexity of the situation. For example in transcostal applications the intercostal spacing changes in time as the ribs move, or from sliding motion of the lungs against the rib cage.[29, 30] Another approach is to compute the deformation due to external (such as motion or acoustic radiation force) and internal (such as tissue compression or expansion due to heating) effects and apply this on to the computational domain and then interpolate the updated field onto the computational grid.[31]

An associated problem is that it may be time consuming to treat large volumes. Lorton et al. derived an approach to exploit the motion of the target to increase the volume of a lesion, to reduce treatment times.[32] Note that drift of organ position may lead to targeting errors.[33] Furthermore, for treatments at low intensities for long durations, the expression of heat shock proteins[34] may inhibit treatment.

6.2.2 Material Properties

Another significant source of uncertainty in planning which can lead to errors in treatment delivery lies in the values for the material properties (density, speed of sound, nonlinearity, attenuation parameters, thermal conductivity and specific heat parameter, etc.) that are needed for the governing equations.

Tissue types must be identified from pre-operative planning images, (typically either CT or MR). For CT images, in the simplest case, this may be performed by thresholding the images, then mapping from Hounsfield units to density, which are then semi-automatically assigned a tissue type with corresponding acoustic and thermal properties, from the literature, e.g. from Duck.[35] For MRI, depending on the sequencing, a similar procedure assigns acoustic and thermal properties based on a look-up table which matches T_1, T_2 relaxation times and spin density to tissue type. Aside from thresholding, there are a plethora of more advanced techniques which can be used to perform the segmentation, such as machine learning, partial differential equations, edge detection, Markov chains, etc.[9]

A significant challenge is that, in contrast to radiotherapy, ultrasound interacts significantly with the propagation medium. Through absorption and nonlinearity, the medium alters the beam, and the beam alters the medium. As mentioned earlier, for computational reasons, this is often neglected, and the material properties are assumed not to change during the exposure. However, the changes in acoustic properties with temperature can be used to monitor treatment delivery. A review article by Lewis et al.[36] discusses techniques for thermometry and dose monitoring and their respective advantages and disadvantages.

Thus, detailed knowledge of the thermal and acoustic properties of soft tissue are required, as well as how they change with temperature. Methods of determining the required patient specific parameters *pre-operatively* are, at present, lacking.

Neufeld,[37] Vaughan and Hynynen[38] and Soumi and Cleveland[39] have all investigated the effect of uncertainty of material properties on simulation. In the context of transcranial ultrasound, Vaughan and Hynynen investigated variations in speed of sound and CT data errors, such as in skull thickness, and found that the predicted pressure can vary by a few percent at the focus. Neufeld investigated variations in attenuation, speed of sound and density for linear propagation through water and found that variations in the speed of sound affected the magnitude and also shape of the focal volume. Recently, using patient data, Soumi and Cleveland[39] found that attenuation from the perinephric fat around the kidneys,[24] and focal splitting due to refraction lead to significant reduction in heat deposition rates. The authors showed that the effect of reflections from soft tissue interfaces was negligible.

While changes in material properties can lead to distortion of the beam through the thermal lensing effect,[5, 40] the most pronounced effects on the beam shape are produced when cavitation occurs in tissue. The presence of bubbles can locally enhance heating rates, potentially reducing sonication times. However, controlling their location is problematic – as large pre-focal echogenic bubbles can distort the focal beam shape.

In some applications, such as transcostal therapies, the effects of the presence of bone can be minimised through ray-tracing, or more advanced methods.[25] However, for transcranial applications, propagation through bone is unavoidable. In such cases, aberration corrections[41] are employed to ensure that the acoustic field has a coherent focus at the intended location.

The presence of bone presents two challenges: Firstly, hard tissues support shear waves, which are readily absorbed. Thus, within treatment planning models, equations which model elastic waves must be coupled to the acoustic wave equations. Secondly, thermometry, especially MR-thermometry, is a challenge in both fat and bone, so that the validation and verification of thermal fields remains a challenge.[42]

A potential challenge for treatment planning in applications in which there is a significant impedance mismatch, such as an air/water interface or soft tissue/bone interface, is the formation of standing waves due to multiple reflections. These are formed by the constructive interference of waves of similar amplitude propagating in opposite directions. Standing waves may lead to localised heating due to constructive interference, or distort the focus as the reflected sound waves affect the vibrations of the transducer. The formation of standing waves presents a challenge in transcranial applications in which they can form[16] (i) between the transducer and the skull (ii) within the calvaria and (iii) within the brain. Techniques such as frequency sweeping[43] or random phase modulation[44] have been employed to suppress their formation.

6.2.3 Vasculature

Thermal therapies may be compromised by the presence of large blood vessels, which advect heat away from the target site.[45] In a review of the safety and efficacy of ablative treatments on the hepatic and biliary systems, Mann et al.[46] stated that vessels larger than 3 mm in diameter acted as a heat sink. Hynynen et al.[47] stated that the presence of large vessels complicates treatment as occlusion of vessels will have an effect on healthy tissue. As mentioned earlier, the acoustic field is time independent. Thus, the effects of the acoustic field on flow, known as acoustic streaming, are neglected. Kamakura[48] investigated the effect of acoustic streaming in an axisymmetric case in which a vessel ran along the axis of propagation, using a finite-difference scheme, and found slight enhancements in mean flow due to the (linear) acoustic field, but a strong dependence on (hydrodynamic) nonlinearity and frequency. The authors stated that high-frequency components from nonlinear propagation would affect flow and heat deposition. Solovchuk[49] investigated clinically relevant vessel configurations, using a linear Westervelt[50] equation and bioheat[51] equations, for the acoustic and thermal fields respectively, coupled to a non-linear Navier-Stokes equation for the flow. This was solved using a finite-element method. These authors found that a large blood vessel can significantly change the temperature field and consequent thermal lesioning close to the vessel walls both by convective cooling and acoustic streaming. However, the effect was highly localised.

6.3 Acoustic Equations

Different applications may require differing governing equations, based on the assumptions that are possible. The central question is, therefore, for a given treatment, 'what is the appropriate governing equation and solution method'?

A common feature is that the initial propagation from the transducer is through water at a single frequency and that in the near field, propagation is linear. Near the focus, the intensities may be sufficiently great that the effects of nonlinear wave propagation cannot be neglected.

The governing equations for the simulation of ultrasound wave propagation can be derived using the Navier-Stokes equations and an appropriate constitutive equation – i.e. an equation which relates a pair of the variables, such as the dependence of the density on the speed of sound.[50, 52] This would be computationally extremely expensive, but would not introduce any approximations into the simulations, and would yield conservation laws which can aid verification of numerical implementations.

The Westervelt and Khokhlov-Zabolskaya-Kuznetsov (KZK) equations can be derived from the Navier-Stokes equations as follows. The first approximation used assumes potential flow, $\vec{v} = \nabla\phi$, where ϕ is the potential function and $\vec{v}$ is the fluid velocity vector. This assumes that vortices and shear waves are negligible. The second step is to consider small perturbations of the variables, and assume that the acoustic Mach number, ε, is small, so that higher-order terms can be neglected. The acoustic Mach number is defined as the ratio of the characteristic particle velocity, $v = |\vec{v}|$, to the speed of sound in the fluid, c, i.e. $\varepsilon = v / c$. This step yields so-called *weakly nonlinear equations*.[53] If the medium is homogeneous, the Kuznetsov equation is derived.[54] Then, discarding thermal effects yields the second-order wave equation.[55] Assuming there are no local effects, then the Westervelt equation results.[56]

If the acoustic field primarily propagates in a single direction, it is reasonable to make a parabolic approximation. This assumption is valid when there are no scatterers in the path of the beam. The parabolic assumption asserts that in the appropriately retarded reference frame $\tau = t - z / c$, the wave profile varies slowly in all directions and extremely slowly in the direction of motion. This is enforced by v being of similar magnitude to the (acoustic) Mach number ε, and writing ϕ as

$$\phi = \phi\left(\tau = t - \frac{z}{c},\, x = x\sqrt{v},\, y = y\sqrt{v},\, z = vz\right) \text{where } v \ll 1,$$

neglecting terms of the order of v^2 and higher. In the above formulations, the transformation assumes that propagation is in the z direction. Note that the change of coordinates is exact, this approximation is the result of discarding $\mathcal{O}(v^2)$ and higher terms.

Due to its relative simplicity, and relatively modest computational cost, the KZK equation, and increasingly the Westervelt equation, are the most commonly used models for simulation of therapeutic ultrasound fields. This is because they represent the simplest acoustic models which capture the three key phenomena of diffraction, nonlinearity and attenuation.

- Diffraction is the spreading of the wave as it propagates through a medium.
- Nonlinearity is the change in the wave form as it propagates through a medium. This is because the speed of sound varies with the magnitude of the pressure. That is, in compression (the positive going portion) the wave speed is greater than in refraction (the negative going portion). This can lead to wave-steepening and shock-like waves.
- Total attenuation is the loss of acoustic energy as the wave propagates through tissue due to absorption and scatter. Attenuation in tissue is known to be dominated by absorption. In the low MegaHertz frequency range, the scatter component of attenuation in soft tissue accounts for about 10% to 15% of the total attenuation.[35] The main mechanisms for absorption, which are dependent on the material, are:
  - Thermo-viscous heating: This is the primary mechanism for absorption in water. It is due to a combination of internal friction in a fluid and heat conduction. The absorption in this case has a quadratic dependence on frequency.
  - Relaxation processes are the dominant mechanism for absorption of ultrasound in tissue.[35] Relaxation refers to the time required for a medium to establish equilibrium in a new thermodynamic state produced by a change in one or more of the internal degrees of freedom, i.e. rotational, vibrational or chemical modes. During each compression cycle, there will be a net transfer of energy from the sound wave to the internal degrees of freedom, thus attenuating the amplitude of the wave.

While both types of absorption are frequency dependent, there is a significant difference: viscous heating follows a quadratic dependency on frequency, whereas the absorption of ultrasound through relaxation processes follows a power-law dependency. The latter is computationally far costlier to model accurately, and influences not only the solution method employed, but also the governing equation.[57]

Accurate computation of the absorption is important in therapeutic applications as the preferential absorption of higher harmonic components means that nonlinearity leads to more concentrated energy deposition in a smaller region, and thus higher focal temperatures. Other consequences are a narrower focus and smaller sidelobes, as well as a restricted ability to steer a phased array electronically.

The therapeutic application under consideration determines the choice of governing equation and the numerical solution employed to solve it. However, the numerical solution essentially determines how the power-law absorption is implemented.

A finite sum of relaxation processes can easily be acquired in finite-difference time-domain simulations[57, 58] whereas for pseudo-spectral methods (either forward-marching in space, or *k*-space methods which step-forward in time) this can be handled by assuming a continuous distribution so that the absorption follows a power-law dependence on frequency.[59] This power-law dependence can yield an operator which may be either a fractional Laplacian in the spatial variables[60] or a fractional operator in the time domain. If a continuous distribution of relaxation processes is assumed in time-domain simulations, an integral or convolution operator[61] can be used to handle the power-law absorption.

A key difference between the KZK and the Westervelt equations is that the KZK equation is rotationally symmetric – the Westervelt equation computes the field in three dimensions, while the KZK equations computes the field in two spatial dimensions. An advantage is that rapid calculations can be made for exposures in homogeneous layered materials from symmetric transducers. However, the simplicity of the KZK approach comes at a cost as the assumption of rotational symmetry severely limits its clinical applicability. For example, it cannot adequately model steered beams from phased arrays.

The paraxial approximation limits the applicability of the model: in theory the KZK equation is valid only for a wave travelling at 16 degrees off the axis of propagation from a focused transducer, i.e. for *f*-numbers above 1.5. Thus, it is less accurate in the near-field and off-axis. However, while in practice the KZK equation has been found[62] to be in good agreement for *f*-numbers as low as 1.0, Soneson[63] performed a sensitivity analysis and found that up to 22 degrees the error is only ~ 5%.

If the medium through which the sound is propagating is weakly inhomogeneous, then reflections are a minor effect[39] and the KZK equation is sufficient. In many applications, especially in the upper abdomen, intervening bone can cause strong reflection and lead to tissue damage far from the focus. For patient safety, the strength of the reflected beam must be estimated. This does not exclude the use of the KZK method – a second field can be introduced to describe the reflected beam – but the formulation becomes more computationally demanding.[64]

While the use of either the Westervelt or KZK equations is widespread, the implementation of the numerical method which is used to predict the acoustic, thermal or intended dose field is thus highly dependent on the application.

For example, for low intensity exposures, nonlinearity can be ignored, whereas for high-intensity exposures, nonlinearity must be included in treatment planning routines. As mentioned previously, the higher harmonic components will be preferentially absorbed. The inclusion of nonlinearity presents a significant computational challenge, as described later.

Exposure duration is also important. For long exposures, a continuous wave can be assumed, whereas when they are short, this is not the case. The assumption of continuous wave exposures allows a range of numerical techniques which can accelerate the computation and provide simplifications in the computation of the absorption.

Two aspects which are, at present, seldom coupled to acoustic computational models are nucleation of inertial cavitation and phase changes, such as boiling or emulsification. The presence of large vaporous echogenic bubbles, which are associated with boiling, has been used for monitoring using B-mode imaging.[36] However, for high void fractions, i.e. over 5%,[65] the effect of the presence of a cloud of bubbles on wave propagation, local absorption and heating is numerically challenging.[66] This is because bubble oscillations and interactions occur on shorter time scales than the frequency of the wave propagation, thus increasing computational requirements. Furthermore, the inclusion of bubble oscillations naturally leads to time-domain computations and the bidirectional coupling of the thermal and acoustic fields.

6.3.1 Shear Waves

In solid tissue such as bone, wave propagation is no longer purely longitudinal, but may support shear waves.[67] Shear waves can be generated at an oblique interface between solid and fluids. They are rapidly absorbed and so do not propagate far in soft tissue. They thus provide a highly localised heat source. Shear wave heating can be used for palliative treatments of bone metastases by damaging periosteal nerves. A pair of elastic moduli, such as Lamé parameters or bulk modulus and shear modulus can be used to characterise the propagation in solid materials.

Poroelastic models, with slow and fast waves may provide more detailed and accurate models of wave propagation through bone than solid materials. McGarry et al.[68] describe the differences between the two models in the context of MR-elastography. A challenge is that the poroelastic properties of bone are dependent on bone density which may be patient specific. Poroelastic modelling requires additional parameters[69] – porosity, hydraulic conductivity and apparent density.

6.3.2 Full-Wave Evolution

Full-wave evolution refers to the ability to compute propagation in all directions. Not all simulations are full-wave either because of the formulation of the governing equations or because of the numerical implementations used to solve them.

Computations can be significantly accelerated by representing some portion of the waves by an orthogonal basis, such as a Fourier series or Chebyshev polynomials. Such methods are referred to as pseudo-spectral. There are two main types of pseudo-spectral methods:

- Pseudo-spectral time-domain methods, also known as k space methods. These methods formulate the governing equation in terms of a time-derivative and represent all of the spatial components of the wave via a Fourier series. For example, the pressure would be written as $p(x,y,z,t)=\hat{p}\,\left(k_x,k_y,k_z,t\right)$, where $\hat{p}=\mathcal{F}(p)$ is the spatial Fourier transform of the pressure and the governing equation would take the form $\frac{\partial \hat{p}}{\partial t}=f\left(\hat{p},k\right)$. The time derivative can then be approximated using finite-differences so that the next time-step can be computed from the previous time steps.
- Pseudo-spectral spatial marching schemes: Those which compute the entire time history in a plane orthogonal to the direction of propagation and march forwards in space.

Hence spatial marching schemes rely on defining the field (pressure and/or velocity) for all times in a particular plane in space. This initial planar field is stepped forward in space to find the solution in a series of planes. The initial source plane is usually determined by holography.[70] A full-wave approach has the field defined everywhere in space at the initial time, and the field then evolves forward in time, with appropriate time-varying boundary conditions at the transducer surface

Propagating in time may be more intuitive and can handle reflections and scatter without too much overhead, whereas propagating in space provides the advantage of being able to handle dispersion and propagation across interfaces efficiently.[71, 72] The primary advantage of spatial marching schemes is that they are efficient for continuous wave exposures as they compute the entire time history of the wave. However, marching forward in space is only applicable in cases for which reflections are not important, and when exposure durations are sufficiently long to assume continuous wave exposure. Continuous wave conditions can be assumed once transient phenomena, such as variations in power due to ramping up have died down, and phenomena associated with continuous wave exposures, such as the formation of standing waves, have stabilised. In the case of continuous wave exposures, forward-marching schemes assume that the material properties do not change in time. For strongly heterogeneous media, Gu and Jing[72] derive phase and amplitude corrections, which are exact in the one-dimensional case, as well as computed multiple reflections.

The primary advantage of pseudo-spectral time-domain methods is that they can stably and accurately compute spatial derivatives with a small number of points per wavelength. However, the presence of discontinuities, such as those between soft tissue and bone requires additional computational techniques, such as Fourier continuation[73] or Gegenbauer reconstruction,[74] to handle discontinuities. Yet for soft tissues, in which local medium properties show small variations, the method is sufficient to compute acoustic fields accurately and efficiently. A computational cost is that the visualisation of the evolution of the acoustic field requires storing the entire state of the acoustic field at each time point.

Pseudo spectral methods require periodic boundary conditions which are inappropriate for therapeutic ultrasound. However, this can be overcome by incorporating Berenger's perfectly matched layer formulation. In contrast to many boundary conditions which impose conditions on points on the boundary, the perfectly matched layer formulation imposes a condition on an artificial domain. The material properties within the domain are chosen so that they fully damp waves which enter into the domain without causing reflections back into the computational domain.[75, 76] The specific implementation of the perfectly matched approach is dependent on the coordinate frame used. Although more computationally expensive than absorbing or reflecting boundary conditions,[77] the perfectly matched layer is perhaps the mostly widely used boundary condition as it allows the implementation of pseudo-spectral methods, and provides physically realistic results without numerical artefacts.

6.4 Thermal Equations

The thermal field, T, is computed using the Pennes bioheat transfer equation

$$c_v \rho_0 \frac{\partial T}{\partial t} = \nabla \cdot \left(k \nabla T \right) + q_a + q_s + q_c + q_m + \omega_p \left(T - T_\infty \right),$$

where c_v is the specific heat capacity, ρ_0 is the ambient density, k is the thermal conductivity, source terms q are heat sources due to absorption, shock-enhanced heating, cavitation and metabolic heating respectively, ω_p is the bulk perfusion parameter and T_∞ is the ambient temperature. The effect of perfusion appears as an isotropic, homogeneous cooling term which reaches instantaneous thermal equilibrium.

One deficiency of this model noted by Pennes is that its assumptions are only true for heat transfer between blood and tissue in the capillaries. This was found to be inaccurate by Chen and Holmes[78] who showed that, in a simplified model, equilibration between blood and tissue occurs primarily in vessels of 0.2 to 0.5 mm diameter, and not in the capillaries (which have diameters in the micron range). Nonetheless, the Pennes model is straightforward to implement, and produces reasonably good agreement with experimental data in regions without large blood vessels. The primary advantage of the Pennes bioheat equation is that the inclusion of a bulk perfusion term simplifies the model significantly, allowing for comparatively rapid simulations to be performed.

All these models are single field. An alternative approach is to consider the evolution of three temperature fields – tissue, venous and arterial. This approach was explored by Keller and Seiler[79], and several modifications have since been proposed. These are expected to be more accurate, but rely on deriving effective medium properties of the blood flow for thermally significant vessels which may not be visible. However, asymptotic homogenisation techniques can rigorously model vascular structures on a scale which is smaller than the resolution provided by medical imaging.[80]

Discrete modelling is possible for thermally significant blood vessels which can be imaged.[81] This is important since vessels greater than 1 mm in diameter can significantly affect the thermal dose delivered during ablative therapies, due to advected heat transfer. This can lead to unwanted tissue sparing (increasing the risk of disease recurrence), asymmetric doses and the over-treatment of healthy tissue. Furthermore, regions with large, thermally significant vessels require a greater ultrasound exposure, involving either higher intensity or longer treatment times. A reduced model, which includes the effects of discrete vasculature without computing the effects of advected blood flow, is simply to assume through a combination of low thermal conductivity and high flow rates, that blood does not heat up and so model vessels as having a fixed temperature. Thus, in this case, like the Pennes' model, the vessels act as heat sinks, but the effect is not isotropic.[82]

6.4.1 Dose Formulations

The primary measure of dose in therapeutic ultrasound is the cumulative equivalent minutes formulation. It is based on a first-order irreversible Arrhenius-type rate equation[83] for protein denaturation. It is assumed that a small element is comprised of tissue which is either alive or dead, and the rate at which tissue is denatured is proportional to the temperature. This yields an integral for a dimensionless, time-dependent irreversible damage function, $\Omega(t)$,

$$\Omega(t) = \int_0^t A e^{\frac{E_a}{RT(\tau)}} d\tau,$$

where R is the universal gas constant, E_α is the activation energy and A is a constant of proportionality which corresponds to the collision frequency. In this case damage refers to denaturation of proteins within cells.[84]

There are extensions to the standard Arrhenius model, for example, by O'Neil et al.[85] or Xu and Qian[86], which include multiple states in which tissue may be alive (reversibly) damaged or (irreversibly) denatured. These more advanced approaches are often used in thermal-deformation models which relate damage to tissue expansion and contraction to tissue denaturation.[87]

A related concept is the cumulative equivalent minutes formulation,[8] which is based on empirical evidence which suggests that there is a relationship between sets of exposure durations and temperatures of the form

$$t_1 = t_2 R_0^{(T_1 - T_2)}.$$

This relationship states that for a given exposure temperature, T_2, and duration, t_2, the equivalent exposure time, t_1, at the new exposure temperature, T_1, is given by the exponential relationship stated earlier. The exponent, empirically derived from the biphasic Arrhenius plot, is given by

$$R_0 = \begin{cases} 0 \text{ for } T < 39^\circ \\ 0.25 \text{ for } 39^\circ \leq T < 43^\circ \\ 0.5 \text{ for } T \geq 43^\circ \end{cases}$$

For time-varying temperatures, the equivalent time is obtained by summing contributions from different temperature-time combinations:

$$\mathrm{CEM}_{T_{\mathrm{ref}}} = \int_0^{t_\infty} R_0^{T_{\mathrm{ref}} - T(t)} dt.$$

The most widely used reference level for thermal ablation is a CEM_{43} of 240, which corresponds to raising the temperature to 43°C for 240 minutes. The relationship between the Arrhenius and CEM formulations is explored by Pierce.[88]

Thus, from the computed thermal field, the dose field computation of the CEM_{43} integral for a small unit of tissue is either above the threshold or below. For thermal therapies, if the dose value is above a threshold, the value of the dose field in this small unit of tissue does not need to be computed at the next time step, whereas if it below the dose, must be updated at the next time step.

For small induced temperature rises, an equivalent minutes formulation which corresponds to the delivery of dose for hyperthermia, rather than ablation, is to heat tissue at 43°C for 90 minutes.[89]

For exposures associated with extreme intensities[62] (i.e. above 20,000W/cm^2), and short exposure times, the time to achieve a CEM_{43} of 240 may be of order of microseconds. The mechanism for cellular damage in such short exposure times is likely to be mechanical damage from boiling.[90, 23] Such short exposure times may negate the effects of two significant sources of uncertainty in treatment delivery of perfusion and tissue motion which occur over longer time scales. However, these high intensities may lead to difficulties in predicting lesion formation due to the random nature of cavitation which distorts the shape of the focus.

6.4.2 Linear Models for Ultrasound Wave Propagation in Tissue

6.4.2.1 Ray Tracing

Perhaps the simplest approach to simulation is to neglect diffraction and nonlinearity and consider ray tracing, i.e. the use of geometrical acoustics. Ray tracing is accurate in the high-frequency limit, which is when the width of the sound beam is much larger than the wavelength. Ray-tracing algorithms are fast, easy to parallelise and can handle inhomogeneous and discontinuous media. Such methods provide a useful measure of transmission losses due to reflection, as well as the influence of shift of the focus due to refraction caused by differences in sound speed between differing media, such as a water/skin interface.[91] However, the precise field in the focal region is difficult to determine. As such they may provide a useful first approximation to iterative nonlinear solvers. Furthermore, ray tracing is a useful approach when considering focusing of phased arrays beyond targets such as the ribs, where the sound from some elements of a phased array is directly incident on the ribs (Figure 6.3). Alaniz et al.[92] used ray tracing to calculate thermal lensing in high-intensity frequency ultrasound (HIFU), i.e. the defocusing of the focal region due to heating (see Figure 6.3).

6.4.2.2 Rayleigh-Sommerfeld Method

The Rayleigh-Sommerfeld method is a time-domain method which, although derived under a number of restrictive assumptions regarding the domain, allows the modelling of a number of transducer geometries. The model is formed under two assumptions: Firstly, that the acoustic field is generated by piezoelectric elements which are planar and within an infinite baffle, and secondly that the waves propagate linearly through an infinite, homogeneous domain. Using these assumptions, a Green's function formulation is employed.

Quadrature methods are typically employed to characterise the source, so that, each element of the phased array is discretised into a finite number of small point sources. The acoustic field at a given point is then computed as being the sum of the contributions from each point source.

To overcome some of the limitations of the Rayleigh-Sommerfeld method a number of modifications have been implemented. For example, it is not possible to compute the acoustic field at the source points since the Green's function is singular, and consequently the computation of the near field is problematic – especially at higher frequencies. To overcome this limitation, fast nearfield methods have been developed for simple transducer geometries. This method replaces the double integral in the Rayleigh-Sommerfeld method with a rapidly converging single integral.[93]

Although the applicability of the model is limited by the restrictions imposed by the use of the Green's function, the Rayleigh-Sommerfeld method is simple to implement, parallelisable and can handle complex transducer geometries and temporal variations in field strength.

The Rayleigh-Sommerfeld method is therefore widely used and can give reasonable agreement with measurements at low pressures.

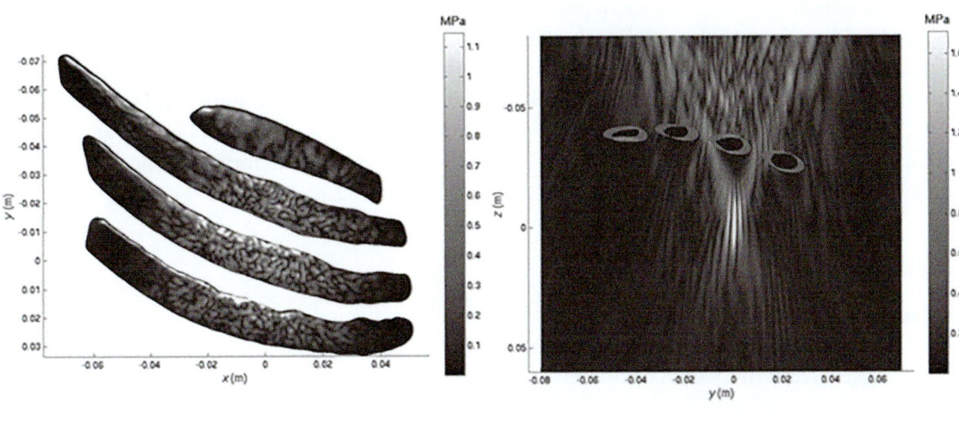

FIGURE 6.3 Acoustic pressure magnitude incident on ribs and at focus using boundary element formulation and constrained optimisation.[25]

6.4.2.3 Angular-Spectrum Methods

The angular-spectrum method is a frequency-domain method which, from a source plane, usually perpendicular to the direction of propagation containing the phase and amplitude of the field, propagates the plane forward (or backwards) in space in the direction of propagation.[94] The source information can be acquired experimentally or computed numerically, i.e. using the Rayleigh-Sommerfeld method. This method naturally handles dispersion and attenuation and is commonly employed to model the diffraction operator in nonlinear simulations which use operator splitting.[95] The method is relatively straight-forward to implement and is computationally efficient, so that large domains can be modelled. However, it implicitly assumes a direction of propagation which may not be relevant for hemi-spherical devices used in transcranial applications. It has been extended to inhomogeneous media[96] for materials which are weakly inhomogeneous, i.e. through computational domains which do not contain any significant discontinuities in acoustic impedance.

6.4.2.4 Finite-Difference Time-Domain Methods

Finite-difference time-domain methods are relatively straight forward to implement and have even been used to simulate large scale models using graphic processing units (GPUs).[97] In order to approximate spatial derivatives, simple first-order accurate differencing schemes typically only require a few terms to be stored in memory. However, finite-difference methods require high spatial resolution, typically 10 points per wave length.[98] This becomes computationally expensive when nonlinear wave propagation needs to be included. Due to the preferential absorption of high-frequency components of a nonlinear wave, it is likely that a linear simulation, or not computing all harmonic components, may underestimate the thermal field. Soneson and Myers[99] calculated thresholds at which nonlinearity became significant using the KZK equation, and so provided guidance as to when nonlinear simulations must be performed in order for accurate computation of the thermal field.

6.4.2.5 Boundary Integral Equations

Boundary element methods exploit the fact that the linear wave equation has a Green's function which, in some cases, can be used to derive a solution over a given surface rather than a volume. That is, from a given incident field, the total acoustic field from the incident and scattered fields can easily be post-processed from the field which has been computed on the surface of the scatterer. This is naturally performed in the frequency domain, so that the governing equation is actually the Helmholtz rather than the linear wave equation. This has been performed, and incorporated into a constrained optimisation scheme to perform treatment planning in the case of transcostal surgery for a phased array.[25] In this case the phase and magnitude of each element of a phased array was determined so that the spatial-peak intensity was maximised at the intended focus, while the energy deposited on the ribs was minimised using a nonlinear least-squares method (Figure 6.3). The formulation assumes homogeneous media, but it is possible to couple boundary element and finite element models, to account for tissue inhomogeneity and thermal fields. However, by solving the Helmholtz equation, it is assumed that there is continuous wave exposure, so that pulsed or short tone-bursts cannot be modelled.

Although the boundary element method solves a linear system of equations, Groth et al.[100] coupled a system of harmonic equations within a series of nested domains to solve for a nonlinear acoustic field. A cascade of Helmholtz equations can be solved successively at each harmonic of the fundamental frequency with source terms which are products of lower harmonics.

6.4.2.6 Machine Learning Methods

Another approach is to develop a neural network which is trained to approximate the solution of the acoustic field given by a propagation equation.[101] Within the context of therapeutic ultrasound, such physics-informed neural networks have been used to model the linear, continuous-wave two-dimensional acoustic fields which propagate through a skull model,[102] but are not necessarily limited to linear propagation. An advantage of such an approach is that the model can be trained to approximate the acoustic field based on a large set of training data, and then applied to patient data to rapidly predict the acoustic field without computing the full acoustic field.

6.4.3 Nonlinear Models for Ultrasound Wave Propagation in Soft Tissue

When the peak pressure in the wave is high, energy will be transferred from the fundamental to higher harmonics. As has been described previously, the absorption of ultrasound is frequency-dependent, so that the higher frequency components will be preferentially absorbed by the medium, leading to higher temperatures. As with linear simulations, the contribution to the thermal field from absorption uses the plane wave assumption, but is given by the sum of the N-harmonics computed

$$q_a = 2\sum_i^N \frac{\alpha_i p_i^2}{c_0 \rho_0},$$

where p_i are the harmonic components of the pressure field of the nonlinear wave and a is the frequency-dependent absorption. A difficulty for the computation of nonlinear wave propagation in three-dimensional simulations is the determination of the number of harmonics to compute *a priori,* to provide efficient memory allocation (or, equivalently, the spatial resolution required). One approach is, if possible, to average the initial source condition around the axial direction, so that it is rotationally symmetric and to use the KZK equation, which is far more computationally tractable, to provide an estimate for the number of harmonics required in three-dimensional simulations. However, this approach assumes layered media, so may not be applicable in highly complex media.

Neglecting dissipative terms, and considering an integral form of the energy conservation equation around the shock front yields[52]

$$q_s = \frac{\beta}{6\rho_0^2 c_0^2}(\Delta P)^3,$$

where β is the nonlinearity parameter and ΔP is the shock-height of the pressure wave. Note that the contribution to heating from shock enhancement is *independent* of the attenuation of the medium. For a discussion of this see Pearce.[52]

Shock-enhanced heating can play a significant role in thermal therapies, such as boiling histotripsy,[62] as it is proportional to the cube of the pressure, rather than the square.[62, 103] Note that as tissue is a heavily attenuating medium, the shocks have a finite rise-time, rather than an infinite rise-time and discontinuity in pressure. This scenario is less computationally demanding, as the shock can be defined over a few grid points, relaxing restrictions on the spatial resolution.

A key difference between shock-enhanced heating and heating due to nonlinearity is that the shock-enhanced heating is a highly localised effect, whereas, although it may only be significant in the vicinity of the focus, the absorption of nonlinear ultrasound is, strictly speaking, a global effect. That is why we must determine whether a shock-like wave has formed, or not, in order to compute any thermal contributions from shock-enhanced heating. The defining feature is that above a threshold initial pressure, the rise time is independent of the driving voltage.

There are two approaches to computing shock-like waves in therapeutic ultrasound: the first is to employ operator-splitting[104] and handle the nonlinearity operator using a high-resolution shock capturing scheme[71, 105]; the second is to compute both the density, ρ, and velocity vector, $\overline{v}$ fields, and formulate the governing equations as a hyperbolic equation by retaining the second-order Lagrangian density[106]

$$\frac{\partial \rho}{\partial t} + \nabla \cdot (\rho \vec{v}) = 0,$$

$$\frac{\partial (\rho \vec{v})}{\partial t} + \nabla \cdot \left(\rho_0 \vec{v} \times \vec{v} + \underline{I} \left(c_0^2 \rho + \frac{c_0^2}{\rho_0} (\beta - 1)(\rho - \rho_0)^2 \right) \right) = \rho_0 \nabla^2 \vec{v},$$

where $\underline{I}$ is the identity matrix. An advantage of the first approach is that the number of variables required does not change from standard models, nor are any additional material properties required. Another advantage is that by retaining the structure of the Westervelt equation, computationally efficient forward propagation methods can be used for attenuation and diffraction. However, a disadvantage is that the use of operator-splitting techniques may reduce the overall spatial accuracy of the scheme unless techniques such as Strang-splitting[104, 107] are employed, but these may increase the computational cost.

Shock-capturing methods usually exploit the hyperbolic structure of the governing equation. The benefit of this is that many modern high-resolution shock-capturing schemes exploit the conservation laws inherent in the hyperbolic formulation. Such approaches use upwind-type differencing schemes, which perform differencing based on local wave speeds, to discretise the equations with the high spatial resolution required for steep gradients associated with shock-like waves. Another advantage is that the computation of the absorption term no longer relies on the quasi-plane wave assumption which may break down at interfaces in which there is a significant change in impedance. Also, through the inclusion of the second-order Lagrangian density term, the governing equation can be considered in a sense more general than the Westervelt equation, with the ability to model the interaction between waves of differing frequency. However, although there are some uses of parametric arrays in therapeutic ultrasound,[108] they are not widespread.

One caveat is that many of therapeutic applications which exploit shock-enhanced heating do so in order to harness the mechanical damage caused by clouds of inertially collapsing bubbles. At present, there are no established measures of dose to describe fractionation cause by bubble clouds. Care is needed in modelling the interaction between the bubble cloud and the acoustic field, as the shockwave scatterer and reflection can lead to prefocal constructive interference, which can initiate nucleation.[66]

6.5 Summary

This chapter discusses the range of factors which influence the selection of numerical scheme for acoustic wave simulations. Table 6.1 summarises the factors which influence the selection of a numerical scheme for acoustic simulation.

There are three key factors to consider for modelling:

- The degree of spatial and temporal inhomogeneity in the medium and the source. This determines whether approximations, such as the paraxial approximation, can be made to reduce the computational complexity of the simulations.
- The intensity of the source. This determines whether nonlinear propagation needs to be modelled, or whether linear models suffice.
- The duration of the exposure time, which determines whether continuous wave exposures, modelled in the frequency domain, or finite duration exposures, modelled in the time domain, are used.

A confounding factor is that these features cannot be considered in isolation. Consider, for example, the case in which short pulsed, high intensities are applied through soft tissue. The first feature means that simulations must be performed in the time domain, the second means that nonlinearity must be considered. Thus, these two features combined require that power law frequency dependent attenuation must be handled in the time domain. As mentioned, this can be applied through a fractional Laplacian operator[60] or by using a distribution of relaxation processes.[57]

TABLE 6.1

Summary of the Factors Which Influence Choice of Numerical Schemes

	Duration	Motion Management	Intensity	Domain
Histotripsy	Short: time-domain simulation	Exposure durations may be sufficiently short to assume during exposure target is essentially stationary.	High: nonlinear, shock-capturing methods required.	Acoustic wave
Thermal Ablation	Long: continuous-wave simulations	This is target specific, but a judgement on whether motion management is employed must be made.	Moderate: computation of higher harmonics required	Acoustic wave
Transcranial	Moderate: however geometry and techniques to suppress standing waves may restrict assumption of frequency-domain methods which assume continuous wave exposures	No, target may not move a significant amount.	Moderate: however, significant proportion of energy is lost through transmission through the skull. Also transducer design distributes energy over a large area.	Acoustic-elastic wave
Bone Metastases	Long: continuous-wave simulations	Many targets may be considered stationary, however, transcostal applications would require a motion management strategy.	Moderate: computation of higher harmonics required	Acoustic-elastic wave
Hyperthermia	Long: continuous wave simulations	Yes, likely targets will move either due to respiration or drift	Low, linear acoustic simulations may be sufficient	Acoustic wave

Another case is that in which the target may move over the duration of a long hyperthermia treatment. The second factor suggests linear continuous wave methods can be employed, however, the first factor means that solutions should potentially be computed in the time domain. Thus, some analysis must be performed to assess the times at which the continuous wave acoustic field should be recomputed to model the change in the position of the target and how this changes the propagation path and consequently the acoustic field. This is both patient and exposure specific.

Table 6.1 outlines which clinical procedures have which features and the potential numerical approaches.

The advantage of frequency-domain simulation methods is that power law absorption can easily be modelled, although pseudo-spectral time stepping schemes can handle power law absorption. Note that if intensity levels are low, nonlinear propagation may be neglected, so frequency dependence of absorption can also be neglected. However, a limitation of many pseudo-spectral schemes (specifically those which use Fourier basis functions) is that a combination of irregular interfaces and discontinuities in density, such as between soft and hard tissues, poses a numerical challenge.

REFERENCES

1. A. E. Lujan, E. W. Larsen, J. M. Balter and R. K. Ten Haken, "A method for incorporating organ motion due to breathing into 3D dose calculations," Med. Phys., vol. 26, no. 5, pp. 715–720, 1999.
2. P. Wust, J. Gellermann, J. Beier, S. Wegner, W. Tilly, J. Tröger, D. Stalling, H. Oswald, H. C. Hege, P. Deuflhard and R. Felix, "Evaluation of segmentation algorithms for generation of patient models in radiofrequency hyperthermia," Phys. Med. Biol., vol. 43, pp. 3295–3307, 1998.
3. L. van Wijngaarden, "One-dimensional flow of liquids containing small gas bubbles," Annu. Rev. Fluid Mech., vol. 4, no. 1, pp. 369–396, 1972.

4. W. Wiedemair, Z. Tukovic, H. Jasak, D. Poulikakos and V. Kurtcuoglu, "On ultrasound-induced microbubble oscillation in a capillary blood vessel and its implications for the blood-brain barrier," Phys. Med. Biol., vol. 57, no. 4, p. 1019, 2012.
5. I. M. Hallaj, R. O. Cleveland and K. Hynynen, "Simulations of the thermo-acoustic lens effect during focused ultrasound surgery," J. Acoust. Soc. Am., vol. 109, pp. 2245–2253, 2001.
6. L. Curiel, F. Chavrier, B. Gignoux, S. Pichardo, S. Chesnais and J.-Y. Chapelon, "Experimental evaluation of lesion prediction modelling in the presence of cavitation bubbles: Intended for high-intensity focused ultrasound prostate treatment," Med. Bio. Eng. Comp., vol. 42, no. 1, pp. 44–54, 2004.
7. C. H. Farny, R. G. Holt and R. A. Roy, "The correlation between bubble-enhanced HIFU heating and cavitation power," IEEE Trans. Biomed. Eng., vol. 57, no. 1, pp. 175–184, 2010.
8. S. A. Sapareto and W. C. Dewey, "Thermal dose determination in cancer therapy," Int. J. Radiat. Oncol. Biol. Phys, vol. 10, no. 6, pp. 787–800, 1984.
9. J. Rogowska, "Overview and fundamentals of medical image segmentation," in Handbook of Medical Imaging, 2000.
10. S. Giles, "MR-guided HIFU for pain palliation of bone," Rad. Magazine, vol. 41, pp. 15–16, 2015.
11. Y.-F. Zhou, "High intensity focused ultrasound in clinical tumor ablation," World J. Clin. Oncol., vol. 2, no. 1, pp. 8–27, 2011.
12. C. M. C. Tempany, N. J. McDannold, K. Hynynen and F. A. Jolesz, "Focused ultrasound surgery in oncology: Overview and principles," Radiology, vol. 259, no. 1, pp. 39–56, 2011.
13. G. Malietzis, L. Monzon, J. Hand, H. Wasan, E. Leen, M. Abel, A. Muhammad, P. Price and P. Abel, "High-intensity focused ultrasound: Advances in technology and experimental trials support enhanced utility of focused ultrasound surgery in oncology," Br. J. Radiol., vol. 86, no. 1024, p. 20130044, 2013.
14. J. F. Aubry, "High-intensity therapeutic ultrasound: Metrological requirements versus clinical usage," Metrologia, vol. 49, no. 5, p. S259, 2012.
15. K. Hynynen and R. M. Jones, "Image-guided ultrasound phased arrays are a disruptive technology for non-invasive therapy," Phys. Med. Biol., vol. 61, no. 17, p. R206, 2016.
16. A. Pulkkinen, B. Werner, E. Martin and K. Hynynen, "Numerical simulations of clinical focused ultrasound functional neurosurgery," Phys. Med. Biol., vol. 59, no. 7, p. 1679, 2014.
17. A. Scherrer, S. Jakobsson, A. Belyaev, A. Hoffmann, M. Bortz, X. R. Reit and K. H. Küfer, "A hybrid optimization method for focused ultrasound plan computation," Berichte des Fraunhofer ITWM (Reports of Fraunhofer ITWM), vol. 249, 2016.
18. A. Scherrer, S. Jakobsson and K.-H. Küfer, "On the advancement and software support of decision-making in focused ultrasound therapy," J. Multi.-Crit. Decis. Anal., vol. 23, no. 5–6, pp. 174–182, 2016.
19. C. Uhler and S. J. Wright, "Packing ellipsoids with overlap," SIAM Rev., vol. 55, no. 4, pp. 671–706, 2013.
20. R. J. Fedewa, R. Seip, R. F. Carlson, W. Chen, N. T. Sanghvi, M. A. Penna, K. A. Dines and R. E. Pfile, "Automated treatment planning for prostate cancer HIFU therapy," in 2005 IEEE Int. Ultrasonics Symp. Proc., 2005.
21. J. Coon, A. Payne and R. Roemer, "HIFU treatment time reduction in superficial tumours through focal zone path selection," Int. J. Hyperthermia, vol. 27, p. 465–481, 2011.
22. M. Malinen, T. Huttunen, J. P. Kaipio and K. Hynynen, "Scanning path optimization for ultrasound surgery," Phys. Med. Biol., vol. 50, no. 15, p. 3473, 2005.
23. T. D. Khokhlova and J. H. Hwang, "HIFU for palliative treatment of pancreatic cancer," J. Gastrointest. Oncol., vol. 2, no. 3, pp. 175–184, 2011.
24. R. Ritchie, J. Collin, C. Coussios and T. Leslie, "Attenuation and de-focusing during high-intensity focused ultrasound therapy through peri-nephric fat," Ultrasound Med. Biol., vol. 39, no. 10, pp. 1785–1793, 2013.
25. P. Gélat, G. ter Haar and N. Saffari, "Modelling of the acoustic field of a multi-element HIFU array scattered by human ribs," Phys. Med. Biol., vol. 56, pp. 5553–5581, 2011.
26. F. Marquet, J.-F. Aubry, M. Pernot, M. Fink and M. Tanter, "Optimal transcostal high-intensity focused ultrasound with combined real-time 3D movement tracking and correction," Phys. Med. Biol., vol. 56, pp. 7061–7080, 2011.
27. Z. Wu, E. Rietzel, V. Boldea, D. Sarrut and G. C. Sharp, "Evaluation of deformable registration of patient lung 4DCT with subanatomical region segmentations," Med. Phys., vol. 35, no. 2, pp. 775–781, 2008.
28. K. K. Brock, M. B. Sharpe, L. A. Dawson, S. M. Kim and D. A. Jaffray, "Accuracy of finite element model-based multi-organ deformable image registration," Med. Phys., vol. 32, no. 6, pp. 1647–1659, 2005.

29. A. Al-Mayah, J. Moseley, M. Velec and K. K. Brock, "Sliding characteristic and material compressibility of human lung: Parametric study and verification," Med. Phys., vol. 36, no. 10, pp. 4625–4633, 2009.
30. A. Schmidt-Richberg, R. Werner, H. Handels and J. Ehrhardt, "Estimation of slipping organ motion by registration with direction-dependent regularization," Med. Image Anal., vol. 16, no. 1, pp. 150–159, 2012.
31. M. Schwenke, J. Georgii and T. Preusser, "Fast numerical simulation of focused ultrasound treatments during respiratory motion with discontinuous motion boundaries," IEEE Trans. Biomed. Eng., vol. 64, p. 1455–1468, 2017.
32. O. Lorton, P. C. Guillemin, N. Möri, L. A. Crowe, S. Boudabbous, S. Terraz, C. D. Becker, P. Cattin, R. Salomir and L. Gui, "Self-scanned HIFU ablation of moving tissue using real-time hybrid US-MR imaging," IEEE Trans. Biomed. Eng., vol. 66, p. 2182–2191, 2018.
33. D. Fontanarosa, S. Van der Meer, J. Bamber, E. Harris, T. O'Shea and F. Verhaegen, "Review of ultrasound image guidance in external beam radiotherapy: I. Treatment planning and inter-fraction motion management," Phys. Med. Biol., vol. 60, no. 3, p. R77, 2015.
34. F. Wu, Z.-B. Wang, Y.-D. Cao, Q. Zhou, Y. Zhang, Z.-L. Xu and X.-Q. Zhu, "Expression of tumor antigens and heat-shock protein 70 in breast cancer cells after high-intensity focused ultrasound ablation," Ann. Surg. Oncol., vol. 14, no. 3, pp. 1237–1242, 2007.
35. F. A. Duck, Physical Properties of Tissue: A Comprehensive Reference Book, London: Academic Press, 1990.
36. M. A. Lewis, R. M. Staruch and R. Chopra, "Thermometry and ablation monitoring with ultrasound," Int. J. Hyperthermia, vol. 31, no. 2, pp. 163–181, 2015.
37. E. Neufeld, A. Kyriacou, W. Kainz and N. Kuster, "Approach to validate simulation-based distribution predictions combining the Gamma-method and uncertainty assessment: Application to focused ultrasound," J. Verif. Valid. Uncert., vol. 1, no. 3, p. 031006, 2016.
38. T. E. Vaughan and K. Hynynen, "Effects of parameter errors in the simulation of transcranial focused ultrasound," Phys. Med. Biol., vol. 47, no. 1, p. 37, 2001.
39. V. Suomi, J. Jaros, B. Treeby and R. Cleveland, "Nonlinear 3-D simulation of high-intensity focused ultrasound therapy in the kidney," in 8th Annual International Conference of the IEEE Engineering in Medicine and Biology Society (EMBC) 2016 Aug 16, pp. 5648–5651, IEEE, 2016.
40. C. W. Connor and K. Hynynen, "Bio-acoustic thermal lensing and nonlinear propagation in focused ultrasound surgery using large focal spots: A parametric study," Phys. Med. Biol., vol. 47, pp. 1911–1928, 2002.
41. G. T. Clement and K. Hynynen, "A non-invasive method for focusing ultrasound through the human skull," Phys. Med. Biol., vol. 47, no. 8, p. 1219, 2002.
42. A. Payne, R. Chopra, N. Ellens, L. Chen, P. Ghanouni, S. Sammet, C. Diederich, G. ter Haar, D. Parker, C. Moonen, J. Stafford, E. Moros, D. Schlesinger, S. Benedict, K. Wear, A. Partanen and K. Farahan, "AAPM Task Group 241: A medical physicist's guide to MRI-guided focused ultrasound body systems," Med. Phys., vol. 48, pp. e772–e806, 2021.
43. T. N. Erpelding, K. W. Hollman and M. O'Donnell, "Bubble-based acoustic radiation force using chirp insonation to reduce standing wave effects," Ultrasound Med. Biol., vol. 33, no. 2, pp. 263–269, 2007.
44. S. C. Tang and G. T. Clement, "Acoustic standing wave suppression using randomized phase-shift-keying excitations," J. Acoust. Soc. Am., vol. 126, no. 4, pp. 1667–1670, 2009.
45. W. M. Whelan, D. R. Wyman and B. C. Wilson, "Investigations of large vessel cooling during interstitial laser heating," Med. Phys., vol. 22, pp. 105–115, 1995.
46. C. D. Mann, M. S. Metcalfe, D. M. Lloyd, G. J. Maddern and A. R. Dennison, "The safety and efficacy of ablative techniques adjacent to the hepatic vasculature and biliary system," ANZ J. Surg., vol. 80, no. 1-2, pp. 41–49, 2010.
47. K. Hynynen, A. H. Chung, V. Colucci and F. A. Jolesz, "Potential adverse effects of high-intensity focused ultrasound exposure on blood vessels in vivo," Ultrasound Med. Biol., vol. 22, no. 2, pp. 193–201, 1996.
48. T. Kamakura, K. Matsuda, Y. Kumamoto and M. A. Breazeale, "Acoustic streaming induced in focused Gaussian beams," J. Acoust. Soc. Am., vol. 97, no. 5, pp. 2740–2446, 1995.
49. M. A. Solovchuk, T. W. H. Sheu, W. L. Lin, I. Kuo and M. Thiriet, "Simulation study on acoustic streaming and convective cooling in blood vessels during a high-intensity focused ultrasound thermal ablation," Int. J. Heat Mass Transfer, vol. 55, pp. 1261–1270, 2011.

50. M. F. Hamilton and D. T. Blackstock, Nonlinear Acoustics, San Diego: Academic Press, 1998.
51. H. H. Pennes, "Analysis of tissue and arterial blood temperatures in the resting human forearm," J. Appl. Physiol., vol. 1, no. 2, pp. 93–122, 1948.
52. A. D. Pierce, Acoustics: An Introduction to its Physical Principles and Applications, New York: American Institute of Physics, 1989.
53. I. Christov, C. I. Christov and P. M. Jordan, "Modeling weakly nonlinear acoustic wave propagation," Quart. J. Mech. Appl. Math., vol. 60, no. 4, pp. 473–496, 2007.
54. V. P. Kuznetsov, "Equations of nonlinear acoustics," Sov. Phys. Acoust., vol. 16, pp. 467–470, 1971.
55. S. I. Aanonsen, T. Barkve, J. Naze-Tjøtta and S. Tjøtta, "Distortion and harmonic generation in the nearfield of a finite amplitude sound beam," J. Acoust. Soc. Am., vol. 75, pp. 749–768, 1984.
56. P. J. Westervelt, "Parametric acoustic array," J. Acoust. Soc. Am., vol. 35, pp. 535–537, 1963.
57. G. Pinton, J. Dahl, S. Rosenzweig and G. Trahey, "A heterogeneous nonlinear attenuating full-wave model of ultrasound," IEEE Trans. Ultrason. Ferroelect. Freq. Contr., vol. 56, no. 3, pp. 474–488, 2009.
58. A. A. Doinikov, A. Novell, P. Calmon and A. Bouakaz, "Simulations and measurements of 3-D ultrasonic fields radiated by phased-array transducers using the Westervelt equation," IEEE Trans. Ultrason. Ferroelect. Freq. Contr., vol. 61, p. 1470–1477, 2014.
59. W. Chen and S. Holm, "Fractional Laplacian time-space models for linear and nonlinear lossy media exhibiting arbitrary frequency power-law dependency," J. Acoust. Soc. Am., vol. 115, no. 4, pp. 1424–1430, 2004.
60. B. E. Treeby and B. T. Cox, "Modeling power law absorption and dispersion for acoustic propagation using the fractional Laplacian," J. Acoust. Soc. Am., vol. 127, pp. 2741–2748, 2010.
61. T. L. Szabo, "Time domain wave equations for lossy media obeying a frequency power law," J. Acoust. Soc. Am., vol. 96, no. 1, pp. 491–500, 1994.
62. M. S. Canney, M. R. Bailey, L. A. Crum, V. A. Khokhlova and O. A. Sapozhnikov, "Acoustic characterization of high intensity focused ultrasound fields: A combined measurement and modeling approach," J. Acoust. Soc. Am., vol. 124, no. 4, pp. 2406–2420, 2008.
63. J. E. Soneson, "A parametric study of error in the parabolic approximation of focused axisymmetric ultrasound beams," J. Acoust. Soc. Am., vol. 131, no. 6, pp. EL481-EL486, 2012.
64. E. G. Lobanova, S. V. Lobanov and V. A. Khokhlova, "Counterpropagation of waves with shock fronts in a nonlinear tissue-like medium," Acoust. Phys., vol. 60, no. 4, pp. 387–397, 2014.
65. A. S. Sangani, "A pairwise interaction theory for determining the linear acoustic properties of dilute bubbly liquids," J. Fluid Mech., vol. 232, pp. 221–284, 1991.
66. K. J. Pahk, S. Lee, P. Gélat, M. O. de Andrade and N. Saffari, "The interaction of shockwaves with a vapour bubble in boiling histotripsy: The shock scattering effect," Ultrason. Sonochem., vol. 70, p. 105312, 2021.
67. P. J. White, G. T. Clement and K. Hynynen, "Longitudinal and shear mode ultrasound propagation in human skull bone," Ultrasound Med. Biol., vol. 32, no. 7, pp. 1085–1096, 2006.
68. M. D. J. McGarry, C. L. Johnson, B. P. Sutton, J. G. Georgiadis, E. E. W. Van Houten, A. J. Pattison, J. B. Weaver and K. D. Paulsen, "Suitability of poroelastic and viscoelastic mechanical models for high and low frequency MR elastography," Med. Phys., vol. 42, no. 2, pp. 947–957, 2015.
69. P. R. Perriñez, F. E. Kennedy, E. E. W. Van Houten, J. B. Weaver and K. D. Paulsen, "Modeling of soft poroelastic tissue in time-harmonic MR elastography," IEEE Trans. Biomed. Eng., vol. 56, no. 3, pp. 598–608, 2009.
70. O. A. Sapozhnikov, S. A. Tsysar, V. A. Khokhlova and W. Kreider, "Acoustic holography as a metrological tool for characterizing medical ultrasound sources and fields," J. Acoust. Soc. Am., vol. 138, no. 3, pp. 1515–1532, 2015.
71. P. V. Yuldashev and V. A. Khokhlova, "Simulation of three-dimensional nonlinear fields of ultrasound therapeutic arrays," Acoust. Phys., vol. 57, no. 3, pp. 334–343, 2011.
72. J. Gu and Y. Jing, "A modified mixed domain method for modeling acoustic wave propagation in strongly heterogeneous media," J. Acoust. Soc. Am., vol. 147, p. 4055–4068, 2020.
73. O. P. Bruno, Y. Han and M. M. Pohlman, "Accurate, high-order representation of complex three-dimensional surfaces via Fourier continuation analysis," J. Comp. Phys., vol. 227, no. 2, pp. 1094–1125, 2007.
74. Y. Jing and G. T. Clement, "On the use of Gegenbauer reconstructions for shock wave propagation modeling," J. Acoust. Soc. Am., vol. 130, pp. 1115–1124, 2011.

75. J. P. Berenger, "A perfectly matched layer for the absorption of electromagnetic waves," J. Comput. Phys., vol. 114, pp. 185–200, 1994.
76. Q.-H. Liu and J. Tao, "The perfectly matched layer for acoustic waves in absorptive media," J. Acoust. Soc. Am., vol. 102, pp. 2072–2082, 1997.
77. G. Mur, "Absorbing boundary conditions for the finite-difference approximation of the time-domain electromagnetic-field equations," IEEE Trans. Electromagn. Compat., no. 4, pp. 377–382, 1981.
78. M. M. Chen and K. R. Holmes, "Microvascular contributions in tissue heat transfer," Ann. NY Acad. Sci., vol. 335, no. 1, pp. 137–150, 1980.
79. K. H. Keller and L. Seiler, "An analysis of peripheral heat transfer in man," J. Appl. Physiol., vol. 30, pp. 779–786, 1971.
80. P. Deuflhard and R. Hochmuth, "Multiscale analysis of thermoregulation in the human microvascular system," Math. Meth. Appld Sci., vol. 27, no. 8, pp. 971–989, 2004.
81. G. M. J. V. Leeuwen, A. Kotte, B. W. Raaymakers and J. J. W. Lagendijk, "Temperature simulations in tissue with a realistic computer generated vessel network," Phy. Med. Biol., vol. 45, pp. 1035–1049, 2000.
82. S. Weinbaum and L. M. Jiji, "A new simplified equation for the effect of blood flow on local average tissue temperature," ASME J. Biomech. Eng., vol. 107, p. 131–139, 1985.
83. K. R. Diller and J. A. Pearce, "Issues in modeling thermal alterations in tissues," Ann. NY Acad. Sci., vol. 888, no. 1, pp. 153–164, 1999.
84. P. Leuenberger, S. Ganscha, A. Kahraman, V. Cappelletti, P. J. Boersema, C. von Mering, M. Claassen and P. Picotti, "Cell-wide analysis of protein thermal unfolding reveals determinants of thermostability," Science, vol. 355, no. 6327, p. eaai7825, 2017.
85. D. P. O'Neill, T. Peng, P. Stiegler, U. Mayrhauser, S. Koestenbauer, K. Tscheliessnigg and S. J. Payne, "A three-state mathematical model of hyperthermic cell death," Ann. Biomed. Eng., vol. 39, p. 570–579, 2011.
86. Y. Xu and R. Qian, "Analysis of thermal injury process based on enzyme deactivation mechanisms," J. Biomech. Eng., vol. 117, p. 462–465, 1995.
87. S. Singh and R. Melnik, "Coupled thermo-electro-mechanical models for thermal ablation of biological tissues and heat relaxation time effects," Phys. Med. Biol., vol. 64, p. 245008, 2019.
88. J. A. Pearce, "Relationship between Arrhenius models of thermal damage and the CEM 43 thermal dose," in V 2009 Feb 23, Vol. 7181, pp. 35–49, SPIE, 2009.
89. E. L. Jones, J. R. Oleson, L. R. Prosnitz, T. V. Samulski, Z. Vujaskovic, D. Yu, L. L. Sanders and M. W. Dewhirst, "Randomized trial of hyperthermia and radiation for superficial tumors," J. Clin. Oncol., vol. 23, p. 3079–3085, 2005.
90. A. D. Maxwell, T.-Y. Wang, C. A. Cain, J. B. Fowlkes, O. A. Sapozhnikov, M. R. Bailey and Z. Xu, "Cavitation clouds created by shock scattering from bubbles during histotripsy," J. Acoust. Soc. Am., vol. 130, no. 4, pp. 1888–1898, 2011.
91. X. Fan and K. Hynynen, "The effect of wave reflection and refraction at soft tissue interfaces during ultrasound hyperthermia treatments," J. Acoust. Soc. Am., vol. 91, pp. 1727–1736, 1992.
92. A. Alaniz, F. Kallel, E. Hungerford and J. Ophir, "Variational method for estimating the effects of continuously varying lenses in HIFU, sonography, and sonography-based cross-correlation methods," J. Acoust. Soc. Am., vol. 111, pp. 468–474, 2002.
93. R. J. McGough, "Rapid calculations of time-harmonic nearfield pressures produced by rectangular pistons," J. Acoust. Soc. Am., vol. 115, no. 5, pp. 1934–1941, 2004.
94. X. Zeng and R. J. McGough, "Optimal simulations of ultrasonic fields produced by large thermal therapy arrays using the angular spectrum approach," J. Acoust. Soc. Am., vol. 125, pp. 2967–2977, 2009.
95. R. J. Zemp, J. Tavakkoli and R. S. C. Cobbold, "Modeling of nonlinear ultrasound propagation in tissue from array transducers," J. Acoust. Soc. Am., vol. 113, pp. 139–152, 2003.
96. U. Vyas and D. Christensen, "Ultrasound beam simulations in inhomogeneous tissue geometries using the hybrid angular spectrum method," IEEE Trans. Ultrason. Ferroelect. Freq. Contr., vol. 59, p. 1093–1100, 2012.
97. J. Georgii, C. von Dresky, S. Meier, D. Demedts, C. Schumann and T. Preusser, "Focused ultrasound-efficient GPU simulation methods for therapy planning," in VRIPHYS 2011, pp. 119–128, 2011.
98. J. Gu and Y. Jing, "Modeling of wave propagation for medical ultrasound: A review," IEEE Trans. Ultrason. Ferroelect. Freq. Contr., vol. 62, no. 11, pp. 1979–1992, 2015.

99. J. E. Soneson and M. R. Myers, "Thresholds for nonlinear effects in high-intensity focused ultrasound propagation and tissue heating," IEEE Trans. Ultrason., Ferroelect., Freq. Contr., vol. 57, no. 11, pp. 2450–2459, 2010.
100. S. P. Groth, P. Gélat, S. R. Haqshenas, N. Saffari, E. van't Wout, T. Betcke and G. N. Wells, "Accelerating frequency-domain numerical methods for weakly nonlinear focused ultrasound using nested meshes," J. Acoust. Soc. Am., vol. 150, p. 441–453, 2021.
101. M. Raissi, P. Perdikaris and G. E. Karniadakis, "Physics-informed neural networks: A deep learning framework for solving forward and inverse problems involving nonlinear partial differential equations," J. Comput. Phys., vol. 378, p. 686–707, 2019.
102. A. Stanziola, S. R. Arridge, B. T. Cox and B. E. Treeby, "A Helmholtz equation solver using unsupervised learning: Application to transcranial ultrasound," J. Comp. Phys., vol. 441, p. 110430, 2021.
103. O. V. Bessonova, V. A. Khokhlova, M. S. Canney, M. R. Bailey and L. A. Crum, "Focusing of high power ultrasound beams and limiting values of shock wave parameters," Acoust. Phys., vol. 55, no. 4, pp. 463–473, 2009.
104. W. Hundsdorfer and J. G. Verwer, Numerical Solution of Time-Dependent Advection-Diffusion-Reaction Equations, Berlin: Springer, 2003.
105. A. Kurganov and E. Tadmor, "New high-resolution central schemes for nonlinear conservation laws and convection-diffusion equations," J. Comput. Phys., vol. 160, no. 1, pp. 241–282, 2000.
106. R. Velasco-Segura and P. L. Rendón, "A finite volume approach for the simulation of nonlinear dissipative acoustic wave propagation," Wave Motion, vol. 58, pp. 180–195, 2015.
107. G. Strang, "On the construction and comparison of difference schemes," SIAM J. Numer. Anal., vol. 5, no. 3, pp. 506–517, 1968.
108. E. Konofagou, J. Thierman and K. Hynynen, "A focused ultrasound method for simultaneous diagnostic and therapeutic applications – A simulation study," Phys. Med. Biol., vol. 46, no. 11, p. 2967, 2001.

7

Ultrasound Monitoring Techniques for Focused Ultrasound Therapy

Ian Rivens and John Civale

7.1 Introduction

A major advantage that ultrasound therapy has over surgery, is that extra-corporeal devices can deliver treatment. This means, however, that radiological techniques are required to guide and monitor treatment before, during and after to ensure safe and effective delivery. The two main techniques used for monitoring non-invasive focused ultrasound therapy during and after delivery are ultrasound (US) and magnetic resonance (MR) imaging, as they are non-ionising and thus avoid the X-ray dose associated with computed tomography scanning. Ultrasound can deliver treatment (i.e. damage tissue) by heating (typically thermal ablation[1]), by mechanical means (e.g. by tissue liquefaction due to acoustic cavitation[2] – known as histotripsy) or by a combination of the two since cavitation can enhance heating rates.[3] Treatment monitoring may involve identification of the position and size of each region of damage in addition to ensuring that no damage occurs in regions where unwanted effects would be particularly deleterious. It should also provide feedback so that the operator can manually or automatically move to the next exposure position, or simply end treatment once it has been delivered in the required way.

MR imaging has the main advantage of allowing thermometry (in tissues other than bone and fat) and providing images with exquisite soft tissue contrast. Ultrasound has the main advantage of being faster, with imaging rates of up to 60 Hz providing "real-time" information at or above the rate of human perception. US devices are small, making them more mobile and cheaper than MR scanners. Ultrasound is also particularly good at monitoring flow using various Doppler techniques, with and without ultrasound contrast agents (microbubbles).

Diagnostic ultrasound works by sending out pulses of sound from an array of transducers (each signal being known as an A-line) and then receiving back the echoes reflected from boundaries or scattered from small objects in the field. These backscattered signals are converted into so called B-mode images by using the time at which a signal arrives to identify the position in space from which the signal was reflected, and the intensity of the signal (to determine the strength of reflection and represented by a grey scale pixel in the relevant position). Beamforming to produce diagnostic quality images involves complex data analysis and filtering which are not described here, but can be found in the medical ultrasound imaging literature.[4, 5] The use of standard B-mode diagnostic ultrasound, and in particular the image grey-scale has been shown to provide only limited focused ultrasound therapy guidance and monitoring information, related to changes in tissue echogenicity[6–9] with bubble formation causing hyperechoes and tissue structure loss causing hypoechoic regions. This can be quite marked when bubble formation is due to boiling of the interstitial water,[10] but is much less obvious if acoustic cavitation occurs in the absence of boiling, or as hot tissue cools.[11] This is discussed in greater depth in Chapter 8, while other techniques for forming ultrasound images or collecting acoustic data that have been investigated more thoroughly as methods for monitoring (and guiding) high-intensity focused ultrasound exposures are described in detail below. The topics covered include passive cavitation detection, elasticity imaging, ultrasound thermography, reflex transmission imaging and Doppler imaging.

DOI: 10.1201/9780429162671-7

7.2 Passive Cavitation Detection

Passive cavitation detection often attempts to differentiate key types of acoustic cavitation. Inertial or collapse (transient) cavitation in which the restoring forces within the bubble are unable to balance the compression of the peak negative pressure leads to bubble implosion, and the production of "white" or broadband noise.[12] This is generally accepted as being a unique indicator, and therefore detection of broadband signals may confidently be related to there being sufficient numbers of imploding bubbles that their detection above background noise is possible. In the absence of any broadband signal, it is generally accepted that harmonics of the drive frequency are created and/or amplified by non-inertial (stable) bubble oscillation. The confounding issue here is that non-linear ultrasound propagation resulting from high amplitude ultrasound signal propagation (typical in high-intensity focused ultrasound) also produces harmonics of the drive signal.[10] Signals from bubbles may be identified either by subtracting a signal that includes non-linear propagation in the absence of bubble formation, or from the transient (chaotic) nature of a signal, typical of bubbles and atypical of non-linear propagation. Alternatively, in the absence of broadband, a subharmonic signal cannot come from non-linear propagation, but may arise from surface waves on a bubble.[13–15]

As the name suggests, passive cavitation detection involves listening to ultrasound signals[16, 17] associated with acoustic bubble activity using a sensor which does not transmit an interrogating pulse. The aim is then to separate those of interest, those emitted or reflected from acoustic cavitation bubbles, from background noise that includes those signals scattered by tissue or coming directly from a therapy source.[18] The pulse that stimulates the cavitation bubbles is generally from a therapy field (see Figure 7.1). If microbubbles or nanodroplets are introduced into the blood stream systemically, pressures below 1 MPa are usually sufficient to stimulate bubble oscillation (i.e. stable or non-inertial cavitation) or bubble collapse (inertial cavitation).[19] In their absence, much higher pressures are required, and the shorter the stimulating pulse the higher the pressure needed. For single-cycle or half-cycle pulses, the peak negative pressures required to create bubbles may be on the order of 100 MPa.[20]

7.2.1 Monitoring Techniques

The simplest monitoring method is perhaps to record the high intensity frequency ultrasound (HIFU) drive as a function of time and to analyse the signals for changes. If the drive voltage and current are

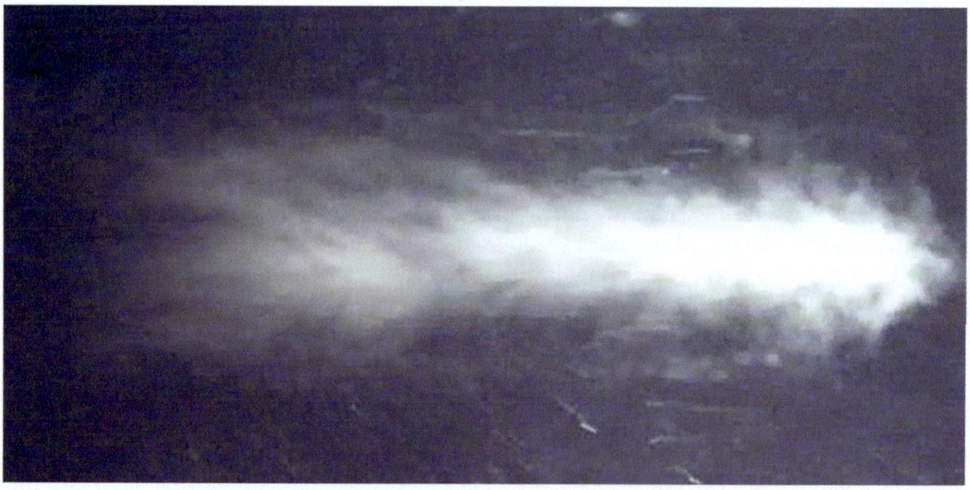

FIGURE 7.1 A cloud of highly energetic bubbles generated proximal to the focus of a high-intensity focused ultrasound beam propagating from right to left in degassed water. Photograph courtesy of the Institute of Cancer Research.

measured independently, they can be combined to calculate the drive power (by multiplying the two time-varying signals together), or the impedance (the time varying voltage divided by the current). Electrical drive power represents the combination of transmitted power going to the transducer and reflected power coming back down the line from it. Placing a reflector (interface) or scatterers such as bubbles in the beam, particularly within the focal region, will alter the reflected signal. Dynamic changes in scattering can produce time variations in the measured drive. The onset or presence of such variations can indicate bubble formation. Since the amplitude of variation due to signals from individual bubbles is small relative to the amplitude of the drive voltage, detection sensitivity is not high and depends on the formation of a sufficiently large cloud of bubbles to create a detectable change. However, if variations are detected, it is highly likely they are due to bubble activity. This is active cavitation detection since the focused ultrasound transducer used to drive the bubbles is also used for detection.

The next simplest passive cavitation monitoring method is to use a single transducer (or hydrophone) to detect signals emitted from acoustic cavitation bubbles. An early study of this suggested that if submarines wanted to avoid detection they needed to travel more slowly than the speed at which their propellers caused cavitation bubbles.[21] Interest in this technique for medical ultrasonics surfaced around the mid-1980s.[17, 22] For therapy ultrasound, commercial devices are available that will slot into apertures in the centre of therapeutic transducers and provide passive detection with automatic registration with the focal region. For therapy applications at a few MHz, sensors are usually wide bandwidth (0 to 20 MHz) single-element devices with a relatively smooth and flat frequency response. This sensor arrangement works well for single-element transducers with a fixed focal position, or for annular arrays that steer the focus only along the sound axis. Their utility for more complex field distributions and lateral beam steering is less clear.

A passive cavitation sensor is usually connected to an electronic (hardware) filter, either a notch, high-pass or low-pass filter, to remove the drive signal, which may be orders of magnitude higher than cavitation signals, without affecting other frequencies of interest. These might be harmonics and ultraharmonics or only subharmonics of the drive. The disadvantage of a high-pass filter compared to a notch filter is that it will remove the therapy's fundamental frequency plus any subharmonics, whilst low-pass filters will only preserve subharmonics. After filtering, the residual signal may be amplified using a low-noise amplifier to give e.g. 20 dB gain in voltage. The signal is then usually passed to a high frequency and high bit-rate data acquisition system. The frequency of acquisition determines the highest frequency that can be resolved from a fast Fourier transform (FFT) of the data. According to the Nyquist theorem, the limit for that value is half the sampling rate. Therefore if 1 MHz therapy ultrasound is being used and harmonic or broadband data up to 10 MHz is of interest, the sampling rate should be a minimum of 20 MHz. Since this will yield only two data points per cycle for 10 MHz data, using higher sampling rates is also beneficial. Once voltages are detected, digital acquisition systems will log the voltage into a quantised range of "voltage bins" depending on the bit-rate of the device, which usually ranges from 8 to 16 bit. An 8-bit system provides 2^8 (256) levels, while a 12-bit system provides 2^{12} (4096) and so on, so the higher the bit rate, the smaller any quantisation errors and the better the quality of the data. Data acquisition may be achieved using a good quality digital oscilloscope or a data acquisition card installed into a computer. After digitisation, data usually needs to be streamed, at high speed, to storage. This is often done on the hard disk of a computer via memory (random access memory [RAM]) on the data acquisition card, which has to deal with input and output data simultaneously. It can be beneficial to have a dual-bus computer, to provide simultaneous logging of cavitation data and drive data (e.g. power or voltage). Data logging limitations may require the sampling frequency to be reduced from the maximum capability or may put an upper limit on the duration for which data can be recorded.

Once acquired, data can be processed/displayed either off-line (post-acquisition) or in real time if manual (user) or automated feedback are required to control exposures. If potentially computationally expensive real-time processing is required, this can be achieved using a dedicated graphics processing unit (GPU) which will not store the raw data but will provide rapid analysis of that data which can be used, for example, in a feedback loop controlling the ultrasound exposure power level and/or exposure duration in order to either stop or sustain acoustic cavitation as soon as it occurs. For example, in blood-brain barrier opening studies, stable oscillation of the bubbles is believed to achieve opening without causing damage, but the onset of bubble collapse can cause haemorrhage, so monitoring for the presence of harmonic signals in the absence of broadband can be an effective feedback control method.

The aim of data processing may be to evaluate whether bubble activity can be detected, by identification of broadband and/or half harmonic signals. The steps to achieve this from the acquired voltage versus time data are segmentation (breaking data into manageable or optimised chunks), fast Fourier transformation (to calculate the frequency spectrum of each chunk) and quantification of frequencies of interest such as half harmonic and/or broadband, usually by the use of software filtering or software masks to select or deselect frequency bands of interest.

Segmentation usually requires a compromise between frequency and temporal resolution. Too small a segment produces low resolution spectra which are difficult to interpret, but too long a segment may average over different types of bubble activity, thus reducing the detection sensitivity. If FFTs are to be performed, they can be improved by ensuring that an integer number of cycles are analysed. At 1 MHz, 20 cycles or more are usually sufficient, but short pulses of 1 to 10 cycles are not well suited to this type of processing. Here it may be possible to exploit the S-transform[23] (based on an improvement to the short-time Fourier transform) or use the Winger-Ville distribution (WVD) function to obtain bilinear time frequency signals.[24] By computing an FFT for each segment, the time variation of signal may be obtained from plots of the FFT of each segment as a function of time. Figure 7.2 shows an example of FFT analysis of short (21 cycle) pulse data for exposures of multiple (38) pulses delivered within multiple (125) bursts, presented as emission "heat maps".

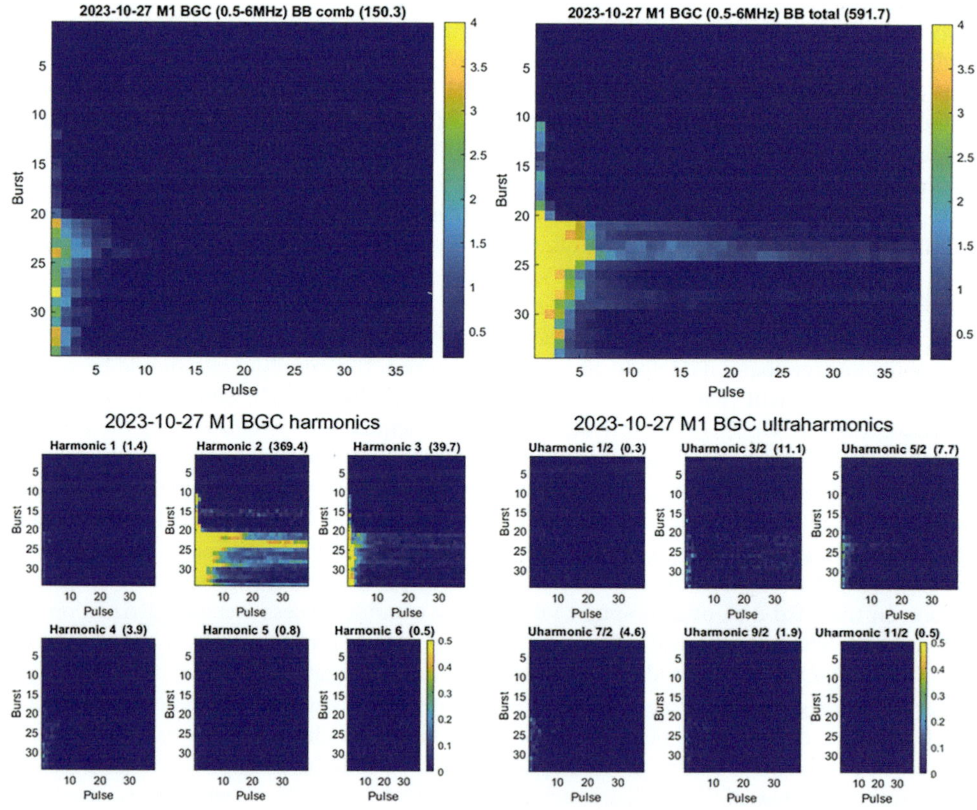

FIGURE 7.2 Example of passive cavitation detection data analysis. Ultrasound exposures of intravenously injected microbubbles in mouse brain using 34 bursts of 38 pulses of 21-cycle 1-MHz focused ultrasound with a pulse repetition frequency of 1.25 kHz and a burst repetition frequency of 0.5 Hz. (Top panels) Data are shown for the broadband emissions in the range of 0.5 to 6.0 MHz without filtering (right) and after comb filtering all integer and half-integer harmonics. (Bottom panels) Emissions detected in the frequency bands of the harmonics 1 (drive) to 6 (left) and ultra-harmonics from ½ (half harmonic) to 11/2 (right). Data courtesy of Institute of Cancer Research in collaboration with Dr James Choi, Imperial College, London.

Additional data processing may be useful in order to achieve better human readability. The presence of the drive frequency (if it hasn't been hardware filtered out) and/or its harmonics within the broadband spectrum increases the complexity of processing required to assess whether inertial cavitation is occurring. To remove those signals which are not exclusively broadband, a "comb" filter is often used. This is a simple software filter (or mask) in which all the harmonic data to be removed are multiplied by zero. The challenge comes in defining the width of the signal (which is usually drive power dependent). Once this has been done, integrated broadband per data segment can be obtained by summing the remaining data within an upper and lower band (e.g. 0.1 to 10 MHz).

The half harmonic is potentially easier to quantify, by summing amplitude over a narrow bandwidth centred on this frequency. For a 1.5 MHz HIFU signal the half harmonic is at 750 kHz. How close to this value data should be taken depends on the frequency resolution of the FFTs. FFT frequency resolution is inversely proportional (reciprocal) to the temporal duration of the signal. For example, if data segments of 200 μs (300 cycles) are used, the frequency resolution is 5 kHz, so data could be summed over 3 frequency bins from 745 to 755 kHz. If the levels of noise in that frequency range are unknown it can be useful to compare the subharmonic to data from the same sized, non-overlapping, band at slightly higher (e.g. 765 kHz) and lower (e.g. 745 kHz) centre frequencies. If specific harmonics are of interest, a similar filtering/mask approach can be used, but usually using a much wider bandwidth especially for the 2nd harmonic.

For completeness several important points should be noted: Subharmonic is only indicative of stable bubble oscillation in the absence of broadband, but non-detection of broadband does not guarantee that there was none, knowledge of the detection threshold levels is relevant here; when broadband is present, it contributes to all harmonic amplitudes; as therapy exposure levels increase, the height and width of harmonics increase, which can lead to leakage of harmonic signal into broadband ranges if appropriate care with software filtering is not taken, this can render the frequencies available for broadband assessment very small; harmonic signals can arise from non-linear propagation of the therapy beam as well as from bubble activity; cavitation signals emanating from depth within tissue will be subject to frequency dependent attenuation, affecting high frequencies more strongly; detectors with wider apertures will be more sensitive due to a larger detection area, however they will also be more susceptible to phase cancellation effects rendering their response highly dependent on the spectral content of cavitation signals and the spatial location of the cavitating bubbles.

A solution to cavitation monitoring for highly steerable array therapy systems (see Chapter 4) is dual-mode arrays in which the same elements are used for therapy and passive cavitation detection.[25–28] A more popular alternative to dual-mode arrays is the use of standard diagnostic imaging equipment, but with zero pulse output, so that it works in receive only mode. Array imaging probes allow image reconstruction that indicates the most likely origin of bubble emissions, based on analysis of the signals detected at multiple transducer elements. This technique is often known as passive acoustic mapping (PAM).[29, 30] Challenges with this technique include beamforming to identify the source of acoustic signals. Methods have evolved from time exposure acoustic (TEA) beamforming[29] through to the robust Capon beamformer (RCB) method,[31] with the best results from either requiring accurate array calibration, correction for tissue attenuation[32] and array element diffraction[33] and arrays lens refraction.[34] Improved mapping has also been demonstrated using 2 linear imaging arrays imaging the same plane from orthogonal angles[35] wide aperture curve arrays.[25, 36–38]

7.2.2 Monitoring Applications

Passive cavitation detection has been successfully deployed in a wide range of applications. The design and implementation of such a system was published in 2006.[18] Its use has been investigated for the detection of acoustic (micro)cavitation,[16] monitoring or optimisation of the destruction of stones using lithotripsy[39] and HIFU studies of platelet aggregation, activation and adhesion[40]; thrombolysis[41–43]; endothelial cell damage[44]; to elucidate the mechanism of HIFU-induced hyperecho in B-mode ultrasound[6, 7, 45, 46]; and interaction with microbubble contrast agents including Optison,[47–49] Definity[42, 50, 51] and Sonovue.[52] Blood-brain barrier (BBB) opening or disruption,[51, 53, 54] including using it for feedback control[55] and more recently for pulsed HIFU-induced immunotherapy, is another area of study.[56] The use of dual-mode HIFU arrays for transcranial exposures with cavitation monitoring,[27, 28] including the use of CMUT transducers[26] (see Chapter 4), has also been reported.

7.3 Elasticity Imaging

Whilst tissue palpation (in which the clinician uses their hands to probe for regions of different stiffness in the body) was one of the earliest methods of medical diagnosis (its use being documented as early as 1500 BC), the use of devices to aid this method only came to the fore in the 1990s when ultrasound was used to perform the palpation (a technique referred to as ultrasound elastography),[57, 58] followed shortly afterwards by MR elastography in the 2000s.[59]

7.3.1 Fundamentals of Elastography

The fundamental principle of elastography is to use a form of imaging to track the motion of tissue in response to an applied force. Soft tissue will deform more easily and transmit the force less well, whereas stiffer tissue maintains its shape better, but moves more, due to the force. The required compression can be generated using manual palpation by, or making use of, changes within the body, with the imaging probe being held as still as possible, with distortions being measured as a result of normal physiological processes such as pulsatile blood flow. There are 4 main elastography methods: strain (or strain rate) elastography, shear wave elastography, acoustic radiation force imaging (ARFI) and transient elastography. The differences in techniques come from (i) how the mechanical stimulus applied to the tissue is produced and (ii) how the resulting elastogram is obtained.

Strain (rate) elastography (SE) may also be referred to as quasi-static elastography or just "elastography" because it was the first method developed by Ophir et al.[60] Compression of the tissue can be obtained by the operator simply applying pressure on the tissue using the imaging probe. Pre- and post-compression images are compared, with image features (i.e. speckle in US B-mode images) being tracked to quantify local tissue displacements in response to the applied compression. Strain rate, that is the rate of change of displacement in space, is then calculated to produce an axial strain image. Stiff tissues, which distort less, will display a lower strain rate than softer regions. Typically the applied stress will not be uniform across the tissue being imaged, and cannot be measured, so it is not possible to estimate stiffness properties such as the Young's modulus, for example, and therefore cannot be considered as a quantitative technique. The technique is also limited due to difficulties in transmitting the mechanical compression to deeper tissues, and to movement of tissues out of the imaging plane as a result of the applied stress. The technique is, however, clinically useful for detecting abnormalities, such as stiff tumours, using ultrasound imaging,[61] and has been implemented by a number of manufacturers on clinical scanners.

In ARFI, an ultrasound impulse is used to induce tissue deformation by providing a push inside the tissue using the radiation force associated with the beam.[62] Momentum transfer from the wave occurs as it is absorbed or reflected, resulting in a force on the local tissue. A focused beam is used with sufficient intensity and duration that the push produces detectable deformations. Short pulses (typically 0.03 to 3 ms long) are used to generate movements of ~1 to 10 μm. As with SE, only relative strain can be measured. By sequentially pushing at many different locations, 2D images can be obtained.[63] This technique has been implemented with both ultrasound and MR.[64] One of its disadvantages is the long time required to build up a detailed image due to the number of ARFI pushes that are required, and the risk of tissue heating due to the greater energy transmitted than used with standard B-mode imaging.

Shear wave elastography (SWE) is achieved when an ARFI push is applied to a volume. Ultrasound imaging is used to track the shear waves generated by this ARFI push. The shear waves propagate away from the location of the push, and providing the imaging frame rate is adequate (>a few kHz), the shear wave displacements can be tracked and associated shear wave speed can be measured. Measurement of shear wave speed is quantitative, and under a number of assumptions (isotropic, linear and incompressible material) can be used to estimate quantitative mechanical properties such as the Young's modulus E (using $E=3\rho c^2$).[65] The advent of SWE therefore represents a shift from qualitative to quantitative elastography. The growth in computing power has also heralded faster image reconstruction, which can now be performed digitally, allowing implementation of ultrafast imaging techniques on commercial ultrasound scanners. This development has been crucial in shear wave elastography where planar wave sonications can be used to reconstruct the entire field of view at frame rates of several kHz. Shear wave speed can thus be measured across a wide region of the field of view from one or more ARFI pushes. A further evolution consists in rapidly sweeping the ARFI focal point in the axial direction. This is made possible by electronically steering the focal position of the ARFI push to increasingly greater depth. This can be achieved at a faster speed than that of the shear wave in soft tissue (<10 m/s), the result being a mechanical impulse resembling a "Mach" cone which generates a near-plane wave in the imaging plane for improved characterisation of shear waves over a greater area.[66]

Transient elastography (TE) uses a short mechanical impulse from the transducer on the skin to produce shear waves in the tissue. Ultrasound echo data is then tracked to monitor the speed through which the impulse propagates into the tissue. Again, shear wave speed is dependent on tissue stiffness allowing calculation of the Young's modulus estimates. A good example of transient elastography in a clinical setting is the Fibroscan system, which is designed to assess liver fibrosis in patients with chronic liver disease.[67, 68]

7.3.2 Radiation Force Imaging

ARFI is a technique in which an ultrasound beam is used to supply the force pushing on the tissue. First proposed in 1990,[69] this can be from a relatively high-amplitude imaging pulse or a pulse from a therapy system. Whilst it is possible to perform MR ARFI, this section concentrates on ultrasound elastography imaging using ARFI.

7.3.3 Vibroacoustography

Vibroacoustography uses a dynamic acoustic radiation force (through the use of pulsed or amplitude modulated ultrasound) to characterise the acoustic properties of tissue using a speckle-free technique. Quantitative elastic properties of tissues are obtained when ultrasound frequencies are converted to acoustic frequencies (2 or more orders of magnitude lower). The emissions are usually recorded with a hydrophone. The ultrasound beam used is usually focused. There are 2 methods of obtaining the imaging information. One method is to use two co-focused beams at slightly different frequencies. The other is to use an amplitude modulated single frequency beam where the modulation frequency is much smaller than the carrier frequency. The detected acoustic signal is generated primarily at the focal region of the transducer and is therefore not dependent on the random distribution of scatterers that is responsible for the speckle patterns typically observed in US imaging. The amplitude of the detected acoustic signals is dependent on the stiffness of the tissue, and depth due to attenuation of the ultrasound beam.

7.3.4 Application of Elasticity Imaging to Focused Ultrasound Therapy

Elastography and other elasticity imaging systems have been evaluated for several biomedical applications: imaging of healthy and diseased tissues, such as breast,[57, 70] liver,[71] kidney,[72] muscle,[73] prostate,[74] noncalcified and calcified arteries,[75] imaging of the vitreous body,[76] intravascular ultrasound (IVUS) elastography[77] and monitoring of lesions, such as HIFU-induced lesions[71–73, 78] and real-time monitoring of HIFU.[79–81]

7.4 Ultrasound Backscatter Thermography

Ultrasound thermometry can exploit a pulse-echo interrogation of the heated region (backscatter thermometry) with analysis of the acquired images used to look at (i) speckle displacement due to sound speed changes, (ii) backscattered energy, (iii) statistical parameters, (iv) non-linearity and (v) attenuation.

Ultrasound imaging of temperature is based on the characteristic of soft tissues that the speed of sound propagation within them is roughly linearly temperature dependent[82] up to around 50°C. Sound speed temperature dependence is well characterised in water[83] and in many soft tissues.[84] Ultrasound scanners assume a constant, fixed sound speed when processing ultrasound echoes to generate an image. If sufficient heating occurs, image speckle arising from tissue will appear to move[85] due to a reduction in echo arrival time, a consequence of the increase in sound speed. This is the underlying mechanism which forms the basis of ultrasound thermography. Radio frequency (RF) echo tracking algorithms similar to those employed in elastography can be used to track small apparent (~μm) displacements in tissue, from which temperature change images may be estimated.

7.4.1 Physical Basis for Backscatter Thermography

Ultrasound echo arrival time is dependent on the sound speed profile in the path between the imaging probe and a region of interest. Echoes arriving from a distal part of the image are therefore subject to larger apparent absolute displacement towards the imaging transducer than those originating from proximal regions, if the sound speed is increased due to heating. Echo strain can then be computed from apparent axial displacement, in a manner similar to that used in strain (static) elastography methods, where tissue mechanical strain is computed from tissue displacements in response to an applied stress. Echo strain in US backscatter thermography indicates the rate of change in apparent displacement with depth, a property directly proportional to the underlying change in sound speed. Echo strain can therefore be related to absolute temperature if both the start reference temperature and sound speed temperature dependence are known. The latter is the source of most of the limitations of ultrasound thermography. For example, while sound speed increase has a relatively linear dependence on temperature increase between 37° and around 50°C in most soft tissues, the dependence then plateaus and reverses, limiting the useful temperature range to a few degrees. The exact sound speed dependence on temperature is also problematic as attempts to calibrate heating induced echo strain as a function of temperature have shown significant variance.[86] Human and mammalian tissue is usually heterogeneous either in terms of its cellular makeup or because of variations in vascularity within organs. The temperature dependence of the speed of sound in tissue is relatively inconsistent between samples of the same tissue type and between different tissue types, making prediction of the tissue temperature from measurements of sound speed variation less than unreliable. Another complication comes from the alignment of the imaging probe with respect to the HIFU transducer. A co-axial alignment is commonly found in clinical US-guided therapy systems, where the heated region extends much farther in the axial direction, with steeper temperature gradients in the lateral direction. This arrangement favours thermoacoustic refractive effects (also known as thermal lensing[87]), whereby tissue displacement measurement precision is decreased due to decorrelation in the speckle pattern.[88] For these reasons ultrasound thermography is somewhat limited in practice to applications requiring low temperature rises, or for siting exposures where a non-therapeutic sonication is used to ascertain the correct targeting location.[89] Finally, this technique is also highly sensitive to noise arising from tissue movement which may be physiological (breathing or cardiac motion) or due to the patient movement.

7.4.2 Application of Backscatter Thermography to Focused Ultrasound

Despite some of the limitations outlined earlier, backscatter thermography (see Figure 7.3) has been shown to provide potential benefit for the delivery of focused ultrasound therapies in the form of treatment guidance. In 1995, Seip and Ebbini proposed a spectral processing technique[90] to measure the echo shift for temperature estimation. Their algorithm tracked the frequency variation in the echo components in the spectral domain and estimated the echo spectrum using an autoregressive model.[91] Since processing data in the time domain has greater computational efficiency, other investigators have used the kinds of time domain cross-correlation strain estimators that had been developed for use in elastography.[82, 88, 89, 92] The cross-correlation algorithm searches for the maximum correlation between a segment window in a preheated A-line and in a postheated one. The shift in the search window yielding the maximum correlation coefficient corresponds to the echo shift caused by the local temperature

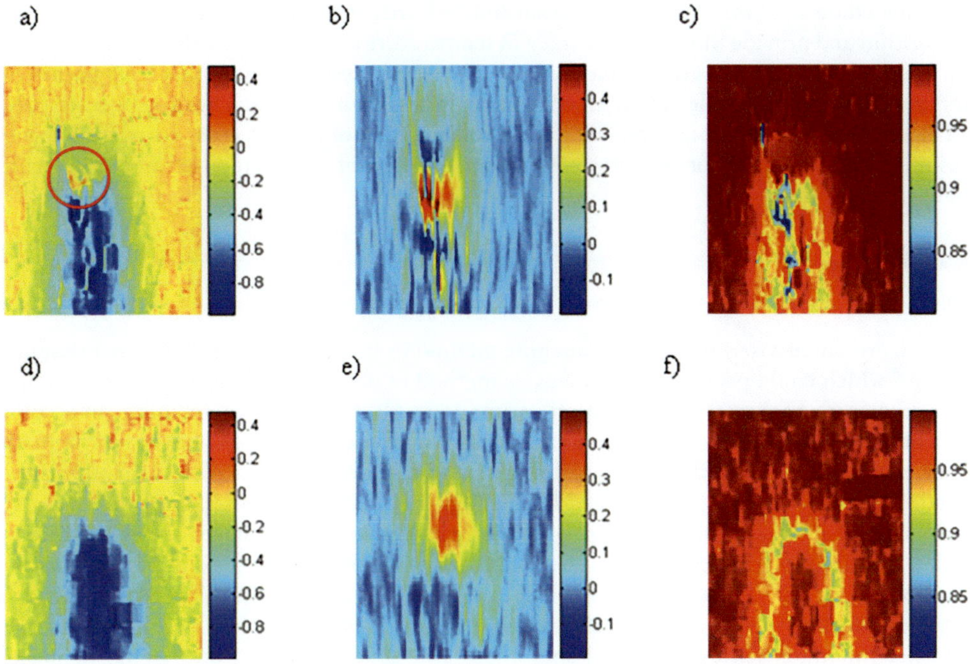

FIGURE 7.3 Axial displacement, strain and correlation images for a 210 W/cm^2 I_{sp} exposure of ex vivo bovine liver at 1.7 MHz with the thermocouple in place (a, b and c, respectively) and with the thermocouple removed (d, e and f). US temperature imaging in the HIFU focal plane using a trans-axial probe alignment. The red circle shows a displacement artefact created by the thermocouple. Displacement images (a, d) are 1.9 × 1.6 cm, with displacement in units of RF samples. Strain images (b, c) are 1.5 × 1.6 cm, in units of percentage) and correlation images (c, f) are 1.9 × 1.6 cm in units of correlation coefficient.

change. Although computationally efficient, the cross-correlation calculation still requires extensive processing. Souchon et al. demonstrated the ability to monitor echo strain in liver tissue samples using a perpendicular alignment of therapy and ultrasound imaging probes.[93] These authors accounted for tissue expansion effects on echo strain by measuring strain between successive image frames during heating and demonstrating good correlation between the regions of thermal coagulation and regions of increased echo strain due primarily to thermal expansion. Thermography approaches have also been used to demonstrate monitoring methods, where RF data can be streamed and processed in real time on GPUs to provide real-time temperature images.[94] A similar approach implemented on a dual mode array uses the same phased array for therapy and imaging, demonstrating real-time implementation where focal position, focal temperature can be controlled.[95, 96]

In a different approach, changes in backscattered energy have been used for ultrasound thermometry.[97] Predicted energy changes were matched by ex vivo measurements in bovine liver, turkey breast and pork muscle. Tissue regions with collections of individual scatterers demonstrated the best potential. Backscatter energy was measured with a focused circular 7.5-MHz transducer. The standard deviation of backscattered energy from 75 to 125 tissue regions from 0.3 to 0.5 cm^3 increased nearly linearly from 37°C to 50°C. Although the slopes were different, the curve for each tissue type fitted a second-degree polynomial, with a correlation coefficient of 0.99, suggesting the potential for future clinical use. The zero-crossing tracking (ZCT) technique, borrowed from US elastography, has also been demonstrated to be applicable to US thermometry.[98] Here, echo shifts are obtained by tracking the shifts in the zero-crossing instants of a pair of A-lines, followed by converting the echo shift gradient to the corresponding temperature variations. Zero-crossing detection is relatively simple, allowing processing time to be reduced, and acquiring zero crossings instead of whole A-line signals can also substantially reduce amount of data that needs to be acquired.

A hybrid method combining cross correlation and zero crossing tracking to exploit the advantages of each algorithm and provide improved accuracy in temperature estimation has also been investigated in ex vivo porcine muscle and in vivo rabbit muscle.[99] The ex vivo results showed that *temperature estimation differed from* thermocouple measurement usually by less than 1°C, when heating by up to 10°C. The hybrid algorithm's computational efficiency was similar to that of the fast cross correlation algorithm, but has improved accuracy. For the interested reader, a review of ultrasound thermometry techniques was published in 2012.

7.5 Reflex Transmission Imaging

Green et al. presented a new ultrasound imaging method in 1985 known as reflex transmission imaging (RTI)[100] which could provide a non-invasive method of obtaining tissue attenuation (sometimes also referred to as backscatter attenuation estimation). US transmission imaging, like computed tomography (CT or CAT) X-ray imaging, allows tomographic (sectional) images of attenuation to be obtained. Using augmented B-mode imaging equipment, orthographic transmission images were obtained. The technique avoided the need for through-body transmission images and could be performed using standard diagnostic imaging equipment. Transmission images are created in a plane normal to the direction of the beam (known as a C-scan) by integrating the signals from beyond the focal zone. The signals act as an incoherent sound source located behind the focal plane. Proof of principle was demonstrated with a rectilinear scanner which produced time-gated C-scans in which back-scatter inhomogeneities were well smoothed, and good resolution and signal to noise were obtained. Such scans could be obtained simultaneously with B-scans and displayed on a scanner. RTI has been used to characterise calculi to be treated with lithotripsy.[101, 102] Later the performance of a linear array imaging probe and the effect of dynamic receive focusing were assessed.[103, 104] It was also investigated for use in the detection and diagnosis of skin cancer[105, 106] and for skull bone aberration correction prior to HIFU exposure of the brain.[107, 108] Since it is well known that HIFU lesions have raised attenuation,[109] this technique has been investigated as a method of monitoring focused ultrasound treatment.[110]

7.5.1 Theory

Reflex transmission imaging integrates the backscattered echoes obtained from a tissue volume lying beyond the focal region of a strongly focused ultrasonic beam (see Figure 7.4) which is scanned through the tissue to be imaged. An image pixel is obtained at each position. The signal obtained is dominated by the attenuation of the tissue within the focal volume.

The technique requires a suitably uniform volume of tissue beyond the focal plane with the intervening tissue being relatively homogeneous. Originally demonstrated in 1985 by Green and Arditi,[100] the technique has largely been under-exploited but interest has recently been revived, and its potential is now being more actively investigated, particularly when combined with other approaches, the performance of which may be enhanced by being able to compensate for attenuation. The original method relied on using a strongly focused transducer to act as a confocal transmitter and receiver. Scanning the device in two dimensions at a constant depth (a so-called C scan) provided an image, by summing the magnitude of echoes from tissue occupying a gate (range of depths) beyond the focus, signals from which pass through the focal region both on their way to the region and after backscattering from it, whose signal was strongly dependent on the attenuation in the focus. Thus, the tissue in the gate is used as a reference that is assumed to be homogenous. Widening of the beam beyond the focus results in spatial averaging over the gated tissue, reducing the impact of homogeneities and providing useful speckle reduction. Similarly the wider beam anterior to the focus will average out any minor fluctuations in attenuation of the tissue overlying the focus. Performing RTI measurements before and after heating (e.g. using HIFU) provides the potential to monitor changes in focal temperature or heat induces attenuation changes.

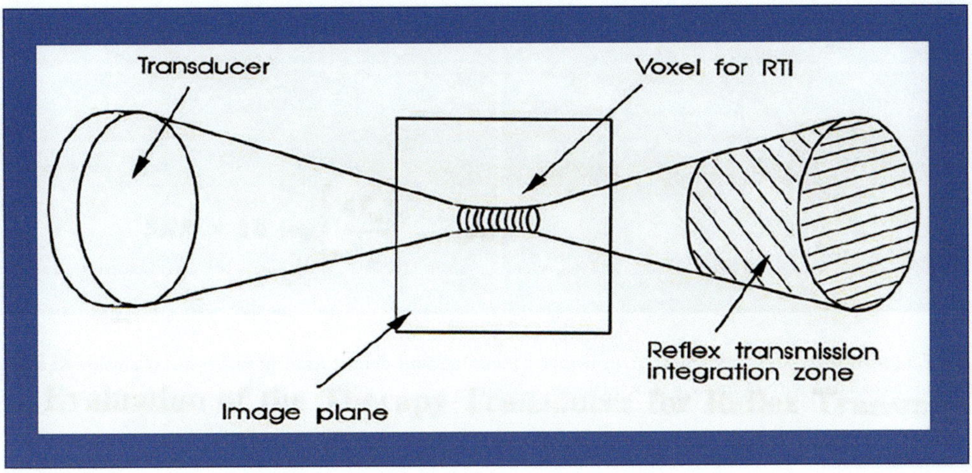

FIGURE 7.4 Principle behind reflex transmission imaging as a method of obtaining attenuation data for a region of homogeneous material. Taken from Malcolm A. PhD thesis, Institute of Cancer Research.

7.5.2 Practice

RTI has not been widely used. The potential to use it at higher frequencies (~20 MHz) for the clinical diagnosis of pigmented skin lesion[105, 106, 111, 112] and at lower frequencies for visualising calculi for targeting with lithotripsy[101, 113] has been demonstrated. RTI for HIFU induced thermal lesion monitoring at 3 to 5 MHz has been investigated by a number of teams, including[114] Baker[103, 104] and Farney.[110, 115] Early application using a single, strongly focused transducer in pulse echo mode showed the potential for obtaining attenuation measurements of homogeneous regions of tissue from pulse-echo data.[116] Later, RTI using a more clinically relevant 1D linear array probe to assess attenuating tiles in a uniformly scattering background showed an average speckle to noise ratio of 5.6, with a value of 4.4. for an attenuation contrast of −62%. Spatial resolution on the order of 2 to 2.5 mm was demonstrated, which has the potential to image focused ultrasound thermal lesions. Numerical simulation demonstrated RTI using a 1-MHz focused transducer was able to detect a 3-mm-diameter water plume kept 7° to 10°C above the temperature of the surrounding water and the spatial temperature distribution of the plume.[117] This was also verified experimentally by comparison with an unheated reference measurement. Heated and unheated measurements made with a 0.2-mm-diameter needle hydrophone and numerical backward projection of the data were used as a surrogate for B-mode imaging with an array probe. The technique was then applied to steady-state focused ultrasound heating (at 1.1 MHz) of a tissue phantom using a 1.68-MHz focused transducer and needle hydrophone. Hydrophone scans performed to obtain the reflex transmission signal before and during heating were numerically back-projected to the region of heating, integrated along the propagation axis, and tomographically reconstructed to obtain the phase change, from which the sound speed and temperature change was determined. For 42°C temperature rises, temperature was reconstructed to within 2°C of that measure by MR thermometry. Thermal lensing effects visible in the images, could be corrected for by applying a moving average filter. The result is a method which can visualise the temperature change over a spatial region sufficient for monitoring thermal ablation treatments.[115] The lengthy hydrophone scanning can be readily replaced by ultrasound imaging and the RTI spatial resolution (0.3 × 0.3 × 0.3 mm) compares favourably with the 0.625 × 0.625 × 1.5-mm MR spatial resolution.[110] A more traditional, but less clinically relevant, transmission approach using a planar 10-MHz ultrasound source co-aligned with an acoustic camera was used to study image intensity during and after (2.0 MHz) HIFU.[108] Although good results were found with lesion size correlation between US transmission imaging and size measured on subsequent dissection (R^2 of the linear correlation was 0.9), the system was not developed further, possibly due to the challenges involved with the experimental configuration, making it difficult to use in a clinical setting.

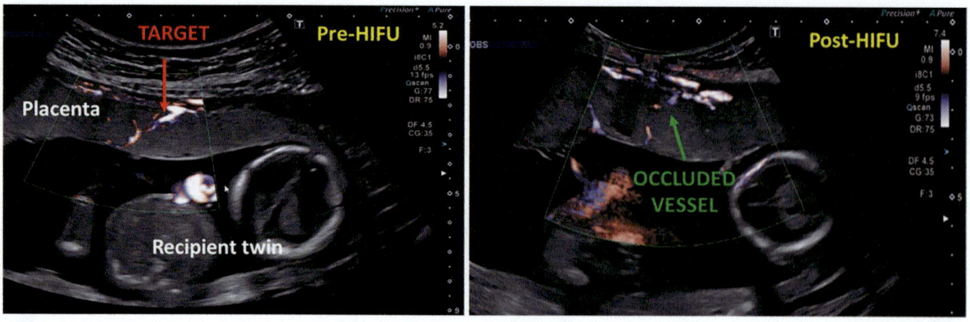

FIGURE 7.5 Advanced dynamic flow (ADF) Doppler measurement demonstrating successful occlusion of a placental anastomosis associated with twin-twin transfusion syndrome.

7.6 Doppler Imaging

Most recently, the use of Doppler (flow) imaging to guide and monitor HIFU-induced vascular occlusion has been demonstrated. Ultrasound reflected from particles (blood cells) that are moving in opposite directions is frequency shifted in opposite directions. The amount of frequency shift and its direction can therefore be used to estimate the velocity and direction of blood flow. This has been an essential diagnostic imaging tool in fetal medicine for many years, but it also offers the opportunity to treat conditions affecting identical (monochorionic) twins who share a placenta noninvasively. In twin-twin transfusion syndrome (TTTS), unwanted blood vessels (anastomoses) can shunt blood from one twin to the other causing an imbalance that affects the donor and recipient twins resulting in poor outcomes if untreated. In twin reversed arterial perfusion (TRAP), anastomoses that connect the arteries of both twins together cause a flow reversal in the acardiac recipient's artery. The continued survival of the non-viable twin adversely affects survival of the otherwise healthy twin.

The ability to occlude blood vessels was demonstrated at the turn of the millennium,[118, 119] but early work in fetal medicine using standard Doppler techniques (spectral, colour and flow Doppler) had some, but rather limited, success.[120, 121] However, recent advances in more sensitive Doppler techniques such as the ADF and superb microvascular imaging (SMI) developed by Toshiba Medical (now Canon Medical Systems) have allowed successful pre-clinical studies[122, 123] to lead to a phase I clinical trial. An example of successful occlusion of a placental anastomosis (shunt vessel) is shown in Figure 7.5.

REFERENCES

1. Fry WJ, Mosberg W, Barnard J, Fry F. Production of focal destructive lesions in the central nervous system with ultrasound. Journal of Neurosurgery. 1954;11(5):471–8.
2. Graham E, Hedges M, Leeman S, Vaughan P. Cavitational bio-effects of 1.5 MHz. Ultrasonics. 1980;18(5):224–8.
3. Hynynen K. Demonstration of enhanced temperature elevation due to nonlinear propagation of focussed ultrasound in dog's thigh in vivo. Ultrasound in Medicine & Biology. 1987;13(2):85–91.
4. Göbl R. Receive beamforming in medical ultrasound – A review of aperture data processing. Authorea Preprints. 2023 Oct 30.
5. Demi L. Practical guide to ultrasound beam forming: Beam pattern and image reconstruction analysis. Applied Sciences. 2018;8(9):1544.
6. Rabkin BA, Zderic V, Vaezy S. Hyperecho in ultrasound images of HIFU therapy: Involvement of cavitation. Ultrasound Med Biol. 2005;31(7):947–56.
7. Rabkin BA, Zderic V, Crum LA, Vaezy S. Biological and physical mechanisms of HIFU-induced hyperecho in ultrasound images. Ultrasound Med Biol. 2006;32(11):1721–9.
8. Yu T, Xu C. Hyperecho as the indicator of tissue necrosis during microbubble-assisted high intensity focused ultrasound: Sensitivity, specificity and predictive value. Ultrasound Med Biol. 2008;34(8):1343–7.

9. Fukuda H, Numata K, Nozaki A, Kondo M, Morimoto M, Tanaka K, et al. Hyperecho in ultrasound images during high-intensity focused ultrasound ablation for hepatocellular carcinomas. Eur J Radiol. 2011;80(3):e571–5.
10. McLaughlan J, Rivens I, Leighton T, ter Haar G. A study of bubble activity generated in ex vivo tissue by high intensity focused ultrasound. Ultrasound Med Biol. 2010;36(8):1327–44.
11. Marquez S, Leija L, Vera A. Influence of temperature variations on the average grayscale of B-mode images of HIFU-induced lesions. Conf Proc IEEE Eng Med Biol Soc. 2010;2010:5983–6.
12. Niemczewski B. A Comparison of Ultrasonic Cavitation Intensity in Liquids. Ultrasonics. 1980;18(3):107–10.
13. Ramble DG, Phelps AD, Leighton TG. On the relation between surface waves on a bubble and the subharmonic combination-frequency emission. Acustica. 1998;84(5):986–8.
14. Vykhodtseva NI, Hynynen K, Damianou C. Histologic effects of high intensity pulsed ultrasound exposure with subharmonic emission in rabbit brain in vivo. Ultrasound Med Biol. 1995;21(7): 969–79.
15. Johnston K, Tapia-Siles C, Gerold B, Postema M, Cochran S, Cuschieri A, et al. Periodic shock-emission from acoustically driven cavitation clouds: A source of the subharmonic signal. Ultrasonics. 2014;54(8):2151–8.
16. Madanshetty SI, Roy RA, Apfel RE. Acoustic microcavitation – Its active and passive acoustic detection. Journal of the Acoustical Society of America. 1991;90(3):1515–26.
17. Atchley AA, Frizzell LA, Apfel RE, Holland CK, Madanshetty S, Roy RA. Thresholds for cavitation produced in water by pulsed ultrasound. Ultrasonics. 1988;26(5):280–5.
18. McLaughlan J, Rivens I, ter Haar G, Shaw A, Leighton T, Humphrey V, et al. The design and implementation of a passive cavitation detection system for use with ex vivo tissue. Therapeutic Ultrasound. 2006;829:338-+.
19. Morse SV, Pouliopoulos AN, Chan TG, Copping MJ, Lin JL, Long NJ, et al. Rapid short-pulse ultrasound delivers drugs uniformly across the murine blood-brain barrier with negligible disruption. Radiology. 2019;291(2):458–65.
20. Lin KW, Kim Y, Maxwell AD, Wang TY, Hall TL, Xu Z, et al. Histotripsy beyond the intrinsic cavitation threshold using very short ultrasound pulses: Microtripsy. IEEE Trans Ultrason Ferroelectr Freq Control. 2014;61(2):251–65.
21. Richardson E. Supersonic vibrations and their applications. Journal of the Royal Society of Arts. 1947;95(4734):90–105.
22. Roy RA, Atchley AA, Crum LA, Fowlkes JB, Reidy JJ. A precise technique for the measurement of acoustic cavitation thresholds and some preliminary results. The Journal of the Acoustical Society of America. 1985;78(5):1799–805.
23. Stockwell RG, Mansinha L, Lowe RP. Localization of the complex spectrum: The S transform. IEEE T Signal Proces. 1996;44(4):998–1001.
24. Boashash B, Black PJ. An efficient real-time implementation of the Wigner Ville distribution. IEEE T Acoust Speech. 1987;35(11):1611–8.
25. Crake C, Brinker ST, Coviello CM, Livingstone MS, McDannold NJ. A dual-mode hemispherical sparse array for 3D passive acoustic mapping and skull localization within a clinical MRI guided focused ultrasound device. Physics in Medicine and Biology. 2018;63(6).
26. Kilinc MS, Lee H, Arvanitis CD, Degertekin FL. Dual mode CMUT array operation for skull imaging and passive acoustic monitoring in transcranial ultrasound. 2021 IEEE International Ultrasonics Symposium (IUS) 2021 Sep 11 (pp. 1–4). IEEE.
27. Lin HC, Yeh CK, Liu HL. Strategy in passively reconstructing and correcting transcranial focal beam via dual-mode ultrasound phased array. 2021 IEEE International Ultrasonics Symposium (IUS) 2021 Sep 11 (pp. 1–4). IEEE.
28. Hoang TN, Lin HC, Tsai CH, Jan CK, Liu HL. Passive cavitation enhancement mapping via an ultrasound dual-mode phased array to monitor blood-brain barrier opening. J Med Biol Eng. 2022;42(6):757–66.
29. Gyongy M, Coussios CC. Passive spatial mapping of inertial cavitation during HIFU exposure. IEEE Trans Biomed Eng. 2010;57(1):48–56.
30. Salgaonkar VA, Datta S, Holland CK, Mast TD. Passive cavitation imaging with ultrasound arrays. J Acoust Soc Am. 2009;126(6):3071–83.
31. Coviello C, Kozick R, Choi J, Gyongy M, Jensen C, Smith PP, et al. Passive acoustic mapping utilizing optimal beamforming in ultrasound therapy monitoring. J Acoust Soc Am. 2015;137(5):2573–85.

32. Gray MD, Coussios CC. Broadband ultrasonic attenuation estimation and compensation with passive acoustic mapping. IEEE T Ultrason Ferr. 2018;65(11):1997–2011.
33. Gray MD, Lyka E, Coussios CC. Diffraction effects and compensation in passive acoustic mapping. IEEE T Ultrason Ferr. 2018;65(2):258–68.
34. Gray MD, Coussios CC. Compensation of array lens effects for improved co-registration of passive acoustic mapping and B-mode images for cavitation monitoring. Journal of the Acoustical Society of America. 2019;146(1):El78–El84.
35. Gray MD, Elbes D, Paverd C, Lyka E, Coviello CM, Cleveland RO, et al. Dual-array passive acoustic mapping for cavitation imaging with enhanced 2-D resolution. IEEE T Ultrason Ferr. 2021;68(3):647–63.
36. Jones RM, O'Reilly MA, Hynynen K. Transcranial passive acoustic mapping with hemispherical sparse arrays using CT-based skull-specific aberration corrections: A simulation study. Physics in Medicine and Biology. 2013;58(14):4981–5005.
37. Lu SK, Zhao Y, Li RY, Wang DY, Yu XB, Zhang B, et al. Enhanced hemispherical-array passive acoustic mapping utilizing dual apodization with cross-correlation. 2020 IEEE International Ultrasonics Symposium (IUS) 2020 Sep 7 (pp. 1–4). IEEE.
38. Zhu H, Huang YM, Jin GF, Cai XR. Ring array passive acoustic mapping using hybrid heterogeneous angular spectrum method. 2022 IEEE International Ultrasonics Symposium (IUS) 2022 Oct 10 (pp. 1–4). IEEE.
39. Bailey MR, Pishchalnikov YA, Sapozhnikov OA, Cleveland RO, McAteer JA, Miller NA, et al. Cavitation detection during shock-wave lithotripsy. Ultrasound Med Biol. 2005;31(9):1245–56.
40. Poliachik SL, Chandler WL, Mourad PD, Ollos RJ, Crum LA. Activation, aggregation and adhesion of platelets exposed to high-intensity focused ultrasound. Ultrasound Med Biol. 2001;27(11):1567–76.
41. Datta S, Coussios CC, McAdory LE, Tan J, Porter T, De Courten-Myers G, et al. Correlation of cavitation with ultrasound enhancement of thrombolysis. Ultrasound Med Biol. 2006;32(8):1257–67.
42. Wu J, Xie F, Kumar T, Liu J, Lof J, Shi W, et al. Improved sonothrombolysis from a modified diagnostic transducer delivering impulses containing a longer pulse duration. Ultrasound Med Biol. 2014;40(7):1545–53.
43. Yang W, Zhou Y. Effect of pulse repetition frequency of high-intensity focused ultrasound on in vitro thrombolysis. Ultrason Sonochem. 2017;35(Pt A):152–60.
44. Hwang JH, Tu J, Brayman AA, Matula TJ, Crum LA. Correlation between inertial cavitation dose and endothelial cell damage in vivo. Ultrasound Med Biol. 2006;32(10):1611–9.
45. Zhang S, Wan M, Zhong H, Xu C, Liao Z, Liu H, et al. Dynamic changes of integrated backscatter, attenuation coefficient and bubble activities during high-intensity focused ultrasound (HIFU) treatment. Ultrasound Med Biol. 2009;35(11):1828–44.
46. Zhou Y, Gao XW. Variations of bubble cavitation and temperature elevation during lesion formation by high-intensity focused ultrasound. J Acoust Soc Am. 2013;134(2):1683–94.
47. Tu J, Hwang JH, Matula TJ, Brayman AA, Crum LA. Intravascular inertial cavitation activity detection and quantification in vivo with Optison. Ultrasound Med Biol. 2006;32(10):1601–9.
48. Tu J, Matula TJ, Brayman AA, Crum LA. Inertial cavitation dose produced in ex vivo rabbit ear arteries with Optison by 1-MHz pulsed ultrasound. Ultrasound Med Biol. 2006;32(2):281–8.
49. Ammi AY, Cleveland RO, Mamou J, Wang GI, Bridal SL, O'Brien WD. Double passive cavitation detection of Optison™ shell rupture. Ultrason. 2005:846–9.
50. Tung YS, Choi JJ, Baseri B, Konofagou EE. Identifying the inertial cavitation threshold and skull effects in a vessel phantom using focused ultrasound and microbubbles. Ultrasound Med Biol. 2010;36(5):840–52.
51. Tung YS, Vlachos F, Choi JJ, Deffieux T, Selert K, Konofagou EE. In vivo transcranial cavitation threshold detection during ultrasound-induced blood-brain barrier opening in mice. Phys Med Biol. 2010;55(20):6141–55.
52. Lin Y, Lin L, Cheng M, Jin L, Du L, Han T, et al. Effect of acoustic parameters on the cavitation behavior of SonoVue microbubbles induced by pulsed ultrasound. Ultrason Sonochem. 2017;35(Pt A):176–84.
53. McDannold N, Vykhodtseva N, Hynynen K. Targeted disruption of the blood-brain barrier with focused ultrasound: Association with cavitation activity. Phys Med Biol. 2006;51(4):793–807.
54. Konofagou EE, Tung YS, Choi J, Deffieux T, Baseri B, Vlachos F. Ultrasound-induced blood-brain barrier opening. Curr Pharm Biotechnol. 2012;13(7):1332–45.
55. Kamimura HAS, Flament J, Valette J, Cafarelli A, Badin RA, Hantraye P, et al. Passive cavitation detection-based feedback control for ultrasound-mediated blood-brain barrier opening in non-human primates. 2017 IEEE International Ultrasonics Symposium (IUS) 2017 Sep 6 (pp. 1–4). IEEE.

56. Mouratidis PXE, Costa M, Rivens I, Repasky EE, ter Haar G. Pulsed focused ultrasound can improve the anti-cancer effects of immune checkpoint inhibitors in murine pancreatic cancer. Journal of the Royal Society Interface. 2021;18(180).
57. Cespedes I, Ophir J, Ponnekanti H, Maklad N. Elastography – Elasticity imaging using ultrasound with application to muscle and breast in-vivo. Ultrasonic Imaging. 1993;15(2):73–88.
58. Miller NR, Bamber JC, Doyley MM, Leach MO. Visual detectability of elastic contrast in real-time ultrasound images. P Soc Photo-Opt Ins. 1997;3036:264–72.
59. Wu T, Felmlee JP, Greenleaf JF, Riederer SJ, Ehman RL. MR imaging of shear waves generated by focused ultrasound. Magn Reson Med. 2000;43(1):111–5.
60. Ophir J, Cespedes I, Ponnekanti H, Yazdi Y, Li X. Elastography – a quantitative method for imaging the elasticity of biological tissues. Ultrasonic Imaging. 1991;13(2):111–34.
61. Parker KJ, Doyley MM, Rubens DJ. Imaging the elastic properties of tissue: The 20 year perspective. Phys Med Biol. 2011;56(1):R1-R29.
62. Nightingale KR, Palmeri ML, Nightingale RW, Trahey GE. On the feasibility of remote palpation using acoustic radiation force. The Journal of the Acoustical Society of America. 2001;110(1):625–34.
63. Melodelima D, Bamber JC, Duck FA, Shipley JA. Transient elastography using impulsive ultrasound radiation force: A preliminary comparison with surface palpation elastography. Ultrasound Med Biol. 2007;33(6):959–69.
64. Souchon R, Salomir R, Beuf O, Milot L, Grenier D, Lyonnet D, et al. Transient MR elastography (t-MRE) using ultrasound radiation force: Theory, safety, and initial experiments in vitro. Magn Reson Med. 2008;60(4):871–81.
65. Sarvazyan AP, Rudenko OV, Swanson DS, Fowlkes BJ, Emelianov SY. Shear wave elasticity imaging: A new ultrasonic technology of medical diagnostics. Ultrasound in Medicine & Biology. 1998 24(9):1419–35.
66. Bercoff J, Pernot M, Tanter M, Fink M. Monitoring thermally-induced lesions with supersonic shear imaging. Ultrason Imaging. 2004;26(2):71–84.
67. Castera L, Vergniol J, Foucher J, Le Bail B, Chanteloup E, Haaser M, et al. Transient elastography (FibroScan®) a novel, non-invasive sensitive method for the assessment of liver fibrosis in chronic hepatitis C.: A prospective evaluation in comparison with liver biopsy, Fibrotest and APRI. Hepatology. 2004;40(4):679a–a.
68. Oeda S, Tanaka K, Oshima A, Matsumoto Y, Sueoka E, Takahashi H. Diagnostic accuracy of FibroScan and factors affecting measurements. Diagnostics. 2020;10(11).
69. Sugimoto T, Ueha S, Itoh K. Tissue hardness measurement using the radiation force of focused ultrasound. Ultrason. 1990:1377–80.
70. Hiltawsky KM, Krüger M, Starke C, Heuser L, Ermert H, Jensen A. Freehand ultrasound elastography of breast lesions: Clinical results. Ultrasound in Medicine and Biology. 2001;27(11):1461–9.
71. Righetti R, Kallel F, Stafford RJ, Price RE, Krouskop TA, Hazle JD, et al. Elastographic characterization of HIFU-induced lesions in canine livers. Ultrasound Med Biol. 1999;25(7):1099–113.
72. Stafford JR, Kallel F, Price RE, Cromeens DM, Krouskop TA, Hazle JD, et al. Elastographic imaging of thermal lesions in soft tissue: A preliminary study in vitro. Ultrasound Med Biol. 1998 24(9):1449–58.
73. Kallel F, Stafford RJ, Price RE, Righetti R, Ophir J, Hazle JD. The feasibility of elastographic visualization of HIFU-induced thermal lesions in soft tissues. Image-guided high-intensity focused ultrasound. Ultrasound Med Biol. 1999;25(4):641–7.
74. Lorenz A, Ermert H, Sommerfeld HJ, Garcia-Schürmann M, Senge T, Philippou S. Ultrasound elastography of the prostate: An innovative technique for tumour-detection. Ultraschall in Der Medizin. 2000;21(1):8–15.
75. Fatemi M, Manduca A, Greenleaf JF. Imaging elastic properties of biological tissues by low-frequency harmonic vibration. Proceedings of the IEEE. 2003;91(10):1503–19.
76. Walker WF, Negron LA, Mondzelewski TJ, McAllister MJ, Fernandez FJ, Toth CA. Imaging the stiffness of the vitreous body with acoustic radiation force. Ultrason. 1999:1635–9.
77. de Korte CL, Céspedes EI, van der Steen AFW, Norder B, te Nijenhuis K. Elastic and acoustic properties of vessel mimicking material for elasticity imaging. Ultrasonic Imaging. 1997;19(2):112–26.
78. Parker KJ, Fu D, Graceswki SM, Yeung F, Levinson SF. Vibration sonoelastography and the detectability of lesions. Ultrasound in Medicine & Biology. 1998;24(9):1437–47.
79. Xia R, Thittai AK. Real-time monitoring of high-intensity focused ultrasound treatment using axial strain and axial-shear strain elastograms. Ultrasound Med Biol. 2014;40(3):485–95.

80. Zhang M, Castaneda B, Christensen J, Saad WE, Bylund K, Hoyt K, et al. Real-time sonoelastography of hepatic thermal lesions in a swine model. Med Phys. 2008;35(9):4132–41.
81. Marigliano C, Panzironi G, Molisso L, Pizzuto A, Ciolina F, Napoli A, et al. First experience of real-time elastography with transvaginal approach in assessing response to MRgFUS treatment of uterine fibroids. Radiol Med. 2016;121(12):926–34.
82. Maass-Moreno R, Damianou CA, Sanghvi NT. Noninvasive temperature estimation in tissue via ultrasound echo-shifts. Part II. In vitro study. J Acoust Soc Am. 1996;100(4 Pt 1):2522–30.
83. Bilaniuk N, Wong GSK. Speed of sound in pure water as a function of temperature. Journal of the Acoustical Society of America. 1993;93(3):1609–12.
84. Bamber JC, Hill CR. Ultrasonic attenuation and propagation speed in mammalian tissues as a function of temperature. Ultrasound Med Biol. 1979;5:149–57.
85. Seip R, VanBaren P, Cain CA, Ebbini ES. Noninvasive real-time multipoint temperature control for ultrasound phased array treatments. IEEE T Ultrason Ferr. 1996;43(6):1063–73.
86. Civale J, Rivens I, ter Haar G, Morris H, Coussios C, Friend P, et al. Calibration of ultrasound backscatter temperature imaging for high-intensity focused ultrasound treatment planning. Ultrasound Med Biol. 2013;39(9):1596–612.
87. Connor CW, Hynynen K. Bio-acoustic thermal lensing and nonlinear propagation in focused ultrasound surgery using large focal spots: A parametric study. Phys Med Biol. 2002;47:1911–28.
88. Miller NR, Bamber JC, Meaney PM. Fundamental limitations of noninvasive temperature imaging by means of ultrasound echo strain estimation. Ultrasound in Medicine and Biology. 2002;28(10):1319–33.
89. Anand A, Savery D, Hall C. Three-dimensional spatial and temporal temperature imaging in gel phantoms using backscattered ultrasound. IEEE Trans Ultrason Ferroelectr Freq Control. 2007;54(1):23–31.
90. Seip R, Ebbini ES. Noninvasive estimation of tissue temperature response to heating fields using diagnostic ultrasound. IEEE T Bio-Med Eng. 1995;42(8):828–39.
91. Wear KA, Wagner RF, Insana MF, Hall TJ. Application of autoregressive spectral-analysis to cepstral estimation of mean scatterer spacing. IEEE T Ultrason Ferr. 1993;40(1):50–8.
92. Miller NR, Bamber JC, ter Haar GR. Imaging of temperature-induced echo strain: Preliminary in vitro study to assess feasibility for guiding focused ultrasound surgery. Ultrasound Med Biol. 2004;30(3):345–56.
93. Souchon R, Bouchoux G, Maciejko E, Lafon C, Cathignol D, Bertrand M, et al. Monitoring the formation of thermal lesions with heat-induced echo-strain imaging: A feasibility study. Ultrasound Med Biol. 2005;31(2):251–9.
94. Liu DL, Ebbini ES. Real-time two-dimensional temperature imaging using ultrasound. 2009 Annual International Conference of the IEEE Engineering in Medicine and Biology Society, Vols 1–20. 2009:1971-+.
95. Ballard JR, Casper AJ, Ebbini ES. Image-guided refocusing of dual-mode ultrasound arrays (DMUAs). Ultrason. 2008:1183–6.
96. Ballard JR, Casper AJ, Ebbini ES. Monitoring and Guidance of HIFU Beams with Dual-Mode Ultrasound Arrays. Annual International Conference of the IEEE Engineering in Medicine and Biology Society, Vols 1–20. 2009:137–40.
97. Arthur RM, Straube WL, Starman JD, Moros EG. Noninvasive temperature estimation based on the energy of backscattered ultrasound. Medical Physics. 2003;30(6):1021–9.
98. Ju KC, Liu HL. Zero-crossing tracking technique for noninvasive ultrasonic temperature estimation. J Ultrasound Med. 2010;29(11):1607–15.
99. Huang CW, Lien DH, Chen BT, Shieh J, Tsui PH, Chen CS, et al. Ultrasound thermal mapping based on a hybrid method combining cross-correlation and zero-crossing tracking. J Acoust Soc Am. 2013;134(2):1530–40.
100. Green PS, Arditi M. Ultrasonic reflex transmission imaging. Ultrason Imaging. 1985;7(3):201–14.
101. Marich KW, Stein A, Pell JW, Jensen JF, Schattner P, Green PS. Reflex transmission imaging improves ultrasonic visualization and characterization of calculi for lithotripsy applications. Journal of Stone Disease. 1992;4(1):46–51.
102. Green PS, Ostrem JS, Whitehurst TK. Combined reflection and transmission ultrasound imaging. Ultrasound Med Biol. 1991;17(3):283–9.
103. Baker LAS, Bamber JC. Performance of reflex transmission imaging (RTI) using a linear array. Ultrason. 2001:1551–4.

104. Baker LAS, Bamber JC. Effect of dynamic receive focusing on reflex transmission imaging (RTI). Ultrason. 2002:1581–4.
105. Rallan D, Dickson M, Bush NL, Harland CC, Mortimer P, Bamber JC. High-resolution ultrasound reflex transmission imaging and digital photography: Potential tools for the quantitative assessment of pigmented lesions. Skin Research and Technology. 2006;12(1):50–9.
106. Bamber JC, Bush NL, Haddock MC, Ott RJ, Rallan D, Harland CC. Combining high frequency ultrasound reflex transmission imaging and imaging spectrophotometry for the diagnosis of skin cancer. IEEE Ultrasonics Symposium Proceedings. 2007;1–6:248-+.
107. Hayner M, Hynynen K. Numerical analysis of ultrasonic transmission and absorption of oblique plane waves through the human skull. The Journal of the Acoustical Society of America. 2001;110(6):3319–30.
108. King RL, Clement GT, Maruvada S, Hynynen K. Preliminary results using ultrasound transmission for image-guided thermal therapy. Ultrasound Med Biol. 2003;29(2):293–9.
109. Bush NL, Rivens I, ter Haar GR, Bamber JC. Acoustic properties of lesions generated with an ultrasound therapy system. Ultrasound Med Biol. 1993;19(9):789–801.
110. Farny CH, Clement GT. Ultrasound phase contrast thermal imaging with reflex transmission imaging methods in tissue phantoms. Ultrasound in Medicine and Biology. 2009;35(12):1995–2006.
111. Rallan D, Bush NL, Bamber JC, Harland CC. Quantitative discrimination of pigmented lesions using three-dimensional high-resolution ultrasound reflex transmission imaging. Journal of Investigative Dermatology. 2007;127(1):189–95.
112. Guittet CM, Bamber JC, Bush NL, Bell DS, Mortimer PS. High frequency reflex transmission imaging: Feasibility for eventual application to the diagnosis of skin tumours. Acoust Imag. 2000;25:325–30.
113. Marich KW, Stein A, Pell JW, Jensen JF, Schattner P, Green PS. Reflex transmission imaging improves ultrasonic visualization and characterization of calculi for lithotripsy applications. J Stone Dis. 1992;4(1):46–51.
114. Malcolm AL. An investigation into ultrasonic methods of imaging the tissue ablation induced during focused ultrasound surgery. Institute of Cancer Research, Sutton: University of London; 1997.
115. Farny CH, Clement GT. Thermal imaging with ultrasound reflex transmission methods. Ultrason. 2008:2088–91.
116. Schattner P, Whitehurst TK, Jensen JF, Shah AS, Green PS. Three-dimensional ultrasonic reflection and attenuation imaging. IEEE Trans Ultrason Ferroelectr Freq Control. 1992;39(1):102–11.
117. Farny CH, Clement GT. Towards a reflex transmission method for ultrasound thermometry. Ultrason. 2007:1796–9.
118. Rivens I, Rowland IJ, Denbow M, Fisk NM, ter Haar GR, Leach MO. Vascular occlusion using focused ultrasound surgery for use in fetal medicine. European Journal of Ultrasound. 1999;9:89–97.
119. Denbow ML, Rivens IH, Rowland IJ, Leach MO, Fisk NM, ter Haar GR. Preclinical development of noninvasive vascular occlusion with focused ultrasonic surgery for fetal therapy. American Journal of Obstetrics and Gynecology. 2000;182(2):387–92.
120. Ichizuka K, Hasegawa J, Nakamura M, Matsuoka R, Sekizawa A, Okai T, et al. High-intensity focused ultrasound treatment for twin reversed arterial perfusion sequence. Ultrasound Obstet Gynecol. 2012;40(4):476–8.
121. Okai T, Ichizuka K, Hasegawa J, Matsuoka R, Nakamura M, Shimodaira K, et al. First successful case of non-invasive in-utero treatment of twin reversed arterial perfusion sequence by high-intensity focused ultrasound. Ultrasound Obstet Gynecol. 2013;42(1):112–4.
122. Shaw CJ, ter Haar GR, Rivens IH, Giussani DA, Lees CC. Pathophysiological mechanisms of high-intensity focused ultrasound-mediated vascular occlusion and relevance to non-invasive fetal surgery. J R Soc Interface. 2014;11(95):20140029.
123. Shaw CJ, Civale J, Botting KJ, Niu Y, ter Haar G, Rivens I, et al. Noninvasive high-intensity focused ultrasound treatment of twin-twin transfusion syndrome: A preliminary in vivo study. Sci Transl Med. 2016;8(347):347ra95.

8

Extracorporeal Ultrasound-Guided HIFU Devices – Clinical Application, Treatment Planning and B-mode Ultrasound for Real-Time Monitoring and Control of Treatment

Feng Wu and Fa-Qi Li

8.1 Introduction

The use of heat to destroy human tumours has a long history. Five thousand years ago, ancient Egyptians reported that they used cautery with heated implements for the treatment of superficial tumours in medical practice.[1] The concept of using high intensity focused ultrasound (HIFU) for destroying diseased tissues dates back more than 80 years. In 1942, Lynn and colleagues[2] found for the first time that HIFU could destroy tissue at depth without any damage to overlying tissues. The brothers William and Frank Fry[3, 4] in the United States did much of the early laboratory work related to therapeutic ultrasound (US) in the 1950s. They found that HIFU-induced lesions were well circumscribed and that a deep brain lesion could be successfully produced in animals after removing a piece of the skull. In collaboration with Russell Meyers, a neurosurgeon, they developed a prototype HIFU neurosurgery device and conducted the first ultrasonic surgery on a human brain in 1957.[5] A total of 87 patients, including those with Parkinson's disease, cerebral palsy, stroke, phantom images, and pain following amputation, received HIFU afterwards.[6] Of these, 50 patients with Parkinson's disease were treated under local anaesthetic following the craniotomy.[7] Although the procedure took 14 hours, it was claimed that the symptoms were eliminated immediately in some patients. Unfortunately, this treatment could not continue at that time due to the concurrent development of the drug L-dopa, which appeared to be a more acceptable option for Parkinson's disease. In addition, the requirement to remove a section of the skull bone, in combination with the technical complexity, also limited the progress of the HIFU neurosurgery.

In the 1980s, HIFU was also used in ophthalmology to treat patients with glaucoma. Lizzi and Coleman developed an extracorporeal HIFU device in the United States, the Sonocare CST-100 therapeutic ultrasound system.[8] This was the first HIFU device to receive pre-market approval from the U.S. Food and Drug Administration (FDA).[9] They treated 880 glaucoma patients with encouraging clinical results. Of these, 79.3% of patients showed a significant decrease of intra-ocular pressure after 1 year.[10] They also used this ophthalmological device to explore the possibility of treating choroidal melanomas and capsular tears, and their early results seemed promising.[11, 12] However, the advent of laser surgery occurred simultaneously in clinical ophthalmology. The laser has superseded HIFU in terms of its wider success and application, presumably due to its apparently simpler technology and application.

Based on a shock-wave lithotripsy technique, Vallancien and colleagues in France constructed an extracorporeal ultrasound-guided HIFU (USgHIFU) device for the treatment of superficial bladder tumours in the 1990s. In the first phase I trial, five patients underwent HIFU treatment, followed by cystoscopic examination. They found that the treated tumour disappeared in 2 cases and coagulation

DOI: 10.1201/9780429162671-8

necrosis was observed in the remaining 3 patients.[13] Subsequently, 25 patients with low-grade superficial bladder tumours were recruited in a phase II trial. After HIFU treatment, 67% of the patients were tumour free at 1 year and no invasion or metastasis was detected during follow-up of 3–21 months.[14] They used the same device to treat 2 patients with metastatic liver cancer prior to surgical resection. Unfortunately, the results were unsatisfactory, including one with no visible thermal effects in the treated lesion, and another with extensive tissue laceration and patchy necrosis.[15]

ter Haar in the UK reported an USgHIFU prototype device in the 1990s. This device used a spherical ceramic transducer 10 cm in diameter. It was driven at a frequency of 1.7 MHz and operated at free field spatial intensities between 1000 W. cm^{-2} and 4660 W. cm^{-2}.[16] The device treated 68 patients in a phase I trial, and the results showed that the HIFU treatment was well tolerated. Some moderate local pain was observed, but only in a few patients.[17]

The team at Chongqing Medical University in China started their HIFU project in 1988. At the beginning the focus was on in vitro studies to investigate the biological effects of focused ultrasound on different tissues and cells, and this then moved to in vivo studies in implanted-tumour models of small animals, particularly in rabbit VX_2 tumours. A prototype extracorporeal USgHIFU device was constructed for a large animal study in 1995. Pigs, goats and monkeys were treated in an attempt to simulate a clinical HIFU procedure. Based on the results of the large animal study, successful clinical strategies for performing real-time B-mode ultrasound imaging for HIFU planning, targeting, monitoring and tumour response assessment were established, as was feedback control of therapeutic ultrasound energy. In 1997, the first clinical USgHIFU device was built, and recruitment of cancer patients for several clinical trials started. From 1997 to 2001 this device was used to treat 1,038 patients with solid tumours in 10 Chinese hospitals, including those of the liver, breast, pancreas, kidney, uterus, bone and soft tissues.[18] It became the first China Food and Drug Administration (CFDA) approved HIFU device for solid tumours and gained Conformité Européenne (CE) approval in Europe in 2005.

Due to rapid development of the HIFU device manufacture and clinical use in China, three important national documents were published in 2005, including a manufacturer's standard, quality assurance for USgHIFU devices and HIFU clinical applications. In March 2005, the Chinese Medical Association published the first clinical guideline for HIFU therapy "Guidelines for clinical applications of high intensity focused ultrasound cancer therapy system".[19] This guideline clarified the clinical requirements for USgHIFU devices and operators, indications and contraindications, the determination of therapeutic dosage and radiological and clinical assessments of HIFU therapy. In September 2005, China also promulgated a national standard GB/T 19890–2005 "Acoustics – high intensity focused ultrasound (HIFU) measurements of acoustic power and field characteristics". This was the first national standard for quality assurance of HIFU devices in the world, and the International Electrotechnical Commission issued it afterwards as an annex in its technical report IEC/TR 62649:2010 "Requirements for measurement standards for high intensity therapeutic ultrasound (HITU) devices". In December 2005, CFDA issued the national industry standard YY0592–2005 "High intensity focused ultrasound therapy system" for manufacturing USgHIFU devices. This standard specified HIFU therapy system terminology and definitions, classification, requirements, test methods, inspection rules and signs, packaging, transport and storage. These 3 national standards have significantly promoted the development of HIFU device manufacture and clinical use in China, where the greatest number of patients have received HIFU treatment in the world so far.

An extracorporeal USgHIFU device is generally used to treat tumours of the abdomen, pelvis, limbs and breast. It requires an appropriate acoustic window on the skin that allows access to the treatment site for which there is no gas in the propagation path. It is also important to couple the ultrasound energy to the skin surface using a water path, coupling gel, water balloon or other suitable material of similar acoustic impedance to that of the skin. Several commercial USgHIFU devices have been described for the treatment of patients with benign and malignant tumours in clinical settings. They are all similar in concept and integrate a B-mode ultrasound imaging probe into a therapeutic transducer for guidance and monitoring of the HIFU procedure.

8.2 Main System Components

An extracorporeal USgHIFU device mainly comprises the following components: (1) operator console, (2) motion scanning device, (3) treatment bed, (4) high-frequency generator, (5) integrated transducer (HIFU transducer combined with B-mode imaging probe) and (6) power and water control unit. The operator console has a treatment workstation and ultrasound imaging device, providing an operating platform, and real-time imaging guidance capability during HIFU procedure. The motion scanning device provides multiple dimensional movement of both HIFU transducer and ultrasound imaging probe. The main function of the treatment bed IS to support the patient. The generator provides high-frequency electrical signals that drive the HIFU transducer. The integrated treatment head includes a HIFU transducer and an ultrasound imaging probe that is embedded in its centre for real-time guidance and monitoring of the HIFU procedure. The main functions of the power and water control device are to distribute electric power to the system and to provide the degassed water for acoustic coupling required for the treatment. In what follows, examples are taken from the Chongqing HAIFU extracorporeal systems.

8.2.1 Operator Console

The operator console includes a diagnostic ultrasound scanner and a treatment computer with therapeutic software (Figure 8.1). The imaging device is mainly used for guiding the HIFU procedure in real time, such as targeting a tumour, making a treatment plan, observing the response of the treated tumour and controlling the exposure, based on greyscale changes at the focus on B-mode ultrasound image. The treatment software comprises a treatment planning system, digital evaluation of greyscale changes within the target tumour before and immediately after a HIFU exposure, treatment data storage, and data analysis.

8.2.2 Scanning Motion Device

Located under the treatment bed and controlled by the therapeutic software, the motion device can scan the integrated transducer in 3-dimensions (3-D). The exact nature of this depends on the device. For

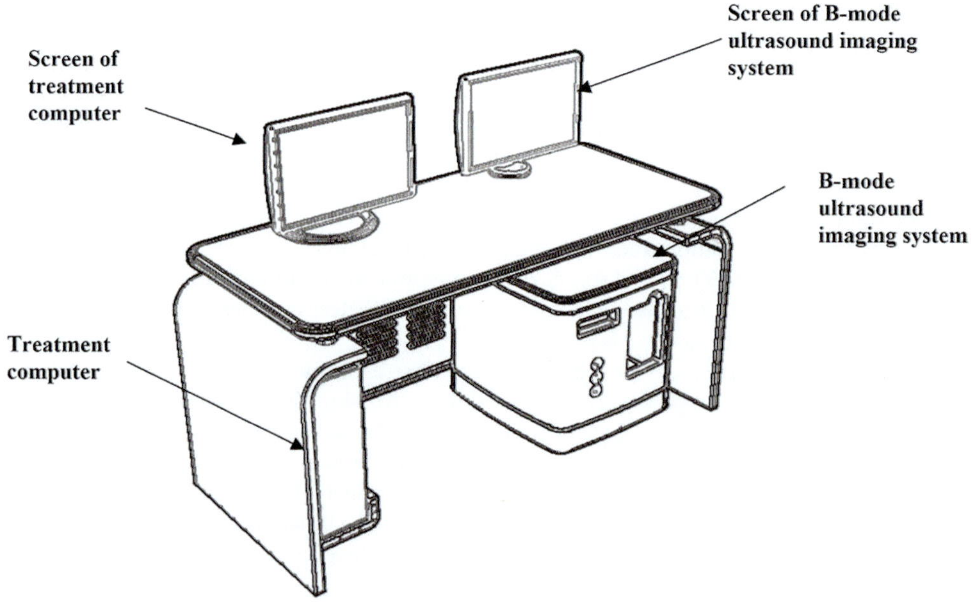

FIGURE 8.1 Schematic diagram of a central operator console.

example, the Chongqing HAIFU system has 2 components: (1) the imaging probe can be rotated in 360 degrees and moved vertically (up to down) and (2) the integrated transducer can be driven linearly in 3 directions including the X-, Y- and vertical axis. The relationship between the movement of the HIFU transducer and ultrasound imaging probe in this case is shown in Figure 8.2.

In this system, the imaging probe can move along a PZ axis and rotates around a PZ axis (PR movement). With the PZ movement, the imaging probe is above the HIFU transducer. The PR motion is a rotary motion around the PZ axis, leading to axis X and Y to rotate simultaneously. This can help to adjust the scanning plane of the imaging probe and make the target tumour easily accessible. Simultaneous linear motion of the HIFU transducer and imaging probe along the three axes X, Y and Z is possible. Movement in these three directions can change the spatial location of the HIFU focus directly.

8.2.3 Treatment Bed

The treatment bed is used to support patients for the treatment. In the Chongqing HAIFU system, there is a water reservoir under the bed, that contains degassed and temperature-controlled water, supplied from the water and power control unit, and circulated during HIFU procedures.

8.2.4 High Frequency Generator

The high frequency generator supplies electrical power to drive the HIFU transducer for treatment. To ensure greatest output efficiency, the high frequency generator requires appropriate matching to the transducer. As each transducer has its own frequency, the values for matching and feedback differ. When replacing the transducer, it is essential to adjust matching and feedback parameters, using the settings in the therapeutic software.

8.2.5 Integrated Transducer

As shown in Figure 8.3, for the Chongqing system, the integrated transducer consists of a HIFU transducer and a B-mode ultrasound imaging probe that is placed at its centre. It sits in a rubber water

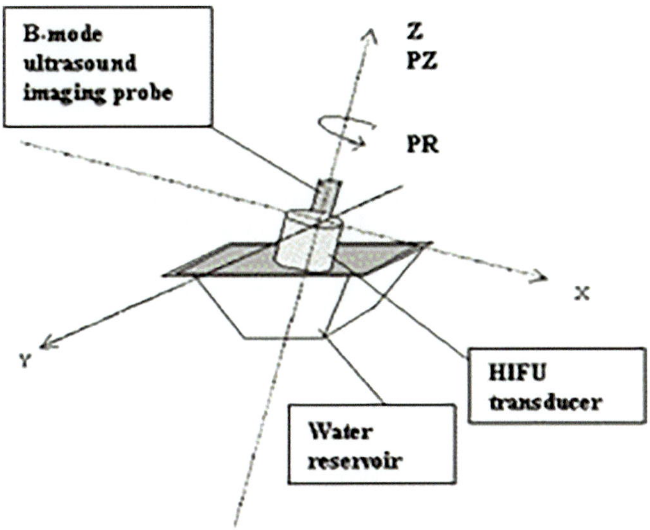

FIGURE 8.2 Schematic diagram showing all scanning motions. Arrows in the figure are in the direction of "positive" motion. The 3 linear movements, X, Y and Z, are perpendicular to each other. The 2 linear motions, PZ and Z, overlap completely with the same direction. PR is the rotary motion around the PZ axis.

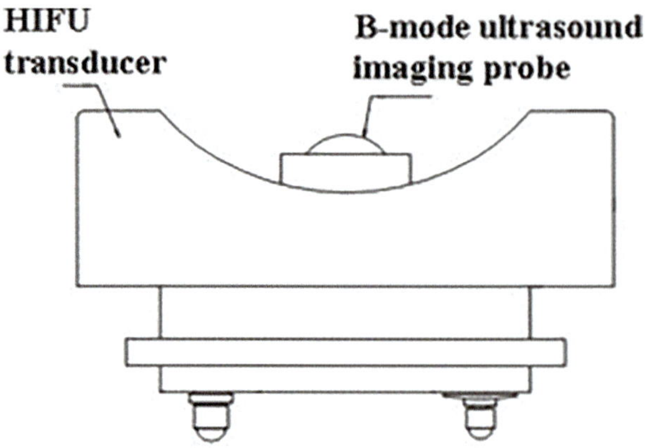

FIGURE 8.3 Schematic diagram of an integrated transducer consisting of a HIFU transducer with a B-mode ultrasound probe in the centre.

reservoir, which is filled with circulating degassed and temperature-controlled water. The focal region of the HIFU transducer lies within the scanning volume of the imaging probe to provide real-time guidance and monitoring of HIFU treatments and provide clear greyscale changes at the focus on real-time images during HIFU exposures. The imaging probe can move vertically and rotate, thus providing clear sectional images of the target tumour.

8.2.6 Power and Water Control Unit

Water provides acoustic coupling and allows the focused ultrasound beam to propagate from the transducer to the skin of a treated patient. If there are air bubbles in the coupling water, they can interfere and scatter focused ultrasound waves. If the bubbles gather on the surface of the skin, they can cause a skin burn during a HIFU procedure. Therefore, degassed and temperature-controlled water with dissolved oxygen less than 3.0 ppm is used. The electrical power can also be controlled in this unit, providing power to the HIFU system in a safe way.

8.3 HIFU Therapy Planning

The aim of HIFU treatments is to deliver focused ultrasound energy to a well-defined target volume at depth through the intact skin, and thus induce complete destruction of the tumour with no damage to overlying or surrounding tissues. The spatial distribution of the energy delivered depends mainly on a well-designed treatment plan, the therapeutic device and the doctor's expertise. The tumour geometry is specific for each patient in terms of location, size and shape. Based on the pretreatment images of the target tumour, a well-designed, 3-D HIFU therapy plan is essential to achieving successful treatment. In this section the processes of HIFU therapy planning, clinical and technical considerations for the treatment are introduced.

8.3.1 Aims of the HIFU Treatment

Most cancer patients receive a combination of local and systemic treatments in routine clinical practice. For example, patients with breast cancer receive local therapies such as surgery and radiation therapy which may be combined with systemic therapies including chemotherapy and hormone therapy. These are usually provided in tandem because clinical results show that the combination of these treatments can provide better survival benefit than one used in isolation. As HIFU is a local therapy (similar to the surgery), it requires combination with other therapies in clinical application.

The aims of HIFU therapy depend on the location and grade of the malignant tumour, the stage of the disease and the general performance of the patient. There are two main aims. For patients with early-stage, localised cancer, the intention of HIFU is to provide a curative option, an alternative to surgical removal of an entire tumour. To achieve this, HIFU should induce complete destruction of the target tumour including a tumour-free margin of healthy tissues. This is the surgical principle that has been used for a long time in the treatment of malignant tumours to prevent local recurrence, and may allow HIFU to replicate the success of surgical resection in the future. HIFU ablation margins can be visualised on post-treatment contrast-enhanced CT and MR images, which show an entire target tumour and healthy tissues surrounding it (Figure 8.4).

The second aim is to provide a debulking option for patients with advanced, late-stage cancer. These are usually those who have unresectable disease and for whom conventional therapies have failed to control tumour growth and metastasis. HIFU can be used clinically to debulk tumours, prolong survival time and improve quality of life. Most HIFU-treated cancer patients have advanced-stage diseases that are beyond the scope of conventional treatments. In these circumstances, HIFU has been successfully performed as a tumour debulking approach in clinical applications.

8.3.2 Pretreatment Images for Planning

Radiological examination provides the detailed characteristics of the target tumour, including its size, shape, margin, location, adjacent large blood vessels and nerves, as well as vital organs that might be at risk of injury by the HIFU treatment. Using contrast-enhanced techniques, tumour vascularity can be assessed in order to help determine the spatial distribution of the focused ultrasound energy delivered to the target tumour.

Images taken for HIFU treatment planning are usually different from those for diagnosis. Apart from imaging aspects of the tumour, adjacent organs, and vital structures such as large blood vessels and nerves, require more attention for safety reasons. Using available imaging techniques, the relationship between the tumour and its surrounding vital structures should be evaluated before and during therapy planning. For example, a hepatic tumour in the lower part of the left liver may be near to the stomach, duodenum, and colon. Ultrasonography, magnetic resonance imaging (MRI) and computed tomography (CT) imaging are important for assessing the relationship between the tumour and adjacent gastrointestinal tracts.

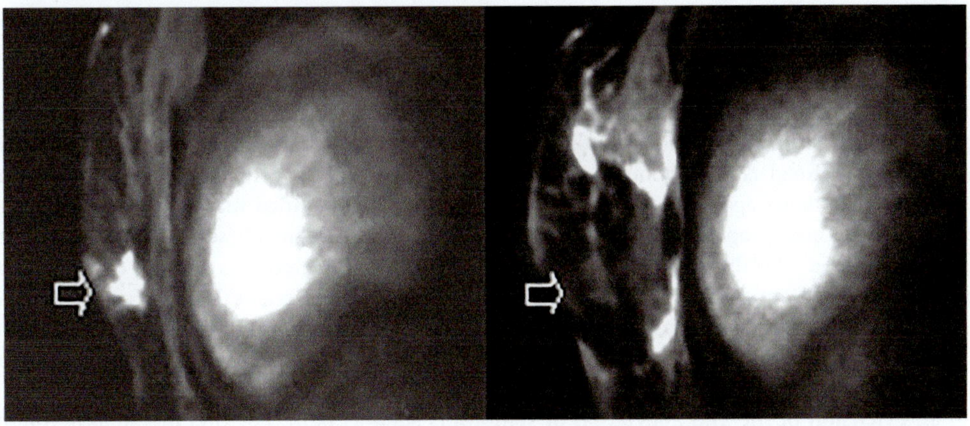

FIGURE 8.4 Sagittal contrast-enhanced T1-weighted MR images before and after USgHIFU treatment in a 36-year-old patient with breast cancer. Before HIFU (left), contrast enhancement is seen within the tumour in the left breast (arrow). However, 2 weeks after HIFU treatment (right), there is no enhancement in the treated tumour and healthy breast tissue surrounding the tumour (arrow), indicating that a surgical margin is achieved by the treatment. (From Wu F, et al. Ultrasound Med Bio 2004; 30:245–260.)[20]

Ultrasound imaging may be in B-mode, colour or power Doppler and microbubble contrast-enhanced imaging mode. MRI/CT examination includes non-contrast-enhanced and contrast-enhanced scans. They all provide tumour characteristics and can be used for essential therapy planning. In addition, both non-enhanced and enhanced MRI/CT scans can compensate for some of the shortcomings of ultrasound imaging, such as its lower sensitivity in predicting the tumour margin, and occasional poor detection of small liver tumours because of overlying ribs. Before establishing a therapeutic plan for each individual patient, a routine examination is required to compare the differences in scan appearances. The operators must mentally register a reference data set from MRI/CT scan and a working data set from ultrasound imaging. However, this may be challenging when the tumour is located behind the ribs, due to the deformation and displacement of the liver by respiration and by the limited acoustic window due to the ribcage and colon. Therefore, an ultrasound technique that entails fusion of B-mode ultrasound and MRI/CT imaging can help detect liver tumours with poor conspicuity and those shielded by the ribs, and reduce technique errors by accurate localisation of the target tumour.[21, 22] This image registration technique can also be used for clarifying the tumour margin, as will be described in Section 8.4.2.

8.3.3 Definition of Target Volume

The target volume is defined as the macroscopic extent of a target tumour, which may be palpable or be visible on radiological imaging. As the determination of the target volume is dependent on CT/MRI scans and ultrasound imaging, it is important to know which radiological images have been used prior to treatment planning.

The definition of the target volume is based on knowledge from surgical and postmortem specimens, radiological imaging, and the patterns of tumour recurrence, as well as from clinical experience. Because cancer cells probably extend beyond the visible tumour margins into normal tissues, surgery often involves removal of the entire tumour along with a border of the normal tissue around it. The pathologist examines the edge of the removed tissue, called the surgical margin, to ensure that it is clear of cancer cells. If they are absent, the margin is described as being negative, suggesting that all cancer cells have been removed surgically. If the margin is described as being positive, this suggests that not all tumour cells have been removed and further treatment, such as additional surgery or radiation therapy, may be required.

The most challenging aspect of the planning process is the definition of the target volume. This is due to the lack of advanced radiological images that can accurately circumscribe a clear tumour-free margin. In addition, there is no standard definition of how wide "a clear margin" should be in minimally invasive ablation approaches. It is therefore clear that the definition of the target volume becomes problematic, and the failure to ablate a satisfactory margin may lead to a local recurrence after treatment.

To ensure the removal of nearby micro-satellites, and to allow for the uncertainty that exists regarding the exact location of tumour margins, HIFU has adopted the surgical principles used for curative treatments of patients with early-stage cancer and aims to ablate the entire visible target tumour and an estimated extent of the microscopic spread surrounding it. For example, although the definition of an adequate tumour-free margin depends on the tumour's histological type, the surgical margin for hepatocellular carcinoma (HCC) has been defined as being about 2 cm (but no less than 1 cm) of normal liver. However, several factors, such as the patient's age and considerations of normal tissue tolerance, may affect the maximum volume considered to be appropriate for HIFU treatment, since HCC is frequently seen in the setting of hepatic cirrhosis with partial liver dysfunction. Definition of the target volume requires cautious determination for each patient. If the extent of ablation is the same as that for surgical resections, HIFU may be equally effective, but with a considerably decreased risk of morbidity and mortality in this high-risk patient population.

If a treatment cannot be curative, HIFU may be a tumour debulking option in patients with advanced, late-stage cancer. The treatment aim is to reduce the tumour burden and to slow its progress, thus leading to an extension of life and alleviation of symptoms such as pain. For this therapeutic intent, the HIFU target volume is not as aggressive as for a curative treatment. When it is difficult to treat an entire tumour with HIFU, it is recommended to debulk the tumour as much as possible, with the least risk of adverse events that would negatively impact the quality of life. As HIFU is not a risk-free therapy, the risks versus potential benefits must be carefully considered case by case in clinical application.

8.3.4 HIFU Beam Path

The HIFU beam path is defined as the best route between the transducer and a target tumour along which the beam can be transmitted to the skin (through a coupling medium if required) and then through overlying tissue to the target. When the beam path is obstructed by bone and air-filled organs such as the bowels and lungs, the propagation and focusing of ultrasound waves becomes complex and may lead to a shift in the focal position, and unpredictable distribution of ultrasound energy delivered to the target. Reflection of the beam by structures in the pre-focal region may cause a significant drop in focal intensity, thus reducing the therapeutic energy deposited in the target. This may result both in undertreatment of the target, and in unwanted effects due to absorption in front of the focus.

The selection of an appropriate beam path is an important process during treatment planning. Because the ultrasound energy is attenuated as it penetrates tissue, the beam path chosen is usually the shortest route from the skin to the target tumour. It may be important to have a large acoustic window on the skin, in order that sufficient focusing can be obtained in the target. In clinical use it is important to reduce the intervening effects in overlying tissue as much as possible. For example, in patients with uterine fibroids, pretreatment scans (MRI/CT/US) can identify whether any bowel loops are interposed between the target fibroid and the expected path of the ultrasound beam. If a safe beam path to the target cannot be found, a HIFU procedure should be avoided because of potential risks of visceral organ injury that will lead to bowel perforation.

8.3.5 Ultrasonic Properties of Overlying Tissue

One of the challenges in HIFU treatments is the need to transmit sufficient energy through the overlying tissues to ablate a target tumour at depth. A focused ultrasound beam is attenuated by absorption, scattering and reflections while it propagates through the overlying tissues. The attenuation and reflection coefficients are dependent upon the ultrasonic properties of the overlying tissues. For example, when HIFU ablates a liver tumour through the ribcage, the ribs both absorb and reflect parts of the ultrasound beam, resulting in decreased ultrasound energy to below an ablation threshold at the focus and to overheating of the bone. Furthermore, the heterogeneity of the overlying tissues may change beam propagation direction, as well as the location, shape, and size of the focus. Thus, it is important to know the ultrasonic properties of the overlying tissues during therapy planning in order to achieve successful ablation and to avoid undesirable adverse events.

Ultrasound attenuation is a sum of the losses from absorption and scattering. Each tissue has a characteristic attenuation coefficient. For example, the amplitude attenuation coefficients in lung and bone are approximately 0.43–0.48 and 0.15–0.35 Np cm^{-1} MHz^{-1}.[23–25] Adipose tissue has lower values, ranging from 0.05 to 0.09 Np cm^{-1} MHz^{-1}, and soft tissue values are generally about 0.1 Np cm^{-1} MHz^{-1}.[26–28] The attenuation of solid tumours is often higher than for the relevant normal tissue. For example, the attenuation is higher in brain tumours than in the normal brain,[29] and a similar difference is also observed between breast cancer and normal breast tissue.[30] It should be remembered that when the deep part of a target tumour is treated, the overlying tissues usually include not only the normal tissue in front of the tumour but also the superficial part of the tumour.

The thermal properties of overlying tissues are also important during therapy planning. These depend primarily on a tissue's composition, but several factors can influence the heat flow path. Both thermal conductivity and diffusivity are essential for characterising the thermal properties of tissues. This is particularly important for therapeutic applications based on local tissue heating. Among mammalian skin, fat, muscle and bone, subcutaneous fat has the lowest value of thermal conductivity (0.233 Wm^{-1} K^{-1}), while muscle has the highest value (0.46 $Wm^{-}1$ $K^{-}1$).[31] Skin with subcutaneous fat has the lowest thermal diffusivity (0.11 mm^2 $s^{-}1$), while muscle has the highest value (0.16 mm^2 $s^{-}1$).[31] However, although the thermal properties of ex vivo tissues are available in the published literature, the values of thermal parameters of living biological tissues with circulating blood in vivo are still unknown.

MRI/CT images used to provide a diagnosis can offer useful information about the structure of the overlying tissues. An USgHIFU device can be used to reassess this by using its real-time imaging ability during therapy planning. The composition and thickness of the overlying tissue are recorded with a patient lying on the bed in the treatment position. Ultrasound attenuation in the overlying tissues may be estimated simply and should be documented in writing, with a diagram. The ultrasonic properties of the overlying tissues, the interface between two-layer tissue structures, and the incident beam angle have significant influence on the attenuation of ultrasound energy. These may vary with the location of target tumours and the patient treatment position. For example, when a liver tumour is being treated through the ribcage, significant energy reflection occurs as the beam propagates from the muscle layer to the rib surface. This results in the loss of energy at the focus, which may then be below the ablation threshold. In contrast, the high attenuation coefficient in the bone leads to a significant local temperature increase at the bone surface. There are large variations between individual patients in the thickness of tissue overlying different organs.

There is little energy reflection between two soft tissue interfaces because the difference in their acoustic impedances is small. The greatest difference is for the interface between the fat and muscle, but this only leads to 1–2% reflection.[23–25] However, there are some exceptional cases in clinical use. For example, when HIFU is used to treat pancreatic cancer and uterine fibroids, the overlying tissues include the rectus abdominis muscle, a paired muscle running vertically on each side of the anterior wall of the abdomen. This muscle is in the rectus sheath that consists of the anterior and posterior abdominal aponeuroses, which are layers of flat broad tendons. As there is a stronger reflection of the ultrasound beam at the interface between the aponeurosis and fat, it may cause a temperature rise up to 15 °C with sustained heating of more than 10 °C, resulting in thermal injury to the skin, subcutaneous fat, and muscles.[32, 33]

8.3.6 Patient Positioning

Patient positioning must be carefully considered during therapy planning. It must be comfortable, reproducible and suitable for the acquisition of clear images both for planning and for subsequent treatment. Position selection depends on the location and size of the target tumour, as seen on pretreatment imaging. It may be supine, prone, right or left lateral. The ideal position gives either the shortest beam path, or the largest available area for the transmission of the acoustic beam for the treatment of the target. The position is confirmed by the HIFU device during the planning session.

It is recommended that a patient lies in a single treatment position during the procedure. Any change in position may lead to changes in internal and external anatomy, risk of mis-targeting and over- or under-treatment. However, if positional change is needed for the purpose of treatment, it must be decided in advance and carefully recorded, in order that these risks are minimised.

The patient position, positioning aids and anatomical measurements should be accurately documented in writing with a diagram and digital photos to ensure reproducibility through all stages of the planning session and subsequent treatment. The position may sometimes be constrained by equipment limitations. For example, the arm position may be restricted by the limited size of the treatment bed.

8.3.7 Selection of Anaesthesia

The selection of anaesthetic technique depends on the target organ, patient position and treatment time. These include sedation/analgesia, regional and general anaesthesia (GA). Full monitoring is required during the anaesthetic period. Monitoring lines, intravenous infusion and airway tubing should be of sufficient length, as access to patients is limited once they are in position for treatment.

Sedation/analgesia is usually used in the treatment of uterine fibroids and pelvic tumours. These can ease the sympathetic response such as pain and discomfort during the procedure and afterwards. Effective communication between the patient and operator during treatment is important to ensure its safety. Although sedated patients are instructed to remain still, they are encouraged to inform the operator about where any pain occurring during HIFU exposure originates from. This helps to optimise the exposure used for ablation and to change the location of the focus to avoid skin burn or sciatic nerve injury. Regional anaesthesia includes local or epidural anaesthesia. These can be used in the treatment of breast cancer, osteosarcoma and soft tissue sarcoma.

General anaesthesia is usually used when treating intra-abdominal tumours including those of the liver, kidney and pancreas. As respiratory motion is significant for these organs, ventilation must be controlled well during a HIFU procedure, which requires minimal movement of the target tumour. There are several types of mechanical ventilation used in GA procedures for HIFU treatment. Conventional ventilation is performed with a single-lumen endotracheal tube. If respiration must be halted, an intermittent breath-hold for up to 30s will be conducted at sustained airway pressures during the treatment. One-lung ventilation with a double-lumen tracheal tube is a suitable alternative. This is a standard approach for facilitating surgical exposure for pulmonary surgery and allows mechanical ventilation of only one lung while the other is permitted to deflate passively. High-frequency jet ventilation has recently been performed in the treatment of intra-abdominal organs in Oxford. This uses frequencies of 110–400/min created by an air jet stream where the expiration is passive, and can significantly reduce organ movement to near static conditions.[34] This thus provides a motion management technique for minimising target movement during HIFU procedures.

8.4 HIFU Treatment

8.4.1 Positioning

Once the anaesthetic procedure is completed, the patient is transferred from a tilting trolley to the HIFU bed and placed in the position selected during the therapy planning. This position varies, depending on the location of the target tumour. It may be prone/supine, or lateral. Co-ordinated effort is important when moving and turning the patient under GA.

Once the patient is correctly positioned, immobilisation with physical restraint is required to protect the patient who is receiving either anaesthesia or sedation. This can be achieved using a number of fixation aids such as cushioned straps, pillows, leg restraints and footrests. Proper cushioning at pressure points can avoid nerve injury or backache. Patients must feel comfortable during the treatment if they are under sedation. It must be ascertained that the respiration of the patient is free while the immobilisation is performed, with no pressure on the chest or abdomen. In a prone position, the patient is placed face down with arms abducted in a swimmer's position. In a lateral position, the upper arm is strapped to the side of the body and the lower arm is outstretched. As with the prone position, care must be taken to avoid nerve injury. Blood perfusion to the lower arm should be monitored as vessels can be compromised during HIFU procedure.

8.4.2 Treatment Planning

Once the patient has been correctly positioned and immobilised, the skin overlying the target tumour is brought into contact with the degassed water or water balloon in order that the ultrasound beam is coupled into the body. Using the device's B-mode ultrasound imaging, the location of the target tumour and surrounding tissues are visualised. The HIFU beam path is then determined by rotating the ultrasound imaging probe from 0- to a 90-degree angle, as necessary. This provides an appropriate acoustic window of treatment. The beam cross section at the skin should be as large as possible (Figure 8.5). Air-filled organs such as the bowel, lung and stomach must be avoided in the beam path in order to reduce the risk of inadvertent damage.

Adjacent ultrasound images are recorded across the tumour, thus segmenting the entire tumour in one direction (Figure 8.6). The slice thickness varies, ranging from 2 to 10 mm, its selection being dependent on the type, structure and blood perfusion of the target tumour, and on clinical experience. The settings for each slice on the X, Y and Z coordinate axes and the relevant ultrasound images are

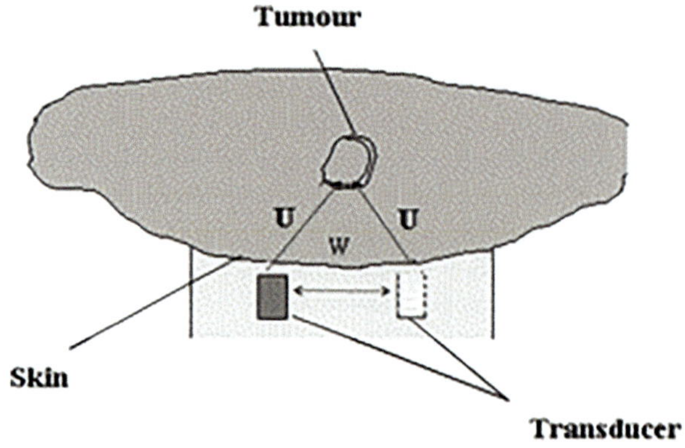

FIGURE 8.5 Schematic diagram of the HIFU beam path. The surface area (W) between focused ultrasound beams (U) is the HIFU beam path.

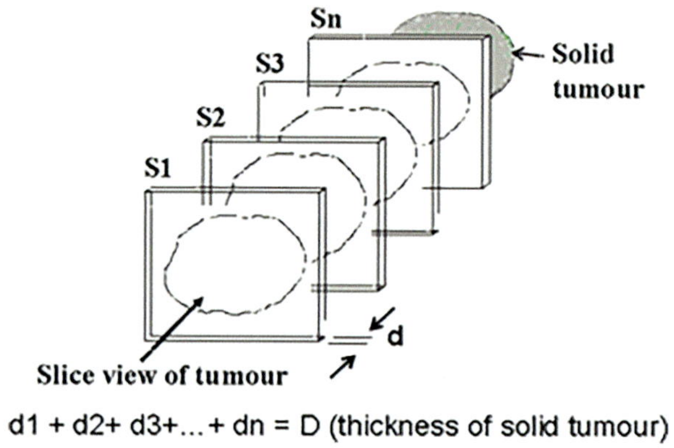

FIGURE 8.6 Schematic diagram showing that an entire tumour is segmented into slices on B-mode ultrasound imaging.

recorded (Figure 8.7) and are not changed during the planning and subsequent treatment. Although each slice provides a 2D image, 3D imaging of the entire target tumour can be achieved using sequential scans of the treatment volume.

The most challenging aspect of the treatment plan is drawing the contour of the region to be treated on each slice. Since MRI/CT scans provide high-quality imaging with better resolution than ultrasound, they can be used to compensate for the shortcomings of B-mode ultrasound imaging in predicting the tumour margin. The operator can mentally register real-time ultrasound images with pretreatment contrast-enhanced MRI/CT scans when the margin is vague. Manual registration that crops and rotates the MRI/CT images to the same orientation as ultrasound images of the treatment slice can also demonstrate the clear margin of the target tumour (Figure 8.8). However, the use of fusion imaging, if available, during treatment planning is strongly recommended, whether or not the margin of the target tumour is clear on B-mode ultrasound imaging. This allows the operator not only to visualise the clear margin of the target tumour on each slice but also to understand complex 3D relationships between the target tumour, peri-tumoural structures, and overlying tissues (Figure 8.9). It can also help the operator to perform HIFU procedures with greater confidence and accuracy for challenging target volumes.

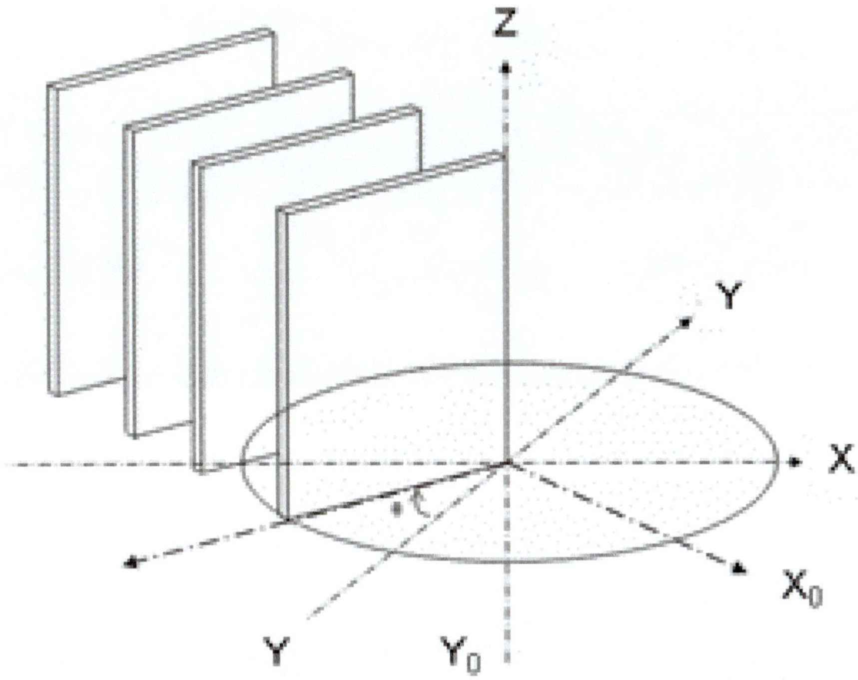

FIGURE 8.7 Schematic diagram showing segmented slices on the X, Y and Z coordinate axes in USgHIFU device. The orientation of the B-mode imaging probe can be any value between 0 and 90 degrees. X and Y coordinate axes are dynamic but X_0 and Y_0 are fixed.

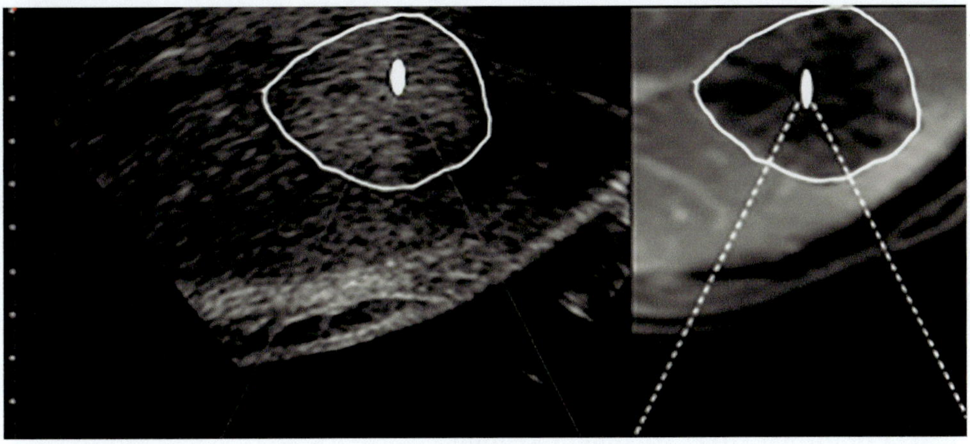

FIGURE 8.8 Real-time B-mode ultrasound imaging (right) manually fused with contrast-enhanced TI-weighted MR imaging (left) shows the clear margin of the liver tumour on the treatment slice.

Once the target tumour has been segmented into slices using B-mode ultrasound imaging, the target contour is drawn manually using the cursor on each treatment slice (Figure 8.10). The target region on each slice is then recorded using the device's software. Finally, the treatment planning software calculates the treatment volume, therapeutic dose and number of HIFU exposures required to completely ablate the defined volume of the target tumour, as well as the total treatment time.

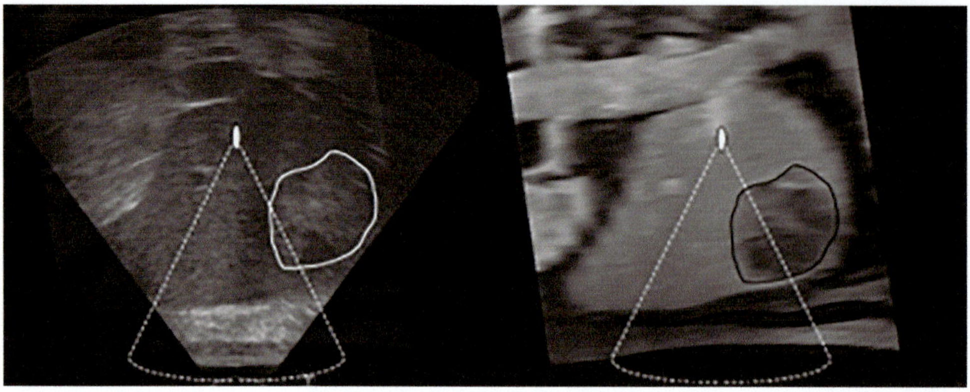

FIGURE 8.9 Using image registration techniques, real-time B-mode ultrasound imaging (right) automatically fused with contrast-enhanced TI-weighted MRI scan (left) shows the clear margin of the liver tumour on the treatment slice.

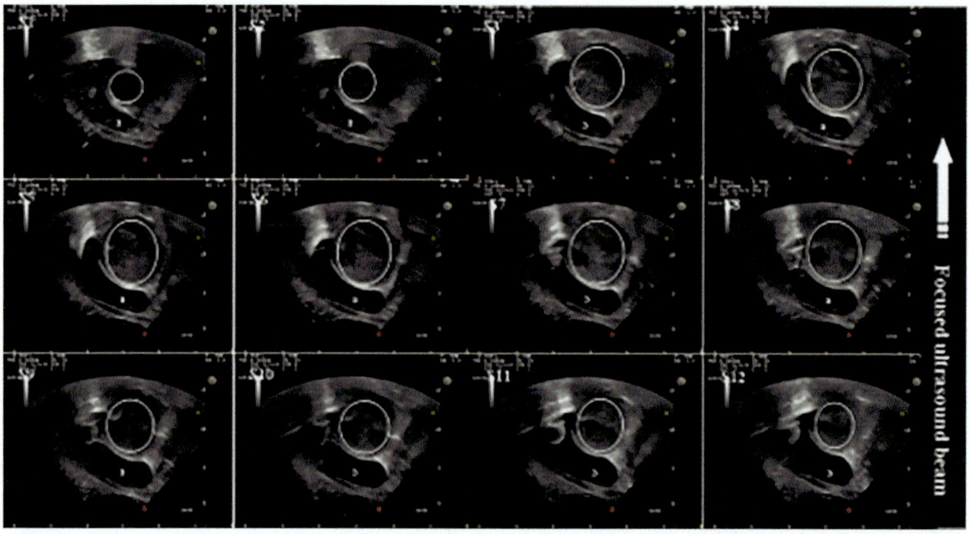

FIGURE 8.10 The contour of a target fibroid (outlined) is drawn manually on sagittal B-mode ultrasound scans during HIFU planning in a patient with uterine fibroid. The entire fibroid is continuously segmented into 12 treatment slices from one edge of the tumour to the other, and the thickness between 2 slices is 5 mm. S: slice; B: bladder.

8.4.3 3D Conformal HIFU Treatment Regime

The basic unit of a HIFU treatment is a single exposure. The ablated tissue volume produced by a single exposure is a HIFU lesion. The focal volume from a HIFU transducer is ellipsoidal, with typical dimensions in the low MegaHertz frequency range of 10–20 mm along the beam axis and 1–2 mm in the transverse direction. So, the single exposure can produce cigar-shaped thermal necrosis at the focus. Although the lesion induced by a single exposure is small, a confluent ablation volume can be achieved by using multiple single exposures. The acoustic power, exposure duration and cooling duration between two single exposures are the main therapeutic parameters to be determined for multiple single exposures. They can either be repeated after predetermined cooling times in the same position to produce a larger cigar-shaped lesion, or placed side by side as multiple single exposures in a linear track to produce a lesioned line. Each single exposure can partially overlap the next one or be separated with no overlap. Multiple single exposures can be repeated from the deepest to the most superficial part of the target region to produce a lesioned slice in the perpendicular direction (Z axis).

To ablate a clinically relevant volume of a target tumour, many of these small HIFU lesions should be systematically positioned side by side to "paint out" or cover the entire target volume, with no surviving cancer cells between each lesion. Figure 8.11 shows that multiple single exposures in ox liver can produce coagulation necrosis ex vivo, which spells out "HIFU". The linear necrosis in each letter consists of many necrotic spots that are induced by "one-by-one" single exposures. This demonstrates that if an appropriate treatment plan is made, HIFU can ablate various shapes and sizes of target tumours in a conformal fashion.

Conformal HIFU treatments can be clinically defined as precise procedures which ablate an entire tumour by moving the high-energy concentrated focus in a 3-D fashion. By scanning the focus in successive sweeps from the deep/distal to shallow/proximal regions of the target area, the tumour can be successfully destroyed on each slice. This process is repeated slice by slice to achieve a complete ablation of the target volume (Figure 8.12).

8.4.4 Dose Delivery

The effects of HIFU exposures are dependent on the acoustic power, exposure regime, exposure time, and cooling duration, as well as on the structure and vascularity of the target tumour. When therapeutic parameters are appropriately selected for a single exposure, the tissue temperature can rise rapidly to 85 °C at the focus, resulting in a cigar-shaped region of coagulation necrosis. Acoustic cavitation can also contribute to tissue damage, and tissue boiling may occur during the exposures. Changing the therapeutic parameters modulates the amount of tissue ablation, but may increase the risk of thermal damage to overlying and adjacent tissues.

After selecting a single exposure and duration, HIFU therapeutic procedures begin by delivering a low power test exposure to the deepest part of the target tumour. The test power varies, depending on the target depth (that is, the distance between the skin and the focus). A short test exposure time is also

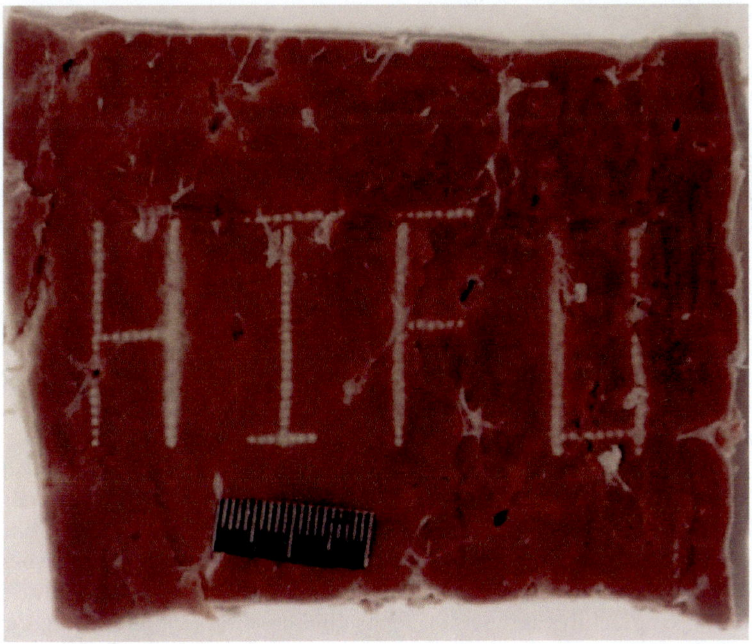

FIGURE 8.11 Multiple single exposures can achieve coagulation necrosis of in vitro ox liver that spells out "HIFU", indicating that HIFU is a 3-dimensional conformal treatment. (From Wu F, et al. Ultrasound Med Bio 2004; 30:245–260.)[20]

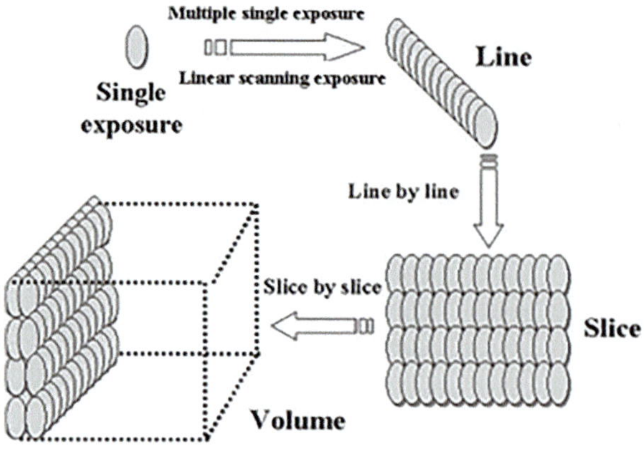

FIGURE 8.12 Schematic diagram showing a conformal HIFU treatment plan to ablate the entire volume of a solid tumour using multiple single exposures. (From Wu F, et al. Radiology 2005;235:659–67.)[35]

important. As an example, exposure durations may start from 1s, and are gradually increased to 5s. Both exposure power and duration can be gradually increased until a focal tissue reaction is clearly seen on real-time B-mode ultrasound imaging (instantaneous hyperechoic changes or greyscale changes in the focus immediately after each exposure). Thus, the acoustic power and exposure duration that cause bright echoes are considered as appropriate for the target tumour. They can be used to treat the entire tumour but need to be modulated when ablating the superficial regions of the target volume.

8.4.5 Real-Time B-mode Ultrasound Imaging for Assessment of Tumour Response During HIFU Procedures

8.4.5.1 B-mode Ultrasound Imaging

The use of ultrasound visualisation for the guidance and monitoring of HIFU procedure usually relies on the appearance of a hyperechoic region immediately following HIFU exposure on B-mode ultrasound images.[36, 37] A hyperechoic region is an area of increased echogenicity that appears as a bright increase in greyscale at the focus. This is a direct tissue response to focused ultrasound energy deposition in a target tumour, and reflects bubble formation rather than the temperature rise that MRgHIFU devices measure with MR thermometry techniques.

The bright echoes observed during a HIFU exposure result from effects of focused ultrasound on the target tissues. Their appearance depends on the ultrasound intensity used for ablation. If this is below the threshold for lesion formation, no hyperechogenicity is seen on B-mode ultrasound. However, when the ablative threshold intensity is reached, it occurs immediately on exposure, becomes gradually less evident, and may disappear within a few minutes, although in a few cases it may persist for a long period. The amplitude of echoes can be compared between pre- and post-exposure images to determine the spatial extent of thermal necrosis in the treated region. Figure 8.13 shows greyscale changes on B-mode ultrasound imaging during a HIFU procedure in a patient with a uterine fibroid. While the HIFU focus is moved from the deep to superficial part of the tumour, progressive hyperechogenicity is clearly seen on ultrasound imaging in the treated tumour.

It is generally believed that the appearance of the hyperechoic region results from bubble activity generated during HIFU exposure. Both thermal and mechanical mechanisms are involved in the formation of tissue boiling and acoustic cavitation bubbles. Absorption of transmitted ultrasound energy can induce tissue boiling temperatures at the HIFU focus, thus creating vapour bubbles. Using passive cavitation detection techniques, inertial cavitation can be detected during the formation of a hyperechoic region at the focus.[39] It typically occurs prior (within 0.5s) to the appearance of a hyperechoic region, suggesting that the initial formation of bubbles at the HIFU focus seems due to acoustic cavitation.[40]

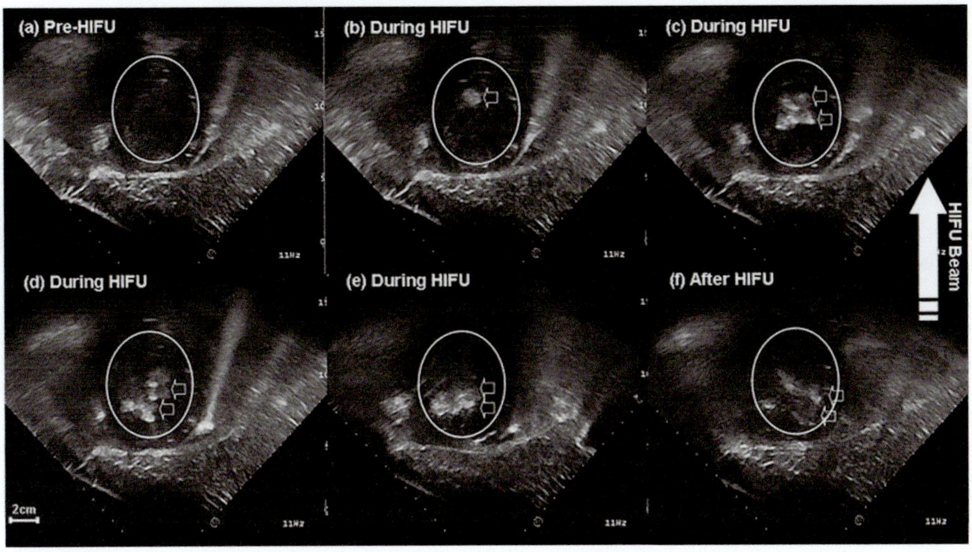

FIGURE 8.13 B-mode ultrasound images before and immediately following USgHIFU exposures in a patient with uterine fibroids. Greyscale changes are seen on real-time ultrasound images in an axial-slice during the HIFU procedure. (a) Ultrasound image obtained before HIFU shows a large uterine fibroid, indicated by a white circle. (b)–(e) Ultrasound images obtained during the HIFU procedure show progressive hyperechogenicity in the treated area of the fibroid (arrows). (f) US images obtained immediately after the HIFU procedure show persistant (but somewhat reduced) hyperechogenicity in the treated fibroid (arrows). (From Lyon PC, et al. Ultraschall Med 2020; 41:550–556.)[38]

There is a strong correlation between the onset of inertial cavitation and a rapid rise in temperature at the focus.[41, 42]

HIFU-induced acoustic cavitation accelerates tissue heating through absorption of broadband emissions.[43] However, as the ambient temperature is increased and the properties of tissue change, inertial cavitation gradually shuts down and can give rise to larger, boiling bubbles that play a significant thermal role through scattering.[38, 43, 44] These boiling bubbles contribute to the hyperechoic region on B-mode ultrasound images. The hyperechoic area has been shown to correspond to the spatial extent of the thermal necrosis, and so assessment of thermal lesions is based on hyperechoic changes seen using B-mode ultrasound imaging, which is thus used to provide real-time feedback in clinical practice to monitor and control acoustic energy delivery to the target tumour.[45–48]

8.4.5.2 Contrast-Enhanced Ultrasonography

Contrast-enhanced ultrasonography (CEUS) combines ultrasound imaging with microbubble contrast agents to show blood flow and perfusion in tissues. These contrast agent microbubbles contain air or gas within a shell, and after intravenous administration, they increase the backscatter of the ultrasound, resulting in high-amplitude echoes from blood vessels. CEUS is a functional imaging technique that provides dynamic imaging of blood flow, allowing quantitative analysis of tissue perfusion throughout vascular phases. CEUS has been recommended as an alternative imaging modality for early detection of residual unablated tumour after thermal ablation and subsequent local tumour recurrence and progression in liver cancer.[49]

CEUS has been used for immediate assessment of therapeutic effect following HIFU procedures. It can distinguish between a complete, partial or equivocal treatment response immediately after HIFU treatment. The lack of any contrast enhancement within an ablated tumour is considered to be an indicator of complete response, as shown in Figure 8.14. The detection of residual viable tumour is indicative of a partial response. It appears as an enhanced nodule on CEUS images. Immediate CEUS assessment

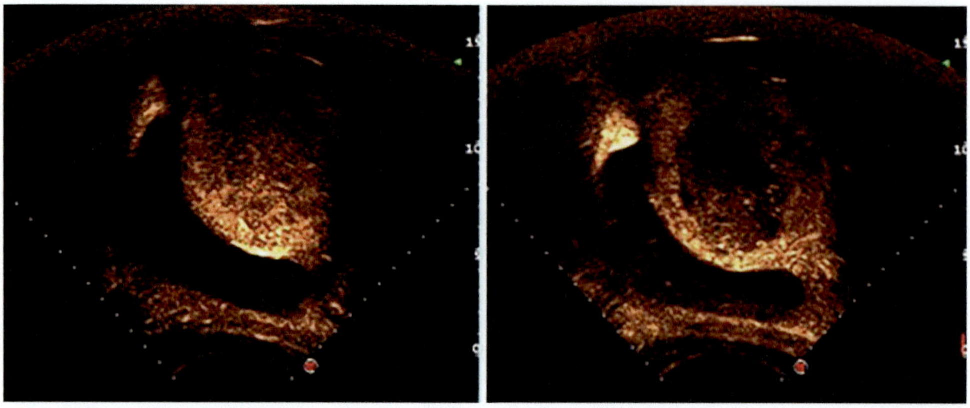

FIGURE 8.14 Sagittal contrast-enhanced ultrasonography before and immediately following USgHIFU treatment in a female patient with uterine fibroids. Before HIFU ablation (left), contrast enhancement is identified within the target fibroid (arrow). However, immediately following HIFU ablation (right), there is an absence of contrast enhancement within the treated tumour (arrow), indicating a good tumour response with complete ablation.

is of critical importance following HIFU in routine clinical practice. It provides immediate feedback as to whether the tumour has been destroyed completely while a patient is still on the treatment bed, and thus gives an opportunity for immediate re-treatment in the same session to reduce the incomplete ablation rate.

8.4.6 Real-Time Imaging Feedback Control

B-mode ultrasound imaging can provide real-time feedback in terms of monitoring and subsequently control of therapeutic dose during HIFU procedure. This feedback control is based on B-mode ultrasound image changes between pre- and post-exposure. It includes (1) monitoring of echo changes in the focus, (2) monitoring of a patient's position, (3) monitoring of skin burn and (4) monitoring of thermal damage in overlying tissues in the HIFU beam path.

B-mode ultrasound changes during HIFU exposure provide real-time information that can be used for feedback control of the energy delivered to the target tumour. This is based on the greyscale changes, which give detailed 2D maps of the tissue reaction to heat at the focus. If the difference between pre- and post-imaging greyscales does not reach a threshold value after a single exposure, the exposure is repeated until the greyscale values reach the level known to indicate thermal necrosis. When sufficient energy is delivered, a hyperechoic area seen on B-mode ultrasound imaging can predict the size and geometry of the thermal lesion. Since each exposure is successfully monitored using real-time imaging, the energy delivery can be controlled dynamically during the treatment. However, although the greyscale changes may be automatically recorded and analysed by the treatment software after each exposure, respiratory motion means that the operator may sometimes need to conduct this imaging-based feedback control.

The patient must remain stationary to maintain spatial immobilisation of the target tumour during HIFU procedure. Any alteration in position can lead to the risk of mis-targeting, over- or undertreatment for the target volume. B-mode ultrasound can provide real-time information about any change in the patient's position during the procedure.

Skin burn is the most common complication of a HIFU treatment. Small air bubbles in the degassed water which serves as the coupling medium, may contribute to this. These small bubbles can remain on the surface of the skin, leading to damage. As they also generate strong echoes, the operator can see them and manually remove them from the skin during a HIFU procedure. Ultrasound imaging can also detect early signs of a skin burn such as small blisters, enabling the operator to adjust therapeutic parameters in order to avoid further thermal skin damage.

Selection of a safe and clear HIFU beam path is essential for successful treatment. This selection can be made using the pretreatment MRI/CT scans and ultrasound imaging. However, the beam path may become inappropriate during the procedure if the bowels move around the target tumour. For example, in the treatment of uterine fibroids, ultrasound imaging can monitor bowel movement in real time and predict when they intervene between the target fibroid and abdominal wall. This allows the operator to perform manoeuvres to manipulate them out of the beam path, so that the potential risk of bowel injury can be avoided.

8.5 Current Clinical HIFU Applications

8.5.1 Overview

Over the past 2 decades HIFU has initiated a change from open surgery to a noninvasive approach for the treatment of solid tumours. Compared to other ablative techniques, HIFU provides a noninvasive treatment option that can precisely and completely ablate an entire tumour in a conformal fashion. Due to its noninvasiveness, lack of skin scarring, reduced pain, and short recovery time, HIFU is becoming more attractive to both patients and clinicians. It has led to an associated reduction in mortality, morbidity, hospital stay and cost, and improved quality of life for cancer patients.[50–52] To date, focused ultrasound therapy including USgHIFU and MRgHIFU has been extensively investigated in preclinical and clinical studies to develop novel treatments for diverse types of diseases. As shown in Figure 8.15,

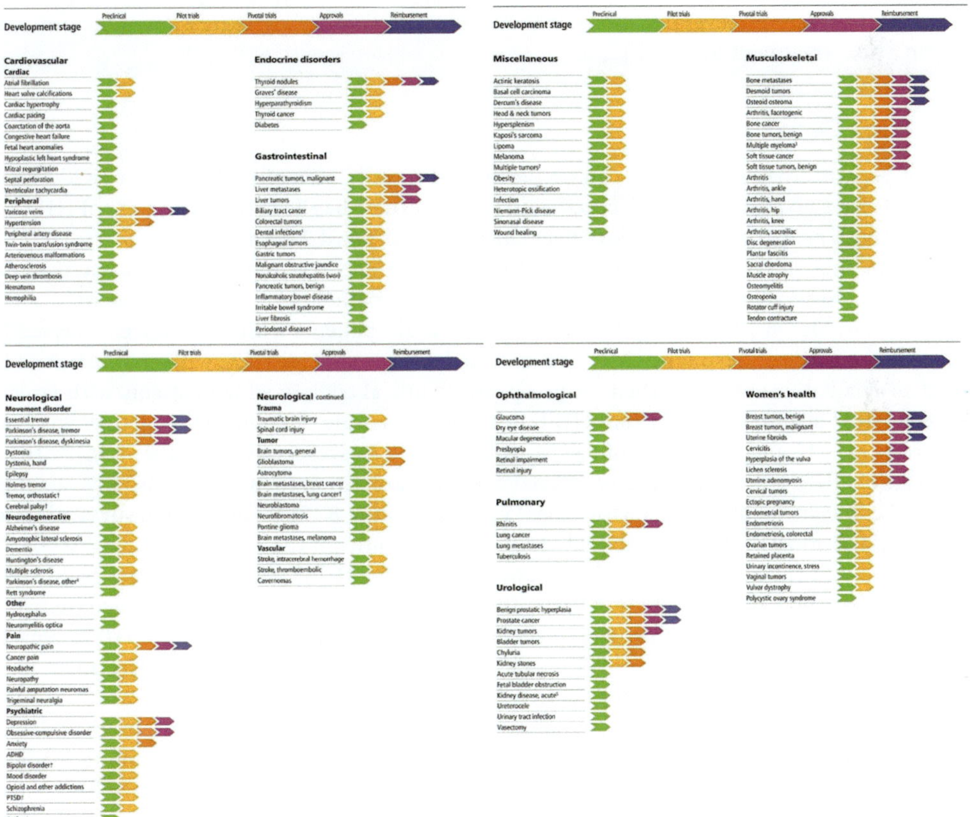

FIGURE 8.15 Clinical indications of focused ultrasound therapy and their development stages. (From Focused ultrasound foundation. 2023 state of the field. https://cdn.fusfoundation.org/2023/07/21125203/FUSF-State-of-the-Field-Report-2023_July-24.pdf#page=9.)

there are currently 166 clinical indications or disorders, of which 32 indications have regulatory approval worldwide, including 8 approved by FDA in the United States.[53]

Since 1997, USgHIFU devices have been used increasingly in routine clinical practice to treat patients with malignant tumours, which include those of the liver, breast, pancreas, kidney, bone and soft tissues. It can also treat benign tumours such as uterine fibroids, breast fibroadenoma and benign thyroid disease. Recently, the treatment indications have expanded to other diseases that are important for women's health. This section summarises the current clinical applications of USgHIFU for malignant and benign tumours, and other diseases.

8.5.2 Malignant Tumours

HIFU treatment for an individual cancer patient requires specialist medical knowledge and a close collaboration between multidisciplinary team members to ensure the accurate accomplishment of a difficult set of procedures. It begins with the pathologic diagnosis of the disease and accurate assessment of the tumour stage using the TNM classification. As there are several choices of therapeutic modality, including local therapies (surgery and radiation therapy) and systemic therapy (chemotherapy), a decision as to whether the planned treatment is curative or palliative should be made by a multidisciplinary team, comprising surgeons, oncologists, radiologists, radiation oncologists and pathologists.

The role, and scheduling, of chemotherapy in relation to a HIFU session must be defined at the beginning of treatment. The location and extent of the tumour relative to the overlying tissues and adjacent organs can be determined by a number of imaging modalities. However, pre-HIFU adjuvant treatments may sometimes influence the shape and size of the target tumour. For example, when a patient with osteosarcoma has received several sessions of neoadjuvant chemotherapy, regression of the tumour may be seen on a post-treatment MRI/CT scan.

8.5.2.1 Liver Cancer

Because of hepatic cirrhosis, surgery can be performed in only 20% of patients with HCC.[54, 55] Most HCC patients have no chance of being cured with surgery. There has been increasing use of HIFU in the treatment of both primary and secondary liver cancer over the past 2 decades.

In 2001, the first successful HIFU treatment of HCC patients was reported. A clearly demarcated coagulation necrosis volume was detected on post-HIFU pathological examination of the treated tumours.[56] From March 1998 to October 2001, a total of 474 patients with liver cancer received HIFU treatment in ten Chinese hospitals.[18] Most patients had advanced-stage HCC with cirrhosis, and HIFU was used as a palliative option for them. A prospective clinical trial, in which patients with large HCC underwent HIFU ablation, showed that HIFU treatment was safe, feasible and effective, with overall survival rates at 6, 12 and 18 months of 86.1%, 61.5% and 35.3%, respectively (Figure 8.16).[57] The combined effects of HIFU with transcatheter arterial chemoembolisation (TACE) was also investigated in a randomised clinical trial in patients with stage IV_A HCC (Figure 8.17).[35] The median survival times for patients were 11.3 months in the combined group, and 4 months in the TACE group ($p = 0.0042$). The 6-month and 1-year survival rates were 80.4% and 42.9% in the HIFU plus TACE group and 13.2% and 0% in the TACE group, respectively ($p < 0.01$). These findings were subsequently verified by two studies which supported the finding that overall survival rates were much better in the HIFU plus TACE group than in the TACE alone group.[58, 59] The safety, feasibility and efficacy of HIFU treatment for HCC patients have been proven by clinical results from a number of groups.[60–63]

HIFU can safely treat HCC patients with poor liver function.[64] It is particularly useful in patients who have poor liver function with clinical ascites, as the ascites itself provides a good coupling medium for ultrasound,[65] as shown in Figure 8.16. The efficacy of HIFU treatment has been proven to be comparable with percutaneous radiofrequency ablation in patients with small HCC lesions (<3 cm),[66] but better than TACE in HCC patients with a median tumour size of 4.8 cm (range 3–8 cm).[67] In addition, its application in recurrent HCC allows the patients to undergo ablation, especially when the abdomen is hostile due to previous surgery, or there is an inadequate liver remnant due to previous major hepatectomy.[68]

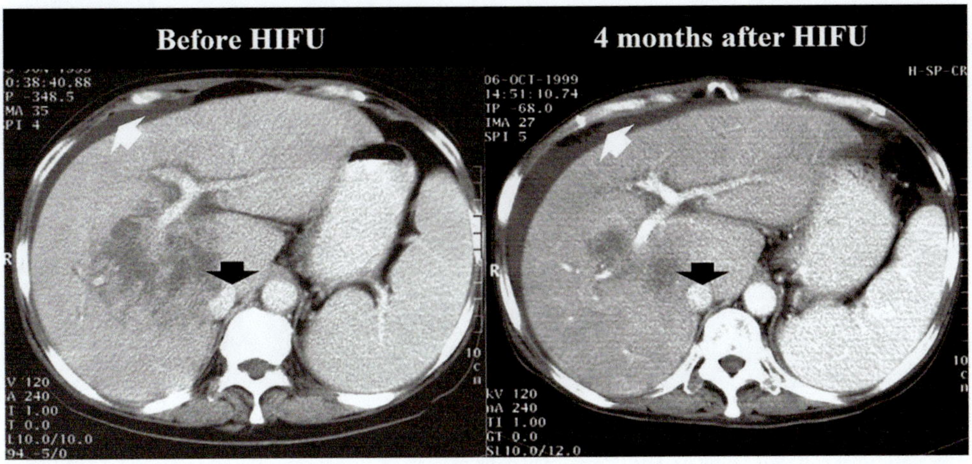

FIGURE 8.16 Contrast-enhanced CT images before and after USgHIFU treatment in a 56-year-old patient with advanced-stage hepatocellular carcinoma. Before HIFU (left), the tumour invades the right branch of the portal vein, and the inferior vena cava is compressed with a change in shape (black arrow). Small amount of ascites is seen (white arrow). (B) Four months after HIFU (right), the treated tumour decreases in size considerably and the vessel compression disappears with the normal shape of the inferior vena cava (black arrow), but a small amount of ascites is still visible (white arrow). (From Wu F, et al. Ann Surg Oncol 2004;11:1061–1069.)[57]

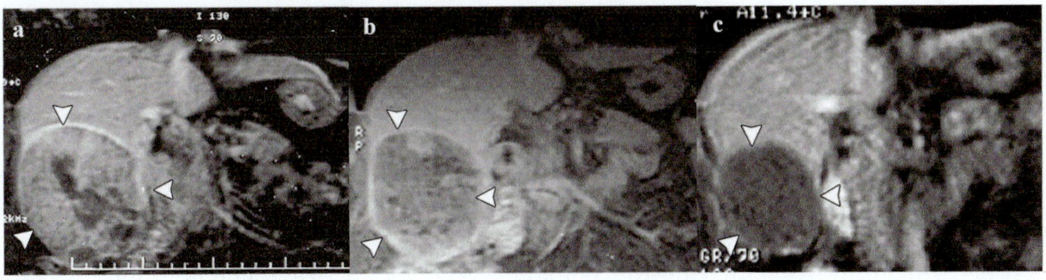

FIGURE 8.17 Coronal contrast-enhanced T-weighted MR images before and after USgHIFU treatment in a 62-year-old patient with hepatocellular carcinoma. (a) Before TACE, rich blood supply is observed in the tumour (arrows). (b) 4 weeks after TACE, just before ablation, tumour blood supply is reduced, but contrast enhancement remains in some areas within the tumour (arrows). (c) 2 weeks after ablation, no contrast enhancement is observed in the treated tumour (arrows), indicative of positive tumour response with complete ablation. (From Wu F, et al. Radiology 2005;235:659–667.)[35]

Furthermore, HIFU can be used as a bridging treatment while awaiting cadaveric liver transplantation. The response rate for these HCC patients who had undergone HIFU was better than for those who underwent TACE treatment.[69] If a target tumour lies close to large blood vessels in the liver such as the portal vein, inferior vena cava or hepatic vein, HIFU is safe and effective with no irreversible injury to the blood vessels.[70] Moreover, HIFU can successfully treat needle-track seeding of HCC, which is one of the complications of tumour biopsy since cancer cells can be deposited along the track of a biopsy needle.[71]

USgHIFU treatment has been also used to treat secondary liver tumours in Europe. Illing and colleagues[72] reported for the first time the results of a prospective HIFU trial for liver metastasis in a Western population. Using radiological and histological examinations, they found that HIFU treatment could produce discrete ablation zones in metastatic liver cancer in all patients (Figure 8.18). Further studies demonstrated that follow-up contrast-enhanced MRI scans could predict zones of coagulative necrosis in liver metastases[73] and that time to maximum enhancement maps and their 3D views on

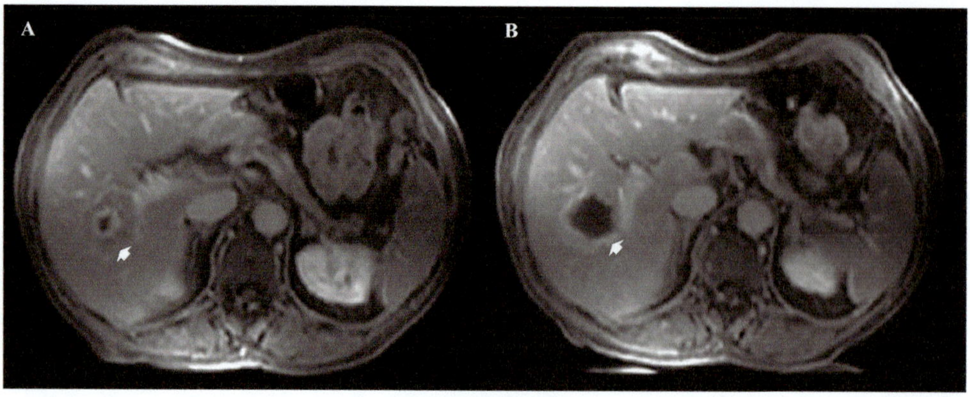

FIGURE 8.18 Contrast-enhanced transverse T-weighted MR images before and after USgHIFU treatment in a patient with metastatic liver cancer. (A) Before HIFU, a right hepatic metastasis shows central necrosis (arrow). (B) 12 days after HIFU, a larger zone consistent with coagulative necrosis (arrow) within the metastasis. (From Illing R, et al. Br J Cancer 2005;92:890–895.)[72]

contrast-enhanced MRI could be used to assess, and potentially to quantify, the success of HIFU treatment.[74] Intra-operative assessment of HIFU ablation can provide an accurate measure of the ablation zone and correlates well with MRI follow-up scan posttreatment.[75] Orsi and colleagues[76] treated metastatic liver cancer in some difficult locations in which the target tumours were close to major blood vessels, the heart, gallbladder, bile ducts, bowel and stomach. After HIFU treatment, PET-CT and/or multidetector computed tomography showed complete ablation in 22/24 liver metastases. Moreover, HIFU combined with TACE has been used successfully to treat children with hepatoblastoma. The median survival time was 14 months, and the 1- and 2-year survival rates were 91.7% and 83.3%, respectively.[77]

Due to the anatomical complexity of the liver, it is difficult to eliminate potential risks during HIFU procedures, but good preparation and training can reduce them. To date, most studies have shown that HIFU is safe for the treatment of liver tumours, with minor adverse events, such as skin burns, subcutaneous oedema and transient pain. However, one study has reported serious complications in a minority of HCC patients after HIFU procedure. These include rib fractures, biliary obstruction, pleural effusion, pneumothorax and fistula formation.[78] This suggests that the selection of suitable patients is crucial for avoiding severe complications, and artificial pleural effusion for creating an adequate acoustic window should be seriously considered in the treatment of hepatic dome lesions.

8.5.2.2 Breast Cancer

Breast cancer is the most frequently occurring female cancer and the leading cause of cancer mortality in women. Radical mastectomy has long been accepted as an appropriate therapy for breast cancer. Breast conserving surgery has been performed as a routine treatment for patients with early-stage breast cancer over the past decades. In the context of this background, HIFU treatments have been explored, with the intention of achieving equivalent efficacy, but with improved cosmesis.

The first clinical trial investigating the safety and feasibility of USgHIFU for the treatment of localised breast cancer was reported in 2003.[79] In this randomised trial, 48 patients were treated with either modified radical mastectomy, or with HIFU followed by modified radical mastectomy. A short-term follow-up radiological study was performed to assess the ablative effect on the tumour, and the result showed that HIFU could ablate an entire tumour and healthy breast tissue surrounding the tumour (Figure 8.19). Using gross examination and triphenyltetrazolium chloride staining, complete coagulation necrosis was confirmed in all HIFU-treated tumours. The mean volume of the HIFU ablated region was 7.4 times greater than the mean volume of breast cancer (124.49 ± 47.84 cm^3 vs. 16.80 ± 13.40 cm^3,

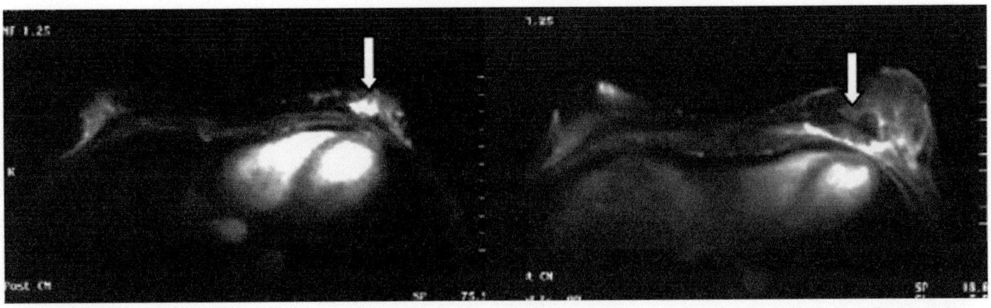

FIGURE 8.19 Compared to the imaging before HIFU (left), post-HIFU contrast-enhanced T1-weighted transverse MR image (right) shows no enhancement in the treated tumour and adjacent healthy breast tissue (arrow) in a breast cancer patient, indicating that a surgical margin is achieved by HIFU treatment. (From Wu F, et al. Br J Cancer 2003; 89:2227–2233.)[79]

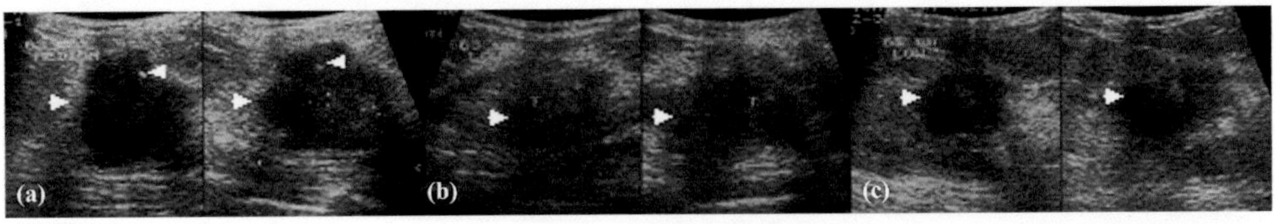

FIGURE 8.20 Colour Doppler ultrasonography before and after USgHIFU treatment in a 62-year-old patient with breast cancer. (a) Before treatment, the tumour is circumscribed (arrow) and blood vessel signals are observed (arrowhead); 6 months (b) and 12 months (c) after HIFU ablation, an obvious decrease of the treated tumour size is seen with no evidence of blood vessel signals. (From Wu F, et al. Breast Cancer Res Treat 2005; 92:51–60.)[84]

P <0.001).[80] Although histological examination showed that typical characteristics of coagulation necrosis were seen in the peripheral region of the ablated tumour in all patients, haematoxylin and eosin staining showed normal cellular structure in the central part of the ablated tumour in 11/23 patients. However, electronic microscopy and nicotinamide adenine dinucleotide-diaphorase staining showed that the normal-appearing cancer cells were not viable, indicating that HIFU could cause the heat fixation of the ablated tumour.[81]

Orsi and colleagues[82] reported an interim result from HIFU treatment of 12 patients with small breast cancers (<1.5 cm). All patients underwent conservative surgery after HIFU to assess histopathological changes in the treated tumours. The results showed that all tumours were completely ablated with no side effects. However, another study showed that the complete ablation rate was low in patients with a mean tumour size of 25.6 mm (range 12–37 mm). Follow-up MRI and histopathological examination showed that HIFU induced complete ablation in 4 (66%) out of 6 patients.[83]

The long-term clinical outcomes of HIFU in the treatment of breast cancer have also been evaluated.[84] Twenty-two patients with biopsy-confirmed breast cancer were treated with HIFU, followed by chemotherapy, radiotherapy or hormone therapy (tamoxifen). Post-treatment imaging showed the regression of the treated lesions in all patients (Figure 8.20) and their disappearance in 8 patients during a median follow-up of 54.8 months. Post-treatment US-guided core needle biopsy showed coagulative necrosis of both tumour cells and adjacent normal tissue at 2 weeks. Partial fibrosis of the treated lesion was seen at 3 months, and complete fibrosis at both 6 months and 12 months (Figure 8.21). Five-year disease-free survival and recurrence-free survival were 95% and 85%, respectively. The cosmetic result was judged as good to excellent in 94% of patients.

The adverse events of HIFU treatment for breast cancer are minor and transient. They include skin burn, mild pain and subcutaneous tissue oedema. No severe complications have been reported in clinical use.

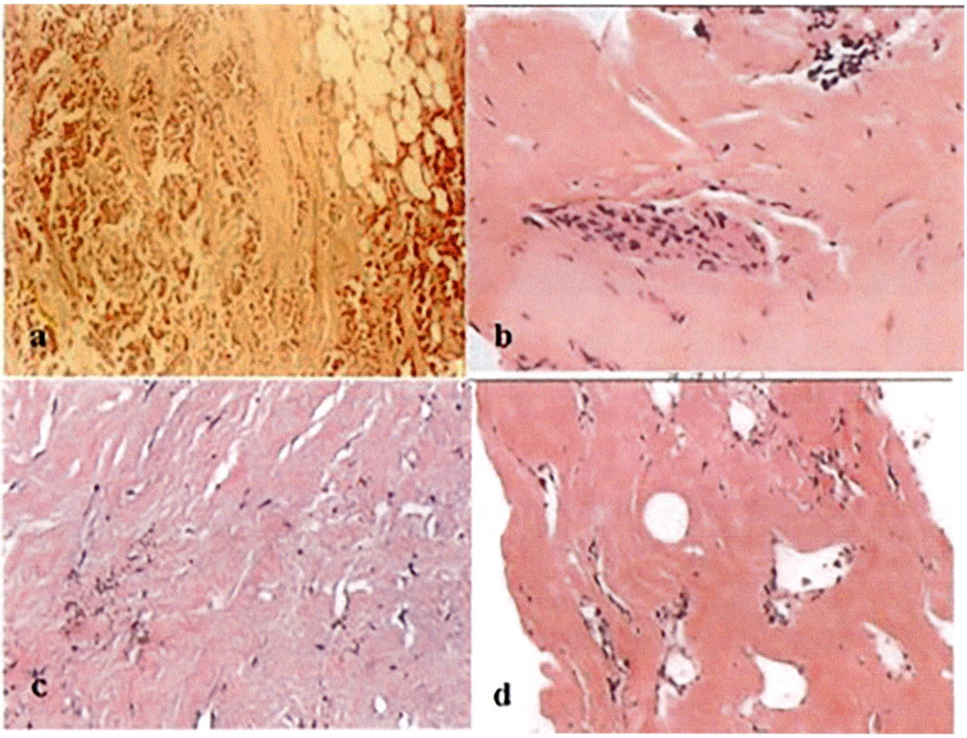

FIGURE 8.21 Follow-up pathological changes in HIFU-ablated tumours in patients with breast cancer. (a) Coagulative necrosis including tumour cells and adjacent healthy breast tissue is observed 2 weeks postoperatively. (b) Fibroblastic scar tissue develops in the treated tumour 3 months after HIFU, but there are necrosed tumour cells among the scar tissue. (c and d) Complete fibrosis of the treated tumour is seen at 6 months (c) and 12 months (d) postoperatively. H&E staining × 200. (From Wu F, et al. Breast Cancer Res Treat 2005; 92:51-60.)[84]

8.5.2.3 Pancreatic Cancer

Pancreatic carcinoma is the fourth leading cause of cancer related death in the Western world. Nearly 80% of patients have unresectable disease at diagnosis. There is no effective therapy for patients with locally advanced disease, and chemo-radiation currently seems the best option although there remains a great deal of debate about this issue. The median survival time is 6–10 months for patients with locally advanced pancreatic cancer and 3–6 months for patients with metastatic disease.

Until now, HIFU treatment has largely been seen as a palliative option for patients with advanced pancreatic cancer. It can be used either alone or in combination with other modalities such as chemotherapy or radiation therapy. In 2005, the first prospective clinical trial using HIFU treatment for locally advanced pancreatic cancer was reported. Follow-up contrast-enhanced CT or MR imaging showed a positive tumour response with no evidence of contrast enhancement in the treated tumour (Figure 8.22). No complications, and both pain control and potential survival benefit, were seen in treated patients during the follow-up period.[85] These results have been repeated in subsequent studies in Asia and Europe. Pain relief in 78–100% patients with a prolonged median survival time has been observed.[86–88] In addition, Wang and colleagues[89] reported the characteristic histological changes seen in 27 of 30 patients with borderline resectable pancreatic cancer after HIFU treatment. They found that typical coagulative necrosis was detected in the HIFU-treated tumour, and that the location and extent of the ablation zone were consistent with those of the non-perfused volume seen on contrast-enhanced CT scan post-treatment. These results strongly support the view that HIFU is safe, feasible and effective in the treatment of patients with advanced-stage pancreatic cancer. However, most clinical evidence to

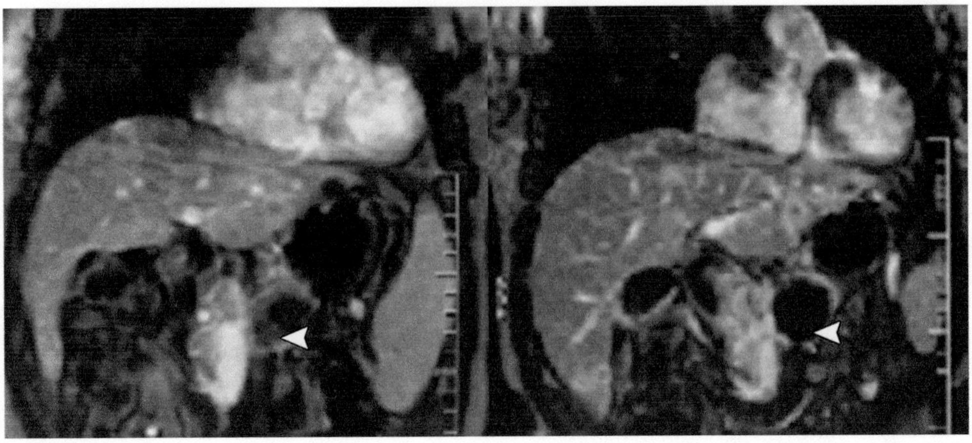

FIGURE 8.22 Coronal contrast-enhanced T1-weighted MR images before and after USgHIFU treatment in a 48-year-old man with advanced pancreatic cancer. Before HIFU (left), there is contrast enhancement in the pancreatic tumour (arrow). Two weeks after HIFU (right), no evidence of contrast enhancement is seen in the treated tumour (arrow), indicative of complete ablation in the pancreatic cancer. (From Wu F, et al. Radiology 2005; 236:1034–1040.)[88]

date has been obtained in retrospective studies. Randomised, controlled prospective clinical trials will be required for assessment of HIFU efficacy on pancreatic cancer in the future.

HIFU combined with either chemotherapy[90–94] or radiotherapy[95] has also been investigated for both locally advanced and metastatic pancreatic cancer. The chemotherapeutic agents include gemcitabine and an S-1 regime consisting of tegafur, gimestat and otastat potassium. The results showed that while HIFU was combined with chemotherapy or radiotherapy, median and overall survival and progression-free survival rates were significantly better in the combined group than those in the single-treatment group. Of them, one study observed an unexpectedly prolonged survival time with a 4-year survival rate of up to 33.5% in the HIFU plus gemcitabine group,[96] suggesting that HIFU might have a synergistic effect with chemotherapy, boosting the drug concentration in the target tumour. However, this claim needs to be confirmed in a randomised, controlled clinical trial.

The most extensive HIFU experience of treating advanced pancreatic cancer has been reported by Ning and colleagues.[97] A total of 689 patients with unresectable pancreatic cancers were analysed retrospectively, including 436 patients who received HIFU treatment alone or in combination with chemotherapy or radiation therapy, and 253 patients treated by conventional chemotherapy or radiotherapy. Median overall survival rate was 7.1 months in the HIFU group and 5 months in the non-HIFU group. A statistical difference between the two groups was also observed in patients with stage II, II and IV tumours, respectively, indicating that HIFU plus conventional therapies could provide survival benefit in the patients with unresectable pancreatic cancer.

Many of the early concerns that surrounded the safety of HIFU treatment for pancreatic cancer have been addressed in pilot studies. However, the incidence of complications caused directly by HIFU is relatively low compared with that for radiation therapy or surgery. Mild complications include abdominal pain, nausea and vomiting, skin burn and subcutaneous fat sclerosis. Patients usually recover within a short time of treatment, with no medication. Wang and colleagues[98] reported a safety analysis of HIFU treatment for 224 patients with advanced pancreatic cancer. Gastrointestinal dysfunction, such as abdominal distension and anorexia with slight nausea, was observed in 10 cases (4.5%) post-treatment. Although no severe complications were observed in any treated patient, one case (with pancreatic head cancer) developed obstructive jaundice. Vertebral injury, identified by MRI scanning, occurred in 2 cases, with no symptoms. However, severe adverse events have also been reported in a few studies. These include portal vein thrombosis, pancreaticoduodenal fistula, obstructive jaundice and pancreatitis with a large pseudocyst, although these are rare. If a target tumour is too close to the duodenum or bile duct, a safe margin should be considered, as HIFU may cause thermal damage to these vital structures, leading to bowel perforation and obstructive jaundice.

8.5.2.4 Kidney Cancer

Renal cell cancer (RCC) has the seventh highest incidence of all cancers in adults. At the time of diagnosis, 75% of tumours are organ confined and thus should be amenable to a local treatment. RCC is both chemotherapy and radiotherapy resistant. The mainstay of treatment for these tumours remains surgery, with 5-year survival rates greater than 80% after surgical resection.[99]

In the early 1990s, Vallancien and colleagues[14] treated 4 RCC patients prior to surgical resection. They found wide variation in the extent of tissue ablation, but encountered a high rate of skin burns in the patients. Susani and colleagues[100] included 2 patients with renal tumours in a phase I trial and claimed accurate placement of HIFU lesions, but reported detail is sparse. Koehrmann and colleagues[101] treated a patient with 3 renal tumours using an experimental hand-held HIFU device. Two of the tumours reduced in size following ablation; however, 1 remained unaffected. A phase II trial was subsequently performed to evaluate the treatment of 14 patients with HIFU prior to surgical resection.[102] Coagulation necrosis was observed in 9 of 14 tumours but the ablation zone measured was much smaller than the original target volume, suggesting incomplete ablation in 9 patients, with no ablation in the remaining 5. Similarly, Häcker and colleagues[103] found thermal ablation in 15 of 19 kidney tumours, but the effects did not correlate with HIFU exposures. Severe complications included grade 3 skin burn in 2 patients and small bowel injury in 1 patient.

In 2003, the first trial using USgHIFU for the palliative treatment of 13 patients with advanced-stage kidney cancer was reported.[104] The results showed that partial ablation was observed in 10 patients and complete ablation in 3 (Figure 8.23). After HIFU, haematuria disappeared in 7 of 8 patients and flank pain of presumed malignant origin disappeared in 9 of 10 patients. An ablation zone was detected on post-treatment imaging, with significant shrinkage of the treated tumour. Of the 13 patients, 7 died (median survival 14.1 months, range 2–27) and 6 were still alive at the time of reporting with median follow-up of 18.5 months (range 10–27).

HIFU has been also used to treat patients with small RCC in several clinical trials in the UK. The first study was designed to evaluate the safety and feasibility of HIFU treatment in a Western population.[72] Eight patients with renal tumours underwent a single HIFU session, followed up with contrast-enhanced MRI and histological assessments after surgical resection of the target tumours. The results showed that discrete zones of the ablation were observed in 67% of the patients. A follow-up study investigated the use of HIFU for the management of small renal tumours over a 3-year period.[105] Fourteen HIFU-treated patients were followed up with contrast-enhanced MRI scan at 12 days, and every 6 months, for a mean of 36 months (ranging from 14 to 55 months). Four patients received other treatments due to incomplete

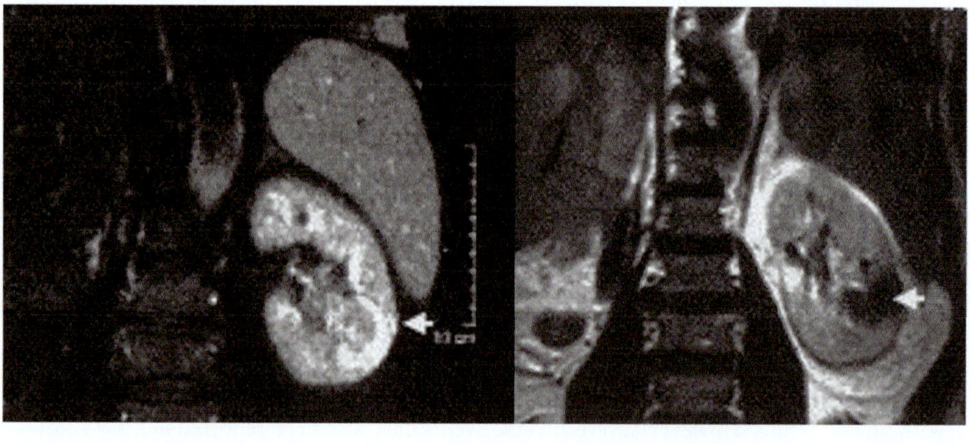

FIGURE 8.23 Coronary contrast-enhanced T1-weighted MR images before and after USgHIFU treatment in a 66-year-old patient with renal cancer of solitary kidney. Before HIFU (left), there is contrast enhancement in the kidney tumour (arrow). Two weeks after HIFU (right), no evidence of contrast enhancement is observed in the treated tumour (arrow), indicative of complete ablation in the kidney cancer. (From Wu F, et al. Ultrasound Med Biol 2004; 30:245–260.)[20]

ablation of the target tumour. However, in the remaining 10 patients there was the appearance of complete ablation post-HIFU on MRI (Figure 8.24), with a mean decrease of 30% in the tumour volume during the follow-up period, indicating that HIFU could create stable lesions in two thirds of patients, with no evidence of local recurrence. As the kidney is surrounded by adipose tissue, the third study explored whether the perinephric fat could influence HIFU ablation in the target tumour.[106] Ten patients with small renal tumours were treated with HIFU prior to surgical resection for histological examination, and the perinephric fat was examined separately to investigate the percentage output drop in energy as the thickness of the fat increased. This showed that the mean attenuation of the perinephric fat was 11.9 ± 0.9 Np/m at 0.8 MHz, the frequency typically used for HIFU kidney ablation. A typical 2 to 4 cm thickness of perinephric fat would result in a reduction in intensity of 3–62% at 0.8 MHz compared with a hypothetical patient with no perinephric fat. This result suggests that perinephric fat may significantly affect the intensity at the HIFU focus and that higher acoustic output is required to compensate for the power loss, which in turn may increase a risk of thermal damage in overlying tissues.

8.5.2.5 Osteosarcoma and Soft Tissue Sarcoma

Osteosarcoma is an aggressive malignant primary bone tumour in children and young adults. Soft tissue sarcomas develop in supporting or connective tissues such as the muscle, nerves, tendons, blood vessels, fat and fibrous tissues. Osteosarcoma requires limb-sparing surgical resection combined with chemotherapy or may require amputation if it is not possible to save the limb. In patients with primary soft tissue sarcoma, the therapeutic choice includes limb-sparing surgical resection, followed by radiation therapy, with or without adjuvant chemotherapy. As a local treatment, HIFU has been used successfully to treat osteosarcoma and soft tissue sarcoma in combination with chemotherapy, indicating that HIFU ablation is safe, feasible and effective in their management. These treatments are introduced in more detail in Chapter 16.

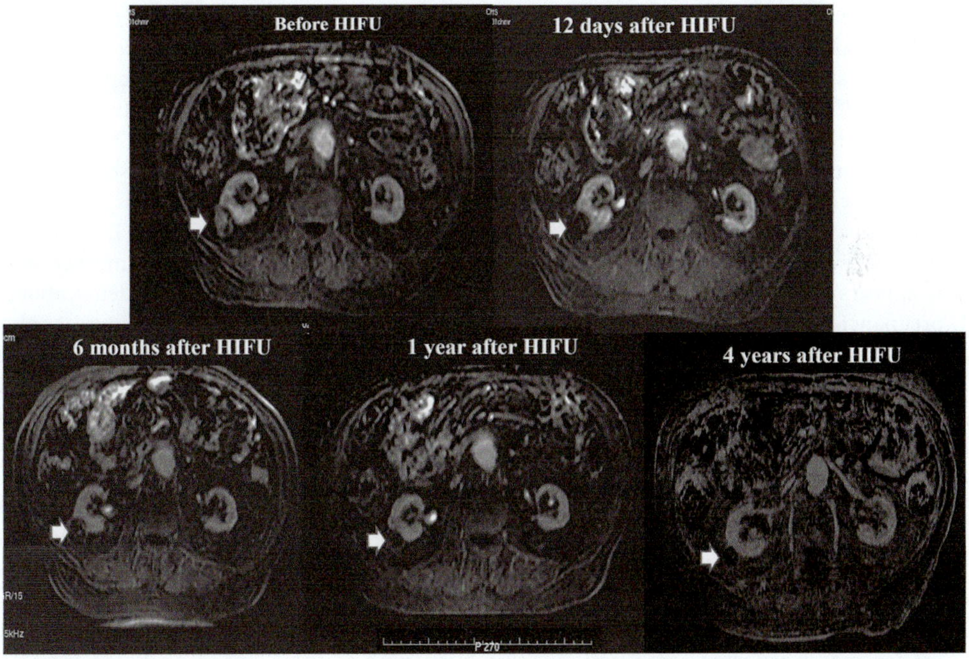

FIGURE 8.24 Transverse contrast-enhanced T1-weighted MR images before and after USgHIFU treatment in a patient with renal cell carcinoma. Before HIFU, there is contrast enhancement in the right kidney tumour (arrow). After HIFU treatment, no evidence of contrast enhancement is observed within the treated tumour (arrow) during a 4-year follow-up, with a decreased size in the treated tumour over time.

8.5.3 Benign Tumours

8.5.3.1 Uterine Fibroids

Uterine fibroids are the most common pelvic tumours, with an incidence of up to 70% in women over 40. They are a significant cause of morbidity for women of reproductive age. Although the majority are asymptomatic, pelvic pain, menorrhagia, dysmenorrhagia, dyspareunia, pelvic fullness, urinary frequency and infertility are reported in approximately 25% of cases. The burden of the diseased uterus has a major impact on health economics and healthcare resources. In the United States, approximately 175,000 hysterectomies are performed annually due to fibroids, at a cost of over $2 billion.[107]

Surgery remains the default clinical management of symptomatic fibroids. Advances in laparoscopic and hysteroscopic instruments, including emerging robotic systems, has allowed the removal of modest sized fibroids with minimally invasive approaches. As a non-invasive modality, HIFU has recently played an increasing role in the clinical management of symptomatic uterine fibroids.

USgHIFU was first used in 1999 to treat symptomatic uterine fibroids in China. From December 1997 to October 2001, 85 patients with symptomatic uterine fibroids underwent HIFU treatment in 10 Chinese hospitals.[18] The results showed that HIFU could significantly improve fibroid-related symptoms with a decreased volume in treated fibroids during the follow-up period. However, transient numbness in the lower limbs was observed in 4 patients, suggesting potential injury to the sciatic nerve.[108] In 2006, a new treatment protocol was established to avoid this complication related to nerve injury. General anaesthesia was replaced by intravenous conscious sedation, thus allowing continuous patient feedback during the HIFU procedure. Since then, USgHIFU treatment has been used successfully in clinical practice, and the results have shown that HIFU is a noninvasive uterus-sparing treatment for patients with uterine fibroids, with improved quality of life and diminished fibroid size.[109–115]

Cheung[116] reviewed 8 articles published from 2005 to 2012 on USgHIFU treatment of uterine fibroids and found that the percentage of the patients who showed symptom improvement was 48.2% 3 months after treatment, and 89.5% at 6 months, with the percentages of fibroid volume reduction at 3-, 6-, and 12-months post-treatment being 27.2%, 47.9%, and 50.3%, respectively. Several clinical trials have recently been performed to compare HIFU with surgical interventions in the management of uterine fibroids. Compared to laparoscopic myomectomy, HIFU was associated with fewer adverse events, shorter hospital stays and no blood loss, although both approaches gave a similar efficacy rate.[117, 118] Chen and colleagues[119] evaluated USgHIFU, myomectomy or hysterectomy in a multicentre patient choice cohort study. A total of 2411 women with symptomatic fibroids were enrolled in 20 Chinese hospitals, including 1353 in HIFU, 472 in hysterectomy and 586 in myomectomy. The results showed that both uterine fibroid score and quality of life improved more rapidly after HIFU than after surgery, but longer-term outcomes were similar. Major adverse events occurred in 3 (0.2%) of HIFU and in 133 (12.6%) of surgical cases, indicating that HIFU led to substantially less morbidity than surgical interventions.

HIFU appears to be a safe option for patients who desire future fertility. Most evidence about post-HIFU pregnancies comes from case reports and series, suggesting that HIFU may not increase obstetric risk. Qin and colleagues[120] followed up 24 women with unintended pregnancies after HIFU treatment. Of these, 7 women completed their pregnancies and delivered term babies by caesarean section, 2 had spontaneous miscarriages and the remaining 15 had elective terminations. Zhou and colleagues[121] reported that 78 of 406 women with uterine fibroids became pregnant after HIFU, including 15 with natural delivery and 56 with caesarean section. Three patients had a miscarriage; 3 patients had full-term normal deliveries after complete curettage of uterine cavity, and 1 patient had induced labour. Li and colleagues[122] reported the largest series of post-HIFU pregnancies, 133 in 131 nulliparous women. Of these, 91 women delivered successfully, 19 were still pregnant at the time of writing, 17 pregnancies ended in spontaneous abortion and 4 elected for abortion.

HIFU is safe for the treatment of symptomatic uterine fibroids, with a small risk of adverse events. The most commonly reported complication is skin burn, with an incidence rate ranging from 0.2% to 1.3%.[119, 123] In a large retrospective review of 9988 HIFU-treated patients, 1062 (10.6%) presented with 1305 adverse events, but most were minor and transient without any medication.[124] They included 874 cases (8.67%) of vaginal secretion, 225 cases (2.23%) of lower abdominal pain 24h after the treatment but requiring no painkillers, 76 cases (0.76%) of melosalgia or buttock pain, 52 cases (0.52%) of odynuria, 20 cases (0.20%) of menstruation-like vaginal bleeding, 2 cases (0.2%) of temporary blurred vision, 26 cases (0.26%) of blisters or tangerine pericarp-like burns in the abdominal skin, 16 cases (0.16%) of urinary retention, 4 cases (0.4%) of fever of 38.5°C, 3 cases (0.3%) of acute renal insufficiency, 2 cases (0.2%) of intestinal perforation and 1 case (0.01%) of long-term lateral ventral syndrome.

8.5.3.2 Breast Fibroadenoma

Fibroadenoma is the most common benign breast tumour in women under the age of 30. It presents with a palpable breast lump, occasionally with local pain. Without any treatment, up to 59% breast fibroadenoma show regression or complete resolution within 5 years. The management of palpable fibroadenoma includes four main treatment options: conservative with reassurance, vacuum-assisted mammotomy, cryoablation and surgical excision. Intervention is normally offered to patients with large fibroadenomas or rapidly growing lesions, or to those who consistently request surgery due to their large size, physical discomfort and anxiety about growth or malignancy. As a minimally invasive treatment, both vacuum-assisted mammotomy and cryoablation have demonstrated excellent efficacy, safety and a high-level satisfaction in clinical use.

In 2015, Kovatcheva and colleagues[125] reported the first clinical experience of using USgHIFU for breast fibroadenoma. It was a multicentric clinical trial in which HIFU was performed in 42 women with 51 breast fibroadenoma, followed by the assessment of B-mode ultrasound imaging. They found that significant mean volume reduction was seen 6- and 12-month post-treatment. This result was further confirmed by Peek's study,[126] suggesting that HIFU is feasible and effective in the treatment of breast fibroadenoma. Peek and colleagues[127] also compared the volume change between 20 patients undergoing HIFU treatment and 20 patients with no treatment. Follow-up ultrasound examination showed a significant mean reduction in lesion volume of 43.5% 6 months post-treatment in the HIFU group compared with 4.6% in the control group.

HIFU appears to be safe for the treatment of breast fibroadenoma. The adverse events include superficial skin burn and subcutaneous oedema, which are transient and resolve spontaneously. Skin hyperpigmentation and asymptomatic subcutaneous induration are also observed during the follow-up period.

8.5.3.3 Benign Thyroid Tumours

Benign thyroid tumours are small and often discovered incidentally when a patient has radiological assessment for conditions unrelated to the thyroid gland. Although more than 95% of thyroid nodules are benign with no treatment required, a small number can grow over time, leading to local pressure symptoms such as neck pain, occasional choking, dyspnoea and dysphagia.

In 2011, Esnault and colleagues[128] reported the first clinical study of USgHIFU treatment of benign thyroid tumours. A total of 25 patients received this treatment, followed by thyroidectomy. Of these, 3 patients discontinued treatment due to pain or skin micro-blisters and the remaining 22 completed treatment with no major complications. Histological examination showed that all HIFU lesions were confined to the target nodules with typical coagulative necrosis. The extent of nodule destruction ranged from 2% to 80%. Subsequently, Korkusuz and colleagues[129] followed up the effect on volume reduction in 12 patients. They found a volume reduction of more than 30% 3 months post-treatment in 9 patients, whilst the remaining 3 did not achieve a 30% of reduction in nodule volume. Similar results were also observed in other studies,[130–132] suggesting that HIFU can significantly reduce nodule size in these tumours. In addition, HIFU relieved local pressure symptoms and shortened the hospital stay, less subclinical hypothyroidism, lower cost and better symptom improvement.[133]

HIFU seems to be safe for the treatment of patients with benign thyroid tumours. There are no severe adverse events such as laryngeal nerve palsy and haematoma. Local pain, skin redness and mild subcutaneous oedema over the nodule area are commonly observed but are transient with no need for medication. However, four patients were reported to suffer from a unilateral vocal cord paresis, although they all recovered fully within 6 weeks of HIFU treatment.[134]

8.5.4 Other Diseases

8.5.4.1 Adenomyosis

Adenomyosis is a disorder of the uterus in which endometrial glands and stroma are present within uterine musculature. Its symptoms of dysmenorrhea and menorrhagia have enormous influence on the quality of life and fertility of women. Treatment of adenomyosis is a challenge. Hysterectomy is a curative option but is not suitable for women who wish to preserve their fertility. Other medication options include levonorgestrel-releasing intrauterine devices, the gonadotropin-releasing hormone analogues, non-steroidal anti-inflammatory drugs and oral contraceptives. However, the effects of these non-surgical treatments are limited, and symptoms recur easily after discontinuation of medication because of side effects.

In 2009, Wang and colleagues[135] reported the first clinical experience of using USgHIFU treatment for 12 patients with adenomyosis. The acoustic powers used for the treatment ranged from 290 W to 420 W. Symptoms were seen to be relieved three months post-treatment, with non-perfused volumes (NPVs) observed on contrast-enhanced ultrasound imaging in all adenomyosis. They found that clinical results seemed much better when high acoustic powers were used for the treatment. Subsequently, Zhou and colleagues[136] reported a retrospective analysis of HIFU treatment for 78 patients with adenomyosis. Of these, 69 patients were followed up for an average of 24 months. The results showed symptom relief in 62 patients, and NPVs on post-treatment MRI in 60 patients, including an NPV ratio more than 50% in 47 patients, and less than 50% in 13 patients.

Since then, several studies have investigated the short- and long-term clinical results of USgHIFU treatment for symptomatic adenomyosis.[137–144] Similar results were observed in more than 2000 patients who received HIFU treatment in these studies, confirming that HIFU is safe, feasible, and effective for the treatment of symptomatic adenomyosis. In addition, they found that the NPV ratio reflected the long-term efficacy of the treatment, with a higher NPV ratio being more likely to achieve long-term clinical success.[138] There were no significant differences in long-term symptom relief between focal and diffuse adenomyosis after treatment.[137] Finally, a gonadotrophin-releasing hormone agonist (GnRH-a) combined with HIFU could significantly decrease uterine and adenomyotic lesion volumes and give symptom relief when compared with HIFU alone.[143]

HIFU is safe for the treatment of adenomyosis. In a total of 10,310 patients who received HIFU treatment from 2011 to 2015 in China, adverse events were reported in 2367 patients (23.0%), but most were minor and transient.[145] The most common adverse event was lower abdominal pain in 2253 patients (21.9%). Minimal vaginal discharge was reported in 1136 (11%) patients and sacrococcygeal pain in 712 (6.9%). Thirteen patients (0.1%) complained of leg pain or numbness that lasted from two weeks to two months posttreatment. Skin burn was found in 21 (0.2%) patients and bowel injury in 2 (0.02%) patients, who developed a bowel perforation 10 and 20 days after the treatment.

8.5.4.2 Caesarean Scar Pregnancy

As a serious complication of caesarean section, caesarean scar pregnancy is an ectopic pregnancy occurring in the scar. If untreated, it may lead to severe haemorrhage and uterine rupture. Current treatments, such as methotrexate, uterine artery embolisation (UAE), hysteroscopic resection and laparoscopic resection, can eliminate the embryo, decrease the risk of bleeding and preserve the uterus to maintain further fertility before gestational sac rupture and haemorrhage.

HIFU has been used increasingly for the treatment of caesarean scar pregnancies. In 2014, Huang and colleagues[146] reported the first successful use of USgHIFU treatment in 4 patients. They used USgHIFU to stop fetal cardiac activity by heating embryonic tissues, followed by dilatation and curettage for removal of conception products under hysteroscopy. A rapid decline of human chorionic gonadotropin level and disappearance of embryonic cardiac activity were observed after the treatment. Furthermore, HIFU reduced the risk of haemorrhage during the dilatation and curettage procedure because of reduced blood flow in the trophoblast tissue as detected on colour Doppler ultrasound imaging, and a significant reduction of blood loss in suction curettage after HIFU treatment. Similar results were confirmed by two other groups,[147, 148] indicating that HIFU combined with a dilatation and curettage procedure was safe, feasible and effective in the treatment of caesarean scar pregnancy.

In addition, several studies have been conducted to compare the efficacy and safety of HIFU and UAE treatment in combination with suction curettage under hysteroscopy.[149–151] The results showed that although the efficacy was similar in both treatments, HIFU resulted in less pain, and fewer adverse events than UAE treatment. Moreover, HIFU is particularly suitable for women wishing to preserve their fertility.

8.5.4.3 Echinococcosis

Echinococcus is a parasitic, cyst-forming disease caused by the larval stage of the taeniid echinococcus. The liver is the organ that is mostly affected by this parasite, resulting in complicated and multiple forms of hydatid disease. This causes severe and prolonged progressive deterioration of liver function. The cysts consist of a fibrous host-derived outer layer (pericyst), an acellular, laminated membrane (ectocyst) and a nucleated inner layer (endocyst). Surgery remains the mainstay of treatment for large, active, complicated or symptomatic hepatic hydatid cysts.

Due to its non-invasive nature, HIFU can avoid some of the risks associated with percutaneous radiofrequency ablation and surgery, such as infection and biliary complications. Tamarozzi and colleagues[152] reviewed the experiments designed to investigate the destructive effects of HIFU on echinococcus, including in vitro and in vivo studies as well as animal models. The results showed that HIFU was effective in the treatment of echinococcus. Injecting a superabsorbent polymer and/or ultrasound contrast agent into the cyst could enhance the thermal effects of HIFU on the parasite.

Imankulov and colleagues[153] reported the first retrospective study of the use of USgHIFU for the treatment of 62 patients with hepatic hydatid cysts. Forty-two patients were followed up after treatment. Histological examination showed at the subcellular level that HIFU could destroy the protoscolexes, cyst germinal layer and embryos of the parasite elements. Post-treatment imaging identified positive clinical responses, including the disappearance, calcification, and size reduction (more than 50%) in treated cysts. No patients had a local recurrence during 3-year follow-up. The authors suggested that HIFU treatment could be applied as a first-line therapy, but further clinical trials will be required to evaluate the long-term results of HIFU for hepatic hydatid cyst.

8.5.4.4 Hypersplenism

Hypersplenism is a clinical syndrome characterised by splenomegaly, a variable combination of anaemia, leucopoenia and/or thrombocytopaenia, compensatory bone marrow hyperplasia and reduced immunity. The conventional treatment is splenectomy. Partial splenic embolisation enables treatment of this condition, but complications appear frequently. Radiofrequency and microwave ablation also have a clear effect on hypersplenism. However, since secondary hypersplenism often occurs with hyperkinesis of the portal vein and fragile splenic tissues, the risk of splenic injury is high due to needle puncture.

HIFU appears to be safe, feasible and effective for the treatment of hypersplenism. Zhu and colleagues[154] reported interim results of HIFU treatment for 9 patients with HCC and secondary hypersplenism, a common manifestation in cirrhotic patients with portal hypertension. This was the first clinical experience and the HCC lesion and spleen were treated simultaneously. Later, they reported the results from 28 patients with secondary hypersplenism, including the previous 9 HCC patients.[155] All patients had splenomegaly with portal hypertension, leucopenia and thrombocytopaenia. The lower pole and the hilum of the spleen were targeted. They found that the HIFU treatment induced a significant reduction in splenic volume from 1307.3 cm^3 to 949.5 cm^3 (measured using MRI) 12 months post-treatment, with an average NPV ratio of 27.2%. The levels of peripheral white blood cells and platelets increased significantly after treatment. Liver function and symptoms such as epistaxis and gingival bleeding were improved during the 12-month follow-up. There were no severe adverse events except hydrothorax (n=2) and pleural plus peritoneal effusions (n = 1) due to hypoproteinaemia. Compared to splenectomy or partial splenic embolisation, HIFU was relatively safe and less invasive, suggesting that it may be a good alternative option for patients at high surgical risk.[156]

8.6 Summary

As a non-invasive approach, HIFU therapy has been shown to be technically and clinically safe, feasible and effective for the local treatment of solid tumours. It can be offered as a curative treatment to destroy an entire tumour or as a salvage treatment to debulk a target tumour. The non-invasive nature of HIFU has already made it more attractive to patients and clinicians, because of its lowered morbidity, low cost and a shorter hospital stay. Where clinically appropriate, HIFU should give at least the same result as surgery. After its clinical use for 2 decades, it has become truly clear that HIFU should take its place in the multidisciplinary management of cancer patients in the future.

Apart from optimisation of technical parameters, HIFU therapy should be undertaken only with a precise knowledge, not only of the number and location of the tumours, but also of the biological characteristics and natural history of cancer cells. The goal of cancer therapy is to kill all cancer cells in each patient. The therapeutic strategy for cancer patients should be multidisciplinary, and so should include surgery, chemotherapy and radiation therapy. Since HIFU is a local treatment, as is surgery, it is important to combine it with other therapeutic options such as chemotherapy. However, it is still unclear how to select the sequencing of combinations in the multidisciplinary therapies for each cancer, especially where HIFU is to be used clinically.

After HIFU ablation, the treated tumour becomes dead tissue. It is left in place and the tumour debris will slowly be reabsorbed as the normal process of healing. This will take months to few years. Recent studies have provided academic evidence that HIFU ablation can elicit a systemic antitumour immune response and the host immune system can become more responsive to the cancer cells. It is not surprising that there is great interest in the relationship between ablation and antitumour immune response since local HIFU treatment has the potential to trigger systemic immunity. This may lead to a post-ablative immune response that eliminates distant disease and prevents local recurrence in HIFU-treated patients, who had dysfunctional antitumour immunity pretreatment. If the destruction of the tumours releases tumour antigens or improves tumour immunogenicity, a therapeutic strategy that combines HIFU with immunotherapies, such as immune checkpoint inhibitors, may augment the efficacy of HIFU-induced antitumour immunity specifically against the target cancer cells. This combined approach may become an important aspect in the HIFU treatment of solid malignancy in the future.

HIFU therapy continues to develop both technically and clinically. More supplementary studies are needed to determine factors that influence HIFU energy deposition in the target tumour, such as tissue structure, movement, function, and blood perfusion. For example, animal studies have shown that when tissue blood perfusion is manipulated by mechanical and pharmacological means, perfusion-mediated tissue cooling can directly affect the shape and size of HIFU-induced lesions, and a decrease of blood perfusion could lead to an increase in the volume of coagulation necrosis in the target tissues. Based on a better understanding of the perfusion effects, novel strategies will be investigated to enhance HIFU's effect and reduce the treatment time in the clinical application.

Imaging techniques are arguably more important in HIFU therapy than in surgery. They can help identify the margin of a unifocal tumour and of adjacent microsatellites to provide accurate determination of the extent of a target tumour before the treatment, assess whether HIFU has destroyed the entire target immediately after the treatment, and observe the shrinkage of the treated tumour over time, as well as to provide an early sign of local recurrence during the follow-up period.

The aim of this chapter has been to focus on extracorporeal USgHIFU and its clinical use. However, HIFU devices do not only use an extracorporeal route, but can also be applied transrectally, laparoscopically and endoscopically. Instead of thermal ablation, focused ultrasound can be used as a hyperthermia tool to deliver a chemotherapeutic agent directly to a target tumour, so that chemotherapeutic dosage can be significantly reduced. Until now, HIFU has been used to treat malignant and benign tumours as well as other diseases. With the development of the technique, it should be considered to be a good candidate for more widespread clinical applications.

REFERENCES

1. Breasted, J. H. 1930. *The Edwin Smith Surgical Papyrus.* Chicago: Chicago University Press.
2. Lynn, J. G., Zwemer, R. L., Chick, A. J., and A. G. Miller. 1942. A new method for the generation and use of focused US in experimental biology. *J Gen Physiol* 26:179–93.
3. Fry, W. J., Mosberg, W. H., Barnard, J. W., and F. J. Fry. 1954. Production of focal destructive lesions in the central nervous system with ultrasound. *J Neurosurg* 11:471–8.
4. Fry, W. J., Barnard, J. W., Fry, F. J., Krumins, R. F., and J. F. Brennan. 1955. Ultrasonic lesions in the mammalian central nervous system. *Science* 122:517–8.
5. Fry, F. J. 1958. Precision high intensity focusing ultrasonic machines for surgery. *Am J Phys Med* 37:152–6.
6. O'Brien, W., and F. Dunn. 2015. An early History of high intensity focused ultrasound. *Physics Today* 68:40–5.
7. Fry, W. J., and F. J. Fry. 1960. Fundamental neurological research and human neurosurgery using intense ultrasound. *IRE Trans Biomed Electronics* ME-7:166–81.
8. Lizzi, F. L. 1993. High-precision thermotherapy for small lesions. *Eur Urol* 23 (Suppl 1):23–8.
9. Muratore, R. 2006. A history of the sonocare CST-100: The first FDA-approved HIFU device. In *Therapeutic Ultrasound: 5th International Symposium on Therapeutic Ultrasound*, ed. G. T. Clement, N. J. McDannold, and K. Hynynen, 508–512. American Institute of Physics. USA.
10. Silverman, R. H., Vogelsang, B., Rondeau, M. J., and D. J. Coleman. 1991. Therapeutic ultrasound for the treatment of glaucoma. *Am J Ophthalmol* 111:327–37.
11. Rosecan, L. R., Iwamoto, T., Rosado, A., Lizzi, F. L., and D. J. Coleman. 1985. Therapeutic ultrasound in the treatment of retinal detachment: Clinical observations and light and electronmicroscopy. *Retina* 5:115–22.
12. Coleman, D. J., Lizzi, F. L., Burgess, S. E., et al. 1986. Ultrasonic hyperthermia and radiation in the management of intraocular malignant melanoma. *Am J Ophthalmol* 101:635–42.
13. Vallancien, G., Chartier-Kastler, E., Harouni, M., Chopin, D., and J. Bougaran. 1993. Focused extracorporeal pyrotherapy: Experimental study and feasibility in man. *Semin Urol* 11:7–9.
14. Vallancien, G., Harouni, M., Guillonneau. B., Veillon, B., and J. Bougaran. 1996. Ablation of superficial bladder tumors with focused extracorporeal pyrotherapy. *Urology* 47:204–7.
15. Vallancien, G., Chartier-Kastler, E., Bataille, N., Chopin, D., Harouni, M., and J. Bougaran. 1993. Focused extracorporeal pyrotherapy. *Eur Urol* 23 (Suppl 1):48–52.
16. ter Haar, G. R., Clarke, R. L., Vaughan, M. G., and C. R. Hill. 1991 Trackless surgery using focussed ultrasound: Technique and case report. *Min Inv Ther* 1:13–9.
17. Visioli, A. G., Rivens, I. H., ter Haar, G. R., et al. 1999. Preliminary results of a phase I dose escalation clinical trial using focused ultrasound in the treatment of localized tumours. *Eur J Ultrasound* 9:11–8.
18. Wu, F., Wang, Z. B., Chen, W. Z., et al. 2004. Extracorporeal high intensity focused ultrasound ablation in the treatment of 1038 patients with solid carcinomas in China: An overview. *Ultrason Sonochem* 11:149–54.
19. Chinese Medical Association. 2005. Guidelines for clinical applications of high intensity focused ultrasound cancer therapy system (Article in Chinese). *Natl Med J China* 85:796–797.
20. Wu, F., Wang, Z. B., Chen, W. Z., et al. 2004. Extracorporeal focused ultrasound surgery for treatment of human solid carcinomas: Early Chinese clinical experience. *Ultrasound Med Biol* 30:245–260.
21. Minami, Y., and M. Kudo. 2014. Ultrasound fusion imaging of hepatocellular carcinoma: A review of current evidence. *Dig Dis* 32:690–5.
22. Lee, M. W. 2014. Fusion imaging of real-time ultrasonography with CT or MRI for hepatic intervention. *Ultrasonography* 33:227–39.
23. Dunn, F. 1974. Attenuation and speed of ultrasound in lung. *J Acoust Soc Am* 56:1638–1639.
24. Wells, P. N. T. 1977. *Biomedical Ultrasonics.* London: Academic Press Inc.
25. Hill, C. R., Bamber, J. C., and G. R. ter Haar. 2004. *Physical Principles of Medical Ultrasound.* 2nd ed. Chichester: John Wiley & Sons Ltd.
26. Goss, S. A., Frizzell, L. A., and F. Dunn. 1979. Ultrasonic absorption and attenuation in mammalian tissues. *Ultrasound Med Biol* 5:181–6.
27. Goss, S. A., Johnson, R. L., and F. Dunn. 1978. Comprehensive compilation of empirical ultrasonic properties of mammalian tissues. *J Acoust Soc Am* 64:423–57.
28. Goss, S. A., Johnson, R. L., and F. Dunn. 1980. Compilation of empirical ultrasonic properties of mammalian tissues. *J Acoust Soc Am* 68:93–108.

29. Kikuchi Y., Uchida R., Tanaka K., and T. Wagai. 1957. Early cancer diagnosis through ultrasonics. *J Acoust Soc Am* 29:824–833.
30. Calderon, C., Vilkomerson, D., Mezrich, R., Etzold, K. F., Kingsley, B., and M. Haskin. 1976. Differences in the attenuation of ultrasound by normal, benign, and malignant breast tissue. *J Clin Ultrasound* 4:249–54.
31. El-Brawany, M. A., Nassiri, D. K., ter Haar, G., Shaw, A., Rivens, I., and K. Lozhken. 2009. Measurement of thermal and ultrasonic properties of some biological tissues. *J Med Eng Technol* 33:249–56.
32. Ozhinsky, E., Kohi, M. P., Ghanouni, P., and V. Rieke. 2015. T2-based temperature monitoring in abdominal fat during MR-guided focused ultrasound treatment of patients with uterine fibroids. *J Ther Ultrasound* 3:15.
33. Kim, Y., Kim, J. H., Rhim, H., et al. 2012. Volumetric MR-guided high-intensity focused ultrasound ablation with a one-layer strategy to treat large uterine fibroids: Initial clinical outcomes. *Radiology* 263:600–9.
34. Galmén, K., Harbut, P., Freedman, J., and J. G. Jakobsson. 2017. High frequency jet ventilation for motion management during ablation procedures, a narrative review. *Acta Anaesthesiol Scand* 61:1066–74.
35. Wu, F., Wang, Z. B., Chen, W. Z., et al. 2005. Advanced hepatocellular carcinoma: Treatment with high-intensity focused ultrasound ablation combined with transcatheter arterial embolization. *Radiology* 235:659–667.
36. Vaezy, S., Shi, X., Martin, R. W., et al. 2001. Real-time visualization of high-intensity focused ultrasound treatment using ultrasound imaging. *Ultrasound Med Biol* 27:33–42.
37. Rabkin, B. A., Zderic, V., and S. Vaezy. 2005. Hyperecho in ultrasound images of HIFU therapy: Involvement of cavitation. *Ultrasound Med Biol* 31:947–956.
38. Nandlall, S. D., Jackson, E., and C. C. Coussios. 2011 Real-time passive acoustic monitoring of HIFU-induced tissue damage. *Ultrasound Med Biol* 37:922–934.
39. McLaughlan, J., Rivens, I., Leighton, T., and G. ter Haar. 2010. A study of bubble activity generated in ex vivo tissue by high intensity focused ultrasound. *Ultrasound Med Biol* 36:1327–1344.
40. Rabkin, B. A., Zderic, V., Crum, L. A. et al. 2006. Biological and physical mechanisms of HIFU-induced hyperecho in ultrasound images. *Ultrasound Med Biol* 32:1721–1729.
41. Holt, R. G., and R. A. Roy. 2001. Measurements of bubble-enhanced heating from focused, MHz-frequency ultrasound in a tissue-mimicking material. *Ultrasound Med Biol* 27:1399–1412.
42. Sokka, S. D., King, R., and K. Hynynen. 2003. MRI-guided gas bubble enhanced ultrasound heating in in vivo rabbit thigh. *Phys Med Biol* 48:223–241.
43. Coussios, C. C., Farny, C. H., Haar, G. T, and R. A. Roy. 2007. Role of acoustic cavitation in the delivery and monitoring of cancer treatment by high-intensity focused ultrasound (HIFU). *Int J Hyperthermia* 23:105–20.
44. Haworth, K. J., Salgaonkar, V. A., Corregan, N. M., Holland, C. K., and T. D. Mast. 2015. Using passive cavitation images to classify high-intensity focused ultrasound lesions. *Ultrasound Med Biol* 41:2420–2434.
45. Lyon, P. C., Rai, V., Price, N., Shah, A., Wu, F., and D. Cranston. 2020. Ultrasound-guided high intensity focused ultrasound ablation for symptomatic uterine fibroids: Preliminary clinical experience. *Ultraschall Med* 41:550–556.
46. Lang, B. H. H., Woo, Y. C., and K. W. Chiu. 2018. Significance of hyperechoic marks observed during high-intensity focused ultrasound (HIFU) ablation of benign thyroid nodules. *Eur Radiol* 28:2675–2681.
47. Wu, F., Wang, Z. B., Chen, W. Z., et al. 2004. Extracorporeal high intensity focused ultrasound ablation in the treatment of patients with large hepatocellular carcinoma. *Ann Surg Oncol* 11:1061–1069.
48. Fukuda, H., Numata, K., Nozaki, A., et al. 2011. Hyperecho in ultrasound images during high-intensity focused ultrasound ablation for hepatocellular carcinomas. *Eur J Radiol* 80:e571–575.
49. Lencioni, R., and J. M. Llovet. 2010. Modified RECIST (mRECIST) assessment for hepatocellular carcinoma. *Semin Liver Dis* 30:52–60.
50. Timmerman, R. D., Bizekis, C. S., Pass, H. I., et al. 2009. Local surgical, ablative, and radiation treatment of metastases. *CA Cancer J Clin* 59:145–170.
51. Liapi, E., and J. F. Geschwind. 2007. Transcatheter and ablative therapeutic approaches for solid malignancies. *J Clin Oncol* 25:978–986.
52. Hong, K., Georgiades, C. S., and J. F. Geschwind. 2006. Technology insight: Image-guided therapies for hepatocellular carcinoma – intra-arterial and ablative techniques. *Nat Clin Pract Oncol* 3:315–324.

53. Focused Ultrasound Foundation. 2023 state of the field. https://cdn.fusfoundation.org/2023/07/21125203/FUSF-State-of-the-Field-Report-2023_July-24.pdf#page=9
54. Lin, D., Lin, S. M., and Y. F. Liaw. 1997. Non-surgical treatment of hepatocellular carcinoma. *J Gastroenterol Hepa* 12:S319–328.
55. Zibari, G. B., Riche, A., Zizzi, H. C., et al. 1998. Surgical and nonsurgical management of primary and metastatic liver tumors. *Am Surg* 64:211–221.
56. Wu, F., Chen, W. Z., Bai, J. et al. 2001. Pathological changes in human malignant carcinoma treated with high-intensity focused ultrasound. *Ultrasound Med Biol* 27:1099–1106.
57. Wu, F., Wang, Z. B., Chen, W. Z., et al. 2004. Extracorporeal high intensity focused ultrasound ablation in the treatment of patients with large hepatocellular carcinoma. *Ann Surg Oncol* 11:1061–1069.
58. Li, C., Zhang, W., Zhang, R., Zhang, L., Wu, P., and F. Zhang. 2010. Therapeutic effects and prognostic factors in high-intensity focused ultrasound combined with chemoembolisation for larger hepatocellular carcinoma. *Eur J Cancer* 46:2513–2521.
59. Kim, J., Chung, D. J., Jung, S. E., Cho, S. H., Hahn, S. T., and J. M. Lee. 2012. Therapeutic effect of high-intensity focused ultrasound combined with transarterial chemoembolisation for hepatocellular carcinoma < 5 cm: Comparison with transarterial chemoembolisation monotherapy-preliminary observations. *Br J Radiol* 85:e94094–6.
60. Li, C. X., Xu, G. L., Jiang, Z. Y., et al. 2004. Analysis of clinical effect of highintensity focused ultrasound on liver cancer. *World J Gastroenterol* 10:2201–2204.
61. Li, Y. Y., Sha, W. H., Zhou, Y. J., and Y. Q. Nie. 2007. Short and long term efficacy of high intensity focused ultrasound therapy for advanced hepatocellular carcinoma. *J Gastroenterol Hepatol* 22:2148–2154.
62. Numata, K., Fukuda, H., Ohto, M., et al. 2010. Evaluation of the therapeutic efficacy of high-intensity focused ultrasound ablation of hepatocellular carcinoma by three-dimensional sonography with a perflubutane-based contrast agent. *Eur J Radiol* 75: e67–75.
63. Ng, K. K., Poon, R. T., Chan, S. C., et al. 2011. High-intensity focused ultrasound for hepatocellular carcinoma: A single-center experience. *Ann Surg* 253:981–987.
64. Cheung, T, T., Chu, F. S., Jenkins, C. R., et al. 2012. Tolerance of high intensity focused ultrasound ablation in patients with hepatocellular carcinoma. *World J Surg* 36:2420–2427.
65. Chok, K. S., Cheung, T. T., Lo, R. C., et al. 2014. Pilot study of high intensity focused ultrasound ablation as a bridging therapy for hepatocellular carcinoma patients wait-listed for liver transplantation. *Liver Transpl* 20:912–921.
66. Cheung, T. T., Fan, S. T., Chu, F. S., et al. 2013. Survival analysis of high intensity focused ultrasound ablation in patients with small hepatocellular carcinoma. *HPB (Oxford)* 15:567–573.
67. Cheung, T. T., Poon, R. T., Jenkins, C. R., et al. 2014. Survival analysis of high-intensity focused ultrasound therapy vs. transarterial chemoembolization for unresectable hepatocellular carcinomas. *Liver Int* 34:e136–143.
68. Chan, A. C., Cheung, T. T., Fan, S. T., et al. 2013. Survival analysis of high-intensity focused ultrasound therapy versus radiofrequency ablation in the treatment of recurrent hepatocellular carcinoma. *Ann Surg* 257:686–692.
69. Cheung, T. T., Fan, S. T., Chan, S. C., et al. 2013. High-intensity focused ultrasound ablation: An effective bridging therapy for hepatocellular carcinoma patients. *World J Gastroenterol* 19:3083–3089.
70. Zhang, L., Zhu, H., Jin, C., et al. 2009. High-intensity focused ultrasound (HIFU): Effective and safe therapy for hepatocellular carcinoma adjacent to major hepatic veins. *Eur Radiol* 19:437–445.
71. Wang, Y., Wang, W., Wang, Y., and J. Tang. 2010. Ultrasound-guided high-intensity focused ultrasound treatment for needle track seeding of hepatocellular carcinoma: Preliminary results. *Int J Hyperthermia* 26:441–447.
72. Illing, R. O., Kennedy, J. E., Wu F., et al. 2005. The safety and feasibility of extracorporeal high-intensity focused ultrasound (HIFU) for the treatment of liver and kidney tumours in a Western population. *Br J Cancer* 93:890–895.
73. Leslie, T. A., Kennedy, J. E., Illing, R. O., et al. 2008. High-intensity focused ultrasound ablation of liver tumours: Can radiological assessment predict the histological response? *Br J Radiol* 81:564–571.
74. Noterdaeme, O., Leslie, T. A., Kennedy, J. E., Phillips, R. R., and M. Brady. 2009. The use of time to maximum enhancement to indicate areas of ablation following the treatment of liver tumours with high-intensity focused ultrasound. *Br J Radiol* 82:412–420.

75. Leslie, T, Ritchie, R, Illing, R, et al. 2012. High-intensity focused ultrasound treatment of liver tumours: Post-treatment MRI correlates well with intra-operative estimates of treatment volume. *Br J Radiol* 85:1363–1370.
76. Orsi, F., Zhang, L., Arnone, P., et al. 2010. High-intensity focused ultrasound ablation: Effective and safe therapy for solid tumors in difficult locations. *Am J Roentgenol* 195:W245–252.
77. Wang, S., Yang, C., Zhang, J., et al. 2014. First experience of high-intensity focused ultrasound combined with transcatheter arterial embolization as local control for hepatoblastoma. *Hepatology* 59:170–177.
78. Jung, S. E., Cho, S. H., Jang, J. H., and J. Y. Han. 2011. High-intensity focused ultrasound ablation in hepatic and pancreatic cancer: Complications. *Abdom Imaging* 36:185–195.
79. Wu, F., Wang, Z. B., Cao, Y. D., et al. 2003 A randomised clinical trial of high-intensity focused ultrasound ablation for the treatment of patients with localised breast cancer. *Br J Cancer* 89:2227–2233.
80. Wu, F., Wang, Z. B., Cao, Y. D., et al. 2007. "Wide local ablation" of localized breast cancer using high intensity focused ultrasound. *J Surg Oncol* 96:130–136.
81. Wu, F., Wang, Z. B., Cao, Y. D., et al. 2006. Heat fixation of cancer cells ablated with high-intensity focused ultrasound in patients with breast cancer. *Am J Surg* 192:179–184.
82. Orsi, F, Arnone, P, Chen, W., and L. Zhang. 2010. High intensity focused ultrasound ablation: A new therapeutic option for solid tumors. *J Cancer Res Ther* 6:414–420.
83. Kim, S. H., Jung, S. E., Kim, H. L., et al. 2010. The potential role of dynamic MRI in assessing the effectiveness of high-intensity focused ultrasound ablation of breast cancer. *Int J Hyperthermia* 26:594–603.
84. Wu, F., Wang, Z. B., Chen, W. Z., et al. 2005. Extracorporeal high intensity focused ultrasound treatment for patients with breast cancer. *Breast Cancer Res Treat* 92:51–60.
85. Wu, F., Wang, Z. B., Zhu, H., et al. 2005. Feasibility of US-guided high-intensity focused ultrasound treatment in patients with advanced pancreatic cancer: Initial experience. *Radiology* 236:1034–1040.
86. Orsi, F., Zhang, L., Arnone, P., et al. 2010. High-intensity focused ultrasound ablation: Effective and safe therapy for solid tumors in difficult locations. *AJR Am J Roentgenol* 195: W245–252.
87. Wang, K., Chen, Z., Meng, Z., et al. 2011. Analgesic effect of high intensity focused ultrasound therapy for unresectable pancreatic cancer. *Int J Hyperthermia* 27:101–107.
88. Sung, H. Y., Jung, S. E., Cho, S. H., et al. 2011. Long term outcome of high-intensity focused ultrasound in advanced pancreatic cancer. *Pancreas* 40:1080–1086.
89. Wang, G., and D. Zhou. 2015. Preoperative ultrasound ablation for borderline resectable pancreatic cancer: A report of 30 cases. *Ultrason Sonochem* 27:694–702.
90. Gao, H. F., Wang, K., Meng, Z. Q., et al. 2013. High intensity focused ultrasound treatment for patients with local advanced pancreatic cancer. *Hepatogastroenterology* 60:1906–1910.
91. Zhao, H., Yang, G., Wang, D., et al. 2010. Concurrent gemcitabine and high-intensity focused ultrasound therapy in patients with locally advanced pancreatic cancer. *Anticancer Drugs* 21:447–452.
92. Li, X., Wang, K., Zheng, L., and Z. Meng. 2015. Retrospective analysis of high intensity focused ultrasound combined with S-1 in the treatment of metastatic pancreatic cancer after failure of gemcitabine. *Am J Cancer Res* 6:84–90.
93. Strunk, H. M., Henseler, J., Rauch, M., et al. 2016. Clinical use of high-intensity focused ultrasound (HIFU) for tumor and pain reduction in advanced pancreatic cancer. *Rofo* 188:662–670.
94. Lv, W., Yan, T., Wang, G., Zhao, W., Zhang, T., and D. Zhou. 2016. High-intensity focused ultrasound therapy in combination with gemcitabine for unresectable pancreatic carcinoma. *Ther Clin Risk Manag* 12:687–691.
95. Li, Y. J., Huang, G. L., Sun, X. L., Zhao, X. C., and Z. G. Li. 2016. The combination therapy of high-intensity focused ultrasound with radiotherapy in locally advanced pancreatic carcinoma. *World J Surg Oncol* 14:60.
96. Vidal-Jove, J., Perich, E., and M. A. Del Castillo. 2015. Ultrasound guided high intensity focused ultrasound for malignant tumors: The Spanish experience of survival advantage in stage III and IV pancreatic cancer. *Ultrason Sonochem* 27:703–706.
97. Ning, Z. Y., Cheng, C. S., Xie, J., et al. 2016. A retrospective analysis of survival factors of high intensity focused ultrasound (HIFU) treatment for unresectable pancreatic cancer. *Discov Med* 21:435–445.
98. Wang, K., Zhu, H., Meng, Z., et al. 2013. Safety evaluation of high-intensity focused ultrasound in patients with pancreatic cancer. *Onkologie* 36:88–92.
99. Reddan, D. N., Raj, G. V., and T. J. Polascik. 2001. Management of small renal tumors: An overview. *Am J Med* 110:558–562.

100. Susani, M., Madersbacher, S., Kratzik, C., Vingers, L., and M. Marberger. 1993. Morphology of tissue destruction induced by focused ultrasound. *Eur Urol* 23(Suppl 1):34–38.
101. Kohrmann, K. U., Michel, M. S., Gaa, J., Marlinghaus, E., and P. Alken. 2002. High intensity focused ultrasound as noninvasive therapy for multilocal renal cell carcinoma: Case study and review of the literature. *J Urol* 167:2397–2403.
102. Marberger, M., Schatzl, G., Cranston, D., and J. E. Kennedy. 2005. Extracorporeal ablation of renal tumours with high-intensity focused ultrasound. *BJU Int* 95(Suppl 2):52–55.
103. Häcker, A., Michel, M. S., Marlinghaus, E., Köhrmann, K. U., and P. Alken. 2006. Extracorporeally induced ablation of renal tissue by high-intensity focused ultrasound. *BJU Int* 97:779–785.
104. Wu, F., Wang, Z. B., Chen, W. Z., Bai, J., Zhu, H., and T. Y. Qiao. 2003. Preliminary experience using high intensity focused ultrasound for the treatment of patients with advanced stage renal malignancy. *J Urol* 170(6, Pt 1):2237–2240.
105. Ritchie, R. W., Leslie, T., Phillips, R., et al. 2010. Extracorporeal high intensity focused ultrasound for renal tumours: A 3-year follow-up. *BJU Int* 106:1004–1009.
106. Ritchie, R., Collin, J. C., Coussios, and T. Leslie. 2013. Attenuation and de-focusing during high intensity focused ultrasound therapy through prinephric fat. *Ultrasound Med Biol* 39:1785–1793.
107. Flynn, M., Jamison, M., Datta, S., and E. Myers. 2006. Health care resource use for uterine fibroid tumors in the United States. Am J Obstet Gynecol 195:955–964.
108. Zhang, L., Zhang, W., Orsi, F., et al. 2015. Ultrasound-guided high intensity focused ultrasound for the treatment of gynaecological diseases: A review of safety and efficacy. *Int J Hyperthermia* 31:280–284.
109. Ren, X. L., Zhou, X. D., Yan, R. L., et al. 2009. Sonographically guided extracorporeal ablation of uterine fibroids with high-intensity focused ultrasound: Midterm results. *J Ultrasound Med* 28:100–103.
110. Zhao, W. P., Chen, J. Y., Zhang, L., et al. 2013. Feasibility of ultrasound-guided high intensity focused ultrasound ablating uterine fibroids with hyperintense on T2-weighted MR imaging. *Eur J Radiol* 82:e43–49.
111. Wang, W., Wang. Y., Wang, T., Wang, J., Wang, L., and J. Tang. 2012. Safety and efficacy of US-guided high-intensity focused ultrasound for treatment of submucosal fibroids. *Eur Radiol* 22:2553–2258.
112. Peng, S., Xiong, Y., Li, K., et al. 2012. Clinical utility of a microbubble-enhancing contrast ("SonoVue") in treatment of uterine fibroids with high intensity focused ultrasound: A retrospective study. *Eur J Radiol* 81:3832–3838.
113. Zhang, L., Chen, W. Z., Liu, Y. J., et al. 2010. Feasibility of magnetic resonance imaging-guided high intensity focused ultrasound therapy for ablating uterine fibroids in patients with bowel lies anterior to uterus. *Eur J Radiol* 73:396–403.
114. Isern, J., Pessarrodona, A., Rodriguez, J., et al. 2015. Using microbubble sonographic contrast agent to enhance the effect of high intensity focused ultrasound for the treatment of uterine fibroids. *Ultrason Sonochem* 27:688–693.
115. Xie, B., Zhang, C., Xiong, C., He, J., Huang, G., and L. Zhang. 2015. High intensity focused ultrasound ablation for submucosal fibroids: A comparison between type I and type II. *Int J Hyperthermia* 31:593–599.
116. Cheung, V. Y. 2013. Sonographically guided high-intensity focused ultrasound for the management of uterine fibroids. *J Ultrasound Med* 32:1353–1358.
117. Liu, Y., Ran, W., Shen, Y., Feng, W., and J. Yi. 2017. High-intensity focused ultrasound and laparoscopic myomectomy in the treatment of uterine fibroids: A comparative study. *BJOG* 124 (Suppl 3):36–39.
118. Wang, F., Tang, L., Wang, L., et al. 2014. Ultrasound-guided high-intensity focused ultrasound vs laparoscopic myomectomy for symptomatic uterine myomas. *J Minim Invasive Gynecol* 21:279–284.
119. Chen, J., Li, Y., Wang, Z., et al. 2018. Committee of the clinical trial of HIFU versus surgical treatment for fibroids. Evaluation of high-intensity focused ultrasound ablation for uterine fibroids: An IDEAL prospective exploration study. *BJOG* 125:354–364.
120. Qin, J., Chen, J. Y., Zhao, W. P., et al. 2012. Outcome of unintended pregnancy after ultrasound-guided high-intensity focused ultrasound ablation of uterine fibroids. *Int J Gynaecol Obstet* 117:273–277.
121. Zou, M., Chen, L., Wu. C., Hu, C., and Y. Xiong. 2017. Pregnancy outcomes in patients with uterine fibroids treated with ultrasound-guided high-intensity focused ultrasound. *BJOG* 124 (Suppl 3):30–35.
122. Li, J. S., Wang, Y., Chen, J. Y., and W. Z. Chen. 2017. Pregnancy outcomes in nulliparous women after ultrasound ablation of uterine fibroids: A single-central retrospective study. *Sci Rep* 7:3977.
123. Lee, J. S., Hong, G. Y., Park, B. J., and T. E. Kim. 2015. Ultrasound-guided high-intensity focused ultrasound treatment for uterine fibroid & adenomyosis: A single center experience from the Republic of Korea. *Ultrason Sonochem* 27:682–688.

124. Chen, J., Chen, W., Zhang, L., et al. 2015. Safety of ultrasound-guided ultrasound ablation for uterine fibroids and adenomyosis: A review of 9988 cases. *Ultrason Sonochem* 27:671–676.
125. Kovatcheva, R., Guglielmina, J. N., Abehsera, M., Boulanger, L., Laurent, N., and E. Poncelet. 2015. Ultrasound-guided high-intensity focused ultrasound treatment of breast fibroadenoma – a multicenter experience. *J Ther Ultrasound* 3:1.
126. Peek, M. C. L., Ahmed, M., Scudder, J., et al. 2017. HIFU-F Collaborators. High-intensity focused ultrasound in the treatment of breast fibroadenomata (HIFU-F trial). *Int J Hyperthermia* 2:1–8.
127. Peek, M. C., Ahmed, M., Scudder, J., Baker, R., Pinder, S. E., and M. Douek. 2016. HIFU-F Trialists' Group. High intensity focused ultrasound in the treatment of breast fibroadenomata: Results of the HIFU-F trial. *Int J Hyperthermia* 32:881–888.
128. Esnault, O., Franc, B., Ménégaux, F., et al. 2011. High-intensity focused ultrasound ablation of thyroid nodules: First human feasibility study. *Thyroid* 21:965–973.
129. Korkusuz, H., Sennert, M., Fehre, N., Happel, C., and F. Grünwald. 2015. Localized thyroid tissue ablation by high intensity focused ultrasound: Volume reduction, effects on thyroid function and immune response. *Rofo* 187:1011–1015.
130. Lang, B. H., Woo, Y. C., and K. W. Chiu. 2017. Single-session high-intensity focused ultrasound treatment in large-sized benign thyroid nodules. *Thyroid* 27:714–721.
131. Kovatcheva, R. D., Vlahov, J. D., Stoinov, J. I., and K. Zaletel. 2015. Benign solid thyroid nodules: Us-guided high-intensity focused ultrasound ablation-initial clinical outcomes. *Radiology* 276:597–605.
132. Lang, B. H., Woo, Y. C., and C. K. Wong. 2017. High intensity focused ultrasound (HIFU) treatment for symptomatic benign thyroid nodules: A prospective study. *Radiology* 284:897–906.
133. Lang, B. H. H., Wong, C. K. H., and E. P. M. Ma. 2017. Single-session high intensity focused ablation (HIFU) versus open cervical hemithyroidectomy for benign thyroid nodule: Analysis on early efficacy, safety and voice quality. *Int J Hyperthermia* 24:1–7.
134. Lang, B. H. H., Woo, Y. C., and K. W. Chiu. 2017. Vocal cord paresis following single-session high intensity focused ablation (HIFU) treatment of benign thyroid nodules: Incidence and risk factors. *Int J Hyperther*mia 33:888–894.
135. Wang, W., Wang, Y., and J. Tang. 2009. Safety and efficacy of high intensity focused ultrasound ablation therapy for adenomyosis. *Acad Radiol* 16:1416–1423.
136. Zhou, M., Chen, J. Y., Tang, L. D., Chen, W. Z., and Z. B. Wang. 2011. Ultrasound guided high-intensity focused ultrasound ablation for adenomyosis: The clinical experience of a single center. *Fertil Steril* 95:900–905.
137. Zhang, X., Li, K., Xie, B., He, M., He. J., and L. Zhang. 2014. Effective ablation therapy of adenomyosis with ultrasound-guided high intensity focused ultrasound. Int J *Gynaecol Obstet* 124:207–211.
138. Liu, X., Wang, W., Wang, Y., Wang, Y., Li, Q., and J. Tang. 2016. Clinical predictors of long-term success in ultrasound-guided high intensity focused ultrasound ablation treatment for adenomyosis. *Medicine (Baltimore)* 95:e2443.
139. Xiong, Y., Yue, Y., Shui, L., Orsi, F., He, J., and L. Zhang 2015. Ultrasound guided high intensity focused ultrasound (USgHIFU) ablation for the treatment of patients with adenomyosis and prior abdominal surgical scars: A retrospective study. *Int J Hyperthermia* 31:777–783.
140. Gong, C., Yang, B., Shi, Y., et al. 2016. Factors influencing the ablative efficiency of high intensity focused ultrasound (HIFU) treatment for adenomyosis: A retrospective study. *Int J Hyperthermia* 32:496–503.
141. Huang, X., Yu, D., Zou, M., Wang, L., Xing, H. R., and Z. Wang. 2017. The effect of exercise on high-intensity focused ultrasound treatment efficacy in uterine fibroids and adenomyosis: A retrospective study. *BJOG* 124 (Suppl 3):46–52.
142. Gong, C., Setzen, R., Liu, Z., et al. 2017. High intensity focused ultrasound treatment of adenomyosis: The relationship between the features of magnetic resonance imaging on T2 weighted images and the therapeutic efficacy. *Eur J Radiol* 89:117–122.
143. Guo, Y., Duan, H., Cheng, J., and Y. Zhang. 2017. Gonadotrophin-releasing hormone agonist combined with high-intensity focused ultrasound ablation for adenomyosis: A clinical study. *BJOG* 124 (Suppl 3):7–11.
144. Shui, L., Mao, S., Wu, Q., et al. 2015. High-intensity focused ultrasound (HIFU) for adenomyosis: Two-year follow-up results. *Ultrason Sonochem* 27:677–681.

145. Zhang, L., Rao, F., and R. Setzen. 2017. High intensity focused ultrasound for the treatment of adenomyosis: Selection criteria, efficacy, safety and fertility. *Acta Obstet Gynecol Scand* 96:707–714.
146. Huang, L., Du. Y., and C. Zhao. 2014. High-intensity focused ultrasound combined with dilatation and curettage for cesarean scar pregnancy. *Ultrasound Obstet Gynecol* 43:98–101.
147. Xiao, J., Zhang, S., Wang, F., et al. 2014. Cesarean scar pregnancy: Noninvasive and effective treatment with high intensity focused ultrasound. *Am J Obstet Gynecol* 211:356.e1–7.
148. Zhu, X., Deng, X., Wan, Y., et al. 2015. High-intensity focused ultrasound combined with suction curettage for the treatment of cesarean scar pregnancy. *Medicine (Baltimore)* 94:e854.
149. Hong, Y., Guo, Q., Pu, Y., Lu, D., and M. Hu. 2017. Outcome of high-intensity focused ultrasound and uterine artery embolization in the treatment andmanagement of cesarean scar pregnancy: A retrospective study. *Medicine (Baltimore)* 96:e7687.
150. Xiao, J., Shi, Z., Zhou, J., et al. 2017. Cesarean scar pregnancy: Comparing the efficacy and tolerability of treatment with high-intensity focused ultrasound and uterine artery embolization. *Ultrasound Med Biol* 43(3):640–647.
151. Zhu, X., Deng, X., Xiao, S., Wan, Y., and M. Xue. 2016. A comparison of high-intensity focused ultrasound and uterine artery embolisation for the management of caesarean scar pregnancy. *Int J Hyperthermia* 32:144–150
152. Tamarozzi, F., Vuitton, L., Brunetti, E., Vuitton, D. A., and S. Koch. 2014. Non-surgical and non-chemical attempts to treat echinococcosis: Do they work? *Parasite* 21:75.
153. Imankulov, S. B., Fedotovskikh, G. V., Shaimardanova, G. M., Yerlan, M., and N. K. Zhampeisov. 2015. Feasibility study of high intensity focused ultrasound (HIFU) for the treatment of hydatid cysts of the liver. *Ultrason Sonochem* 27:712–716.
154. Zhu, J., Zhu, H., Mei, Z., et al. 2013. High-intensity focused ultrasound ablation for treatment of hepatocellular carcinoma and hypersplenism: Preliminary study. *J Ultrasound Med* 32:1855–1862.
155. Zhu, J., Zhu, H., Mei, Z., et al. 2014. High-intensity focused ultrasound ablation: An effective and safe treatment for secondary hypersplenism. *Br J Radiol* 87:20140374.
156. Zhu, J., Chen, X., Hu, X., Zhu, H., and C. He. 2016. A comparative study of surgical splenectomy, partial splenic embolization, and high-intensity focused ultrasound for hypersplenism. *J Ultrasound Med* 35:467–474.

9

Imaging Assessment of Tumour Response and Treatment Outcome after High Intensity Focused Ultrasound Ablation

Feng Wu

9.1 Introduction

Medical imaging is essential in the clinical management of cancer patients at many stages during their illness. It is used as a clinical tool for screening and characterising lesions, staging the disease, assessing tumour response post-treatment, and for follow-up for tumour recurrence and progression. Imaging is also performed in routine clinical practice for guiding tumour biopsies and treatments such as tumour ablation and external beam radiotherapy.

Imaging used for cancer patients falls into two categories: anatomical and functional ("molecular"). The most established imaging methods are based on anatomical imaging. These include radiography, ultrasonography, angiography, computed tomography (CT), and magnetic resonance imaging (MRI). These (in particular CT and MRI) provide unparalleled anatomical details about tumour location, number, size, morphology, and structural alterations in adjacent organs and tissues. However, they present little insight into tumour biology and physiology, although a few methods offer functional components. Functional imaging includes single photon emission computed tomography (SPECT) and positron emission tomography (PET). Using radiolabelled compounds, these provide molecular and physiological information on the metabolism and function of tumours.

Both anatomical and functional imaging have strengths and limitations. Anatomical imaging provides excellent anatomical structural information about the tumour but gives little insight into tumour physiology. On the other hand, functional imaging is rich in tumour function but less informative about tumour morphology. However, when both imaging types are combined to form fusion images, many of their limitations are addressed by the creation of hybrid images such as single photon emission computed tomography-computed tomography (SPECT-CT), positron emission tomography-computed tomography (PET-CT), and positron emission tomography-magnetic resonance imaging (PET-MRI), where anatomical precision and functional information are provided simultaneously in a single image set.[1, 2] These hybrid images are used extensively in clinical practice and are becoming particularly valuable tools for assessment of tumour response after treatment.

Imaging is of utmost importance in high intensity focused ultrasound (HIFU) ablation. Recent developments in medical imaging technology have led dramatically to significant advances in HIFU procedures and have continuously improved the ability to plan and implement ablation procedures, and post-treatment assessments. Briefly, both anatomic and functional images are used for each step in the HIFU process, including pre-, peri-, and post-procedural assessment. They involve disease diagnosis, lesion measurement, treatment planning, guidance and assessment of tumour response, follow-up, and outcome evaluation.

Both US and MRI scanners can be incorporated into HIFU devices and serve to guide and monitor treatment procedures. MR-guided HIFU (MRgHIFU) devices use MR temperature-sensitive imaging

DOI: 10.1201/9780429162671-9

sequences to provide a focal temperature rise relative to baseline during the treatment procedure. These sequences involve proton resonance frequency (PRF), the diffusion coefficient, T1 and T2 relaxation times, magnetisation transfer, or proton density.[3,4] Of these, PRF-based temperature mapping provides high temporal and spatial resolution imaging. It has been clinically accepted as a good sequence for monitoring thermal ablation, thus ensuring treatment safety and efficacy. However, technical challenges, such as motion and susceptibility artifacts for targets in the abdomen and chest, remain for the clinical use of MR thermometry. With the development of MR thermometry techniques, novel and advanced sequences will overcome these technical limitations in the future. As Chapter 17 introduces MRgHIFU devices, the technical principles, and clinical applications, these will not be described in detail here.

Using pulse-echo B-mode imaging, ultrasound-guided HIFU (USgHIFU) monitors the direct response of a tumour to focused ultrasound energy rather than relying on a temperature measurement during an ablative procedure. This is achieved through real-time echo changes in the focal region, with bright echoes observed during HIFU exposure being related to ultrasound effects on the treated tumour in terms of coagulative necrosis. This is a direct tissue reaction when ultrasound energy is deposited in the target and can serve to provide online feedback for monitoring and controlling energy delivery. In this chapter we will initially introduce evaluation criteria for assessments of tumour response post-treatment, including Response Evaluation Criteria in Solid Tumours and Positron Emission Tomography Response Criteria in Solid Tumours. These are relevant to all major imaging modalities used as clinical follow-up tools to evaluate tumour response and treatment outcome. Finally, requirements and standardisation criteria for reporting image-guided tumour ablation will be discussed.

9.2 Tumour Response Evaluation Criteria

The main goal of antitumour treatments is to improve patient survival and quality of life. Treatment-related adverse events and toxicity are generally considered to be ethically acceptable if the patient benefits from the treatments in the end. It is therefore important from an oncological view to determine therapeutic tumour response. As morphologic changes in tumour size are usually related to survival time, monitoring tumour response and time to progression have been considered as valid surrogates for the assessment of therapeutic efficacy and the prediction of survival.

In 1997, World Health Organization (WHO) criteria, based on the measurement of tumour burden, i.e., the tumour size, were proposed for the assessment of tumour response.[5] They established a fundamental standard for the identification of tumour response, and included clinical, radiological, biochemical, or surgical-pathological staging. These criteria were rapidly accepted by the oncological community and have been endorsed as the reference criteria for evaluating tumour response in clinical trials. They can be summarised as follows in 3 steps:

- Tumours are simplified before assessment. The assessment is based on a 2-dimensional measurement of tumours and the size calculated by multiplying the maximum diameter by its longest perpendicular diameter.
- The presence of multiple lesions requires the sum of the cross-products of all measured lesions for estimation of tumour burden.
- The results are used to classify patients into 4 different categories for evaluating overall tumour response: complete response, partial response, stable disease, and progressive disease. These are determined by a percentage range of change in the overall tumour burden.

However, the WHO criteria were found to have limitations in clinical use and improvements have subsequently been made to address their weaknesses. In 2000, the Response Evaluation Criteria in Solid

Tumours (RECIST) guideline was published.[6] It was based on the same philosophy as the WHO criteria but provided certain definitions for "measurable lesions" and "non-measurable lesion". It also included the terms "target lesion" and "non-target lesion". Target lesions involved all measurable lesions up to 5 per organ and 10 in total, and other lesions were identified as non-target lesions. The most important change was that RECIST used a one-dimensional measurement to record the sum of the longest diameters of measurable target lesions, instead of the two-dimensional criteria of the WHO guidelines. Due to clinical requirements, RECIST was revised and updated as RECIST 1.1 in 2009.[7] Major changes were introduced in RECIST 1.1, including the number of maximum target lesions (decreased from 5 to 2 per organ, and 10 to 5 in total), assessment of pathological lymph nodes, redefinition of disease progression, clarification of unequivocal progression of nontarget lesions, and inclusion of ^{18}F-fluorodeoxyglucose positron emission tomography (^{18}F-FDG PET) for the detection of new lesions. The evaluation of overall response in RECIST 1.1 is dependent upon tumour responses in both target and nontarget lesions. For instance, if there is any new lesion, the overall response is always progressive disease. In the absence of a new lesion, complete response is classified as the complete disappearance of all targets and nontarget lesions. RECIST 1.1 has become the most widely used and validated criterion for assessment of therapeutic response in solid tumours worldwide and is particularly suitable for patients treated with conventional chemotherapy.

Based on anatomical and morphological changes, RECIST is the current gold standard for the assessment of therapeutic response in solid tumours. However, it also has limitations, particularly when RECIST is performed as a response assessment in locoregional therapies such as thermal ablation and transarterial chemoembolisation, because these novel therapeutics induce tumour necrosis with no marked reduction in tumour size. A modified version of the RECIST criteria (mRECIST) has thus been developed to consider tumour necrosis rather than lesion shrinkage following locoregional treatment.[8] This new criterion introduces the concept of "viable tumour", which is defined as the portion of tumours showing significant enhancement on arterial/venous phase images using contrast-enhanced computed tomography (CECT) or contrast-enhanced magnetic resonance imaging (CEMRI) after intravenous contrast administration. Therefore, tumour necrosis induced by treatment is considered in response assessment and a measure of tumour enhancement is used as a surrogate imaging characteristic of a viable tumour. mRECIST provides viable tumour size-based criteria, which are built on the unidimensional measurement of the enhanced portions of target tumours on CECT or CEMRI scans. It is simple and easy to use in clinical practice. Clinical studies have shown that, according to mRECIST criteria, tumour response is associated with overall survival of patients with hepatocellular carcinoma after thermal ablation and transarterial chemoembolisation.[9–12]

^{18}F-FDG PET scans appear to be useful for quantitative assessment of metabolic tumour response, rather than tumour size reduction. It is usually used as a clinical tool for the differentiation of benign and malignant tumours, preoperative staging, and local recurrence detection. These scans are included in RECIST 1.1 for the detection of new lesions. In 2009, Positron Emission Tomography Response Criteria in Solid Tumours (PERCIST) version 1.0 was introduced for assessment of metabolic tumour response using ^{18}F-FDG PET-CT scans.[13] These measure metabolic expression of tumours with classifications as follows: complete metabolic response, partial metabolic response, progressive metabolic disease, and stable metabolic disease. The standardised uptake value (SUV) corrected for lean body mass (SUL) provides a quantitative assessment of radiolabelled molecule uptake in a tumour region of interest, and SUV/SUL is based on a ratio between tracer uptake within a tumour and homogeneous distribution of radiotracer in the whole body. PERCIST criteria provide a valuable method of measuring tumour response in the absence of marked anatomical changes. They can provide more rapid response data than morphological measurements at the beginning of treatment. Compared to RECIST 1.1 or other established criteria, the ability to use PERCIST as a tumour response criterion has been demonstrated to predict progression-free survival, response to therapy, and overall survival in clinical studies.[14–16]

9.3 Medical Imaging Modalities for Assessment of Tumour Response after HIFU Ablation

9.3.1 Ultrasonography

9.3.1.1 Technique and Principles

Ultrasonography is a medical imaging modality that uses high-frequency sound (ultrasound) waves to create real-time visual images of organs and tissues within the body. The term includes B-mode, colour and power Doppler (CPDUS), and contrast-enhanced (CEUS) imaging. They all provide real-time high-resolution images for the diagnosis and treatment assessment of cancer patients in routine clinical practice. B-mode gives anatomical images, but CPDUS and CEUS can provide functional information beyond the purely anatomical imaging. Ultrasonography has advantages and disadvantages in clinical use. Compared to CT and MRI scanners, ultrasonography devices are cheap, portable, flexible, and easy to use. As a real-time imaging modality, it is considered as safe. Its disadvantages include limitations to the field of view and its unsuitability for air-filled organs such as the bowels and lungs because ultrasound waves cannot travel through air or gas. It is also difficult to obtain good visualisation of structures obscured by air, bone, and gases.

B-mode scans provide a cross-sectional image which bears a close resemblance to the tissues and organ anatomy inside the body.[17] It is constructed from echoes which are generated by reflection of the ultrasound beam at tissue boundaries and by scattering from small irregular structures within the tissues. Each echo is displayed at a point in the image which corresponds to the relative position of its origin. This leads to a scaled image of echo-producing features in a cross section within the body, with the brightness of the image at each point being related to the amplitude of the echo. B-mode ultrasound imaging is very efficient at distinguishing between solid and cystic structures in tissue.

CPDUS uses ultrasound waves to produce images of blood moving through the vasculature.[18] It provides functional imaging data, particularly about the presence, direction, speed, and concentration of blood flow in tissues. Colour Doppler US shows the direction and speed of blood as it flows through arteries or veins. It usually consists of two components, and the image shows the Doppler mode superimposed on the B-mode image to present the anatomical position of the blood flow. The speed and direction of blood flow are shown in colour in real time.[19] Power Doppler US provides more sensitive imaging than standard colour Doppler in the assessment of blood flow.

As a functional imaging tool, CEUS is a repeatable, cost-effective modality that enables real-time dynamic assessment of tumours throughout the vascular phase. It uses microbubble contrast agents and specialised sensitive imaging techniques to show blood flow and perfusion in tissues.[20] Ultrasound contrast agents consist of stabilised microbubbles that contain air or other gases within a shell. After intravenous administration, contrast agents enhance the backscatter of the ultrasound waves and result in a marked enhancement of the signals from the blood flow within acoustic windows. This allows CEUS to deliver dynamic imaging of blood flow for quantitative analysis of tissue perfusion.[21] Dynamic CEUS can play a similar role as CECT and CEMRI in the evaluation of blood perfusion in organs.[22] For instance, when used in the liver, it has an arterial phase (up to approximately 25 seconds after injection), a portal venous phase (starting approximately 25 to 45 seconds after injection) and a late phase (starting 2 minutes after injection).[23] According to the clinical guidelines published by the World Federation of Ultrasound in Medicine and Biology (WFUMB) and European Federation of Societies for Ultrasound in Medicine and Biology (EFSUMB), CEUS is recommended as an effective alternative for assessing postprocedural tumour response in liver cancer patients who have kidney failure or iodine allergy.[24] Compared to other imaging modalities, CEUS has a much higher temporal resolution, without the associated radiation burden of CECT or the cost and the long examination time of CEMRI.

9.3.1.2 Post-Ablation Assessments

Postprocedural ultrasonography is routinely used as an imaging tool for assessing therapeutic response in clinical practice. Based on a pretreatment baseline assessment, it can evaluate changes in target tumour size and vascularity after treatment. Both B-mode ultrasound and CPDUS are sensitive methods for measuring tumour size, but CPDUS can also provide some clues about tumour viability. However, they are not reliable for assessing the technical success or therapeutic efficacy of tumour ablation, as neither can distinguish the difference between residual viable tumour, coagulation necrosis, and scar tissue in the treated volume.[25] During follow-up, B-mode ultrasound sometimes shows the ablated tumour with heterogeneous hyperechoicity in greyscale (Figure 9.1) which gradually decreases in size over time. CPDUS can discriminate between vascularised and non-vascularised tumours. It is used to assess the changes in tumour vascularity. A significant decrease in tumour blood flow can be observed immediately following HIFU ablation (Figure 9.2). However, if the tumour blood supply is poor, CPDUS is not sufficiently sensitive to detect thermal damage to small blood vessels within the treated tumour.

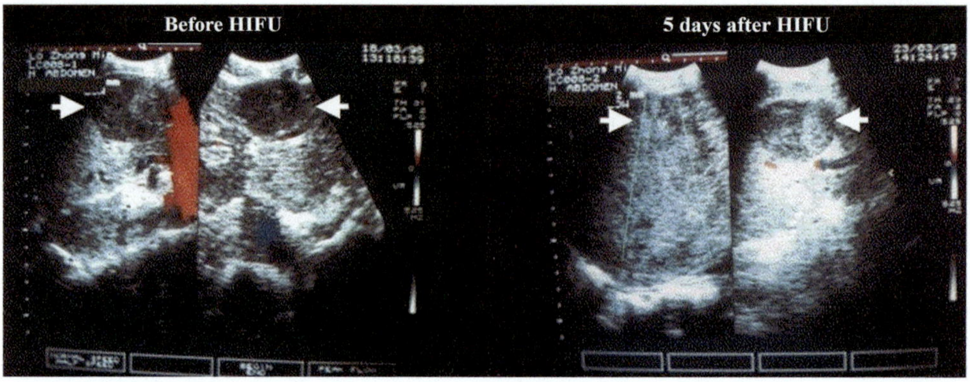

FIGURE 9.1 Colour Doppler ultrasonography before and after USgHIFU treatment in a male patient with hepatocellular carcinoma. The image shows a hypoechoic lesion (arrow) in the right lobe of the liver before treatment. Five days after HIFU, an increased greyscale change (arrow) is seen within the treated tumour. (From Wu F, et al. Ultrasound Med Bio 2004; 30:245–260.)[27]

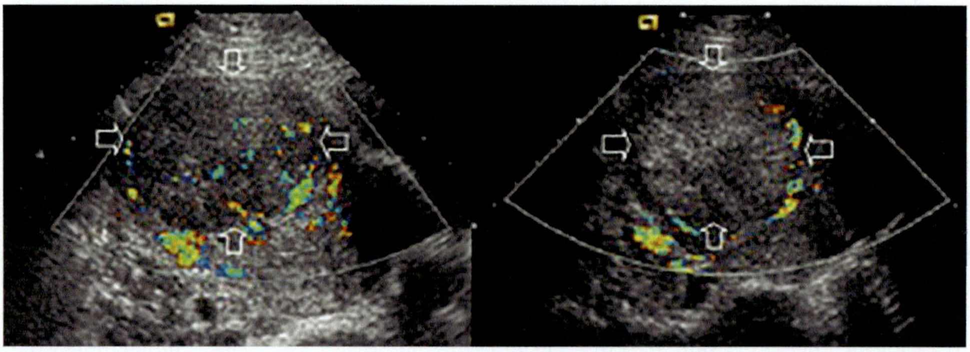

FIGURE 9.2 Colour Doppler ultrasonography before and after USgHIFU treatment in a female patient with uterine fibroid (arrow). Compared to the imaging before HIFU (left), colour Doppler signals (blue or red colour) are obviously decreased in the treated tumour 5 days after HIFU ablation (right), indicating the destruction of tumour vascularity. (From Wu F, Clinical application of high intensity focused ultrasound in the treatment of patients with solid malignancies. In: Wu J, Nyborg W, eds. Emerging therapeutic ultrasound. World Scientific Publishing, Singapore, 2006, page 279–339.)

CEUS is currently used in thermal ablation for early detection of residual viable tumour and subsequent local tumour recurrence and progression. It can distinguish between a complete response, a partial response, and an equivocal treatment response. The lack of any nodular arterially enhanced portion within, or at the edge of the ablated tumour, is considered to be a complete response, as shown in Figure 9.3. In contrast, the detection of residual viable tumour is considered to be a partial response. It usually appears as an enhanced nodule in the arterial phase and washout in the portal vein and delayed phases within the treated tumour.[26]

CEUS has been used for immediate assessment of therapeutic effect in clinical practice in order to reduce incomplete tumour ablations. This is of critical importance following thermal ablation because it gives immediate feedback as to whether the tumour has been destroyed completely and provides an opportunity for immediate retreatment in the same session.[28] During the follow-up period, CEUS has been performed to evaluate new lesions and to monitor for evidence of early recurrence within the ablation zone. It can be used as a secondary surveillance method, normally performed every 3 to 4 months for early detection of recurrence.[29]

9.3.2 Angiography

Angiography is used to examine blood vessels. It requires the insertion of a catheter into the artery in the area being examined, injection of iodinated contrast agent through the catheter, and visualisation of the blood vessels using X-ray based rapid-sequence imaging techniques. Nowadays, most angiography is carried out with digital image-capture devices. This is known as digital subtraction angiography (DSA).

DSA is a high-resolution medical imaging technique, but its invasive nature and the high dose of radiative energy delivered to patients have limited its clinical use. Because rapid-sequence CT scanning techniques have been successfully developed for vascular imaging, non-invasive CT angiography has rapidly replaced DSA for cancer diagnosis.[31, 32] However, the use of DSA as an image-guided tool to deliver vascular treatment has already become important in clinical settings. It allows the use of an arterial catheter for delivery of chemotherapeutic agents, embolisation materials, and radioactive microspheres directly to a target tumour with therapeutic intent.[33–35] It appears that while diagnostic angiography has been used less frequently, DSA-guided cancer treatments are increasingly being performed in routine clinical practice. In our early clinical trials, post-HIFU DSA was used to assess therapeutic effects on tumour blood vessels, and the results showed the complete disappearance of

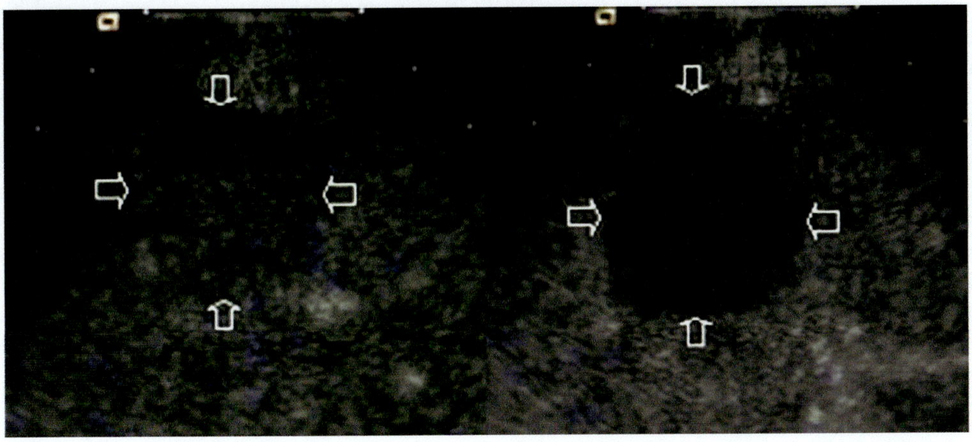

FIGURE 9.3 Contrast-enhanced ultrasonography before and after USgHIFU treatment in a male patient with metastatic liver cancer. Before HIFU ablation, blood perfusion can be identified within the target tumour (left). However, there is an absence of blood perfusion within the treated tumour 1 day after HIFU ablation (right). (From Kennedy JE, et al. Ultrasound Med Bio 2004; 30:851–854.)[30]

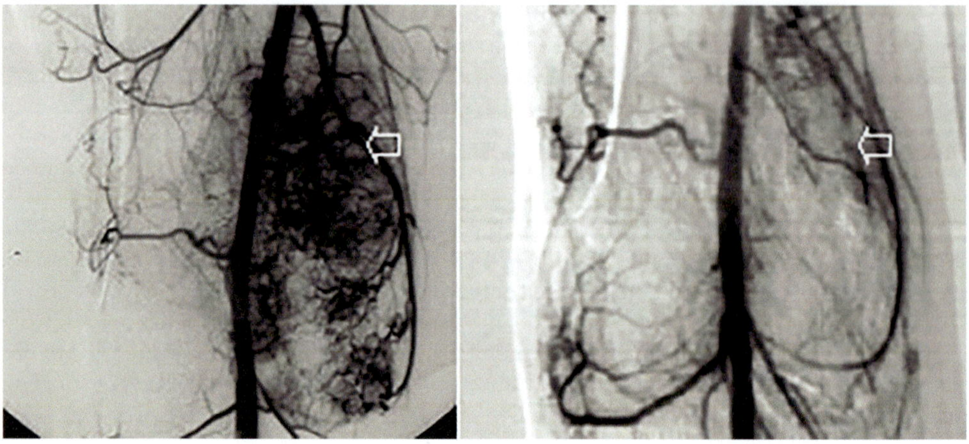

FIGURE 9.4 Digital subtraction angiography images before and after USgHIFU treatment in a male patient with distal femur osteosarcoma. Before treatment (left), persistence of tumour vascularity and capillary stain (arrow) appear in the target tumour. However, 3 months after HIFU (right), complete disappearance of tumour vascularity and stain (arrow) is clearly seen within the treated tumour. (From Wu F, et al. Ultrasound Med Bio 2002; 28:535–542.)[36]

tumour vascularity after HIFU ablation in patients with osteosarcoma (Figure 9.4). However, due to its invasive nature, the use of DSA is now relatively limited for the clinical assessment of tumour response after thermal ablation.

9.3.3 Computed Tomography

9.3.3.1 Technique and Principles

Computed tomography is an imaging modality that uses x-rays and computer processing to generate detailed internal images within the body. During CT scanning, a narrow x-ray beam is rapidly rotated around the patient to produce digital signals, which are immediately processed by a computer to create cross-sectional image slices. These imaging slices can be collected and stacked together by the computer to form a 3-dimensional (3D) image with detailed information about anatomic structures and abnormalities. Using an iodine-based radiocontrast, CECT scanning highlights blood vessels and obtains functional information about tissues. In addition, as CT angiography avoids insertion of a catheter into the artery, it has rapidly taken the place of DSA in clinical diagnosis.

CT has rapidly become the dominant imaging technique in routine clinical practice. It is often performed for disease detection, diagnosis, staging, treatment monitoring and post-treatment follow up in oncology. CT scanning has several advantages over other medical imaging modalities. It requires a short scan time but provides high resolution images in the areas of interest. CT produces 3D images and multiplanar reformatted images, where slice images are visualised in the transverse, coronal and sagittal planes. Compared to MRI scanning, it is faster, cheaper, and less subject to motion artifacts. However, the ionising radiation exposure is a major disadvantage and contrast agents may cause allergic reactions in some patients during CT scanning. Recently, technological innovations have developed high-speed CT scanners that reduce the radiation dose, and large field-of-view CT systems can potentially scan the entire body within 1 minute.[37, 38]

9.3.3.2 Post-ablation Assessment

CT scanning plays an important role in the assessment of tumour response and post-treatment follow-up. It is the second most widely used imaging modality for ablation assessment due to its ability to acquire volumetric datasets rapidly.[39] Compared to baseline pre-treatment imaging, the ablated tumour is mainly hypo-attenuated but frequently heterogeneous on unenhanced CT scan after thermal ablation. However, there may be variability in post-procedural imaging presentation among various types of solid tumours.

Due to the destruction of vascularity, the treated tumour appears as an unenhanced region on CECT images immediately after HIFU ablation. The unperfused region is sometimes surrounded by an enhancing rim that is directly related to local tissue inflammatory reactions to thermal injury. This peripheral rim enhancement is usually uniform in thickness and envelops the ablated tumour, whereas residual unablated tumour shows focal and irregular peripheral enhancement. During follow-up, the ablated region remains unenhanced with a gradual reduction in size over time (Figure 9.5). The presence of a new, peripheral, intra-, or extra-zonal soft-tissue nodule in the ablation zone is suggestive of tumour recurrence after treatment.[40]

9.3.4 Magnetic Resonance Imaging

9.3.4.1 *Technique and Principles*

MRI scanners use powerful magnets to produce a strong magnetic field, which is combined with computer-generated radiofrequency to create detailed internal images within the body. It is established as an advanced technology that excites and detects changes in the direction of protons, the small particles at the centre of each hydrogen atom that are contained in the water molecules in living tissues. During MRI scanning, strong magnetic fields force protons to align in the magnetic direction, and a radiofrequency pulse is then sent to knock the protons out of alignment. When the radiofrequency field turns off, the protons realign with the magnetic field, and MRI sensors receive radiofrequency signals with information

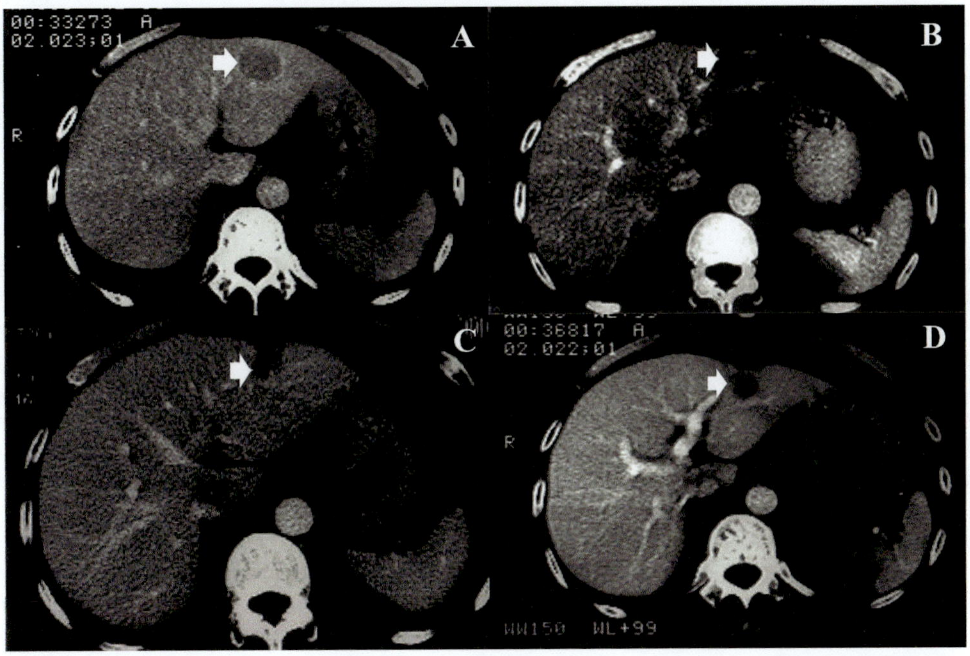

FIGURE 9.5 Transverse contrast-enhanced computed tomography images before and after USgHIFU treatment in a male patient with hepatocellular carcinoma. (A) Before treatment, the tumour is in the left lobe of the liver with contrast enhancement (arrow); (B) 3 months after HIFU, no contrast enhancement is seen in the treated tumour (arrow); (C) 12 months after HIFU, an involution of the treated tumour is seen with an absence of contrast enhancement (arrow); (D) 24 months after HIFU, the treated tumour decreases in size without any blood supply (arrow). (From Wu F, et al. Ann Surg Oncol 2004; 11:1061–1069.)[41]

about the location of the protons and the amount of energy released. Finally, all radiofrequency signals are analysed by the computer and assigned greyscale values to create cross-sectional images based on tissue characteristics.[42] For example, the water is shown as hypointense (dark) and the fat as hyperintense (bright) in T1-weighted images, and various soft tissues are represented as a shade of grey between these. In contrast, in T2-weighted images, water is seen as hyperintense, fat as hypointense and soft tissues lie in the middle.

Like CT imaging, MR imaging is widely used for disease detection, diagnosis, staging, treatment monitoring and post-treatment follow-up for cancer patients. It produces high resolution images of the area of interest with detailed 3D anatomical data that are visualised from various angles, as well as functional information from tissues. In contrast to CT scans, MRI does not use ionising radiation. It provides higher resolution images of the nervous and musculoskeletal systems, making MRI particularly useful in evaluating tumours of the brain, spinal cord, bone, joints, and soft tissues. As MRI scans can be performed with a number of imaging sequences, it offers significant amounts of information with different tissue displays.[43] However, MRI has several disadvantages. It is more expensive than CT and needs longer times to acquire images. MRI is not suitable for patients who have metal implants such as pacemakers, cochlear implants, or artificial joints.

9.3.4.2 Post-Ablation Assessment

MRI scans are the most widely used images for the assessment of thermal ablation in clinical practice. It provides a wide variety of techniques for post-ablation assessment.[39] Conventional T1-weighted/T2-weighted images, and contrast-enhanced T1-weighted images are considered to be the most accurate sequences for the early detection of residual/recurrent tumours after ablation. Additionally, diffusion-weighted imaging (DWI) generates tissue contrast through local differences in the diffusion of water molecules in extracellular spaces and does not require the use of contrast such as gadolinium. Diffusion characteristics are usually quantified using apparent diffusion coefficient (ADC) values for each voxel by fitting to a single exponential, generating an ADC map. DWI and ADC maps have been investigated to evaluate the therapeutic effects of thermal ablation. Clinical results show that tumour ablation can reduce cellularity and perfusion while increasing necrosis. There is a positive correlation between ADC and necrosis,[44] and a negative correlation between ADC and tumour cellularity.[45]

Unenhanced T1- and T2-weighted images have been used extensively for the evaluation of tumour response after HIFU treatment. They show variable signal intensities with no consistent results. Compared to surrounding parenchyma, coagulation necrosis may appear as heterogeneous changes with increased signal on T1- and T2-weighted images within the treated tumour (Figure 9.6) but in some patients there may be no changes. Over time, the treated tumour will slowly reduce in size and the signal may change on T2-weighted image during the follow-up period (Figure 9.7).

The most common MR sequence for assessing HIFU ablation is gadolinium contrast-enhanced T1-weighted imaging. Figure 9.8 shows the MR images pre- and post-HIFU in a hepatocellular carcinoma patient. Compared to the pre-HIFU images, the ablation zone shows an absence of contrast enhancement in the treated region in the hepatic arterial, portal veinous and delayed phases on contrast-enhanced T1-weighted images. This zone is sometimes surrounded by a smooth, thin, continuous rim of peripheral hyperenhancement, which is the result of local inflammation and hyperaemia at the interface between the ablation zone and normal hepatic parenchyma. The hypervascular rim is differentiated from residual tumour by its smooth, thin, continuous morphology. Residual viable tumour usually presents with nodular, thickened, and irregular enhancement around the periphery of the ablation zone.

A diffusion-weighted MR scan provides unique insights into molecular water distribution within a tumour, and therefore indicates tumour viability at a cellular level.[47, 48] After HIFU treatment, coagulation necrosis usually causes less restriction to the motion of water molecules and increases ADC values on DWI images.[49] Figure 9.9 shows DWI images pre- and post-HIFU in a patient with sacral chordoma.

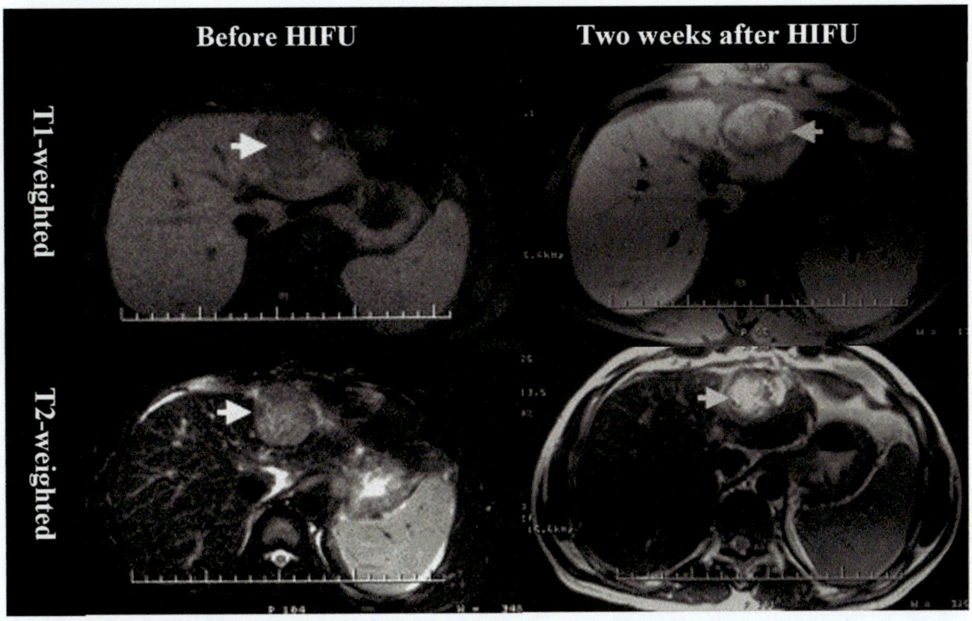

FIGURE 9.6 Transverse unenhanced MR images before and after USgHIFU treatment in a 38-year-old patient with hepatocellular carcinoma in the left lobe of the liver (arrow). Unenhanced T1- and T2-weighted images show hyperintense signals within the treated tumour (arrow) 2 weeks after treatment. (From Wu F, et al. Ultrasound Med Bio 2004; 30:245–260.)[27]

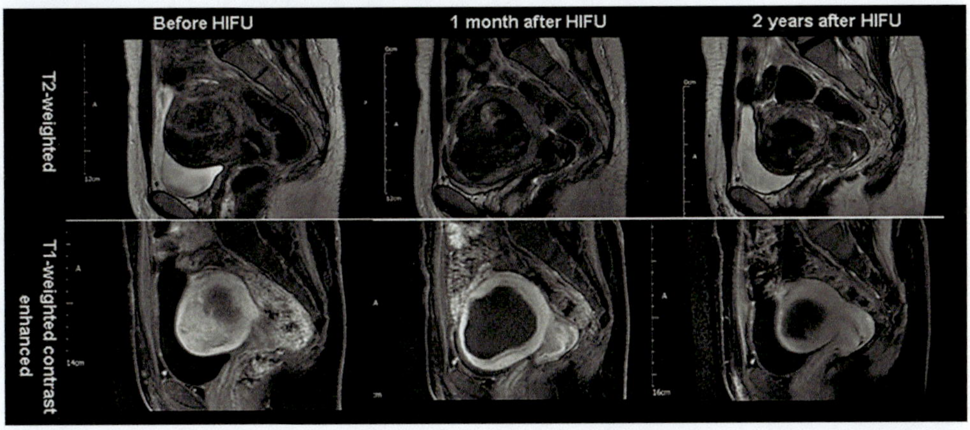

FIGURE 9.7 Sagittal magnetic resonance imaging before and after USgHIFU treatment in a 46-year-old woman with a dominant intramural fibroid during a 2-year follow-up period. T2-weighted image shows a time-dependent decrease in size of the treated fibroid, with 68% volume reduction 2 years post-treatment. T1-weighted contrast-enhanced fat-suppressed image obtained 1 month after treatment shows more than 90% non-perfused volume ratio in the treated fibroid. (From Lyon PC, et al. Ultraschall Med 2020; 41:550–556.)[46]

Compared to the untreated right side of the tumour, the treated left side shows low signal on DWI images and high ADC values, indicating reduced diffusion restriction in the treated tumour. In addition, ^{18}F-FDG PET/CT imaging shows mild FDG avidity within the untreated right side of the sacral chordoma. However, the treated left side is markedly photopenic,[50] in keeping with the tumour necrosis and supporting the previous DWI findings (Figure 9.10).

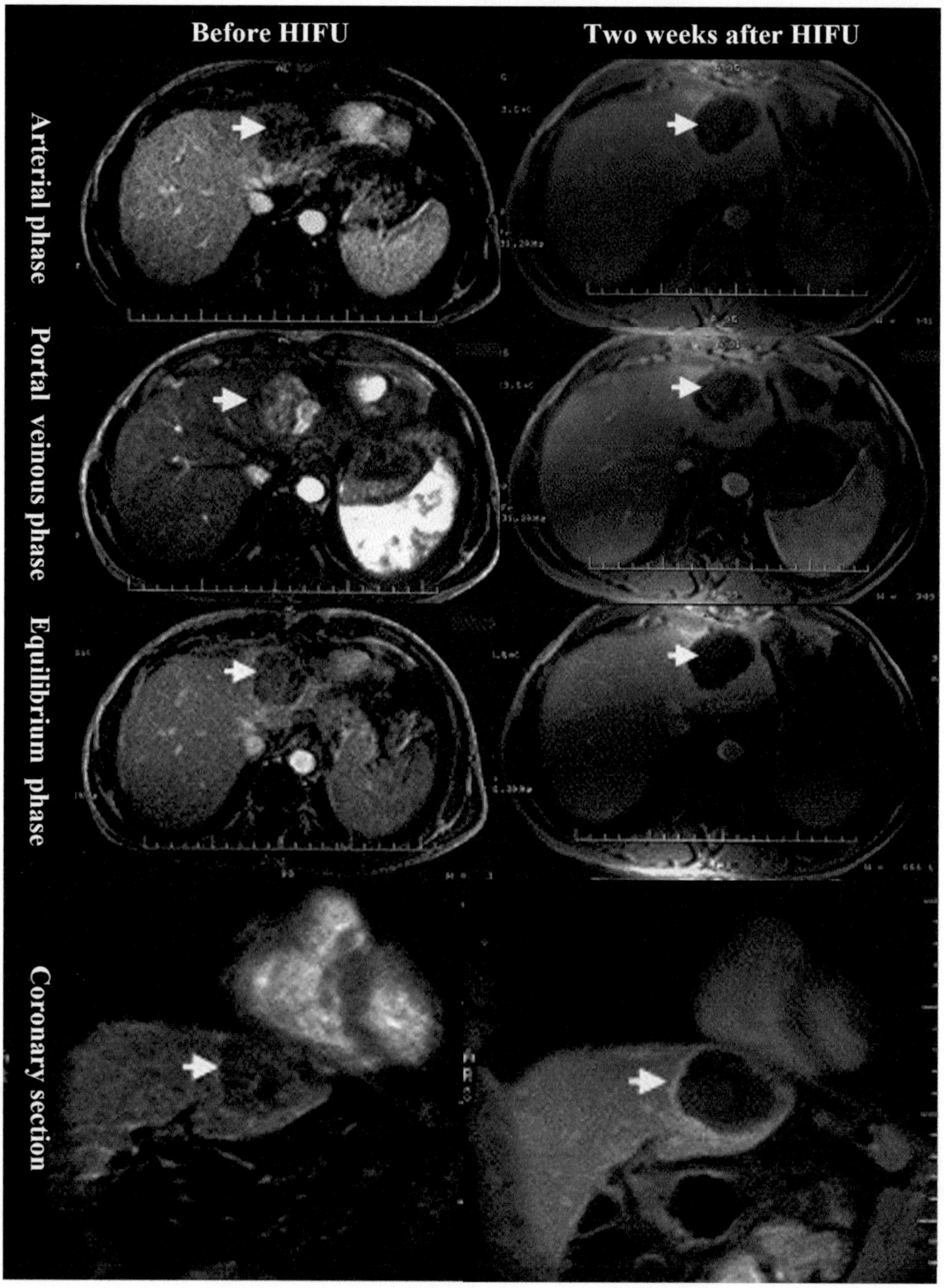

FIGURE 9.8 Gadolinium contrast-enhanced T1-weighted magnetic resonance imaging before and after USgHIFU treatment in a 38-year-old patient with hepatocellular carcinoma in the left lobe of the liver (arrow). Two weeks after HIFU treatment, transverse images show an absence of contrast enhancement in the treated tumour (arrow) during hepatic arterial, portal venous, and equilibrium phases. Coronary images show a thin peripheral rim of contrast enhancement (arrow) on the margin between treated and untreated regions. (From Wu F, et al. Ultrasound Med Bio 2004; 30:245–260.)[27]

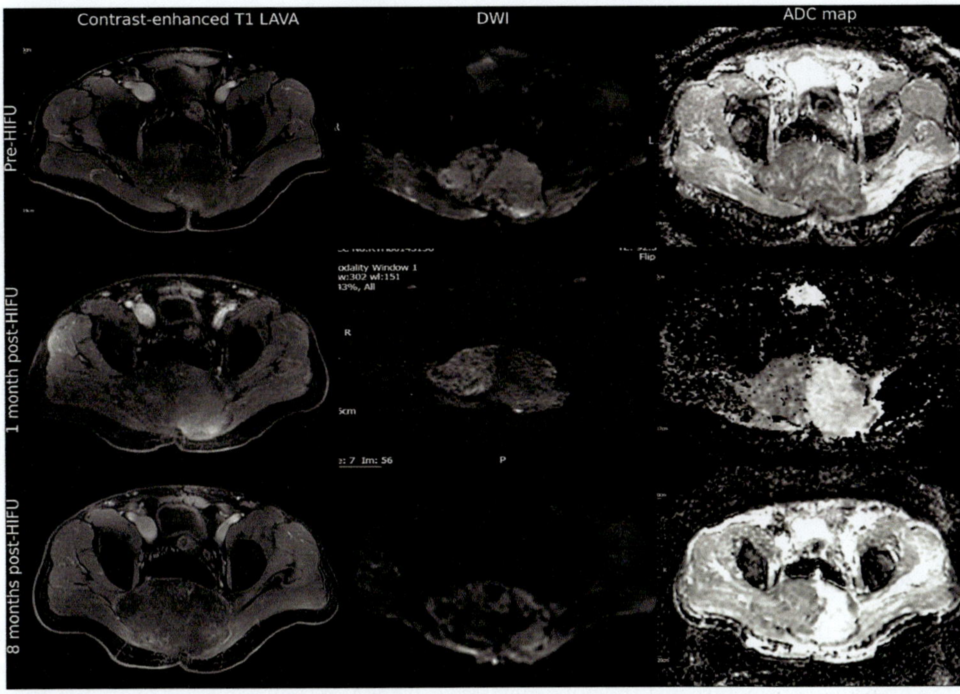

FIGURE 9.9 Transverse diffusion-weighted MR images before and after USgHIFU treatment in a male patient with sacral chordoma. MRI prior to HIFU treatment (top row) and at 1 month (middle row) and 8 months (bottom row) after HIFU treatment. Left column: axial T1-weighted fat-suppressed fast-spoiled gradient echo (LAVA) sequence, venous-phase imaging. Middle and right columns: axial DWI and ADC map at b = 800 (top row), b = 1000 (middle row), b = 700 (bottom row). ADC values are significantly higher on the HIFU-treated left side of the chordoma than the untreated right side, indicating a reduction in diffusion restriction. (From Chetan MR, et al. Radiol Case Rep 2019;14:1197–1201.)[50]

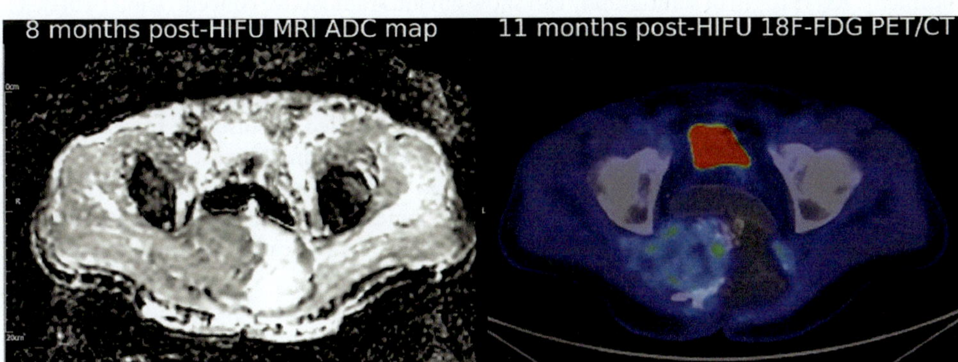

FIGURE 9.10 Diffusion-weighted MR and ^{18}F-FDG PET/CT images before and after USgHIFU treatment in a male patient with sacral chordoma. Axial ADC map 8 months after HIFU treatment (left) and axial fused ^{18}F-FDG PET/CT 11 months after HIFU treatment (right). The HIFU-treated left side of the chordoma shows excellent correlation with high ADC values and no ^{18}F-FDG uptake, indicating tumour necrosis. (From Chetan MR, et al. Radiol Case Rep 2019;14:1197–1201.)[50]

9.3.5 Single Photon Emission Computed Tomography

9.3.5.1 Technique and Principles

SPECT is a radionuclide scanning technique that integrates CT and a radioisotope tracer to provide insight into a tumour's biological functions and its surrounding microenvironment.[1] The radioisotopes, such as ^{99m}technetium sestamibi (^{99m}Tc-MIBI) and ^{99m}technetium methylene diphosphate (^{99m}Tc-MDP), have a high extraction rate in some malignant tumours.[51–53] They emit gamma rays that are collected by a gamma camera to provide physiological imaging information using tomographic images of the radioactivity distribution within the tumour. Interpretation of SPECT images is based on observed intensity relative to expected normal activity. It can either be increased (often called a "hot spot") or decreased (termed "photopenic"). It is customary to describe the severity of the scintigraphic findings as showing intensely or severely, moderately, mildly, slightly increased, or decreased radiotracer uptake.[54]

SPECT has high sensitivity and specificity for the assessment of tumour response after ablation. However, it is limited in clinical use due to its low spatial resolution and inability to provide anatomical information. Recently, SPECT and CT scanners have been integrated to develop a hybrid SPECT-CT system, and clinical studies have shown increased accuracy and reporter confidence with SPECT-CT compared to SPECT alone.[55]

9.3.5.2 Post-Ablation Assessment

^{99m}Technetium is the most frequently used radioisotope in clinical practice due to its desirable imaging properties. Whole body bone scintigraphy with ^{99m}Tc-MDP is routinely used in the management of patients with primary osteosarcoma and bone metastasis. It has also been employed to predict and monitor tumour response after treatments in clinical studies.[56–58] Figure 9.11 shows SPECT images pre- and post-HIFU in an 18-year-old patient with left tibia osteosarcoma. Two weeks after treatment, no abnormal ^{99m}Tc-MDP signal was detected in the treated region, indicating a positive therapeutic response and an absence of residual viable tumour.

^{99m}Tc-MIBI is a radioactive diagnostic agent used to evaluate pathology in breast tissues. It can passively diffuse into the mitochondria through cell membranes. Metabolically active tissues can take up and retain more ^{99m}Tc-MIBI because they contain more mitochondria. In patients with breast cancer, the uptake and accumulation of ^{99m}Tc-MIBI represents the presence of metabolically active breast cancer cells indirectly. As ^{99m}Tc-MIBI scintigraphy can show obvious radioactive concentration in breast lesion, it has been already used as a functional imaging method for evaluating tumour response after treatment.[59, 60] In recent years, breast-specific gamma imaging (BSGI) has been developed for the diagnosis of breast cancer. This is a high-resolution radionuclide imaging modality that uses a small field-of-view gamma camera to visualise breast tissues.[61] BSGI with ^{99m}Tc-labelled radioisotope tracers has proved to be a highly sensitive diagnostic tool with high specificity even for small breast lesions.[62, 63] Figure 9.12 shows ^{99m}Tc-MIBI SPECT images pre- and post-HIFU in a patient with breast cancer. A focal area of increased tracer uptake is seen in the left breast before treatment. However, 1 week after treatment, there is an absence of the tracer uptake within the treated breast region, indicating complete ablation with the absence of residual viable tumour.

9.3.6 ^{18}F-Fluorodeoxyglucose Positron Emission Tomography

9.3.6.1 Technique and Principles

PET is a functional imaging technique that uses a radioactive tracer to visualise and measure changes in metabolic and physiological activity of tissues and organs.[64] It provides detailed 3D images of the whole body, including any abnormal areas, in real time. PET can be combined with a CT on the same gantry, which is known as PET-CT imaging. PET and CT scans are performed at the same time to produce detailed images that contain anatomical and metabolic information about the presence of tumours.

^{18}F-Fluorodeoxyglucose (^{18}F-FDG) is the most frequently used PET agent in oncology.[1] FDG is a glucose analogue that enters cells via glucose transporters, notably Glut-1 and Glut-3 which are upregulated

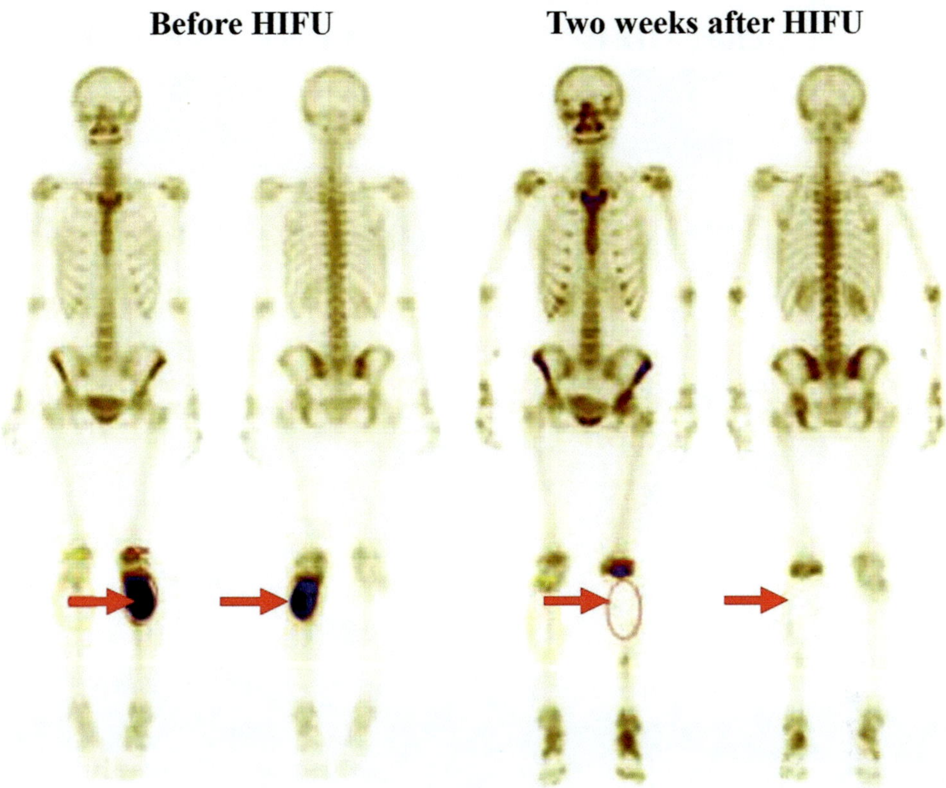

FIGURE 9.11 ^{99m}Technetium methylene diphosphonate SPECT images before and after USgHIFU treatment in an 18-year-old female patient with left tibia osteosarcoma. She received neoadjuvant chemotherapy with good response before HIFU. However, an increased uptake of the radioisotope is still detected in local abnormality (arrow) pre-ablation. Two weeks after HIFU, the tracer uptake disappears completely in the treated tumour (arrow), indicating a radioactive photopenic area. (From Chen W, et al. Radiology 2010; 255:967–978.)[58]

in cancer cell membranes, and remains trapped inside the cells after hexokinase phosphorylation.[65, 66] Metabolic trapping of the ^{18}F-FDG results in the accumulation of the radiotracer with intense radiolabelling in cancer cells; this allows the use of ^{18}F-FDG for assessment of glucose consumption in the body through PET imaging.[67] As upregulated glycolysis is associated with cancer aggressiveness, invasiveness, proliferative activity, and poor prognosis, it is very important to assess the glycolytic activity of tumours with PET-CT scans in the clinical management of cancer patients.[68, 69]

9.3.6.2 Post-Ablation Assessment

^{18}F-FDG PET-CT has played a significant role in the diagnosis, preoperative staging, treatment planning, treatment response monitoring, and local recurrence detection after treatments in oncology. It is a highly accurate tool for assessing the technical success of local treatment, identifying residual or recurrent tumour early after intervention, and providing prognostic and predictive information in cancer patients.[70–73] As a functional imaging tool, ^{18}F-FDG PET-CT is also an accurate tool for determining the efficacy of thermal ablation.[74] Tumours that show increased ^{18}F-FDG uptake on PET-CT become completely photopenic (no ^{18}F-FDG uptake) immediately after ablation, indicating technical success, with complete ablation. An inadequate increase in ^{18}F-FDG uptake, and focal or multifocal areas of increased ^{18}F-FDG uptake within the ablation zone suggest residual viable tumour after treatment. Reactive tissue changes such as inflammation are seen in the periphery of the ablated lesion and show a uniform

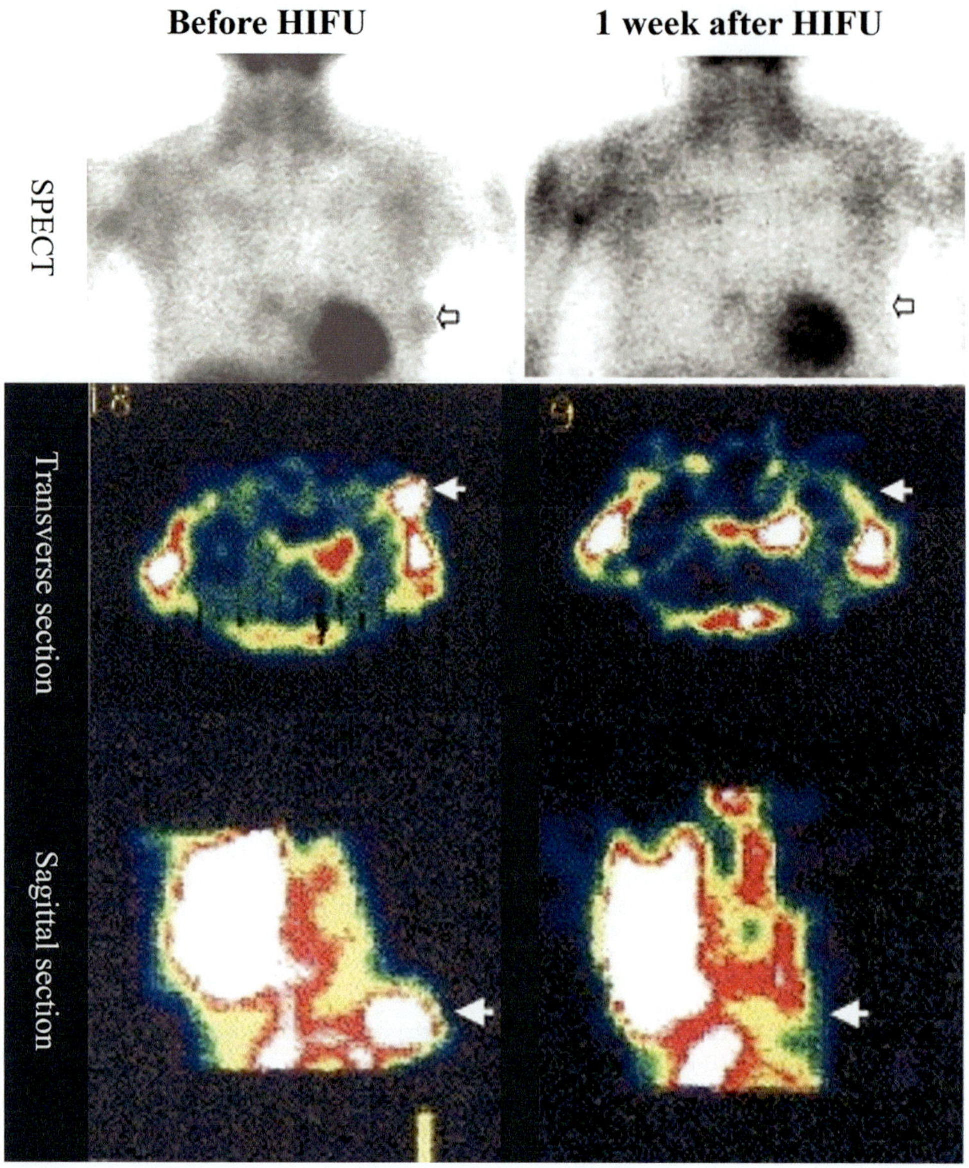

FIGURE 9.12 ^{99m}Tc sestamibi SPECT images before and after USgHIFU treatment in a 62-year-old patient with breast cancer. Images before treatment show a focal area of increased tracer uptake on the left breast, corresponding to a local abnormality (arrow). One week after HIFU, the tracer uptake of the treated breast cancer disappears completely in the treated region (arrow) on the SPECT images including those of transverse and sagittal sections. (From Wu F, et al. Ultrasound Med Bio 2004; 30:245–260.)[27]

low-grade FDG uptake, which can be differentiated from the focal, nodular intense uptake in areas of residual disease.[75]

^{18}F-FDG PET-CT can show residual viable tumour post-ablation and local recurrence earlier than other imaging modalities. Compared to CECT and CEMRI scans, PET-CT has proved to be more accurate, sensitive, and specific for the assessment of tumour response after treatment in cancer patients.[74–76] Figure 9.13 shows images pre- and post-HIFU in a 27-year-old male patient with relapse of osteosarcoma in the right pelvic/ilium region. Before HIFU treatment, he received 6 cycles of chemotherapy, and

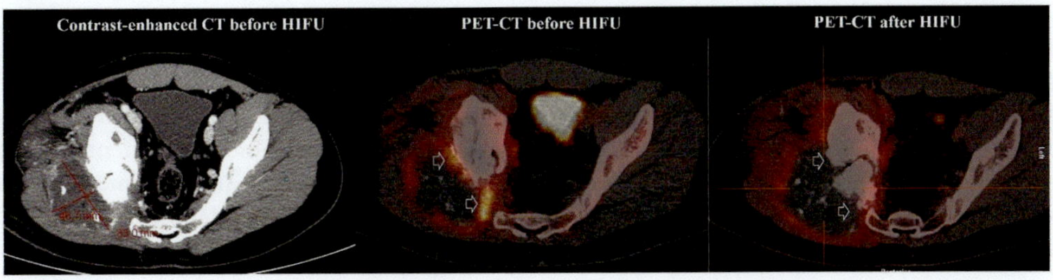

FIGURE 9.13 Transverse ^{18}F-fluorodeoxyglucose PET-CT images before and after USgHIFU treatment in a 27-year-old male patient with relapse of osteosarcoma in right pelvic/ilium region. Before HIFU treatment, he received 6 cycles of chemotherapy with good response on contrast-enhanced CT image. However, an increased uptake of the radiotracer is still detected in local abnormality (arrow) on PET-CT scan. Four weeks after HIFU, the tracer uptake disappears completely in the treated tumour (arrow), indicating technical success with the completeness of ablation.

contrast-enhanced CT imaging showed good tumour response with significant necrosis. However, the PET-CT scan still showed two areas of an increased FDG uptake at the margin of the tumour, suggesting the presence of residual viable tumour. Four weeks after HIFU, the tracer uptake disappeared completely in the treated tumour on PET-CT image, indicating technical success with completeness of ablation.

9.4 Imaging Reporting Requirements for Post-procedural Imaging Assessments

9.4.1 Standardisation of Reporting Criteria for Image-Guided Tumour Ablation

As a minimally invasive treatment, image-guided tumour ablation has been performed increasingly in routine clinical practice. Methods include chemical and thermal ablation, and HIFU is the only non-invasive ablation approach amongst the thermal ablation modalities. In 2003, Standardisation of Terms and Reporting Criteria for Image-Guided Tumour Ablation was proposed by International Working Group on Image-guided Tumour Ablation.[77] The main objective of this proposal was to improve precision and communication in this field, leading to more accurate comparison of technologies and results, and ultimately to improve patient outcomes. It was based on long term discussions among radiologists, who acknowledged that as a new field, image-guided tumour ablation required standardisation of terms and reporting criteria. Their efforts were intended to facilitate effective communication for reporting the various aspects of image-guided tumour ablation, including classification of techniques, procedure terms, descriptors of imaging guidance, terminology of imaging and pathological findings, methods for standardising reporting of technique, follow-up timing, complications, and clinical results. It was reviewed at regular intervals in conjunction with the Technology Assessment Committee, Society of Interventional Radiology (SIR) and republished nearly in original form in 2005[78] and 2009.[79] Since then, image-guided tumour ablation has evolved considerably with the development of new techniques and clinical applications.

The proposal was updated in 2014[80] to incorporate the latest advances in thermal ablation technology. As before, the modified document was approved by the Technology Assessment Committee of SIR. It also received official approval from the Cardiovascular and Interventional Radiological Society of Europe (CIRSE) to attain greater worldwide adoption. The guidelines provided a framework with which to facilitate comparisons of studies and techniques in interventional oncology. However, clear definitions and recommendations on how to use and interpret oncologic outcome measures, such as disease-free and recurrence-free survival, local tumour progression-free survival, organ-specific progression-free survival, distant progression-free survival, time to progression, time to local progression, time to organ-specific progression, were not clearly proposed. There was no consensus regarding preferred clinical outcome measures after tumour ablation or clear definitions of oncologic end points.[81]

In 2021, Puijk and colleagues[82] proposed standardised definitions for a broad range of outcome measures with recommendations on how to uniformly document, analyse, and report oncological outcomes.

This consensus guideline was a collaboration between the SIO and Definition for the Assessment of Time-to-Event End Points in Cancer Trials (DATECAN) and advanced the field of interventional oncology towards more evidence-based clinical medicine. Using the validated 3-step modified Delphi consensus method, recommendations were developed for defining outcome measures for patients who received imaging-guided thermal ablation, including when to assess outcomes per patient, per session, or per tumour, on starting and ending time and survival time definitions, and on time-to-event end points. This guideline provided a framework for key opinion leader recommendations with the intent of facilitating clear interpretation of clinical results and standardising worldwide communication.

9.4.2 Post-procedural Imaging Assessment Criteria for HIFU Tumour Ablation

Just as for pre-treatment imaging, post-procedural imaging assessment is a critical component of HIFU ablation. It provides valuable image information for assessing ablation results and related complications, monitoring changes in the ablated tissues over time and detecting residual tumour and local recurrence. According to the standardisation of terminology and reporting criteria related to image-guided tumour ablation,[78, 80] we here introduce terminology and imaging reporting requirements that have been used in clinical practice for post-HIFU imaging assessment.

9.4.2.1 Ablation Zone

The term "ablation zone" refers to the radiological area or zone of coagulation necrosis that has been induced by the HIFU procedure. This area should encompass the ablated tumour and a circumferential margin of approximately 5 to 10 mm around the tumour, similar to the tumour-free margin for surgical resection. Reporting of the ablation zone should be made in relation to the target tumour. For a successful ablation, the target tumour should be completely covered by the ablation zone plus a 5- to 10-mm margin surrounding the ablated tumour.

On follow-up images, the ablation zone should show changes in signal intensity on MR imaging, echogenicity on US and attenuation on CT scan. Post-procedural CECT and CEMRI scans should reveal that the ablation zone is well demarcated with absent perfusion. Compared to pre-procedural imaging, absence of contrast enhancement indicates successful treatment with a lack of viable tumour. Lack of enhancement can be more confidently assessed on subtraction images. For FDG-avid tumours, an ^{18}F-FDG PET-CT scan can reveal a lack of FDG uptake in the ablation zone.

9.4.2.2 Ablation Margin

The term "ablative margin" is preferable to "surgical margin". It refers to a 5- to 10-mm-wide region that should ideally be ablated along with the target tumour, because an appropriate ablation margin beyond the borders of the tumour is important for achieving complete tumour destruction. The extent of the desired or intended ablation margin should be specifically mentioned in reporting a HIFU treatment. Desirable for curative ablation, an extensive ablation margin is important. However, the ablation margin is different for different tumours. The most common wide margin considered by HIFU investigators is 5 to 10 mm in liver and kidney cancer, and 15 to 20 mm in osteosarcoma. However, there are currently no data to support definitive recommendations regarding the ideal margin size.

Due to inflammatory reactions and granulation tissue formation in the marginal regions of treated tumours immediately after HIFU, peri-ablation oedema can be seen as a sharply marginated, low-attenuation rim on unenhanced CT, or as a subtle hyperintense rim on T2-weighted MR imaging. It appears as an ill-defined, concentric, thin rim of contrast enhancement on both CECT and CEMRI images. This typically measures 1 to 2 mm, but up to 5 mm with smooth inner margins. A peripheral rim of uniform FDG uptake of low to moderate intensity can be also seen on ^{18}F-FDG PET-CT images.

A thick and irregular rim on CECT and CEMRI scans, or irregular and nodular FDG uptake on a PET-CT scan usually represents residual viable tumour at the ablation margin. This enhancing residual tumour indicates incomplete ablation. The irregular peripheral enhancement may be subtle and difficult to detect when compared with the thin peri-ablation rim in complete ablation. Careful comparison of post-procedural imaging with pre-procedural imaging is therefore critical in these equivocal cases. As the residual tumour can continue to grow, close imaging follow-up is necessary in these equivocal patients.

9.4.2.3 Involution of the Ablation Zone

The term "involution" refers to the process by which the body eliminates the zone of induced thermal necrosis over time. As it involves both target tumour and the surrounding tissues, the term "regression" and "shrinkage" should be avoided when describing this process. Pathological findings reveal that the involution is directly related to normal inflammatory reaction to thermal injury within the body, which initiates the formation of granulation tissue at the ablation margins during the acute period. Due to normal repair processes, coagulation is then replaced by fibrous and scar tissues, and the ablation zone gradually becomes smaller over this period, until its complete disappearance. On CECT and CEMRI scans, scar tissue is well marginated and does not enhance on contrast administration. However, the lack of involution does not imply treatment failure if no contrast enhancement remains in the ablation zone.

9.4.2.4 Residual Unablated Tumour

The term "residual unablated tumour" refers to the persistence of a part of the treated tumour on initial follow-up imaging after HIFU ablation. It is caused by incomplete coverage of the ablation zone because of the large size of the tumour, inaccurate targeting, satellite nodules, or inadequate HIFU ablation. Residual unablated tumour appears as an eccentric, irregular, peripheral, enhancing soft tissue nodule on post-procedural CECT and CEMRI scans. PET-CT is an important diagnostic tool for detecting residual unablated tumour. It can be used as the primary method of surveillance after HIFU ablation or when CT or MRI findings are equivocal. For FDG-avid tumours, the residual unablated tumour appears as an eccentric, focal area of FDG uptake against the background of low-grade homogeneous tracer distribution, or irregular FDG uptake at the ablation margin on ^{18}F-FDG PET-CT imaging.

9.4.2.5 Local Tumour Progression

The term "local tumour progression" refers to the appearance of new tumour foci after a tumour has previously been considered as being completely ablated. It occurs in the same place as the original treated tumour, or very close to it, with an increase in size with time. The distinction between local tumour progression and new tumour is important for determining the technical success of HIFU ablation (i.e., local treatment success rate). However, in routine clinical practice, it seems virtually impossible to distinguish whether it is residual unablated tumour that continues to grow, or a new tumour growing from a microscopic tumour satellite that is not detected by preprocedural imaging at the original site.

Recurrent tumour appears as a new, peripheral, intra-, or extra-zonal soft tissue tumour nodule on postprocedural imaging during the follow-up period. In liver cancer, it is seen as soft-tissue density on unenhanced CT, isointense to hypointense on T1-weighted MR imaging, or isointense to moderately hyperintense on T2-weighted MR imaging, and contrast enhancement on CECT or CEMRI scans. It can also appear as an irregular, eccentric, or asymmetric thickening along the margin of the ablation zone with the loss of sharp delineation. FDG PET-CT imaging is the most important tool for the early detection of recurrent tumours in patients with FDG-avid tumours. Recurrent tumours manifest themselves as new, focal, nodular, eccentric, intra-, or extra-zonal FDG uptake on ^{18}F-FDG PET-CT imaging.

9.4.2.6 Complications and Adverse Events

The term "complication" refers to any unexpected variation from a procedural course, and "adverse event" refers to any actual or potential injury related to the treatment. These can occur during the procedure or afterwards.

9.5 Summary

Over the past two decades, HIFU ablation has evolved as an important non-invasive option for the treatment of a wide range of solid tumours throughout the body. The role of HIFU ablation has expanded to include tumours of the prostate, liver, pancreas, kidney, breast, uterus, bone, soft tissues, brain, and thyroid and its clinical applications continue to increase, ranging from malignant to benign tumours, as well as other diseases. Although many published trials describe post-procedural imaging assessment, the lack of standardised definitions and assessments in the HIFU literature limits the use of imaging modalities for post-procedural outcome measures and comparison between clinical studies and results. Therefore, HIFU requires the development of standard reporting criteria for postprocedural imaging assessments.

This chapter has introduced tumour response evaluation criteria for assessment of tumour response after treatment, including RECIST and PERCIST. It addresses major imaging modalities that have been used as follow-up tools in clinical practice to evaluate tumour response and treatment outcome. Of these, CECT and CEMRI are the reference standards for assessment of therapeutic response after tumour ablation. CEUS plays an increasingly important role in early detection of residual unablated tumour immediately following thermal ablation. ^{18}F-FDG PET-CT imaging is more sensitive for assessing metabolic tumour response. Using the published standardisation of terminology and reporting criteria related to image-guided tumour ablation, this chapter introduces the terminology and imaging report requirements for post-ablation imaging assessment.

In conclusion, evaluation of technical success and associated therapeutic efficacy is critical in the clinical management of cancer patients after HIFU ablation. As there is no official widely accepted imaging protocol for post-ablation surveillance, the protocol for assessment of therapeutic response and follow-up varies by institutions and tumour types. In our institution the first post treatment imaging for HIFU ablation is an intraprocedural CEUS scan when the patient is still on the HIFU treatment bed. It is ideally carried out immediately following treatment for the early detection of residual unablated tumour. This allows operators to perform immediate retreatment if residual unablated tumour remains in the treated region. Follow-up CECT or CEMRI scan is performed 2 weeks after ablation and then every 3 months thereafter. The assessments include reporting tumour size, the diameter of the ablation zone, and contrast enhancement in the treated tumour. The absence of contrast enhancement can provide imaging information about tumour response and residual viable tumour after treatment. Follow-up imaging at 6 to 12 months can show obvious involution of the treated tumour and the region of coagulation necrosis. In patients with FDG-avid tumours, ^{18}FDG PET-CT scanning is recommended for the early detection of residual unablated tumour within 1 week of ablation.

REFERENCES

1. Histed, S. N., Lindenberg, M. L., Mena, E., Turkbey, B., Choyke, P. L., and K. A. Kurdziel. 2012. Review of functional/anatomical imaging in oncology. *Nucl Med Commun* 33:349–361.
2. Fatima, N., Zaman, M. U., Gnanasegaran, G., et al. 2015. Hybrid Imaging in Oncology. *Asian Pac J Cancer Prev* 16:5599–5605.
3. Napoli, A., Anzidei, M., Ciolina, F., et al. 2013. MR-guided high-intensity focused ultrasound: Current status of an emerging technology. *Cardiovasc Intervent Radiol* 36:1190–1203.
4. Siedek, F., Yeo, S. Y., Heijman, E., et al. 2019. Magnetic resonance-guided high-intensity focused ultrasound (MR-HIFU): Technical background and overview of current clinical applications (Part 1). *Rofo* 191:522–530.
5. Organization WH. 1979. *WHO Handbook for Reporting Results of Cancer Treatment*. Geneva and Albany, NY: World Health Organization; WHO Publications Centre USA.
6. Therasse, P., Arbuck, S. G., Eisenhauer, E. A., et al. 2000. New guidelines to evaluate the response to treatment in solid tumors. European Organization for Research and Treatment of Cancer, National Cancer Institute of the United States, National Cancer Institute of Canada. *J Natl Cancer Inst* 92:205–216.
7. Eisenhauer, E. A., Therasse, P., Bogaerts, J., et al. 2009. New response evaluation criteria in solid tumours: Revised RECIST guideline (version 1.1). *Eur J Cancer* 45:228–247.

8. Lencioni, R., and J. M. Llovet. 2010. Modified RECIST (mRECIST) assessment for hepatocellular carcinoma. *Semin Liver Dis* 30:52–60.
9. Gillmore, R., Stuart, S., Kirkwood, A., et al. 2011. EASL and mRECIST responses are independent prognostic factors for survival in hepatocellular cancer patients treated with transarterial embolization. *J Hepatol* 55:1309–1316.
10. Memon, K., Kulik, L., Lewandowski, R. J., et al. Radiographic response to locoregional therapy in hepatocellular carcinoma predicts patient survival times. *Gastroenterology* 141:526–535, 535.e1–2.
11. Sato, Y., Watanabe, H., Sone, M., et al. 2013. Tumor response evaluation criteria for HCC (hepatocellular carcinoma) treated using TACE (transcatheter arterial chemoembolization): RECIST (response evaluation criteria in solid tumors) version 1.1 and mRECIST (modified RECIST): JIVROSG-0602. *Ups J Med Sci* 118:16–22.
12. Pallan, P., Wholey, M., Palacios, R., et al. 2018. Transarterial chemoembolization with 40-micron drug-eluting beads: A multicenter study, a San Antonio experience. *J Vasc Interv Radiol* 29: S22.
13. Wahl, R. L., Jacene, H., Kasamon, Y., and M. A. Lodge. 2009. From RECIST to PERCIST: Evolving considerations for PET response criteria in solid tumors. *J Nucl Med* 50(Suppl 1):122s–150s.
14. Min, S. J., Jang, H. J., and J. H. Kim. 2016. Comparison of the RECIST and PERCIST criteria in solid tumors: A pooled analysis and review. *Oncotarget* 7:27848–27854.
15. Ko, C. C., Yeh, L. R., Kuo, Y. T., and J. H. Chen. 2021. Imaging biomarkers for evaluating tumor response: RECIST and beyond. *Biomark Res* 9:52.
16. Sorace, A. G., Elkassem, A. A., Galgano, S. J., et al. 2020. imaging for response assessment in cancer clinical trials. *Semin Nucl Med* 50:488–504.
17. Carovac, A., Smajlovic, F., and D. Junuzovic. 2011. Application of ultrasound in medicine. *Acta Inform Med* 19:168–171.
18. Lagalla, R., Caruso, G., and M. Finazzo. 1998. Monitoring treatment response with color and power Doppler. *Eur J Radiol* 27 (Suppl 2): S149–S156.
19. Hamper, U. M., DeJong, M. R., Caskey, C. I., et al. 1997. Power Doppler imaging: Clinical experience and correlation with color Doppler US and other imaging modalities. *Radiographics* 17:499–513.
20. Jung, E. M., Weber, M. A., and I. Wiesinger. 2021. Contrast-enhanced ultrasound perfusion imaging of organs. *Radiologe* 61(Suppl 1):19–28.
21. Chung, Y. E., and K. W. Kim. 2015. Contrast-enhanced ultrasonography: Advance and current status in abdominal imaging. *Ultrasonography* 34:3–18.
22. Fröhlich, E., Muller, R., Cui, X. W., Schreiber-Dietrich, D., and C. F. Dietrich. 2015. Dynamic contrast-enhanced ultrasound for quantification of tissue perfusion. *J Ultrasound Med* 34:179–196.
23. Kloth, C., Kratzer, W., Schmidberger, J., Beer, M., Clevert, D. A., and T. Graeter. 2021. Ultrasound 2020 – diagnostics & therapy: On the way to multimodal ultrasound: Contrast-enhanced ultrasound (CEUS), microvascular doppler techniques, fusion imaging, sonoelastography, interventional sonography. *Rofo* 193:23–32.
24. Dietrich, C. F., Nolsøe, C. P., Barr, R. G., et al. 2020. Guidelines and good clinical practice recommendations for contrast enhanced ultrasound (CEUS) in the liver – update 2020 – WFUMB in cooperation with EFSUMB, AFSUMB, AIUM, and FLAUS. *Ultraschall Med* 39:187–210.
25. Kelekis, A., and D. Filippiadis. 2016. Computed tomography and ultrasounds for the follow-up of hepatocellular carcinoma ablation: What you need to know. *Diagnostics (Basel)* 6(1):9.
26. Meloni, M. F., Francica, G., Chiang, J., Coltorti, A., Danzi, R., and P. F. Laeseke. 2021. Use of contrast-enhanced ultrasound in ablation therapy of HCC: Planning, guiding, and assessing treatment response. *J Ultrasound Med* 40:879–894.
27. Wu, F., Wang, Z. B., Chen, W. Z., et al. 2004. Extracorporeal focused ultrasound surgery for treatment of human solid carcinomas: Early Chinese clinical experience. *Ultrasound Med Biol* 30:245–260.
28. Gummadi, S., Eisenbrey, J. R., and A. Lyshchik. 2018. Contrast-enhanced ultrasonography in interventional oncology. *Abdom Radiol (NY)* 43:3166–3175.
29. Inzerillo, A., Meloni, M. F., Taibbi, A., and T. V. Bartolotta. 2022. Loco-regional treatment of hepatocellular carcinoma: Role of contrast-enhanced ultrasonography. *World J Hepatol* 14:911–922.
30. Kennedy, J. E., ter Haar, G. R., Wu, F., et al. 2004. Contrast-enhanced ultrasound assessment of tissue response to high-intensity focused ultrasound. *Ultrasound Med Biol* 30:851–854.
31. Rindler, R. S., Allen, J. W., Barrow, J. W., Pradilla, G., and D. L. Barrow. 2020. Neuroimaging of intracerebral hemorrhage. *Neurosurgery* 86: E414-E423.

32. Jadhav, A. P., and T. G. Jovin. 2012. Vascular imaging of the head and neck. *Semin Neurol* 32:401–410.
33. Yu, H., and J. M. Stavas. 2013. The role of interventional radiology in management of benign and malignant gynecologic diseases. *Obstet Gynecol Surv* 68:691–701.
34. Odisio, B. C., and M. J. Wallace. 2014. Image-guided interventions in oncology. *Surg Oncol Clin N Am* 23:937–955.
35. Arnold, M. J., Keung, J. J., and B. McCarragher. 2019. Interventional radiology: Indications and best practices. *Am Fam Physician* 99:547–556.
36. Wu, F., Chen, W. Z., Bai, J., et al. 2002. Tumor vessel destruction resulting from high-intensity focused ultrasound in patients with solid malignancies. *Ultrasound Med Biol* 28:535–542.
37. Seeram, E. 2018. Computed tomography: A technical review. *Radiol Technol* 89:279CT-302CT.
38. Booij, R., Budde, R. P. J., Dijkshoorn, M. L., and M. van Straten. 2020. Technological developments of X-ray computed tomography over half a century: User's influence on protocol optimization. *Eur J Radiol* 131:109261.
39. Fite, B. Z., Wang, J., Ghanouni, P., and K. W. Ferrara. 2022. A review of imaging methods to assess ultrasound-mediated ablation. *BME Front* 2022:9758652.
40. Patel, N., King, A. J., and D. J. Breen. 2017. Imaging appearances at follow-up after image-guided solid-organ abdominal tumour ablation. *Clin Radiol* 72:680–690.
41. Wu, F., Wang, Z. B., Chen, W. Z., et al. 2004. Extracorporeal high intensity focused ultrasound ablation in the treatment of patients with large hepatocellular carcinoma. *Ann Surg Oncol* 11:1061–1069.
42. Kissane, J., Neutze, J., and H. Singh. 2020. *Radiology Fundamentals, Introduction to Imaging & Technology*, 6th ed. Cham, Switzerland: Springer, 32–35p.
43. Yousaf, T., Dervenoulas, G., and M. Politis. 2018. Advances in MRI methodology. *Int Rev Neurobiol* 141:31–76.
44. Chenevert, T., Stegman, L., Taylor, J., et al. 2000. Diffusion magnetic resonance imaging: An early surrogate marker of therapeutic efficacy in brain tumors. *J Natl Cancer Inst* 92:2029–2036.
45. Koral, K., Mathis, D., Gimi, B., et al. 2013. Common pediatric cerebellar tumors: Correlation between cell densities and apparent diffusion coefficient metrics. *Radiology* 268:532–537.
46. Lyon, P. C., Rai, V., Price, N., Shah, A., Wu, F., and D. Cranston. 2020. Ultrasound-guided high intensity focused ultrasound ablation for symptomatic uterine fibroids: Preliminary clinical experience. *Ultraschall Med* 41:550–556.
47. Cox, D. R. A., Chung, W., Grace, J., et al. 2023. Evaluating treatment response following locoregional therapy for hepatocellular carcinoma: A review of the available serological and radiological tools for assessment. *JGH Open* 7:249–260.
48. Mendiratta-Lala, M., Masch, W. R., Shampain, K., et al. 2020. MRI assessment of hepatocellular carcinoma after local-regional therapy: A comprehensive review. *Radiol Imaging Cancer* 2:e190024.
49. Lewis, H. L., Ghasabeh, M. A., Khoshpouri, P., Kamel, I. R., and T. M. Pawlik. 2017. Functional hepatic imaging as a biomarker of primary and secondary tumor response to loco-regional therapies. *Surg Oncol* 26:411–422.
50. Chetan, M. R., Lyon, P. C., Wu, F., et al. 2019. Role of diffusion-weighted imaging in monitoring treatment response following high-intensity focused ultrasound ablation of recurrent sacral chordoma. *Radiol Case Rep* 14:1197–1201.
51. Taillefer, R. 1999. The role of ^{99m}Tc-sestamibi and other conventional radiopharmaceuticals in breast cancer diagnosis. *Semin Nucl Med* 29:16–40.
52. Buckley, O., O'Keeffe, S., Geoghegan, T., et al. 2007. ^{99m}Tc bone scintigraphy superscans: A review. *Nucl Med Commun* 28:521–527.
53. Del Vecchio, S., and M. Salvatore. 2004. ^{99m}Tc-MIBI in the evaluation of breast cancer biology. *Eur J Nucl Med Mol Imaging* 31 (Suppl 1): S88–96.
54. Kissane, J., Neutze, J., H. Singh. 2020. *Radiology Fundamentals, Introduction to Imaging & Technology*, 6th ed. Springer: Cham, Switzerland, 36–43p.
55. Ritt, P. 2022. Recent developments in SPECT/CT. *Semin Nucl Med* 52:276–285.
56. Cai, J., and F. Li. 2013. Single-photon emission computed tomography tracers for predicting and monitoring cancer therapy. *Curr Pharm Biotechnol* 14:693–707.
57. Lee, I., Byun, B. H., Lim, I., et al. 2018. Comparison of 99mTc-methyl diphosphonate bone scintigraphy and 18F-fluorodeoxyglucose positron emission tomography/computed tomography to predict histologic response to neoadjuvant chemotherapy in patients with osteosarcoma. *Medicine (Baltimore)* 97: e12318.

58. Chen, W., Zhu, H., Zhang, L., et al. 2010. Primary bone malignancy: Effective treatment with high-intensity focused ultrasound ablation. *Radiology* 255:967–978.
59. Ren, C., Jin, S., Zhou, Q., Zhu, H., Wang, H., and C. Liang. 2020. Clinical significance of ^{99}mTc-MIBI breast imaging in the diagnosis of early breast cancer. *Asian J Surg* 25:126–129.
60. Li, H., Liu, Z., Yuan, L., et al. 2021. Radionuclide-based imaging of breast cancer: State of the art. *Cancers (Basel)* 13:5459.
61. Narayanan D, Berg WA. 2018. Dedicated breast gamma camera imaging and breast PET: Current status and future directions. *PET Clin* 13(3):363–381.
62. Zhang, A., Li, P., Liu, Q., and D. Song. 2017. Breast-specific gamma camera imaging with 99mTc-MIBI has better diagnostic performance than magnetic resonance imaging in breast cancer patients: A meta-analysis. *Hell J Nucl Med* 20:26–35.
63. De Feo, M. S., Sidrak, M. M. A., Conte, M., et al. 2022. Breast-specific gamma imaging: An added value in the diagnosis of breast cancer, a systematic review. *Cancers (Basel)* 14:4619.
64. Wood, K. A., Hoskin, P. J., and M. I. Saunders. 2007. Positron emission tomography in oncology: A review. *Clin Oncol (R Coll Radiol)* 19:237–255.
65. Buck, A. K., and S. N. Reske. 2004. Cellular origin and molecular mechanisms of 18FFDG uptake: Is there a contribution of the endothelium? *J Nucl Med* 45:461–463.
66. Gatenby, R. A., and R. J. Gillies. 2004. Why do cancers have high aerobic glycolysis? *Nat Rev Cancer* 4:891–899.
67. Miladinova, D. 2019. Molecular imaging in breast cancer. *Nucl Med Mol Imaging* 53:313–319.
68. Neveu, M.-A., De Preter, G., Joudiou, N., et al. 2016. Multi-modality imaging to assess metabolic response to dichloroacetate treatment in tumor models. *Oncotarget* 7:81741–81749.
69. Chun, Y. J., Jeung, H.-C., Park, H. S., et al. 2019. Significance of metabolic tumor volume and total lesion glycolysis measured using 18F-FDG PET/CT in locally advanced and metastatic gallbladder carcinoma. *Yonsei Med J* 60:604–610.
70. Paydary, K., Seraj, S. M., Zadeh, M. Z., et al. 2019. The evolving role of FDG-PET/CT in the diagnosis, staging, and treatment of breast cancer. *Mol Imaging Biol* 21:1–10.
71. Howard, B. A., and T. Z. Wong. 2021. ^{18}F-FDG-PET/CT imaging for gastrointestinal malignancies. *Radiol Clin North Am* 59:737–753.
72. Sheikhbahaei, S., Marcus, C., and R. M. Subramaniam. 2015. ^{18}F FDG PET/CT and head and neck cancer: Patient management and outcomes. *PET Clin* 10:125–145.
73. Wartski, M., and A. Sauvanet. 2019.^{18}F-FDG PET/CT in pancreatic adenocarcinoma: A role at initial imaging staging? *Diagn Interv Imaging* 100:735–741.
74. Aarntzen. E. H. J. G., Heijmen, L., and W. J. G. Oyen. 2018. ^{18}F-FDG PET/CT in local ablative therapies: A systematic review. *J Nucl Med* 59:551–556.
75. Purandare, N. C., Rangarajan, V., Shah, S. A., et al. 2011. Therapeutic response to radiofrequency ablation of neoplastic lesions: FDG PET/CT findings. *Radiographics* 31:201–213.
76. Samim, M., El-Haddad, G. E., Molenaar, I. Q., et al. 2014. $^{[18F]}$ Fluorodeoxyglucose PET for interventional oncology in liver malignancy. *PET Clin* 9:469–495.
77. Goldberg, S. N., Charboneau, J. W., Dodd, G. D. 3rd, et al. 2003. Image-guided tumor ablation: Proposal for standardization of terms and reporting criteria. *Radiology* 228:335–345.
78. Goldberg, S. N., Grassi, C. J., Cardella, J. F., et al. 2005. Image-guided tumor ablation: Standardization of terminology and reporting criteria. *Radiology* 235:728–739.
79. Goldberg, S. N., Grassi, C. J., Cardella, J. F., et al. 2009. Image-guided tumor ablation: Standardization of terminology and reporting criteria. *J Vasc Interv Radiol* 20(7 Suppl): S377–390.
80. Ahmed, M., Solbiati, L., Brace, C. L., et al. 2014. Image-guided tumor ablation: Standardization of terminology and reporting criteria-a 10-year update. *J Vasc Interv Radiol* 25:1691–1705.e4.
81. Liddell, R. P. 2021. Consensus guidelines in image-guided tumor ablation: Toward evidence-based interventional oncology. *Radiology* 301:541–542.
82. Puijk, R. S., Ahmed, M., Goldberg, S. N., et al. 2021. Consensus guidelines for the definition of time-to-event end points in image-guided tumor ablation: Results of the SIO and DATECAN initiative. *Radiology* 301:533–540.

10

Focused Ultrasound Treatment of the Prostate: Devices and Clinical Results

David Cranston

10.1 Introduction

Benign prostatic hypertrophy and prostate cancer are two of the most common diseases of the prostate, both affecting men in their later years. Benign prostatic hypertrophy is characterised by a non-cancerous enlargement of the prostate, and since the prostate envelopes the urethra, it may cause symptoms of bladder outflow obstruction and consequently bothersome urinary symptoms such as poor flow, hesitancy and terminal dribbling.[1] If symptomatic, benign prostatic hypertrophy can often be treated with drug therapy, but if that fails and the symptoms become severe, a number of surgical treatments are now available. Much of the early research into high intensity focused ultrasound (HIFU) for the treatment of prostate disease focused on its use as a treatment for benign prostatic hyperplasia. A number of studies showed HIFU to be effective, at least in the short term, with improvement in urinary flow rate and improved symptomatic relief.[2–5] However, despite this early promise, long-term data tended to show that these effects were short-lived, and many patients required further treatment within four years.[6] Thus HIFU is currently not in use for benign disease, although this may change in the future as the technology improves.

Today the clinical application of HIFU in prostate disease is in the treatment of men with prostate cancer.

The management and treatment of prostate cancer remains controversial. It is the second-most prevalent cancer, after that of the breast, and the fifth leading cause of cancer-related death among men.[7]

In 2020, 200,000 men were diagnosed with prostate cancer in the United States but only 30,000 died. The United Kingdom has similar figures, with 50,000 receiving the diagnosis every year and 12,000 dying. However postmortem data suggest many more men who have the disease, are undiagnosed, and do not die of it. Prostate cancer is graded on the Gleason scale which looks histologically at the greatest number of aggressive cells and grading them 1–6, and then the next most aggressive cells again graded between 1 and 6. In practice, however, the grading ranges from 3–5 with 3 + 3 being the lowest grade, which is often treated by active monitoring, while 5 + 5 is the most aggressive grade.[8]

Since the introduction of prostate specific antigen (PSA) testing the incidence of diagnosis of prostate cancer has increased dramatically, leading to earlier diagnosis and an increased number of men being diagnosed with localised disease.[9]

However, the question remains as to not only what the best treatment is but when treatment is actually necessary. Professor Freddie Hamdy led the ProtecT study which screened over 82,000 men between 50 and 69 for prostate cancer with PSA and diagnosed cancer in 2004. These were then randomly enrolled in a trial to evaluate the effects of treatment by active monitoring, radical prostatectomy or radiotherapy. After 15 years of follow-up, prostate cancer mortality was low regardless of treatment.[10]

Furthermore, the paper showed that it is the *diagnosis* of prostate cancer that has the greatest impact on quality of life, which is one of the reasons why PSA testing remains controversial.[11, 12] However, wherever possible, it remains important to identify the prostate cancers that are life threatening. With

DOI: 10.1201/9780429162671-10

this increasing diagnostic rate, based on the increased use of PSA testing, the search for less invasive treatments has led to the investigation of HIFU as one possible treatment.

Localised disease is usually asymptomatic, and radical treatment with radical prostatectomy or radiotherapy while often being curative, are often associated with significant side effects. HIFU to either the whole prostate, hemi-ablation or even ablation more focally has been proposed as a way of treating the disease while minimising the complications. William Osler (1849–1919), the most famous physician of his day, said, "Diseases that harm require treatments that harm less".[13]

Complications vary, depending on the series. In 2019 patient-reported outcomes for radical surgery and radiotherapy for prostate carcinoma (PCa) were published by the National Prostate Cancer Audit who had received replies from over 25,000 men who underwent treatment between April 2015 and September 2016. In these two years of treatment for localised disease, 1 in 10 men experienced what was described as a severe urinary complication following surgery or a severe bowel complication following external beam radiation. On a scale of 1 (best) to 100 (worst) sexual function post-surgery averaged at 23 and urinary continence at 71. After radiotherapy these were 17 and 85, respectively.

Radical treatment with surgery or radiotherapy for localised disease aims for cure but may be associated with morbidity.[14] This, in turn, may affect mental wellbeing,[15] and high intensity HIFU has been advocated as a treatment that may be equally effective in terms of cancer treatment but with much less in the way of side effects.[16]

Treatment of early-stage, clinically significant disease, which carries the highest risk of progression,[17] requires active treatment, but since whole-gland therapies are associated with serious adverse events in the sexual and urinary domains,[14, 15] focal therapy could be a better option for these patients.

10.2 Clinical Studies

The earliest clinical data that demonstrated that HIFU could successfully treat prostate cancer were published by Madersbacher et al. in Vienna[18] who first reported that HIFU could destroy prostate carcinoma in 1995.[19] Subsequent studies by Beerlage in Nijmegen[20] and Gelet in France[21, 22] confirmed these initial findings. Over the last 20 years there has been an expansion of interest in the use of HIFU as a treatment modality for prostate cancer in the UK, with acceptance of it as an approved procedure by the National Institute of Clinical Excellence (NICE) in 2005.

Over the last two decades HIFU has been expanding its indications, from its early days in patients with localised disease unfit for more radical treatment, to partial ablations for focal disease, and salvage therapy following primary surgery and radiotherapy.[23–25] At the time of writing, prostate cancer treatment using trans-rectal HIFU under general anaesthesia has shown promise in more than 100 sites across the world.[26]

Depending on the volume of the disease, and the localised staging, different treatment regimes have been proposed, including whole gland or focal gland ablation.[27, 28] After the procedure, the type and length of bladder catheterisation has varied significantly among the initial studies.

The first UK series of HIFU treatments for prostatic carcinoma was carried out in 2008 by Ahmed et al. who reported a significant drop in PSA.[29] In 2017, the French Urological Association reported results of a six-year prospective IDEAL[30] multi-institutional study (2009–2015), which evaluated HIFU-hemi-ablation as a primary treatment in 111 patients with medium- or low-grade unilateral localised prostate cancer. The report found that at one year there was a 95% absence of clinically significant cancer, and at two years there was a treatment-free survival rate of 89%.[31]

Medium-term outcomes in 569 men from a national multi-centre registry cohort receiving primary whole-gland HIFU (Sonablate 500) for primary non-metastatic prostate cancer were reported by Dickinson et al.[32] Redo-HIFU was permitted as part of the intervention, leading to a total of 754 interventions. They found that whole-gland HIFU is a repeatable day-case treatment that confers low rates of urinary incontinence, with 12% of the patients who had not previously required pads for incontinence now requiring them. Disease control at a median of just under five years of follow-up demonstrated the potential of whole-gland HIFU as a treatment for non-metastatic prostate cancer. Endoscopic interventions and erectile dysfunction rates were similar to those found with other whole-gland treatments, with 61% having erectile problems post-HIFU. Only one patient developed a recto-urethral fistula (0.13%).

Another group, also using the Sonoblate 500 system,[33] reported the medium-term oncological outcomes following focal treatment in 1032 men, 80% of whom had a Gleason score of 3 + 4 or above. While the overall survival rate of 97% at 96 months is not surprising, they found that freedom from radical treatment was 81% at 96 months and concluded that focal HIFU for prostatic carcinoma is a feasible therapeutic strategy, with acceptable survival and oncological results, and a reduction in the five-year retreatment rates.

Abreu et al. reported the first series of focal HIFU for prostate cancer in 100 men in the United States. Although retrospective in nature, the report did show good results, similar to other studies, in terms of disease control and genitourinary function, with 91% of patients avoiding radical treatment and all patients maintaining full continence after two years with no major adverse events.[34]

HIFU treatment has been used in a number of studies for salvage treatment. In a study limited by its retrospective nature, Crouzet et al. [35] looked at the oncological outcomes from 1995 to 2009 in 418 patients who had undergone salvage high intensity focused ultrasound for locally recurrent prostate cancer after external beam radiotherapy. The study found a seven-year cancer-specific survival of over 80%, but at the price of significant morbidity. However, complication rates of incontinence, outflow obstruction and recto-urethral fistula decreased significantly after 2002, when treatment-specific parameters for post-radiotherapy salvage HIFU were introduced to account for the decreased vascularisation of the prostate gland and peri-prostatic tissue that resulted from radiotherapy-induced fibrosis. Using these amended parameters, the recto-urethral fistula rate decreased from 9% to 0.6%.

Similarly, Houstiou et al.[36] evaluated the oncological and functional outcomes of salvage high intensity HIFU for locally recurrent prostate cancer after low-dose-rate brachytherapy in a clinical Phase II study of 50 patients between 2003 and 2015. They found satisfactory disease control, and the complication rate was decreased with specific post-brachytherapy parameters of the HIFU delivery and hemi-ablation when possible. Kanthabalan et al.[37] found a similar benefit of focal salvage therapy in a study of 150 men.

A few units have looked at transurethral ultrasound ablation of the prostate (TULSA). Bonekamp et al.[38] demonstrated a median 12-month reduction in viable prostatic volume of 88% in 29 patients in a radiology review of the Phase I clinical trial of MRI-guided TULSA in patients with localised prostate cancer.

Although no large randomised clinical trials of HIFU in prostate cancer have been conducted, the "Partial ablation versus radical prostatectomy in intermediate-risk prostate cancer: the PART feasibility RCT study"[39] demonstrated that randomisation of men to an RCT comparing partial ablation with radical treatments of the prostate is feasible. The full study has received funding from the NIHR and is ongoing at the time of writing.

Short-term oncologic results have been reported in the majority of the studies reviewed, while just two studies[40, 41] have reached a postoperative follow-up adequate for intermediate-term results.

In virtually all studies it has taken up to a year for the PSA to reach its lowest level and agreement on the strict definition of biochemical disease control has yet to be reached.

Retreatment possibilities have been reported in some of the studies. Therefore, no data regarding indications for different retreatment strategies, including second focal HIFU or other focal therapies, or for whole-gland treatment options were reported in any of the studies. For low-risk recurrence, a deferred treatment option was offered in the majority of the studies, where up to 35% of patients with PCa after focal HIFU were undergoing active surveillance. The majority of the studies used radical treatment options, such as salvage RP and salvage External Beam Radiotherapy (EBRT) to treat PCa recurrence or progression. Second focal HIFU was initiated in up to 20% of patients with PCa, where in-field recurrence was treated in 11% of patients and out-of-field progression in 13% of patients.

The majority of complications from HIFU are minor in nature with urinary retention, urethral sloughing and urinary tract infections being the most common. Postoperative recto-urethral fistulas have been reported.[42] Bass et al. reported a slightly higher number (3%) of, this complication but the problem was solved by increased cooling time between treatment pulses in the midzone of the prostate.

Gradual recovery during the early postoperative phase was also observed, and 86% of patients retained sufficient erection for sexual intercourse following the procedure.

10.3 Devices

Several HIFU systems designed to treat prostate cancer are currently available, three of which are transrectal and one transurethral (see Figure 10.1).

Typically, the HIFU transducer is integrated into an transrectal imaging ultrasound (TRUS) probe, which is used to image the prostate during HIFU interventions to aid with planning and monitoring. In addition to US-guided HFIU, recently developed systems allow the delivery of prostate HIFU under magnetic resonance (MR) imaging guidance.

The Sonablate-500 (SB-500) system consists of a transrectal probe, console (with monitor and printer) and a chilling device.[43] The SB-500 probe contains two US transducers composed of piezoceramic material that can both provide imaging and deliver HIFU treatment through the acoustic window opening located at the tip of the probe. A cooling device (Sonachill) is connected to the console and probe and circulates cooled, de-gassed water through the probe to ensure the rectal wall and HIFU transducer remain cool, whilst simultaneously relaying temperature information to the console. Custom software is bundled with the SB-500 systems which displays ultrasound images of the prostate on the monitor in both transverse and longitudinal planes. The software enables on-screen planning and allows the

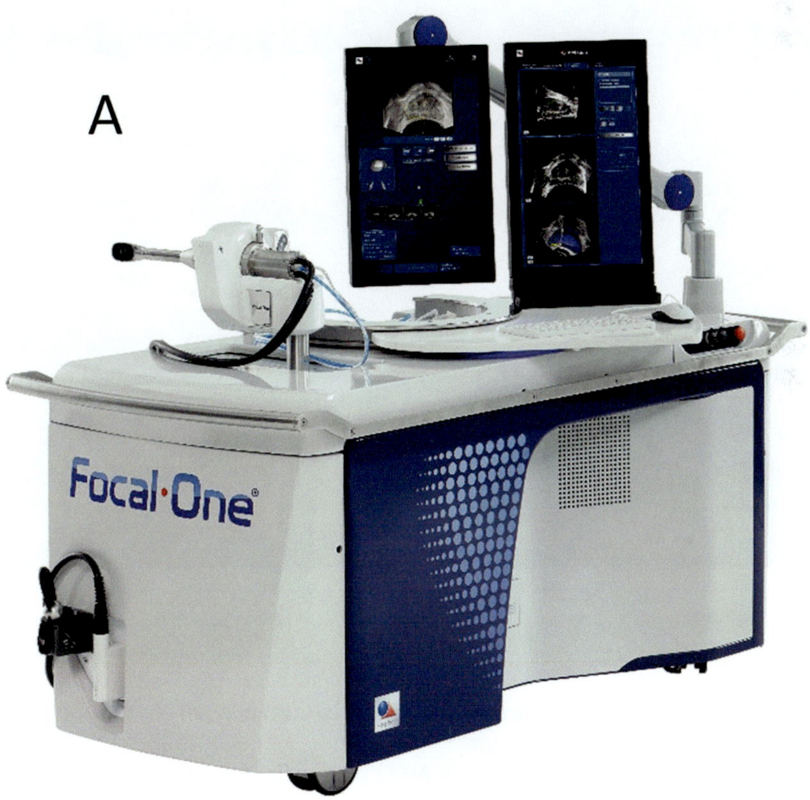

FIGURE 10.1 (a) Focal One device showing the transrectal probe. (Courtesy of Nicholas Guillen Edap-TMS). (b) Representative treatment screen from the Sonablate 500 showing the ultrasound scan, and the delineated treatment volume. (Courtesy of Professor Mark Emberton.)

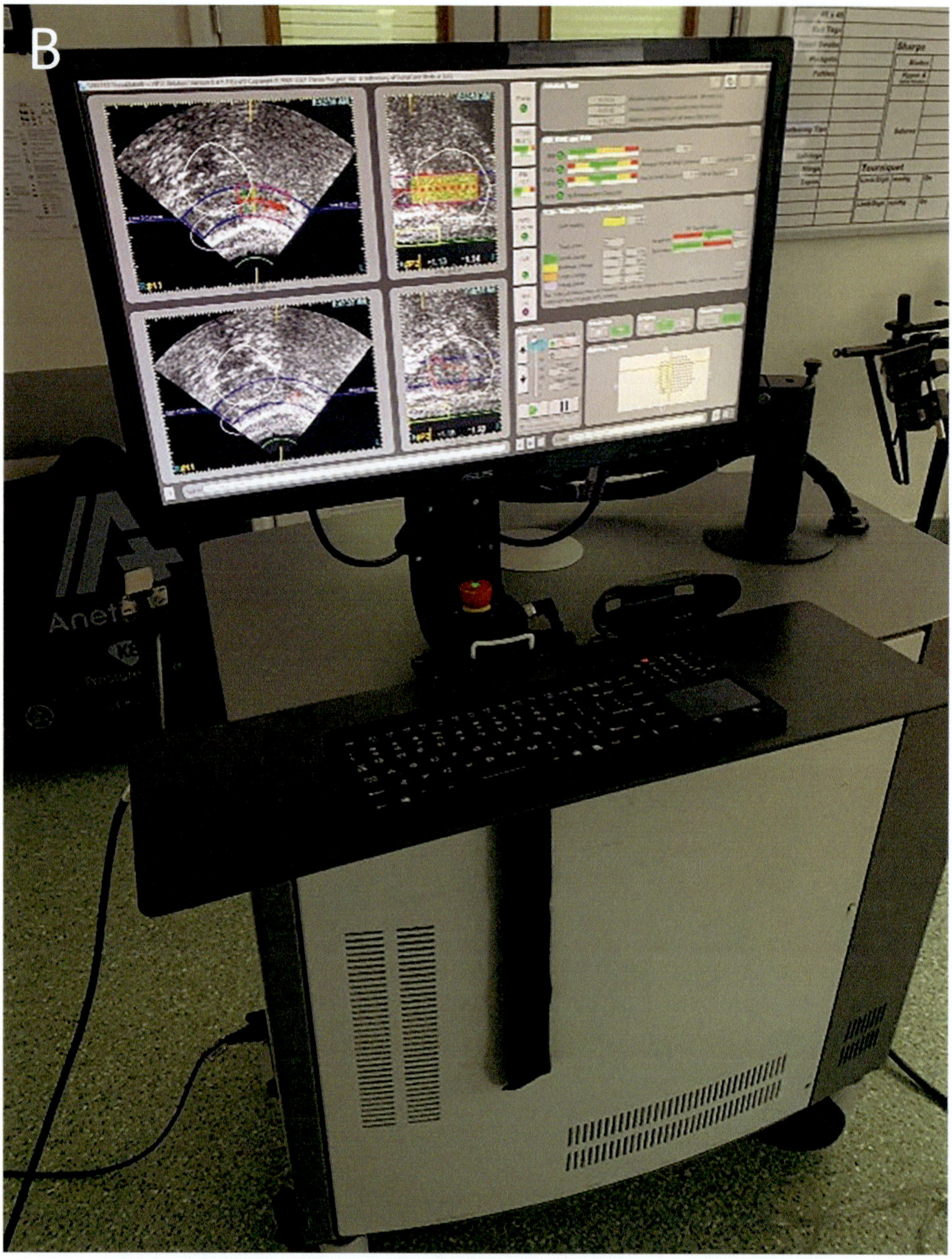

FIGURE 10.1 (Continued)

operator to define treatment zones. The transducer is moved automatically by the software according to the treatment zone(s) defined by the operator.[44]

The Ablatherm system operates on the same principles as the SB-500 device, being a TRUS-based device capable of both imaging the prostate with ultrasound and delivering HIFU treatment.[45] A major difference between the two systems is that the Ablatherm device employs two ultrasound crystals, one for imaging (7.5 MHz) and one for delivering HIFU (3 MHz), whereas the SB-500 system uses a single 4-MHz crystal for both imaging and treatment. Aside from this, the two systems share many commonalities, such as a cooling system to protect the rectal wall and software to facilitate on-screen planning and treatment delivery.[46]

The Ablatherm, and its later incarnation, Focal One devices use coupling liquid to protect the rectum; thus, patients should be placed in a lateral position to allow gas bubbles to rise outside the imaging and therapy fields.

The Sonablate 500 device uses circulating chilled water instead of coupling liquid, thus, a supine patient position is recommended. This features the latest technology, enables more precise pre-treatment planning and shape and size modifications during the procedure (which were not possible with the earlier Ablatherm device) as well as end-of-treatment validation through contrast-enhanced ultrasound (which is not possible with the Sonablate 500 device).[47]

In general, the ultrasound-guided (USg) devices are smaller and more flexible than devices using magnetic resonance imaging (MRg). The combination of imaging and therapy sources into one treatment head allows a wide range of mounting designs, such as devices used in transrectal probes or on robotic arms. The extracorporeal USg device that has been used most frequently to date has this combined head mounted in a water bath below a treatment bed, in a similar geometry to that of MRg devices. Successful ablation is seen on ultrasound images as newly created bright echoes in the target volume. These echoes are due to the production of bubbles, usually resulting from tissue water boiling. MRg-guided systems arguably provide more readily interpretable images than ultrasound, and as temperature-sensitive imaging sequences are available, thermal maps can be produced during treatment. However, these systems are dependent on clinical MRI scanners, which, in some settings denies their use for other diagnostic imaging purposes.

With the exception of the TULSA system for the treatment of prostate cancer, intracavitary devices use ultrasound guidance.

10.4 Conclusions

As mentioned earlier, Sir William Osler, who ended his career as the Regius Professor of Medicine in Oxford and died in 1919, is reputed to have said that "diseases which harm require treatments that harm less". Technology does not go backwards. There is no doubt that HIFU works and is now an accepted treatment for localised prostate cancer. In due course, there will be a new generation of machines for treating prostate cancer including extracorporeal machines. These devices will further minimise the side effects of radical treatment of prostate cancer, and with further research and greater understanding of the genetics of prostate cancer, the right people will be treated in the right way at the right time and for the right reason. Successful non-invasive surgical treatments will become increasingly important in the next decade.

REFERENCES

1. Hegarty NJ, Fitzpatrick JM. High intensity focused ultrasound in benign prostatic hyperplasia. Eur J Ultrasound. 1999;9(1):55–60.
2. Madersbacher S, Kratzik C, Szabo N, Susani M, Vingers L, Marberger M. Tissue ablation in benign prostatic hyperplasia with high-intensity focused ultrasound. Eur Urol. 1993;23 Suppl 1:39–43.
3. Nakamura K, Baba S, Fukazawa R, et al. Treatment of benign prostatic hyperplasia with high intensity focused ultrasound: An initial clinical trial in Japan with magnetic resonance imaging of the treated area. Int J Urol. 1995;2(3):176–80.
4. Uchida T, Yokoyama E, Iwamura M, et al. High intensity focused ultrasound for benign prostatic hyperplasia. Int J Urol. 1995;2(3):181–5.
5. Madersbacher S, Klingler CH, Schatzl G, Schmidbauer CP, Marberger M. The urodynamic impact of transrectal high-intensity focused ultrasound on bladder outflow obstruction. Eur Urol. 1996;30(4):437–45.
6. Madersbacher S, Schatzl G, Djavan B, Stulnig T, Marberger M. Long-term outcome of transrectal high-intensity focused ultrasound therapy for benign prostatic hyperplasia. Eur Urol. 2000;37(6):687–94.

7. Bray F, Ferlay J, Soerjomataram I, Siegel RL, Torre LA, Jemal A. Global cancer statistics 2018: GLOBOCAN estimates of incidence and mortality worldwide for 36 cancers in 185 countries. CA Cancer J Clin. 2018;68:394–424. Erratum in: CA Cancer J Clin. 2020;70:313.
8. Gleason DF, Mellinger GT. The Veterans Administration Cooperative Urological Research Group: Prediction of prognosis for prostatic carcinoma by combined histological grading and clinical staging. J Urol. 1974;111:58–64.
9. Cooperberg MR, Broering JM, Kantoff PW, Carroll PR. Contemporary trends in low risk prostate cancer: Risk assessment and treatment. J Urol. 2007;178(3 Pt 2):S14–9.
10. Hamdy FC, Donovan JL, Lane JA, et al. Fifteen-year outcomes after monitoring, surgery, or radiotherapy for prostate cancer. N Engl J Med. 2023;388(17):1547–8.
11. Martin RM, Donovan JL,. Turner EL, et al. Effect of a low-intensity PSA-based screening intervention on prostate cancer mortality: The CAP randomized clinical trial. JAMA. 2018;319:883–895.
12. Cranston D. PSA testing: A personal view. Br J Gen Pract. 2019;69:562.
13. Cranston D. William Osler and His Legacy to Medicine Words by Design. Oxford University Press. 2017.
14. Haglind E, Carlsson S, Stranne J, et al. Urinary incontinence and erectile dysfunction after robotic versus open radical prostatectomy: A prospective, controlled, nonrandomised trial. Eur Urol. 2015;68:216–25.
15. Sanda MG, Dunn RL, Michalski J, et al. Quality of life and satisfaction with outcome among prostate-cancer survivors. N Engl J Med. 2008;358:1250–61.
16. Valerio M, Ahmed HU, Emberton M, et al. The role of focal therapy in the management of localised prostate cancer: A systematic review. Eur Urol. 2014;66:732–51.
17. Fletcher SA, von Landenberg N, Cole AP, et al. Contemporary national trends in prostate cancer risk profile at diagnosis. Prostate Cancer Prostatic Dis. 2020;23:81–7.
18. Madersbacher S, Pedevilla M, Vingers L, Susani M, Marberger M. Effect of high-intensity focused ultrasound on human prostate cancer in vivo. Cancer Res. 1995;55(15):3346–51.
19. Madersbacher S, Pedevilla M, Vingers L, et al. Effect of High Intensity Focused Ultrasound on human prostate cancer in vivo. Cancer Res. 1995;55:3346–51
20. Beerlage HP, van Leenders GJ, Oosterhof GO, et al. High-intensity focused ultrasound (HIFU) followed after one to two weeks by radical retropubic prostatectomy: Results of a prospective study. Prostate. 1999;39(1):41–6.
21. Gelet A, Chapelon JY, Bouvier R, et al. Treatment of prostate cancer with transrectal focused ultrasound: Early clinical experience. Eur Urol. 1996;29(2):174–83.
22. Gelet A, Chapelon JY, Bouvier R, Pangaud C, Lasne Y. Local control of prostate cancer by transrectal high intensity focused ultrasound therapy: Preliminary results. J Urol. 1999;161(1):156–62.
23. Chaussy CG, Thuroff S. High Intensity Focused Ultrasound for the treatment of prostate cancer, a review. J Endourol. 2017;31:S-30–37.
24. Uddin Ahmed H, Cathcart P, Chalasani V, et al. Whole-gland salvage high-intensity focused ultrasound therapy for localized prostate cancer recurrence after external beam radiation therapy. Cancer. 2012;118(12):3071–8.
25. Kanthabalan A, Peters M, Van Vulpen M, et al. Focal salvage high-intensity focused ultrasound in radiorecurrent prostate cancer. BJU Int. 2017;120(2):246–56.
26. Izadifar Z, Izadifar Z, Chapman D, et al. An Introduction to high intensity focused ultrasound: Systematic review on principles, devices, and clinical applications. J Clin Med. 2020;9:460–82.
27. Stabile A, Moschini M, Montorsi F, Cathelineau X, Sanchez-Salas R. Focal therapy for prostate cancer – index lesion treatment vs. hemiablation. A matter of definition. Int Braz J Urol. 2019;45:873–6.
28. Stabile A, Moschini M, Montorsi F, Cathelineau X, Sanchez-Salas R. Focal therapy for prostate cancer – index lesion treatment vs. hemiablation. A matter of definition. Int Braz J Urol. 2019;45:873–6.
29. Ahmed H, Zacharakis E, Dudderidge T, et al. High-intensity-focused ultrasound in the treatment of primary prostate cancer: The first UK series. Br J Cancer. 2009;101:19–26.
30. McCulloch P, Altman DG, Campbell WB, et al. No surgical intervention without evaluation. The IDEAL recommendations. Lancet. 2009;374:1105–12.
31. Rischmann P, Gelet A, Riche B, et al. Focal high intensity focused ultrasound of unilateral localized prostate cancer: A prospective multicentric hemiablation study of 111 patients. Eur Urol. 2017;71:267–73.

32. Dickinson L, Arya M Afzal N, et al. Medium-term outcomes after whole-gland high-intensity focused ultrasound for the treatment of nonmetastatic prostate cancer from a multicentre registry cohort. Eur Urol. 2016;70:668–74.
33. Stabile A, Orczyk C, Hosking-Jervis F, et al. Medium-term oncological outcomes in a large cohort of men treated with either focal or hemi-ablation using high-intensity focused ultrasonography for primary localized prostate cancer. BJU Int. 2019;124:431–40.
34. Abreu AL, Peretsman S, Iwata A, et al. High intensity focused ultrasound hemi-gland ablation for prostate cancer: Initial outcomes of a United States series. J Urol. 2020;204:741–7.
35. Crouzet S, Blana A, Murat FJ, et al. Salvage high-intensity focused ultrasound (HIFU) for locally recurrent prostate cancer after failed radiation therapy: Multi-institutional analysis of 418 patients. BJU Int. 2017;119:896–904.
36. Hostiou T, Gelet A, Chapelon JY, et al. Salvage high-intensity focused ultrasound for locally recurrent prostate cancer after low-dose-rate brachytherapy: Oncological and functional outcomes. BJU Int. 2019;124:746–57.
37. Kanthabalan A, Peters M, van Vulpen M, et al. Focal salvage high-intensity focused ultrasound in radiorecurrent prostate cancer. BJU Int. 2017;120:246–56.
38. Bonekamp D, Wolf MB, Roethke MC, et al. Twelve-month prostate volume reduction after MRI-guided transurethral ultrasound ablation of the prostate. Eur Radiol. 2019;29:299–308.
39. Hamdy FC, Elliot D, leConte S, et al. Partial ablation versus radical prostatectomy in intermediate-risk prostate cancer: The PART feasibility RCT. Health Technol Assess. 2018;22:1–96.
40. Guillaumier S, Peters M, Arya M, et al. Multicentre study of 5-year outcomes following focal therapy in treating clinically significant nonmetastatic prostate cancer. Eur Urol. 2018;74:422–9.
41. Tourinho-Barbosa RR, Sanchez-Salas R, Claros OR, Collura-Merlier S, Bakavicius A, Carneiro A, et al. Focal therapy for localized prostate cancer with either high intensity focused ultrasound or cryoablation: A single institution experience. J Urol. 2020;203:320–30.
42. Bass R, Fleshner N, Finelli A, Barkin J, Zhang L, Klotz L. Oncologic and functional outcomes of partial gland ablation with high intensity focused ultrasound for localized prostate cancer. J Urol. 2019;201:113–9.
43. Illing R, Emberton M. Sonablate-500: Transrectal high-intensity focused ultrasound for the treatment of prostate cancer. Expert Rev Med Devices. 2006;3(6):717–29.
44. Madersbacher S, Kratzik C, Szabo N, Susani M, Vingers L, Marberger M. Tissue ablation in benign prostatic hyperplasia with high-intensity focused ultrasound. Eur Urol. 1993;23 Suppl 1:39–43.
45. Rewcastle JC. High intensity focused ultrasound for prostate cancer: A review of the scientific foundation, technology and clinical outcomes. Technol Cancer Res Treat. 2006;5(6):619–25.
46. Nakamura K, Baba S, Fukazawa R, et al. Treatment of benign prostatic hyperplasia with high intensity focused ultrasound: An initial clinical trial in Japan with magnetic resonance imaging of the treated area. Int J Urol. 1995;2(3):176–80.
47. Chapelon JY, Rouvière O, Crouzet S, Gelet A. Prostate focused ultrasound therapy. Adv Exp Med Biol. 2016;880:21–41.

11

Ultrasound-Guided Focused Ultrasound Ablation for Uterine Fibroids

Jordi Isern-Quitllet

11.1 Background

Uterine fibroids, myomas or leiomyomas, are the most common gynaecological tumours,[1] with a prevalence of up to 70–80% in women who have reached the age of 50.[2] The prevalence increases with age, peaking in women in their 40s. In 60–70 % of women, myomas are asymptomatic and are diagnosed incidentally on clinical examination or with imaging. In 30% of women, myomas cause significant morbidity, due to menstrual abnormalities, iron deficiency, anaemia, pelvic pressure or obstructive symptoms, and fertility issues.[3–4] The high prevalence of fibroids has a profound impact on health care costs around the world. Uterine fibroids are currently the most common indication for hysterectomy, which is not without significant morbidity and mortality. The social and economic impact of uterine fibroids is consequently considerable.[5–7]

Uterine fibroids are monoclonal tumours arising from uterine smooth muscle tissue. The cells proliferate at a modest rate, and their growth is dependent on the ovarian steroids oestrogen and progesterone. Most fibroids therefore shrink after menopause.[8] Although uterine fibroids tend mainly to be benign, there is some incidence of malignant degeneration. On the malignant spectrum, uterine sarcomas tend to occur more in older patients than do leiomyomas and only account for 3–7% of all uterine malignancies.[9] They often present with the same symptoms as leiomyomas and thus cannot reliably be distinguished clinically.[10] Leiomyosarcomas (LMSs) are the most common uterine sarcomas, with an estimated annual incidence of 0.5–7/100,000 women.[9]

Myomas can be single or multiple and can vary in size, location (intramural, subserosal, submucosal), and perfusion (from low to highly perfused). These various presentations lead to different clinical manifestations which may be important when choosing appropriate treatment. Numerous classifications of myomas can be found in the literature, the most commonly used being the FIGO leiomyoma classification system.[11]

Risk factors for the development of uterine fibroids include nulliparity, early menarche, family history of uterine fibroids, obesity, and age.[8] There are notable racial differences in the prevalence and presentation of fibroids. Fibroids are more common, tend to present at a younger age and are larger in women of African ancestry than in white or Asian women.[12]

11.1.1 Clinical Presentation

The most common symptom of uterine leiomyoma is abnormal uterine bleeding (AUB) which can lead to anaemia. Large fibroids can also result in pressure symptoms (bulk symptoms) that may cause bowel and bladder dysfunction, including urgency, increased daytime urinary frequency, and urinary incontinence.[13] Other symptoms include abdominal distension and hydronephrosis due to pelvic pressure on the ureters. Dysmenorrhea and pelvic pain are frequently encountered. All these symptoms can significantly reduce the quality of life (QoL) of the affected women.[14]

DOI: 10.1201/9780429162671-11

11.1.2 Fibroids and Fertility

Uterine fibroids have a negative impact on fertility and increase the risk of miscarriage.[15–17] Fibroids can affect fertility through several possible mechanisms, including alteration of the local anatomy, anatomic distortion of the cavity, and functional changes. There is a consensus that submucosal fibroids of any size, and intramural fibroids larger than 4 cm, impair fertility and increase the rate of miscarriage up to 20–30%.[15–17] Some reviews have suggested that non-cavity-distorting intramural fibroids, even those of small size, can significantly reduce the implantation rate, clinical pregnancy rate, and live birth rate and significantly increase the miscarriage rate after in vitro fertilisation (IVF) treatment.[18–20] Furthermore, fibroids are associated with obstetric complications such as preterm delivery, breech presentation, placental abruption, placenta previa, caesarean section, postpartum haemorrhage, and lower birthweight infants.[21, 22]

11.1.3 Diagnosis and Imaging

Ultrasonography is the most widely used modality because of its availability, ease of use, and cost-effectiveness. MRI can provide information on the number of fibroids, their size, vascularisation, and relationship with the endometrial cavity and serosa. It has the advantage over ultrasound imaging of not being operator dependent. While MRI findings can suggest a diagnosis of sarcoma, they cannot diagnose malignancy with any certainty.[23, 24]

11.1.4 Treatment

There is increasing consensus on the need for an individual approach when treatment is necessary. Thus, many factors should be taken into account: the patient's desire for future fertility, the desire for organ preservation, the severity of symptoms, the FIGO classification (International Federation of Gynaecology & Obstetrics), the expectation of improvement, and finally the complication rate of each procedure.[25, 26] Actual fibroid treatments range from medical therapies to surgical procedures and less invasive heat-based or ischaemia-based procedures. Medical treatments are classically used to control the symptoms, mainly AUB, and are mostly not designed to cure the fibroids. Among them, anti-fibrinolytic agents, non-steroidal anti-inflammatory drugs (NSAIDs), aromatase inhibitors, anti-progestins, combined hormonal contraceptives or progesterone-only treatments, selective progesterone receptor modulators (SPRMs), and gonadotropin-releasing hormone (GnRH) agonists or antagonists[25] are commonly used. Curative treatments are designed to remove or ablate the fibroids and usually involve surgical intervention. Hysterectomy is the most frequent for symptomatic fibroids and remains the most effective procedure. It is considered to be the gold standard. Despite this, its minor and major complications rates are 28% and 6%, respectively,[27] and surgery is inapplicable in the case of fertility preservation or where there is the desire for organ preservation.[28] The 'uterine sparing' surgical option is myomectomy. The choice between a laparoscopic, laparotomic, or hysteroscopic approach will depend on the size, localisation, and number of fibroids. In laparoscopic or laparotomic myomectomy – minor complications 14%, major complications 5%[29] – a uterine wall incision is mandatory in some cases, and this may also affect the delivery outcomes.

Among the less invasive treatments, uterine artery embolisation (UAE) is an interventional radiological procedure that creates ischaemic necrosis by delivering embolic agents in a chosen catheterised fibroid feeding artery. Despite being less invasive, the procedure is not exempt from major and minor complications (3% and 52%, respectively), and its consequences to fertility are not clear due to the risk of extension of the ischaemia to the rest of the uterus and even to the ovaries.[29, 30]

Recently, thermally based non-invasive or minimally invasive treatments have been introduced into clinical practice with the aim, as in UAE, of ablating the fibroid and improving symptoms through the consequent shrinkage in tumour volume. These non-invasive gynaecological interventions have achieved acceptance, mostly due to their advantages: the possibility of preserving fertility and reducing the risks associated with invasive surgery but with similar results in symptom resolution.[31] Tissue destruction is achieved by increasing the temperature to 60–90 °C locally, causing coagulative necrosis and irreversible damage. The energy needed to ablate the tumour can be delivered through a needle, as in the case of microwaves or radiofrequency treatments,[32] or it can be generated by the confluence of ultrasound waves at a determined focal point: high-intensity focused ultrasound (HIFU).

Microwave and radiofrequency needle placement is usually ultrasound guided for uterine fibroid treatment, and commonly these are performed via an endo-vaginal approach.[33] HIFU is a totally non-invasive treatment in which the therapeutic energy delivery is transcutaneous. The treatment can be guided either by MR or ultrasound imaging.

11.2 HIFU Principles

The basic principle on which HIFU is based is coagulative necrosis arising from a combination of the absorption of ultrasound energy, causing a thermal effect, and tissue damage induced by cavitation, a mechanical effect.[34] The high temperature generated by HIFU can result in immediate and irreversible cell death by coagulative necrosis in exposed tissues when it exceeds 60 °C and lasts longer than 1 s. Focused ultrasound beams allow delivery of energy to a relatively small volume region, which may, for example, be 10 × 3 × 3 mm at the focus.[35] A mechanical effect occurs when high-negative pressure acoustic pulses generate cavitation. Cavitation results in very high local temperatures and creates microscopic streaming and microbubbles which can cause cell apoptosis (see Chapter 3).

The ability to focus HIFU at a distance from its source allows these high frequency, high amplitude pressure waves to pass through overlying skin and tissues without damaging them, with damage restricted to a small focal target volume, that can be positioned deep within tissue.

HIFU delivery systems consist of three main components. The first is a piezoelectric ultrasound transducer that is used to generate (and often focus) the therapeutic ultrasound. The second is a positioning system that allows the movement of the transducer in different axes to place the focal point at the desired location. The third major component of HIFU is the imaging device used for guidance. Ensuring a safe and effective treatment is of great importance, and real-time imaging during a therapeutic procedure is therefore essential. Finally, software is needed to assemble and interpret all the information and provide an understandable display. At present, magnetic resonance imaging (MRI) or ultrasound are used for guiding and monitoring treatment, leading to the definition of two major, different types of (high intensity) focused ultrasound (FUS or HIFU) devices providing ultrasound guided FUS (USgFUS) and MRI guided FUS (MRgFUS).

MRI has good anatomical resolution and its sensitivity for tumour detection is excellent. Also, MRI thermometry offers near real-time temperature monitoring during HIFU treatment, providing control of the energy deposited with a thermal accuracy up to 1 °C. It thus may ensure safety and efficacy during HIFU treatment. Although MRI is good for indicating the temperature in the targeted tissue, it does not detect an ablative thermal dose. On the other hand, its excellent image resolution allows treatment guidance in obese patients, where ultrasound can sometimes not provide images of sufficient quality due to fat attenuation.[36, 37] Regardless, MRgFUS is expensive and laborious, and a radiologist is needed during the whole procedure,[38] while USgFUS could be performed by a gynaecologist, as long as they are trained in ultrasound imaging.

Ultrasonography was the first diagnostic imaging technique used for monitoring HIFU treatment of uterine fibroids. Compared to MRgFUS, it is less costly and provides real-time images of anatomy and blood flow. In addition, USgFUS does not require the patient to be confined in a tube, communication with the medical staff is direct, it is quieter, and special installations are not necessary.[39] The ablated area is visualised thanks to hyper-echogenicity caused by the ultrasonic generation of thermal and cavitation bubbles. This ultrasound greyscale change is a reliable indicator of the tissue response to HIFU treatment.[39, 40]

USgFUS was first used in 1999 to treat malignant tumours in the UK and China. In 2002, the preliminary results from the first patients with uterine fibroids treated with USgFUS were reported and in 2004, Wu et al. published the results of an 85-patient series.[39] Following these preliminary results, published studies have multiplied, with more than 15,000 patients having now been treated.[41] Studies both report longer follow-up series and evaluate new methods of improving treatment efficacy as well as describing studies comparing HIFU with other techniques to treat fibroids.

11.3 Ultrasound-Guided HIFU Clinical Application in Fibroids

The majority of patients with fibroids could potentially be treated with USgFUS. However, HIFU ablation is affected by factors such as fibroid tissue characteristics, vascularisation, size, position, and number. There are, in addition, some technical limitations, such as the presence of scar tissue in the acoustic pathway, the distance between the skin and the focal point, the presence of bowel, and excessive subcutaneous fat.[42] Thus, preoperative evaluation plays an essential role in the efficacy of the treatment. MRI provides the most information, such as histological type, number, and location of fibroids. The most commonly used MR sequences include T1-weighted images (T1WI), T2-weighted images (T2WI), and contrast-enhanced T1WI. Fibroid histology correlates with MRI appearance, with the most common fibroids being hypointense on T2-weighted images due to a high fibrous content, with less common hypercellular fibroids tending to be hyperintense on T2-weighted images. A fibroid is classified as type I when the signal intensity is lower than that of skeletal muscle, type II when it is lower than that of the myometrium but higher than that of skeletal muscle, or type III when is higher than that of the myometrium. T2 hyperintense fibroids usually have poor clinal response, with low nonperfused volumes and less effective volume reduction after the treatment, and thus type III fibroids are generally excluded.[43, 44] Contrast-enhanced T1WI allows assessment of the vascularity of the fibroid. Fibroids can be classified as having low perfusion if their vascularisation is lower than the myometrium and as highly perfused if it is equal to or higher than the myometrium. Highly vascular fibroids, with high blood flow and volume, are less responsive to treatment, with lower rates of non-perfused volume (NPV) and volume reduction.[45]

In addition, MRI is useful for evaluating precisely the distance between the skin and the focal point, and the thickness of abdominal subcutaneous fat. The number of fibroids is not a limitation by itself, the length of the procedure being the limiting factor. In some cases, a multiple session procedure is proposed. The size of the fibroids is, in most protocols, limited to 10–12 cm in the largest direction, due also to the length of the treatment. However, pre-HIFU treatment with GnRH agonists has been demonstrated to decrease fibroid volume and increase ablation efficacy. In addition, large fibroids can be treated in sequential treatment sessions.[46]

MRI allows the evaluation of subcutaneous tissue. Excessively thick subcutaneous fat in the abdominal wall leads to the accumulation of heat in the superficial area due to the absorption of acoustic energy by the tissue, increasing the risk of fat and skin burn, and at the same time diminishing the capacity to ablate the tumour. Thus, obese patients have a worse response to treatment.

11.3.1 HIFU Procedure

Before treatment, patients undergo specific bowel and skin preparation in order to minimise the presence of intestinal gas, and to degrease and degas the skin.

The patients are positioned on the HIFU table lying either face down (e.g. HAIFU JC 200) or in a supine position (e.g. PRO 2008) depending on the device. The anterior abdominal wall must always be free of air, either by immersion in a water tank for a prone-position, or through close contact with a balloon containing degassed water, and the transducer in the case of supine positioning. Water is also used for cooling the skin to prevent superficial thermal lesions. Treatment is performed under conscious sedation in order to minimise patient movement and relieve discomfort and pain, while not preventing communication between the patient and the medical staff.

The safety of the procedure depends on obtaining a safe beam pathway. To prevent intestinal injury, the beam must be free of intervening bowel loops. In order to achieve an unobscured pathway, the uterine position and the sonication window may be changed using different manoeuvres. Bowel and other anatomical structures can be repositioned by filling or emptying the bladder or by positioning a degassed water balloon between the transducer and the skin and adjusting its water content to apply more or less pressure to the skin and internal anatomy. It is also important to verify that the focal point is positioned at a safe distance from sacral bone and adjacent lumbosacral nerves. Special attention must be paid to the presence of abdominal scars in the pathway of the beam that could lead to skin burns, due to their higher rate of energy absorption.

After the target fibroid has been confirmed and a safe beam pathway achieved, it is ablated by high intensity ultrasound energy. Real-time ultrasound imaging is used to monitor the target area and the adjacent tissue. Usually, the treatment is performed from the deepest part of the fibroid to the shallowest, to avoid interference in the sonication pathway due to the gas and microbubbles produced by the ablation of the tissue. The targeted fibroid its treated spot by spot, using sonication times of between 1 and 5 seconds. This process is repeated on a section-by-section basis to achieve complete ablation of the tumour. It is considered that ablation is achieved when significant grayscale changes (hyper echogenicity with a posterior acoustic shadow) are observed with ultrasound imaging. Ultrasound contrast enhanced imaging can be used to confirm the ablated volume. The total sonication time can be very variable depending on the characteristics, size, number and location of the fibroids and the total treatment procedure can reach up to 3 hours in exceptional cases.

11.3.2 Treatment Outcomes

The main indicators of treatment efficacy are resolution of symptoms and reduction in fibroid volume. The reduction of symptoms is intimately related to fibroid shrinkage. This reduction depends mainly on the initial fibroid volume and the non-perfused volume ratio (NPVR) achieved after the treatment. NPVR is defined as the percentage of NPV in the uterine fibroids seen post-USgFUS on MRI divided by original tumour volume targeted. There is a positive relationship between fibroid shrinkage and NPVR; the higher the NPVR, the greater the volume reduction.[19] The NPVR is also a good predictor of re-intervention rates, with fibroids with NPVs greater than 50–60% being less likely to need additional treatments.[47] Thus, the therapeutic goal of HIFU should be to achieve the highest NPVR as possible, without increasing complications and side effects, in order to achieve maximum symptom relief, and the best prognosis for patients. Mean NPV ratio found in the literature ranges from 67% to 100%. In the 2 largest retrospective case series (one with 17,402 patients and the other with 7,438), the median NPV ratios were 85% (interquartile range 75%–94%) and 83.1% ± 15.6%, respectively. There are other published series, prospective or retrospective, with similar results.[48–52] In addition, in one comparative retrospective study of symptomatic fibroids treated with USgFUS or MRgFUS, Wang et al.[52] found that there were more patients (43%) in the USgFUS group with an NPV ratio of 100% at 6 months than in the MRgFUS cohort (23%), and the proportions of patients with an NPV ratio of less than 90% at 6 months were 39% compared to 53%, respectively. These results, consistent with other USgFUS and MRgFUS published series could suggest that USgFUS is more effective for the treatment of uterine fibroids. In the studies with published follow-up data, the mean uterine fibroid volume shrinkage varies from 49% to 70 % at 12 months, with this reduction being maintained or increased in subsequent follow-up (24 months).[52–53] As previously mentioned, it is this volume reduction that mainly leads to clinical improvement and symptom relief in patients – obviously the ultimate goal of the treatment. Symptoms are evaluated using a validated health and symptom-related quality of life questionnaire (UFS-QoL). This is used in most studies of uterine fibroid treatment evaluation, including studies of UAE, radiofrequency thermal ablation, medical therapies, and myomectomy.[54, 55] It is applied before the treatment, at 3 or 6 months, at 12 months, and up to several years after HIFU. All published studies show a significant reduction in the symptom severity score (SSS) and a substantial improvement in the QoL questionnaire after USgFUS. When compared to other techniques, few studies had observed greater symptom relief with USgFUS than with myomectomy,[56, 57] but at least the majority of them show no difference between these techniques. It thus seems that USgFUS is as effective as myomectomy for symptom relief.

The complication rates after HIFU are very low (<1%). Major complications are rare, skin burn being the most frequent (0.005–0.38%). Bowel injury is possible, but infrequent, with a reported incidence of 0.0001–0.0017%. This can happen when the bowel is fixed in the acoustic pathway, for example, due to previous intestinal adhesions. Other major complications described are venous thrombosis, pubic symphysis pain (due to bone heating when treating low-positioned tumours, such as cervical fibroids), and hydronephrosis. The most common minor complications, the majority being as a result of the inflammatory response to the thermal effects of HIFU, are mild lower abdominal pain, sacrococcygeal pain, irradiated leg pain, abnormal vaginal discharge, and uterine bleeding, all receding within few days.[58, 59]

However, and despite these good treatment outcomes, HIFU has higher reintervention rates in the long term than UAE and myomectomy. In a meta-analysis conducted by Xu et al.[60] the intervention rates at 36 months were significantly higher in the HIFU group (up to 49%), than in myomectomy or UAE (up to 20%). The majority of data analysed in this study comes from MRgFUS series. When analysing another meta-analysis conducted by Yu et al.[61] the global reintervention rate for HIFU was 8.1% for fibroids smaller than 300 cm^3, with MRgFUS giving higher rates than USgFUS (13.4% vs. 5.2%). However, the reintervention rate improves for HIFU when stratification is performed. Thus, it is lower in small fibroids (less than 300 cm^3) and in fibroids with hypointense signal on T2 MRI. The reintervention rate seems consistent with the ablation ratio, which depends on the fibroid type and size.[61] That could explain the different results observed between USgFUS and MRgFUS, as the ablation ratio reported with MRgFUS tends to be smaller than for USgFUS.

Patient age could be another factor affecting HIFU efficacy. The results are worst for patients with higher-than-average baseline anti-müllerian hormone level (AMH) with HIFU compared to other techniques, but the reintervention rate at three years in women with low AMH levels was similar in all treatments.[62]

Regarding pregnancy outcomes, studies show that conception after HIFU could occur in more than 67% of women seeking to be pregnant. In a series of 443 patients published by Wu et al.[63] post-intervention pregnancies rates were 68.4 % after USgFUS and 66.7% after myomectomy, with average times to pregnancy being statistically significantly higher after myomectomy (18.9 months vs. 13.6 months). After USgFUS, spontaneous vaginal delivery was more frequent (51.1% vs. 36.4%) and caesarean section rate was lower (41.6% vs. 54.9%) than for myomectomy.

Some pregnancy-related complications were lower after HIFU, including preterm labour, placenta previa, and placenta accreta, but others, such as rates of preterm birth, fetal distress, fetal growth restriction, and puerperal infection, were slightly higher. In one of the few published series of pregnancy outcomes in a Caucasian population after USgFUS, the pregnancy outcomes and complications were similar to those described in the Asiatic population, but with a lower pregnancy rate (34% – 55/160). This could be explained by the high mean age of the group (37 +/– 4 years).[64]

11.4 Expert Commentary

Fibroids are highly prevalent and represent a high health cost. About 30% of women with leiomyomas will request treatment due to morbidities such as heavy menstrual bleeding, abdominal pain, pressure symptoms, and/or infertility. Patient involvement in the decision process, and their greater knowledge of the different options and potential risk of adverse outcomes, has increased their interest in new, less invasive, and more conservative alternatives to classical surgery. It is therefore important to improve access to these safe and effective minimally invasive approaches that increase a woman's chance to preserve her uterus and fertility and, at the same time, to have good cosmetic results. In the last decade, HIFU has been introduced as a promising technology, able to reduce fibroid volume and symptoms. As myomectomy remains the gold-standard procedure for uterus-sparing treatment of fibroids, HIFU has been demonstrated to have similar or better effects on QoL after 36 months, that conception can occur during the first three months in more than 67% of women seeking to be pregnant with the average time to pregnancy shorter than in myomectomy, and that it has low incidence of adverse events, none with permanent sequelae or death. In addition, it seems that the difference in efficacy between HIFU, UEA, and myomectomy treatments is minimal.[64]

Despite this, USgFUS is not widely spread beyond Asian countries. There exist many series published with thousands of patients included, but very few from non-Asiatic populations. This could perhaps be one of the explanations for the low extension into use by the occidental medical community. Besides, it is well known that the introduction of new technologies in medical practice takes a long time from device development to approval by regulatory agencies. Moreover, their acceptance and introduction in guidelines and clinical practice as alternatives to standard therapies can also depend on its understandability and affordability. Currently available USgFUS devices (i.e. Haifu Model JC200/Model JC/Model JC200 from Chongqing Haifu Medical Technology Co. Ltd. or PRO2008 from Shenzhen Pro Hifu Medical Co. Ltd.) require initial high levels of investment, up to €1.8 million in some cases, and specialist installation in a large room. The evolution to less expensive and portable office devices could be of great help to expanding the technology. Since the majority of health professionals involved in fibroid treatments, gynaecologists, are trained in the use of ultrasound imaging, the learning process to achieve the necessary skills to use HIFU technology safely could be short and easy. In this sense, the appearance on the market of new portable or semi-portable devices such as the ALPIUS 900 from Alpinion Medical Systems or PRO300 from Shenzhen Pro Hifu Medical Co. Ltd might open interesting possibilities.

Secondly, the high reintervention rate could play a role. It might be said that the difficulty in predicting the outcomes of the treatment could prevent its indication. That could be true for the global intervention rate, but when identifying the factors influencing HIFU results and correct selection of patients, the reintervention rate becomes similar to myomectomy. In this regard, it has been seen that fibroid T2WI signal type had a linear correlation with the treatment outcomes, because the signal corresponded to different histological structures. The hypointense and isointense fibroids, especially the hypointense, are typically composed of a high proportion of collagen fibres, and so are likely to absorb more ultrasonic energy and can be easily treated. Hyperintense T2WI fibroids which are mostly cellular, with low concentration of collagen, tend to low absorption of ultrasonic energy, and thus to poor results in terms of ablated area.[65] In this regard, different solutions have been proposed to improve results when treating 'bad prognosis' fibroids including those that have a high or hyperintense signal on T2WI MR imaging, are highly vascularised, or are large. The pre-treatment use of GnRH analogues can reduce fibroid size and can potentiate the thermal effects of HIFU, helping the treatment in cases of volumes greater than 300 cm^3.[66, 67] The use of ultrasound enhanced contrast agent, as SonoVue, during the treatment can not only shorten the time to reach massive greyscale changes but also a larger non-perfused volume can be achieved in all type of fibroids,[68–70] thus probably improving the final, long-term results.

However, with the current knowledge and available evidence, USgFUS should be considered as a non-surgical alternative treatment for uterine fibroids. But in order to facilitate the clinical decision making, some considerations are needed:

- It is more difficult to ablate fibroids with a long tissue path from skin to the target. Thus, deep fibroids are less responsive.
- Fibroids with hyperintense signal on T2WI in MRI are relatively not indicated.
- Myoma perfusion: The higher the perfusion, the more difficult to treat.
- In fibroids of volume >300 cm^3 GnRH analogues prior to HIF treatment could be considered.
- In young women, with high levels of AMH, the rate of fibroid re-growth is higher than in older women.
- Women seeking to be pregnant can undergo HIFU treatment if indicated.

By using the inclusion and exclusion criteria and recommendations we have given, the reintervention rate would be similar to other uterus-sparing treatments and, as has been seen before, HIFU treatment will be effective and safe. Nevertheless, high-quality clinical studies are needed in future to further evaluate the re-intervention rate of HIFU using more advanced, and probably more restrictive, protocols. At the same time further research is needed to improve HIFU technology and to implement new strategies for treating fibroids with low response to HIFU.

REFERENCES

1. Stewart EA. Uterine fibroids. Lancet. 2001;357:293–8.
2. Baird D, Dunson DB, Hill MC, Cousins D, Schectman JM. High cumulative incidence of uterine leiomyoma in black and white women: Ultrasound evidence. Am J Obstet Gynecol. 2003;188:100–7.
3. Zimmermann A, Bernuit D, Gerlinger C, Schaefers M, Geppert K. Prevalence, symptoms and management of uterine fibroids:an international internet-based survey of 21,746 women. BMC Womens Health. 2012;12:6.
4. Pritts EA, Parker WH, Olive DL. Fibroids and infertility: An updated systematic review of the evidence. Fertil Steril. 2009;91:1215–23.
5. Soliman AM, Yang H, Du EX, Kelkar SS, Winkel C. The direct and indirect costs of uterine fibroid tumors: A systematic review of the literature between 2000 and 2013. Am J Obstet Gynecol. 2015;213:141–60.
6. Canadian Institute for Health Information, Statistics Canada. Health indicators. Ottawa CIHI; 2010. Available at:https://secure.cihi.ca/free_products/Healthindicators2010_en.pdf. Accessed on November 10, 2014.
7. Boyd LR, Novesky AP, Curtin JP. Effect of surgical volume on route of hysterectomy and short-term morbidity. Obstet Gynecol. 2010;116:909–15.
8. Bulun SE. Uterine fibroids. N Engl J Med. 2013;369:1344–55.
9. del Carmen MG. Uterine leiomyosarcoma. In: del Carmen MG, Young RH, Schorge JO, Birrer MJ, editors. Uncommon gyneco logic cancers. 2014. John Wiley & Sons Incorporated; 2014 Nov 10. UK.
10. Santos P, Cunha TM. Uterine sarcomas: Clinical presentation and MRI features. Diagn Interv Radiol. 2015;21:4–9.
11. Munro MG, Critchley HO, Fraser IS. The two FIGO systems for normal and abnormal uterine bleeding symptoms and classification of causes of abnormal uterine bleeding in the reproductive years: 2018 revisions. Int J Gynecol Obstet. 2018;143:393–408.
12. Baird DD, Dunson DB, Hill MC, Cousins D, Schectman JM. High cumulative incidence of uterine leiomyoma in black and white women: Ultrasound evidence. Am J Obstet Gynecol. 2003;188:100–7.
13. Gupta S, Jose J, Manyonda I. Clinical presentation of fibroids. Best Pract Res Clin Obstet Gynaecol. 2008;22:615–26.
14. Spies JB, Coyne K, Guaou Guaou N, Boyle D, Skyrnarz-Murphy K, Gonzalves SM. The UFS-QOL, a new disease-specific symptom and health-related quality of life questionnaire for leiomyomata. Obstet Gynecol. 2002;99:290–300.
15. Somigliana E, De Benedictis S, Vercellini P, et al. Fibroids not encroaching the endometrial cavity and IVF success rate: A prospective study. Hum Reprod. 2011;26(4):834–9.
16. Galliano D, Bellver J, Díaz-García C, Simón C, Pellicer A. ART and uterine pathology: How relevant is the maternal side for implantation? Hum Reprod Update. 2015;21(1):13–38.
17. Zepiridis LI, Grimbizis GF, Tarlatzis BC. Infertility and uterine fibroids. Best Pract Res Clin Obstet Gynaecol. 2016;34:66–73.
18. Behbehani S, Polesello S, Hasson J, Silver J, Son WY, Dahan M. The effect of intramural myomas without an intracavity component on in vitro fertilization outcomes in single fresh blastocyst transfer cycles. J Minim Invasive Gynecol. 2018;25(7):1241–8.
19. Radhika BH, Naik K, Shreelatha S, Vana H. Case series: Pregnancy outcome in patients with uterine fibroids. J Clin Diagn Res. 2015;9(10):QR01–QR4.
20. Wang X, Chen L, Wang H, Li Q, Liu X, Qi H. The impact of noncavity-distorting intramural fibroids on the efficacy of in vitro fertilization-embryo transfer: An updated metaanalysis. Biomed Res Int. 2018;2018:8924703.
21. Shavell VI, Thakur M, Sawant A, Kruger ML, Jones TB, Singh M, Puscheck EE, Diamond MP. Adverse obstetric outcomes associated with sonographically identified large uterine fibroids. Fertil Steril. 2012;97:107–10.
22. Parazzini F, Tozzi L, Bianchi S. Pregnancy outcome and uterine fibroids. Best Pract Res Clin Obstet Gynaecol. 2015;S1521–6934:00231–0023.
23. Sun S, Bonaffini PA, Nougaret S, Fournier L, Dohan A, Chong J, Smith J, Addley H, Reinhold C. How to differentiate uterine leiomyosarcoma from leiomyoma with imaging. Diagn Interv Imaging. 2019 Oct;100(10):619–34.

24. Lumsden MA, Hamoodi I, Gupta J, Hickey M. Fibroids: Diagnosis and management. BMJ. 2015;351:h4887.
25. Giuliani E, As-Sanie S, Marsh EE. Epidemiology and management of uterine fibroids. Int J Gynaecol Obstet. 2020 Apr;149(1):3–9.
26. Donnez J, Dolmans MM. Uterine fibroid management: From the present to the future. Hum Reprod Update. 2016 Nov;22(6):665–86.
27. Clarke-Pearson DL, Geller EJ. Complications of hysterectomy. Obstet Gynecol. 2013 Mar;121(3):654–73.
28. Practice Committee of American Society for Reproductive Medicine in collaboration with Society of Reproductive Surgeons. Myomas and reproductive function. Fertil Steril. 2008;90:S125–30.
29. Gupta JK, Sinha A, Lumsden MA, Hickey M. Uterine artery embolization for symptomatic uterine fibroids. Cochrane Database Syst Rev. 2014;(12):CD005073
30. Freed MM, Spies JB. Uterine artery embolization for fibroids: A review of current outcomes. Semin Reprod Med. 2010 May;28(3):235–41
31. Wang Y, Zhang S, Li C, Bo L, Ouyang L. Minimally invasive surgery for uterine fibroids. Ginekol Pol. 2020;91:149–57.
32. Knavel EM, Brace CL. Tumor ablation: Common modalities and general practices. Tech Vasc Interv Radiol. 2013 Dec;16(4):192–200.
33. Jiang X, Thapa A, Lu J, Bhujohory VS, Liu Y, Qiao S. Ultrasound-guided transvaginal radiofrequency myolysis for symptomatic uterine myomas. Eur J Obstet Gynecol Reprod Biol. 2014 Jun;177:38–43.
34. Haar GT, Coussios C. High intensity focused ultrasound: Physical principles and devices. Int J Hyperth. 2007;23:89–104.
35. Hill CR, Rivens I, Vaughan MG, ter Haar GR. Lesion development in focused ultrasound surgery: A general model. Ultrasound Med Biol. 1994;20(3):259–69.
36. Yagel S. High-intensity focused ultrasound: A revolution in non-invasive ultrasound treatment? Ultrasound Obstet Gynecol. 2004;23:216–7.
37. Jolesz FA, McDannold N. Current status and future potential of MRI-guided focused ultrasound surgery. J. Magn Reson Imaging. 2008;27:391–9.
38. Zhang CHJ, Ngobese ZE, Setzen Z. Efficacy and safety of ultrasound guided high intensity focused ultrasound ablation of symptomatic uterine fibroids in black women: A preliminary study. BJOG. 2017;124:36–9.
39. Zhang L, Zhang W, Orsi F, Chen W, Wang Z. Ultrasound-guided high intensity focused ultrasound for the treatment of gynaecological diseases: A review of safety and efficacy. Int J Hyperthermia. 2015 May;31(3):280–4.
40. Orsi F, Zhang L, Arnone P, et al. High-intensity focused ultrasound ablation: Effective and safe therapy for solid tumors in difficult locations. Am J Roentgenol. 2010;195:W245–52.
41. Wang Q, Wu X, Zhu X, Wang J, Xu F, Lin Z, Gong C, He M, Zhang L. MRI features and clinical outcomes of unexpected uterine sarcomas in patients who underwent high intensity focused ultrasound ablation for presumed uterine fibroids. Int J Hyperth. 2021;38:39–45.
42. Peng S, Zhang L, Hu L, Chen J, Ju J, Wang X, Zhang R, Wang Z, Chen W. Factors influencing the dosimetry for high-intensity focused ultrasound ablation of uterine fibroids: A retrospective study. Medicine (Baltimore). 2015 Apr;94(13):e650.
43. Funaki K, Fukunishi H, Funaki T, Sawada K, Kaji Y, Maruo T. Magnetic resonance-guided focused ultrasound surgery for uterine fibroids: Relationship between the therapeutic effects and signal intensity of preexisting T2-weighted magnetic resonance images. Am J Obstet Gynecol. 2007;196(2):e1–e6.
44. Zhao WP, Chen JY, Zhang L, et al. Feasibility of ultrasound-guided high intensity focused ultrasound ablating uterine fibroids with hyperintense on T2-weighted MR imaging. Eur J Radiol. 2013;82:e43–49.
45. Keserci B, Nguyen D. The role of T1 perfusion-based classification in magnetic resonance-guided high-intensity focused ultrasound ablation of uterine fibroids. Eur Radiol. 2017;27:5299–308.
46. Smart OC, Hindley JT, Regan L, Gedroyc WG. Gonadotrophin releasing hormone and magnetic-resonance-guided ultrasound surgery for uterine leiomyomata. Obstet Gynecol 2006;108(1):49–54.
47. Verpalen IM, de Boer JP, Linstra M, et al. The Focused Ultrasound Myoma Outcome Study (FUMOS); a retrospective cohort study on long-term outcomes ofMR-HIFU therapy. Eur Radiol. 2020;30:2473–82.
48. Liu YC, Zhang WW, He M, et al. Adverse effect analysis of high-intensity focused ultrasound in the treatment of benign uterine diseases. Int J Hyperthermia. 2018;35(1):56–61.

49. Chen J, Chen W, Zhang L, et al. Safety of ultrasound-guided ultrasound ablation for uterine fibroids and adenomyosis: A review of 9988 cases. Ultrason Sonochem. 2015;27:671–6.
50. Chen J, Li Y, Wang Z, et al. Evaluation of high-intensity focused ultrasound ablation for uterine fibroids: An IDEAL prospective exploration study. Int J Obstet Gynaecol. 2017;125(3):354–64.
51. Zhang W, He M, Huang G, et al. A comparison of ultrasound-guided high intensity focused ultrasound for the treatment of uterine fibroids in patients with an anteverted uterus and a retroverted uterus. Int J Hyperthermia. 2016;32(6):623–9.
52. Wang Y, Wang ZB, Xu YH. Efficacy, efficiency, and safety of magnetic resonance-guided high-intensity focused ultrasound for ablation of uterine fibroids: Comparison with ultrasound-guided method. Korean J Radiol. 2018;19(4):724–32.
53. Recker F, Thudium M, Strunk H, et al. Multidisciplinary management to optimize outcome of ultrasound-guided high-intensity focused ultrasound (HIFU) in patients with uterine fibroids. Sci Rep. 2021 Nov 23;11(1):22768.
54. Spies JB, Coyne K, Guaou Guaou N, Boyle D, Skyrnarz-Murphy K, Gonzalves SM. The UFS-QOL, a new disease-specific symptom and health-related quality of life questionnaire for leiomyomata. Obstet Gynecol. 2002 Feb;99(2):290–300.
55. Harding G, Coyne KS, Thompson CL, Spies JB. The responsiveness of the uterine fibroid symptom and health-related quality of life questionnaire (UFS-QOL). Health Qual Life Outcomes. 2008 Nov 12;6:99.
56. Wang Y, Liu X, Wang W, Tang J, Song L. Long term clinical outcomes of US-guided high intensity focused ultrasound ablation for symptomatic submucosal fibroids: A retrospective comparison with uterus sparing surgery. Acad Radiol. 2020;28:1102–7.
57. Chen J, Li Y, Wang Z, McCulloch P, Hu L, Chen W, Liu G, Li J, Lang J. Evaluation of high-intensity focused ultrasound ablation for uterine fibroids: An IDEAL prospective exploration study. BJOG. 2018;125:354–64.
58. Wang Y, Geng J, Bao H, Dong J, Shi J, Xi Q. Comparative effectiveness and safety of high-intensity focused ultrasound for uterine fibroids: A systematic review and meta-analysis. Front Oncol. 2021 Mar 9;11:600800.
59. Torres-de la Roche LA, Rafiq S, Devassy R, Verhoeven HC, Becker S, De Wilde RL. Should ultrasound-guided high frequency focused ultrasound be considered as an alternative non-surgical treatment of uterine fibroids in non-Asiatic countries? An opinion paper. J Clin Med. 2022 Feb 5;11(3):839.
60. Yu L, Zhu S, Zhang H, Wang A, Sun G, Liang J, Wang X. The efficacy and safety of MRgHIFU and US-HIFU in treating uterine fibroids with volume <300 cm3: A metanalysis. Int J Hyperth. 2021;38:1126–32.
61. Xu F, Deng L, Zhang L, Hu H, Shi Q. The comparison of myomectomy, UAE and MRgFUS in the treatment of uterine fibroids: A metaanalysis. Int J Hyperth. 2021;38:24–9.
62. Laughlin-Tommaso S, Barnard EP, AbdElmagied AM, et al. FIRSTT study: Randomized controlled trial of uterine artery embolization vs. focused ultrasound surgery. Am J Obstet Gynecol. 2018;220:174.e1–e13.
63. Wu G, Li R, He M, Pu Y, Wang J, Chen J, Qi H. A comparison of the pregnancy outcomes between ultrasound guided high intensity focused ultrasound ablation and laproscopic myomectomy for uterine fibroids: A comparative study. Int J Hyperth. 2020;37:617–23.
64. Rodríguez J, Isern J, Pons N, Carmona A, Vallejo E, Cassadó J, De Marcos JA, Paraira M, Giménez N, Pessarrodona A. Pregnancy outcomes after ultrasound-guided high-intensity focused ultrasound (USgHIFU) for conservative treatment of uterine fibroids: Experience of a single institution. Int J Hyperthermia. 2021 Sep;38(2):9–17.
65. Peng S, Zhang L, Hu L, Chen J, Ju J, Wang X, Zhang R, Wang Z, Chen W. Factors influencing the dosimetry for high-intensity focused ultrasound ablation of uterine fibroids: A retrospective study. Medicine (Baltimore). 2015 Apr;94(13):e650.
66. Smart OC, Hindley JT, Regan L, Gedroyc WG. Gonadotrophin-releasing hormone and magnetic-resonance-guided ultrasound surgery for uterine leiomyomata. Obstet Gynecol. 2006 Jul;108(1):49–54.
67. Smart OC, Hindley JT, Regan L, Gedroyc WM. Magnetic resonance guided focused ultrasound surgery of uterine fibroids–the tissue effects of GnRH agonist pre-treatment. Eur J Radiol. 2006;59(2):163–7.
68. Peng S, Xiong Y, Li K et al. Clinical utility of a microbubble-enhancing contrast ("SonoVue") in treatment of uterine fibroids with high intensity focused ultrasound: A retrospective study. Eur J Radiol. 2012;81(12):3832–8.

69. Isern J, Pessarrodona A, Rodriguez J, Vallejo E, Gimenez N, Cassadó J, De Marco JA, Pedrerol A. Using microbubble sonographic contrast agent to enhance the effect of high intensity focused ultrasound for the treatment of uterine fibroids. Ultrason Sonochem. 2015 Nov;27:688–93.
70. Farny CH, Glynn Holt R, Roy RA. The correlation between bubble-enhanced HIFU heating and cavitation power. IEEE Trans Biomed Eng. 2010;57:175–84.

12

Clinical Application of Ultrasound-Guided Focused Ultrasound Ablation for Liver Tumours

Nicholas Kotewall and Tan To Cheung

12.1 Background

12.1.1 Hepatocellular Carcinoma

Hepatocellular carcinoma (HCC) is the most common primary cancer of the liver and the fifth most common cancer in the world. It accounts for the third highest number of cancer-related deaths in Hong Kong.[1] HCC is especially common in Asia, where the hepatitis B viral infection is endemic. Other risk factors for the development of HCC include hepatitis C infection, alcoholic cirrhosis, hereditary hemochromatosis, and primary biliary cirrhosis

Although HCC is a disease primarily affecting Asian countries due to the prevalence of chronic hepatitis B viral infection in the area, its incidence in western countries has been rising in recent years.[2, 3] The annual incidence of HCC in hepatitis B carriers is around 0.5%. The incidence in patients with liver cirrhosis is even higher at around 2.5% annually.[4, 5]

12.1.2 Treatment of HCC

Patients who are hepatitis B virus carriers should be offered regular surveillance in order to identify small tumours that may be potentially resectable. However, most patients with small HCCs do not have symptoms. Hepatic resection forms the cornerstone of the surgical management of HCC. Anatomical resection for HCC as proposed by Makuuchi et al. is the gold standard for treatment for HCC.[6] However, resection is only possible in 25% of patients because the disease is usually very advanced upon presentation. Moreover, HCC is often associated with cirrhosis, making resection difficult, if not impossible. Hence the prognosis for the majority of HCC patients remains dismal.

Even for those who are fit to undergo resection, cure is far from guaranteed. Post-resection tumour recurrence is common, with a 5-year recurrence rate over 50%.[7] Salvage treatment (defined as treatment given for recurrent disease after resection) for recurrent HCC poses several challenges, especially when tumour recurrence occurs in a small and cirrhotic remnant liver. Factors such as inadequate liver reserve (both in terms of volume and function), presence of adhesions from previous operations, and tumour location in the vicinity of major hepatic vessels or bile ducts in the liver remnant are all major impediments to further resection. Alternative treatments are therefore needed.

The advent of local ablation therapy has revolutionised the treatment protocol for HCC over the last decade.[8] With technological advances, local ablation therapy using a variety of energy sources has emerged as an effective treatment alternative for patients for whom conventional surgery is not suitable. These include cryoablation therapy, interstitial laser therapy, microwave coagulation, and radiofrequency ablation (RFA). Recently, high intensity focused ultrasound (HIFU) ablation has emerged as a new form of local ablative therapy.[9, 10] This innovative treatment entails the delivery of intense ultrasonic beams from an extracorporeal energy source into a targeted volume, resulting in heating which in turn leads to coagulative necrosis of tumour cells.

DOI: 10.1201/9780429162671-12

For patients with small unresectable HCC, liver transplantation appears to be the only viable option at the moment. Transplantation has the advantage of eradicating the tumour as well as replacing the native premalignant cirrhotic liver with a new and healthy graft liver. The chance of receiving a liver graft varies worldwide. Liver donation rate is highest in Spain where there are 33.7 donations per 1 million of the population. In contrast, the donation rates in Asia range from 0.05 to 4.3 donations per one million of the population. The general lack of suitable deceased donors make successful liver transplantation for HCC difficult.[11, 12] In order to maximise the benefit when utilising this scarce resource, different liver graft allocation systems have been adopted around the world. The principle of allocation is to prioritise the sickest and also those most likely to benefit from transplantation. The aim when using these allocation systems is to achieve the best results for the most patients. Since the opportunity cost of a liver graft is so high, a healthy liver given to a less deserving recipient often spells doom for another potential candidate. As a corollary, patients with very high Model for End-stage Liver Disease (MELD) scores have priority on the transplant waiting list. In most countries, patients with unresectable HCC (usually small multiple tumours) but lower MELD scores have a low priority.

The results of liver transplantation in its early development were not encouraging, with a 5-year survival rate below 40%. This led to the recognition of poor prognostic factors in liver transplantation for patients with HCC.[13] Mazzaferro et al. showed that a subgroup of patients with radiological evidence of a single tumour smaller than 5 cm in diameter or two to three tumours each smaller than 3 cm in diameter had better survival outcome.[14, 15] The Milan criteria (transplantation for solitary HCC less than 5 cm or 2 to 3 tumours each less than 3 cm) were established in 1996. Better patient selection based on these criteria has led to the improvement of the 5-year survival rate to 83%. At many liver transplant centres, patients with tumour status outside the Milan criteria are not accepted for transplantation and those patients on waiting lists are disqualified (or delisted) if their tumours grow beyond sizes specified by the criteria, ensuring that liver grafts are allocated to patients predicted to have the most favourable outcome after surgery.

In order to make sure patients with growing HCC remain on the waiting list, different appropriate treatments before transplantation, known as bridging therapies, have been tried. Bridging therapy arose out of the need to suspend tumour progression and to enable patients to remain within the transplantation criteria as long as possible in order to receive a graft liver.

12.1.3 High Intensity Focused Ultrasound

The concept of using ultrasound energy as a penetrating energy to destroy tissue from a distance originated in the last century and has been summarised by Kremkau.[16] In the 1950s, researchers such as the Fry brothers in Illinois brought the phenomenon of piezoelectricity to the clinical setting, treating Parkinson's disease and other neurological conditions with focused ultrasonic energy.[17–20] It was not until the 1990s that interest in applying HIFU therapy in the treatment of solid tumours arose again.

HIFU is based on the unique characteristic of sound waves at frequencies between 0.8 and 3.5 MHz which can be focused at a distance from the radiating transducer. The acoustic energy harnessed (up to 10,000 Watt/cm^2) causes intense vibrations of tissue, generating heat which causes necrosis in the target location without collateral damage to the surrounding structures. The benefit of inducing immediate tissue death from a distance using an ultrasonic energy source, without the need for invasive surgery or insertion of ablation instruments, makes HIFU an attractive option for the treatment of HCC. Although data on the efficacy of HIFU is still growing, the initial results obtained from pioneering researchers in Asia have been positive.[10, 21–26]

The mechanism of injury is twofold: thermal and mechanical. Heat is generated due to absorption of the acoustic energy by the target tissue. A lethal temperature of 60°C causes coagulative necrosis within a matter of seconds. At this temperature, water within the body's tissue starts to vaporise followed by microbubble formation. The mechanical process of cavitation then ensues.[27]

Cavitation is a process in which bubbles develop and increase in size to the point at which resonance is achieved. The bubble formation is a consequence of the negative pressure component of the ultrasound wave. As the bubbles expand and collapse, high pressures, ranging from 20,000 to 30,000 bars develop and damage nearby cells. A popcorn effect has been described as being typical of cavitation.[28] With these destructive mechanisms, irreversible cell death occurs by coagulative necrosis and apoptosis.

Since the high intensity energy is focused in such a small volume, the damage to structures between the transducer and the target lesion is minimal because the temperature outside the focal region does not rise significantly. This confers additional advantage over other ablative options such as RFA, in which inadvertent collateral damage is not completely avoidable. Patients with disrupted liver function and thrombocytopenia usually cannot tolerate RFA.[29]

The slow process of heating by HIFU energy propagation followed by intermittent resting results in little collateral tissue destruction beyond the focused target.

The HAIFU machine (JC model Focused Ultrasound Tumour Therapeutic Systems, Chongqing Haifu Technology, Chongqing, China) has been used on patients with HCC in 3 clinical settings: 1) as primary treatment of unresectable disease, 2) a salvage treatment, and 3) as a bridging therapy for liver transplantation. A fourth option, as described in the literature, is to use this technology in combination with other treatment modalities.[30]

The procedure is performed by a dedicated team of hepatobiliary surgeons, interventional radiologists and anaesthetists. All patients receiving HIFU therapy need to be anaesthetised for the procedure as it is necessary to control respiration to minimise the displacement of the liver by the diaphragm, and for adequate pain control since the procedure can take up to 3 hours. The patients are placed over the centre of the water reservoir and turned to a right lateral position if the tumour is located in the right lobe of liver or to a prone position if the tumour is located in the left lobe. The machine comprises a real-time diagnostic imaging unit, a therapeutic unit, a degassed water circulation unit, and a computer unit. The therapeutic unit, which comprises a transducer, lies at the centre of the water reservoir. It is able to move in 3 orthogonal planes along the x, y, and z axes and rotates around 90 degrees to enable tumour localisation. The frequency of the transducer is 0.8 MHz with a focal length ranging from 100 to 160 mm. The tumour location is then ascertained by real-time 2-dimensional liver ultrasonography, and the treatment pathway is determined. It is important to ensure that no adjacent organ, such as the large bowel or gallbladder lies within the treatment pathway, in order to prevent collateral damage to these organs. The degassed water circulation unit provides a coupling medium for ultrasonic transmission outside the body. Artificial pleural effusion and ascites can be created if deemed necessary for improving the efficiency of the acoustic energy transmission. Treatment power ranging from 230 to 466 watts is used. Lastly, the computer unit controls these 3 parts.

Parallel slices of the target tumour with 5-mm separation are planned using ultrasound images and then ablated slice by slice with focused acoustic energy emitted by the transducers. Grey-scale changes in the ablated sites are observed during the ablation process, indicating sufficient temperature rise inside the target lesion. A dose of intravenous antibiotic (Augmentin; Beecham Pharmaceuticals) is given just before starting the procedure, and oral-form antibiotics are continued for 5 days afterwards.([31, 32])

During the treatment, special attention must be paid to possible changes in the tumour location caused by diaphragmatic movement, so as to avoid overshooting or undershooting of the tumour. A rise in temperature at the skin surface may also occur, and regular monitoring of skin changes is crucial to preventing thermal injury. The most common complication of HIFU is skin burn. As the skin and adipose tissue absorb energy easily, any prefocal peak of energy coinciding with reflection of energy from the ribs can cause thermal injury. Although the overall incidence of skin burn is high, the severity is usually very mild. Only a very small percentage of these patients require surgical debridement as a result of a burn.

12.2 Clinical Use

The clinical application of HIFU for HCC is threefold:

1) HIFU ablation can be given as primary treatment of small HCC or of colorectal liver metastases which are not amenable to open resection. For HCC patients who do not have cirrhosis, surgical resection is undoubtedly the treatment of choice with best survival outcomes. On the other hand, the treatment of HCC in patients with cirrhosis is an entirely different story. Patients with HCC, even those smaller than 3 cm in size, may not be able to tolerate a hepatectomy if

they are plagued with advanced liver cirrhosis.[33–35] A large tumour, difficult tumour location, poor underlying liver function, comorbidity, etc., can render a hepatectomy dangerous, if not impossible. In these scenarios, liver transplantation is the ideal, and only, treatment. The post-transplant survival for a patient within Milan Criteria can be as high as 90% at 5 years in the hands of experienced centres.[36, 37] The scarcity of liver grafts means expecting these terrific outcomes is barely realistic. Many patients, while on the waiting list, will have tumour progression which would result in their disqualification.

Ablation is an accepted and standard practice of treatment for unresectable HCC.[31] Hepatectomy is the treatment of choice for small HCCs with normal liver function. RFA should be performed as an alternative in patients with small but unresectable HCC where liver transplantation is not an option. A percutaneous approach should be adopted where technically feasible. Patients with gross ascites, or a tumour located closed to the biliary system, major blood vessels, gallbladder, or diaphragm are not considered suitable for percutaneous RFA. HIFU is an alternative ablation option for this group of patients. Perhaps with time, when more data about the long-term outcome of HIFU becomes available, this treatment modality may replace RFA for small unresectable HCC.

2) HIFU can be used as a salvage treatment for HCC recurrence after resection.

   In the case of recurrent disease, only patients with Child-Pugh class A cirrhosis, and selected patients with Child-Pugh class B cirrhosis, should be considered for re-resection or RFA. The usual indication for re-resection was a solitary or oligonodular tumour within the same single section of the liver in the presence of sufficient future liver remnant. Re-resection should be avoided in the presence of gross ascites, an indocyanine green retention rate more than 15% at 15 minutes or a platelet count lower than 100×10^9/L. Percutaneous RFA should be considered when the recurrent tumour is in a deep-seated location where an anatomical resection will sacrifice a large amount of functional liver parenchyma. RFA should generally be avoided in the presence of gross ascites, a platelet count lower than 50 × 109/L in spite of platelet transfusion, or a tumour located in a difficult position as described earlier. HIFU should be considered as an alternative ablation option for this group of patients in the setting for salvage treatment for HCC. To conclude, for the treatment of HCC smaller than 3 cm (either in the setting of primary or salvage treatment), HIFU ablation offers an excellent oncological outcome which is comparable to the results achieved by RFA, using either an open or a percutaneous approach. This relatively new method can offer hope to patients with poor liver function and advanced cirrhosis when other therapies are not suitable.

3) HIFU can be used as a bridging therapy for patients with HCC on the liver transplantation waiting list. Effective bridging therapy is particularly limited for patients whose treatment options are restricted by poor liver reserve and portal hypertension. Transarterial chemoembolisation (TACE) and RFA are the most popular bridging therapies. TACE is standard at some centres, achieving a rate of tumour down-staging of around 40%. However, about 20% of patients develop tumour progression after TACE, leading to them being delisted.[38–41] RFA is an effective thermal ablative treatment modality and is widely practiced to treat small HCCs. The complete ablation rate achieved by RFA ranges from 75% to 96%.[42, 43] RFA is also used as a bridging therapy. Successful tumour down-staging is observed in 70% to 80% of patients. However, the dropout rate after RFA is around 14%.[44–47] TACE and RFA are reasonable choices for bridging therapies, but are only applicable for selected patients. A bridging therapy must not cause further liver decompensation, and these 2 modalities are not safe for patients with severe cirrhosis in the presence of gross ascites and thrombocytopenia. This is where HIFU as a bridging therapy can prove to be superior.

12.3 Treatment Outcome

The first experience of HIFU on HCC was gained by researchers in China using the JC HAIFU system. In a study by Wu et al. in which 55 patients with large HCC (mean diameter of 8.1 cm, 4 to 14 cm) and concomitant cirrhosis underwent HIFU treatment, no major complications were recorded.[21] Completeness of ablation was assessed in 26 patients and the complete ablation rate was 69%. The overall survival rates were 62% at 12 months and 35% at 18 months. This was one of the first studies to demonstrate the efficacy of HIFU in the treatment of advanced HCC

Several later series have expanded this pioneering work on HCC. Ng et al. reported on the safety and efficacy of HIFU in the treatment of HCC (median tumour size 2.2 cm; range, 0.9 to 8 cm) for a series of 49 patients who were not surgical candidates and concluded that HIFU was an effective modality in this setting, with 1- and 3-year overall survival rates reported as 87.7% and 62.4%, respectively.[31] The study found that tumour size (≥3.0 cm) was a significant risk factor affecting the complete ablation rate. HIFU was shown to be a safe treatment, and none of the patients receiving HIFU as a bridging therapy developed complications due to intolerance after the procedure.[48] The complication rate was 8.2%, with the complications involving mild skin oedema and injury due to energy accumulation in the ultrasound beam pathway. Besides tumour size, the Child-Pugh grading of liver cirrhosis was another prognostic factor which influenced the overall patient survival. This is compatible with the natural course of the disease and a patient's suboptimal liver function may not allow them to receive further treatments.[31]

HIFU has been used in combination with TACE in prior studies. In a randomised trial comparing TACE alone vs TACE + HIFU, Wu et al. showed that the total effective rate for tumour response was 72.8% in the TACE + HIFU group.[10] This response was significantly higher than in the TACE group alone (44.5%, $P < 0.05$). The corresponding 1-, 2-, 3-, and 5-year overall survival rates for the TACE-HIFU group were 72.7%, 50.0%, 31.8%, and 11.4%, respectively. These rates were higher than in the TACE alone group (47.2%, 16.7%, 2.8%, and 0%, respectively, $P < 0.01$).

In a study which compared TACE and HIFU as bridging therapies for transplantation, Cheung et al. demonstrated that 90% of patients receiving HIFU had complete tumour response, while 10% had partial response. There was no complete or partial tumour response in the TACE group. Fourteen (46%) patients had progressive disease, and 14 (46%) patients had stable disease. The overall dropout rate was 24.1%.[49]

Studies investigating the use of HIFU for the treatment of metastatic liver tumours are limited. Most studies do not address outcomes related to this defined subset of patients. Wu et al. reported on the largest series of patients who have undergone HIFU (n = 1,038); however, histological findings and tumour location were variable. In their study, primary and metastatic liver tumours were reported on as a single cohort without analysis of the subgroups.[22] Overall, these studies indicate that HIFU may serve as an excellent local ablation technique for the treatment of HCC; however, technical implementation of the procedure serves as a significant barrier to its more widespread use.

Previous studies have shown that HIFU can improve the quality of life of patients with HCC. In a study involving 145 patients with HCC, symptoms improved or pain was relieved in 84.8%. Additionally, the size of the target tumour shrank by varying amounts. The 2-year survival rate was 80% in patients with stageIb HCC, 51.4% in stage IIa, and 46.5% in stage IIIa.[50]

Moreover, HIFU is safe for the treatment of disease adjacent to, or surrounding, a major liver vessel. The study by Zhang et al enrolled 39 patients with HCC. All of the treated tumours had a distance between the tumour and a main blood vessel (inferior vena cava, main hepatic vein branches, portal vein) of less than 1 cm, and no major blood vessel injury was observed in any of the patients included.[26]

Despite early success, this technology has not gained mainstream popularity. The application of HIFU technology in the management of patients with HCC has been validated with much research. Once considered a Chinoiserie, HIFU ablation is gathering momentum in other parts of the world.[51–53] The feasibility and safety of HIFU for liver tumours were initially demonstrated in the early 1990s. The tolerance and safety limits, both vital information, have been further studied. In a study by Cheung, patient age is the only significant factor for treatment intolerance, as with other operations that require general anaesthesia. Aging is an inevitable physiological phenomenon characterised by degenerative changes in both the structure and the functional capacity of organs. Elderly patients are prone to both dehydration and fluid overload. Chronic obstructive pulmonary disease and pneumonia are very common among the elderly. As a result, risks of pneumothorax, pneumonia, and pleural effusion increase when a Valsalva manoeuvre is applied during general anaesthesia. Poor liver function, which plagues patients with Child-Pugh B or C cirrhosis, often gives rise to more complication after therapies such as TACE, RFA, and hepatectomy. HIFU can, however, deal with poor liver function with a greater margin of safety. No association between treatment intolerance and liver function was found in a group of 100 patients in which 84 had Child-Pugh grade of A, 15 had B, and 1 had C.[32]

Although HIFU has the benefit of being extracorporeal in its administration, the portion of skin and subcutaneous tissue along the path of the acoustic energy is frequently affected, resulting in tissue oedema. As large tumours require longer ablation times, the ensuing skin and subcutaneous oedema reduces the ultrasound imaging targeting accuracy. In other words, the precision of the focused energy will be negatively affected in larger tumours which required longer ablations.[31] Since large tumours are often incompletely ablated, multiple courses of HIFU treatment should be anticipated.

HIFU is not without complications. First- and second-degree burns are especially disturbing. Further technique refinements, such as artificial ascites and intermittent delivery of acoustic energy to allow skin cooling, have been introduced. Since ultrasonic energy requires a fluid medium to propagate, the presence of artificially induced ascites will facilitate energy propagation to the target lesions

It should be emphasised that meticulous techniques are necessary to ensure complete ablation of a tumour using HIFU. It is important to carry out to plan using diagnostic ultrasound to ensure that the liver tumour is clearly visible before administering HIFU. Complete tumour ablation can be achieved by acoustic energy from the HIFU system as long as the margins of the tumour can be clearly defined during the procedure. The difficulty of tumour localisation and of monitoring of the ablation effect initially made this treatment modality less operator-friendly. Recent advances in Doppler ultrasonic imaging and real-time magnetic resonance imaging (MRI) have solved these problems, considerably improving the accuracy of tumour location.[54]

12.4 Expert Commentary

Locoregional methods of ablation for unresectable HCC, especially RFA, are becoming more popular due to the fact that they are effective, simple, and repeatable. The survival outcome from RFA for HCCs smaller than 2 cm is similar to liver resection.[55–57] Nonetheless, it is invasive, and according to a review of reports involving 3670 patients, it has an overall complication rate of 8.9%.[29, 58] Similar to liver resection, RFA may not be well tolerated in patients with cirrhosis. Currently, TACE is a common treatment for unresectable HCC which are not amenable to RFA. The efficacy of TACE has been supported by randomised controlled studies.[59, 60] However, the 2-year survival rate after TACE is less than satisfactory, at only around 30%.[61]

Among all local ablative therapies that use various energy sources, HIFU is the only treatment modality that is totally extracorporeal, making it less invasive and hence less dangerous. HIFU aims to offer a more effective treatment option for the group of patients who cannot tolerate resection and who are marginal candidates for receiving RFA. The unique needleless design of the HIFU system makes this type of ablation superior to RFA, as percutaneous needle penetration may induce torrential haemorrhage from a hypervascular HCC in a patient with coagulopathy and a low platelet count, both common features in patients with cirrhosis.[62] Furthermore, without needle puncture, there is reduced chance of the theoretical risk of tumour dissemination into the systemic circulation from the surrounding major vessels.[63]

For tumours located in difficult positions of the liver, percutaneous RFA is not feasible and an open approach would be required. On the other hand, the application of HIFU is not limited by tumours at the liver dome as the ultrasonic energy can safely be delivered to these target lesions. The feasibility of percutaneous RFA is limited by the location of the lesion. A tumour at the liver dome in section 7 or 8 is a contraindication for percutaneous RFA because of potential injury to the diaphragm. However, HIFU energy can target lesions even in difficult positions, e.g. ones close to the diaphragm or to the heart. While the presence of gross ascites (a sign of severe liver cirrhosis) is an impediment to receiving RFA, it actually facilitates HIFU treatment. As ultrasound energy travels easily through water, ascites encourages energy propagation to the target lesion. In addition, the presence of ascites acts as a cushion of coolant inside the peritoneal cavity and prevents the muscle wall and skin absorbing too much energy from the beam pathway where a subcutaneous tissue burn could happen.

Therefore, the passage of energy without puncture using a physical instrument, its versatility regarding tumours located at difficult positions and its superior performance in patients with ascites, give HIFU treatments superiority over other ablation therapies for HCC, such as RFA.

12.5 Summary

HIFU, which employs acoustic energy as a form of treatment for HCC, is safe and effective. At the moment, HIFU can be used alone or in combination with other systemic treatments such as TACE to treat unresectable HCC not amenable to RFA. It also has a place in a salvage setting for treating recurrent HCC not amenable to resection. Thirdly, it provides hope for those waiting for a liver transplantation as a bridging therapy. It is a safe procedure, with its only complication being occasional mild skin burn. The fact that it is totally extracorporeal, works well in patients with ascites, and has no difficulty tackling tumours in the dome of liver (traditionally seen as a difficult site for ablation) make this modality of treatment very attractive.

Currently, it certainly fills the gap in treatment protocols for those patients with HCC who are not fit to undergo resection or RFA and those for whom TACE is not sufficient. Perhaps, with wider application of HIFU technology and the emergence of more long-term data on survival, this treatment modality will replace RFA as the ablation option of choice.

REFERENCES

1. Hospital Authority. Hong Kong Cancer Registry. http://www3.ha.org.hk/cancereg. Accessed April 2019.
2. El-Serag HB, Lau M, Eschbach K, et al. Epidemiology of hepatocellular carcinoma in Hispanics in the United States. Arch Intern Med. 2007; 167: 1983–1989.
3. El-Serag HB, Epidemiology of hepatocellular carcinoma in USA. Hepatol Res. 2007; 37 (Suppl 2): S88–S94.
4. Poon RT, Fan ST, Lo CM, et al. Longterm prognosis after resection of hepatocellular carcinoma associated with hepatitis B-related cirrhosis. J Clin Oncol. 2000; 18: 1094–1101 [PMID: 10694562]
5. Poon RT, Fan ST, Lo CM, Liu CL, Wong J. Long-term survival and pattern of recurrence after resection of small hepatocellular carcinoma in patients with preserved liver function: Implications for a strategy of salvage transplantation. Ann Surg. 2002; 235: 373–382 [PMID: 11882759 DOI: 10.1097/00000658-200203000-00009].
6. Hasegawa K, Kokudo N, Imamura H, et al. Prognostic impact of anatomic resection for hepatocellular carcinoma. Ann Surg. 2005; 242 (2): 252–259.
7. Poon RT, Fan ST, Wong J. Risk factors, prevention and management of post-operative recurrence after resection of hepatocellular carcinoma. Ann Surg. 2000; 232: 10–24.
8. Chan AC, Poon RT, Ng KK, et al. Changing pattern in the management of hepatocellular carcinoma improves the survival benefit of early detection by screening. Ann Surg. 2008; 247: 666–673.
9. Orsi F, Zhang L, Arnone P, et al. High-intensity focused ultrasound ablation: Effective and safe therapy for solid tumours in difficult locations. AJR AM J Roentgenol. 2010; 195: W245–W252.
10. Wu F, Wang ZB, Chen WZ, et al. Advanced hepatocellular carcinoma: Treatment with high-intensity focused ultrasound ablation combined with transcatheter arterial embolization. Radiology. 2005; 235: 659–667.
11. Lo CM, Fan ST, Liu CL, Chan SC, Wong J. The role and limitation of living donor liver transplantation for hepatocellular carcinoma. Liver Transpl. 2004; 10: 440–447 [PMID: 15004774 DOI: 10.1002/lt.20097]
12. Ríos A, López-Navas A, Ayala-Garcia MA, et al. Donation and transplantation among personnel in the hospital emergency department: A multicenter study conducted in Spain and Mexico. Transplant Proc. 2011; 43: 48–51 [PMID: 21335151 DOI: 10.1016/j.transpr oceed.2010.11.008]
13. Ringe B, Pichlmayr R, Wittekind C, Tusch G. Surgical treatment of hepatocellular carcinoma: Experience with liver resection and transplantation in 198 patients. World J Surg. 1991; 15: 270–285 [PMID: 1851588 DOI: 10.1007/BF01659064]

14. Mazzaferro V, Rondinara GF, Rossi G, et al. Milan multicenter experience in liver transplantation for hepatocellular carcinoma. Transplant Proc. 1994; 26: 3557–3560 [PMID: 7998274]
15. Mazzaferro V, Regalia E, Doci R, et al. Liver transplantation for the treatment of small hepatocellular carcinomas in patients with cirrhosis. N Engl J Med. 1996; 334: 693–699 [PMID: 8594428 DOI: 10.1056/NEJM199603143341104]
16. Kremkau FW. Cancer therapy with ultrasound: A historical review. J Clin Ultrasound. 1979; 7: 287–300 [PMID: 112118 DOI: 10.1002/jcu.1870070410]
17. Barnard JW, Fry WJ, Fry FJ, Krumins RF. Effects of high intensity ultrasound on the central nervous system of the cat. J Comp Neurol. 1955; 103: 459–484 [PMID: 13286367 DOI: 10.1002/cne.901030304]
18. Fry WJ, Barnard JW, Fry EJ, Krumins RF, Brennan JF. Ultrasonic lesions in the mammalian central nervous system. Science. 1955; 122: 517–518 [PMID: 13255886 DOI: 10.1126/science.122.3168.517]
19. Fry WJ, Barnard JW, Fry FJ, Brennan JF. Ultrasonically produced localized selective lesions in the central nervous system. Am J Phys Med. 1955; 34: 413–423 [PMID: 14376518]
20. Fry WJ, Mosberg WH, Barnard JW, Fry FJ. Production of focal destructive lesions in the central nervous system with ultrasound. J Neurosurg. 1954; 11: 471–478 [PMID: 13201985 DOI: 10.3171/jns.1954.11.5.0471]
21. Wu F, Wang ZB, Chen WZ, et al. Extracorporeal high intensity focused ultrasound ablation in the treatment of patients with large hepatocellular carcinoma. Ann Surg Oncol. 2004; 11: 1061–1069.
22. Wu F, Wang ZB, Chen WZ, et al. Extracorporeal high intensity focused ultrasound ablation in the treatment of 1038 patients with solid carcinomas in China: An overview. Ultrason Sonochem. 2004; 11: 149–154.
23. Wu F, Wang ZB, Chen WZ, et al. Extracorporeal focused ultrasound surgery for treatment of human solid carcinomas: Early Chinese clinical experience. Ultrasound Med Biol. 2004; 30: 245–260.
24. Li CX, Xu GL. Jiang ZY, et al. Analysis of clinical effect of high intensity focused ultrasound on liver cancer. World J Gastroenterol. 2004; 10: 2201–2204.
25. Li YY, Sha WH, Zhou YJ, et al. Short and long term efficacy of high intensity focused ultrasound therapy for advanced hepatocellular carcinoma. J Gastoenterol Hepatol. 2007; 22: 2148–2154.
26. Zhang L, Zhu H, Jin C, et al. High-intensity focused ultrasound {HIFU}: Effective and safe therapy got hepatocellular carcinoma adjacent to major hepatic veins. Eur Radiol. 2009; 19: 437–445.
27. Chen H, Li X, Wan M. The inception of cavitation bubble clouds induced by high-intensity focused ultrasound. Ultrasonics. 2006; 44(Suppl 1): e427–e429.
28. Mearini, L. High intensity focused ultrasound, liver disease and bridging therapy. World J Gastroenterol. 2013 Nov 21; 19(43): 7494–7499.
29. Cheung TT, Ng KK, Poon RT, Fan ST. Tolerance of radiofrequency ablation by patients of hepatocellular carcinoma. J Hepatobiliary Pancreat Surg. 2009; 16: 655–660 [PMID: 19370304 DOI: 10.1007/s00534-009-0103-9]
30. Liao MH, Huang JW, Zhang T, et al. Transarterial chemoembolization in combination with local therapies for hepatocellular carcinoma: A meta-analysis. PLoS One. 2013; Jul (7): e68453.
31. Ng KK, Poon RT, Chan SC, et al. High-intensity focused ultrasound for hepatocellular carcinoma: A single center experience. Ann Surg. 2011; 253: 981–987.
32. Cheung TT, Chu FS, Jenkins CR, et al. Tolerance of high-intensity focused ultrasound ablation in patients with hepatocellular carcinoma. World J Surg. 2012; 36: 2420–2427.
33. Fan ST. Surgical therapy of hepatocellular carcinoma in the cirrhotic liver. Swiss Surg. 1999; 5: 107–110.
34. Fan ST, Ng IO, Poon RT, et al. Hepatectomy for hepatocellular carcinoma: The surgeon's role in long-term survival. Arch Surg. 1999; 134: 1124–1130. 19.
35. Belghiti J, Kianmanesh R. Surgical treatment of hepatocellular carcinoma. HPB. 2005; 7: 42–49.
36. Belghiti J, Carr BI, Greig PD, Lencioni R, Poon RT. Treatment before liver transplantation for HCC. Ann Surg Oncol. 2008; 15: 993–1000.
37. Lo CM, Fan ST, Liu CL, et al. Living donor versus deceased donor liver transplantation for early irresectable hepatocellular carcinoma. Br J Surg. 2007; 94: 78–86.
38. Roayaie S, Frischer JS, Emre SH, et al. Long-term results with multimodal adjuvant therapy and liver transplantation for the treatment of hepatocellular carcinomas larger than 5 centimeters. Ann Surg. 2002; 235: 533–539 [PMID: 11923610 DOI: 10.1097/00000658-200204000-00012]
39. Maddala YK, Stadheim L, Andrews JC, et al. Drop-out rates of patients with hepatocellular cancer listed for liver transplantation: Outcome with chemoembolization. Liver Transpl. 2004; 10: 449–455 [PMID: 15004776 DOI: 10.1002/lt.20099]

40. Graziadei IW, Sandmueller H, Waldenberger P, et al. Chemoembolization followed by liver transplantation for hepatocellular carcinoma impedes tumour progression while on the waiting list and leads to excellent outcome. Liver Transpl. 2003; 9: 557–563 [PMID: 12783395 DOI: 10.1053/jlts.2003.50106]
41. Hayashi PH, Ludkowski M, Forman LM, et al. Hepatic artery chemoembolization for hepatocellular carcinoma in patients listed for liver transplantation. Am J Transplant. 2004; 4: 782–787 [PMID: 15084175 DOI: 10.1111/j.1600-6143.2004.00413.x]
42. Francica G, Marone G. Ultrasound-guided percutaneous treatment of hepatocellular carcinoma by radiofrequency hyperthermia with a 'cooled-tip needle'. A preliminary clinical experience. Eur J Ultrasound. 1999; 9: 145–153.
43. Rossi S, Di Stasi M, Buscarini E, et al. Percutaneous RF interstitial thermal ablation in the treatment of hepatic cancer. AJR Am J Roentgenol. 1996; 167: 759–768.
44. Brillet PY, Paradis V, Brancatelli G, et al. Percutaneous radiofrequency ablation for hepatocellular carcinoma before liver transplantation: A prospective study with histopathologic comparison. AJR Am J Roentgenol. 2006; 186: S296–S305 [PMID: 16632691 DOI: 10.2214/AJR.04.1927]
45. Mazzaferro V, Battiston C, Perrone S, et al. Radiofrequency ablation of small hepatocellular carcinoma in cirrhotic patients awaiting liver transplantation: A prospective study. Ann Surg. 2004; 240: 900–909 [PMID: 15492574 DOI: 10.1097/01.sla.0000143301.56154.95]
46. Fisher RA, Maluf D, Cotterell AH, et al. Non-resective ablation therapy for hepatocellular carcinoma: Effectiveness measured by intention-to-treat and dropout from liver transplant waiting list. Clin Transplant. 2004; 18: 502–512 [PMID: 15344951]
47. Pompili M, Mirante VG, Rondinara G, et al. Percutaneous ablation procedures in cirrhotic patients with hepatocellular carcinoma submitted to liver transplantation: Assessment of efficacy at explant analysis and of safety for tumour recurrence. Liver Transpl. 2005; 11: 1117–1126 [PMID: 16123960 DOI: 10.1002/lt.20469]
48. Cheung TT, Poon RT, Lo CM, et al. Survival analysis of high-intensity focused ultrasound therapy vs. transarterial chemoembolization for unresectable hepatocellular carcinomas Liver Int. 2014; 34: e136–e143.
49. Cheung TT, Fan ST, Chan SC, et al. High-intensity focused ultrasound ablation: An effective bridging therapy for hepatocellular carcinoma patients. World J Gastroenterol. 2013 May 28; 19(20): 3083–3089.
50. Xu G, Luo G, He L, et al. Follow-up of high-intensity focused ultrasound treatment for patients with hepatocellular carcinoma. Ultrasound Med Biol. 2011 Dec; 37(12): 1993–1999.
51. Maruyama H, Yoshikawa M, Yokosuka O. Current role of ultrasound for the management of hepatocellular carcinoma. World J Gastroenterol. 2008; 14: 1710–1719.
52. Illing RO, Kennedy JE, Wu F, et al. The safety and feasibility of extracorporeal high-intensity focused ultrasound (HIFU) for the treatment of liver and kidney tumours in a Western population. Br J Cancer. 2005; 93: 890–895. 15.
53. Noterdaeme O, Leslie TA, Kennedy JE, Phillips RR, Brady M. The use of time to maximum enhancement to indicate areas of ablation following the treatment of liver tumours with high-intensity focused ultrasound. Br J Radiol. 2009; 82: 412–420.
54. Hiroyuki F, Kazushi N, Akito N, et al. High-intensity focused ultrasound ablation assisted using color Doppler imaging for the treatment of hepatocellular carcinomas. Abdom Imaging. 2013; 38(6): 1263–1268.
55. Hasegawa K, Kokudo N, Makuuchi M, et al. Comparison of resection and ablation for hepatocellular carcinoma: A cohort study based on a Japanese nationwide survey. J Hepatol. 2013; 58: 724–729.
56. Lam CM, Ng KK, Poon RT, et al. Impact of radiofrequency ablation on the management of patients with hepatocellular carcinoma in a specialized centre. Br J Surg. 2004; 91: 334–338. 7.
57. Toshikuni N, Takuma Y, Goto T, Yamamoto H. Prognostic factors in hepatitis c patients with a single small hepatocellular carcinoma after radiofrequency ablation. Hepatogastroenterology. 2012; 59: 2361–2366.
58. Mulier S, Mulier P, Ni Y, et al. Complications of radiofrequency coagulation of liver tumours. Br J Surg. 2002; 89: 1206–1222.
59. Llovet JM, Real MI, Montana X, et al. Arterial embolisation or chemoembolisation versus symptomatic treatment in patients with unresectable hepatocellular carcinoma: A randomised controlled trial. Lancet 2002; 359: 1734–9. 10.
60. Lo CM, Ngan H, Tso WK, et al. Randomized controlled trial of transarterial lipiodol chemoembolization for unresectable hepatocellular carcinoma. Hepatology. 2002; 35: 1164–71.

61. Doffoel M, Bonnetain F, Bouche O, et al. Multicentre randomised phase III trial comparing tamoxifen alone or with transarterial lipiodol chemoembolisation for unresectable hepatocellular carcinoma in cirrhotic patients (Federation francophone de cancerologie digestive 9402). Eur J Cancer. 2008; 44: 528–38.
62. Mulier S, Mulier P, Ni Y, et al. Complications of radiofrequency coagulation of liver tumours. Br J Surg. 2002; 89: 1206–1222.
63. Nicoli N, Casaril A, Abu Hilal M, et al. A case of rapid intrahepatic dissemination of hepatocellular carcinoma after radiofrequency thermal ablation. Am J Surg. 2004; 188: 165–167 [PMID: 15249243 DOI: 10.1016/j.amjsurg.2003.12.061]

13

Clinical Application of Ultrasound-Guided Focused Ultrasound Ablation for Kidney Tumours

Paul Lyon and David Cranston

13.1 Background

The epidemiology of renal (kidney) cancer, has changed over the last three decades, such that its incidence has risen significantly, and has almost doubled in the over 65s.[1] This is due both to increased rates of diagnosis due to improved abdominal imaging (ultrasound, CT, MRI) and to a real increase in occurrence.[1–3] In the United States, over 70% of all renal cancers are detected incidentally following imaging for unrelated reasons.[4] Currently, renal cancer is one of the commonest urological malignancies. Although in recent years worldwide trends are now demonstrating a plateau in the rising incidence of kidney cancer,[5] it remains a frequently occurring malignancy across the globe. Worldwide, in 2008, 270,000 new cases of renal cancer were diagnosed, representing 2% of all cancers, and the same year saw 111,000 renal cancer-related deaths.[6] Those with advanced kidney cancer have five-year relative survival rates of approximately 11–12%.[7]

Incidental small renal masses of low-grade are slow growing and are associated with synchronous metastatic disease in only 5% of cases for tumours under 3 cm.[8, 9] However as the size increases, so does the chance of synchronous metastatic disease, with the risk doubling with a 3.5 cm increase in the size of the primary tumour.[10] Originating in the renal cortex, renal cell carcinoma (RCC) is the most common form of renal cancer and accounts for over 80–85% of all primary renal neoplasms. The incidence of RCC demonstrates significant regional variation, with Europe and North America having some of the highest rates worldwide.[5] RCC is commonly asymptomatic, particularly in its early course, and thus is typically either diagnosed incidentally or at a late-stage following regional or distant metastatic spread, the latter group being the greatest contributor to the lethality of the malignancy.

RCC is typically resistant to chemotherapy and radiotherapy, although immunotherapies, such as interferons, tyrosine kinase inhibitors and interleukin-2 therapies, have demonstrated limited, but reproducible, efficacy in terms of prolonged survival for metastatic RCC.[11–13]

Surgery is presently the only curative option available for renal cancer and remains the standard of care for clinically localised renal cancers. Nephron-sparing surgery (NSS), or partial nephrectomy, has become the preferred management for early stage renal carcinoma, as outcomes are comparable to those of radical nephrectomy (RN), whilst preserving renal function.[14–17] To take an example, in patients with bilateral renal cancers, NSS would clearly be advantageous, and indeed RN is contraindicated. Surgical cure rates are high, and 10-year cancer-specific survival rates are over 75% for both RN and NSS groups.[18] However surgical intervention is not without significant levels of risk and post-operative medical (renal failure, myocardial infarction, thrombosis, embolism) and surgical complications (urine leakage, haemorrhage) are not uncommon.[19] Furthermore, given that the vast majority of cases of RCC are diagnosed in individuals over 65 years of age,[20] comorbidities exclude a significant proportion of patients from surgery.

In the treatment of small renal malignancies, minimally invasive techniques, such as cryoablation or thermal coagulation by radio-frequency ablation (RFA), are gaining ground due to low morbidity and overall survival rates approaching those of surgical resection.[21–25] One meta-analysis, comprising 1375

DOI: 10.1201/9780429162671-13

renal tumours, noted a local tumour progression rate of 5.2% following cryoablation compared with 12.9% after RFA, with 1.8% overall of ablated patients from both groups going on to develop metastasis.[26] Whilst the outcomes of minimally invasive strategies are very good, local tumour progression means they still do not meet up to surgical oncologic outcomes[23]; this said, they currently have a clear role in selected patient cohorts, for example in those unfit for surgical resection.

Highintensity focused ultrasound (HIFU) has been the subject of medical research for over 60 years, and like chemotherapy and radiotherapy, benefits greatly from being non-invasive. Since Burov first proposed the use of HIFU for oncological treatments in 1956,[27] it has been used for targeted ablation of tumours in many organs including those in liver, kidney, breast, prostate, uterus, bladder, pancreas, testis, brain and the eye.[28] Dissemination of tumour following HIFU ablation was an early concern, raised by Fry et al. (1978), a pioneer of the technology, who demonstrated increased metastatic potential of implanted medulloblastoma tumours in the flanks of hamsters, following intense ultrasound.[29] Several small animal studies have since explored this hypothesis for a variety of tumour types and have failed to confirm it; HIFU ablation of malignant tumours does not result in their dissemination.[30–34] Indeed other pre-clinical[35–37] and clinical studies[38, 39] have demonstrated that ablative therapies, including HIFU, may induce an immune-mediated host response following curative treatment, protecting against further metastatic spread.

HIFU has an advantage over chemo- and radiotherapy in that it offers a very favourable side effect profile, with no upper limit of tissue tolerance following repeated exposures of (non-ionising) ultrasound.[40] Over conventional systemic chemotherapy, it has the added benefit of being highly targeted; due to the tight focusing of ultrasound energy, the non-targeted tissues of the body, even tissues in very close proximity to the target, remain completely unharmed. Safety and feasibility of the extracorporeal approach for HIFU ablation has been demonstrated in China for a wide variety of solid cancers[41] and, in the West, specifically for those of the liver and kidney.[42]

13.2 Pre-clinical Studies in the kidney

For the studies described here, one can assume HIFU was applied in continuous (or 'tone burst') mode unless otherwise specified as a pulsed exposure. Several pre-clinical studies using small and large animal models for ablation of both normal kidney parenchyma and renal tumours have been performed both ex vivo and in vivo. In 1977 Frizzell et al. established thresholds for focal ultrasonic lesions in rabbit kidney, liver, and testicle using a 2-MHz device, but organs were exteriorised through surgical incisions, and thus whilst the experiments were performed using in vivo perfused kidneys, this was not an extracorporeal approach.[43] The device used had a focal length of 5 cm, and was tested at the first and third harmonic of its fundamental frequency using exposures of up to a minute. A 2-MHz frequency was shown to provide near-optimal depth of penetration for localised heating in solid organs. At 6 MHz, much lower-intensity thresholds were found for lesion formation. In this study, tissue damage was presumed to be predominantly by thermal mechanisms, based on another study, which determined an in situ focal intensity threshold of 200 W/cm^2, above which non-thermal effects contribute to tissue destruction.[44]

In the early 1990s, attempts at in vivo extracorporeal HIFU ablation by Vallancien et al.[45] in the porcine kidney and liver used a system of multiple 1-MHz piezo-ceramic elements arranged in a concave dish to target a common focal volume. Derived from piezo-electric lithotripters, these, when combined, generated very high focal intensities of over 10 kW/cm^2, and hence produced lesions using a predominantly cavitation-based, rather than purely thermal, mechanism. Although these large animal studies and ultimately early human trials[46] demonstrated the device's ability to form extracorporeal renal lesions, proceeding with the multiple and sizeable generators required ultimately proved to be impractical and too unreliable for clinical use.

Around the same time, Chapelon et al. looked at HIFU ablation of kidney tissue in rat and canine models using an extracorporeal device (1–2.25 MHz) capable of generating a combination of cavitation and thermal effects.[47] Of the 16 canine kidneys treated, macroscopic lesions were seen in 10 animals following sacrifice within 2–4 hours of treatment, with histological confirmation of coagulative necrosis. However, collateral damage was also observed, with half having injury to the spleen, 3/16 having bowel injury, 1/16 having lung injury and 1/16 having pancreatic injury in addition to 12/16 having skin burns.

Subsequently, Hynynen et al. (1995) used an MR-guided HIFU device (1.5–1.68 MHz, 10 s exposures at up to 142 W_{ac}, free field peak focal intensity of 1.2 kW/cm^2) to target the renal cortex of five rabbits in vivo.[48] Based on earlier work, a T1-weighted spoiled gradient-echo sequence was successfully used to monitor temperature elevations in real time. Histological evaluation demonstrated that kidney necrosis could be achieved consistently without damage to the overlying skin and muscle.

A year later, Adams et al. published a study that used a transrectal HIFU device,[1] intended for use on the prostate, to ablate rabbit VX-2 kidney tumours using direct contact with surgically exteriorised kidneys, and in a subsequent phase, an extracorporeal approach.[49] Exposures of 4 s, followed by 12 s for imaging, were used to provide a 2 × 2 × 10 mm treatment volume over a 16-s cycle. Lesions were stacked together using spacing of 1.8 mm to create longitudinal lesions. In the first phase, ex vivo ablation was performed and in all nine rabbits, macroscopic lesions were observed with well-demarcated histological correlation with the HIFU-ablated regions. In the subsequent in vivo phase, macroscopic evidence of kidney ablation was seen in 7/9 animals, which similarly demonstrated well-demarcated histological correlation. However, only two of these demonstrated successful targeting, thought to be due to the insufficient imaging capability of this early device prototype, when used in combination with respiratory movement during normal ventilation. In addition, 4/9 rabbits had circular skin burns on the abdominal wall where there had been contact with the device.

In 1997, using a single-element device (fundamental 0.56 MHz, run at third harmonic) Watkin et al. performed HIFU ablation in 18 porcine kidneys in vivo. Gross and histologically discrete damage was observed in 13.[50] Nine cases demonstrated skin induration and in one case, a skin burn. Skin toxicity was deemed to be the limiting factor and, in addition, a wide variation in the extent of damage was noted. The study observed that at high spatial peak intensities (I_{SP} over 1.5 kW/cm^2) the rate of heating was rapid and thus conductive heat losses become a negligible factor at the threshold for lesion formation. Indeed other simulation, and small animal, studies have shown that the effects of organ perfusion can be practically eliminated for applications of ablative thermal therapy using exposure times of less than three seconds.[51,52] There is, however, a trade-off between high intensities for rapid lesion formation, which overcome the cooling effect of organ perfusion, and collateral skin damage and unpredictable pre-focal lesions.[53]

Subsequently, towards the end of the century, for the first time, Daum et al. used a continuous-wave 256-element phased ultrasonic array (1.1 MHz, 12 cm diameter) with MR guidance and MR monitoring to generate larger-volume lesions in an in vivo porcine model.[54] In total, seven lesions were created across the kidneys of two pigs. By rapidly cycling a series of multiple focus fields over a 20-s continuous exposure period, using a previously published method they were able to generate a cross-sectional focal region of 0.5 × 0.5 cm^2.[55] Each kidney underwent this sonication protocol once or twice, using an average acoustic power of 210 W_{ac} and estimated peak tissue pressure of 5.1 MPa (calculated using an attenuation coefficient of 5 Np/m/MHz and a tissue depth of 6 cm), resulting in a peak temperature rise of 24 °C. MRI showed lesions in all attempts, whilst autopsy revealed that visible lesions were achieved in 4/7 kidneys. Using this strategy, the study demonstrated the feasibility of achieving ablation volumes of over 0.5 cm^3 with MR thermography feedback.

At a similar time Tu et al. ablated VX2 kidney tumours in rabbits using two 90 s periods at 1.2 kW/cm^2 focal intensity.[56] The time of sacrifice was staggered to study the evolution of histological changes. When compared with a control group, which did not receive HIFU, there was a significant improvement in the control of metastatic spread in the treated group and in the treatment group, in which 4/6 of the primary tumours were completely eradicated.

In 2003, Yu et al. performed a study of therapeutic efficacy in which ablation was attempted in both kidneys of 40 rabbits, using a clinical HIFU device known as the Model-JC Tumour Therapy System (Chongqing HAIFU Company),[57] described later. Ultrasound contrast agents are commonly gas filled microbubbles, typically 3 μm in diameter, and which are used to improve the contrast in diagnostic ultrasound images.[58] In an attempt to improve efficiency of energy disposition in HIFU ablations of the kidney, the study examined whether the presence of systemically circulating microbubbles could modify the acoustic properties of kidney tissue. Animals were randomised to receiving intravenous saline or an isovolumetric microbubble agent prior to insonication. Using the ultrasound-guidance system, microbubbles were seen to distribute rapidly throughout the kidney after administration. For the purposes of this study, a 1-MHz transducer of 15 cm in both diameter and focal length was selected for sonication. HIFU was applied using a linear (moving-beam) scan of 1 cm, 0.5 cm below the renal capsule, at a velocity of 3 mm/s in both groups (spatial average temporal average focal intensity, I_{SATA}, of 14.3 kW/cm^2) and was repeated until therapeutic effects were seen, as determined by greyscale echo changes. Repeated linear scan mode was used to protect near field tissues due to the transient dwell time at any given focal point. Animals were sacrificed after 24 hours, and the kidneys were harvested. All 40 left kidneys were treated but only 26 right ones were due to the presence of structures obstructing the path for ultrasound propagation. All treated kidneys showed evidence of damage with no damage to overlying tissues. The necrosis rate (cm^3/s) was quantified in order to evaluate therapeutic efficacy. This rate was significantly higher in the group of rabbits receiving the microbubble agent. Furthermore, pathological analysis revealed that no tissue was spared within the exposed regions of both groups, and both macroscopic and histological analysis revealed a sharp demarcation between viable and necrotic tissues.

In 2003, a Sonablate 200 (Focus Surgery, Indianapolis, Indiana) HIFU device (4 MHz, 3 cm focal length) was modified for laparoscopic use and used in vivo in a porcine model by Paterson et al.[59] HIFU was applied at 26 W_{ac} power, 5 s on 6 s off, over an average activation time of 18.3 minutes. The results demonstrated reproducible partial kidney ablation, with no collateral damage, and pathological assessment demonstrated well-demarcated lesions with complete and homogeneous tissue destruction.

Around the same time, Damianou demonstrated the capability of an extracorporeal 4-MHz piezoelectric ceramic transducer (PZT4, Etalon, Lebanon, IN) rigidly mounted on a 3D positioning system to perform volumetric ablations of normal renal parenchyma of both ex vivo and in vivo porcine kidneys, using grids of lesions (e.g. 8 × 8 with 3-mm spacing).[60] HIFU lesions were generated using exposures of 5 s, with average in situ spatial average intensity (I_{SA}) of 2 kW/cm^2 at a focal depth of 15 mm. Successful necrosis of the cortex was noted in all 12 kidneys in vivo, with lesions being noted to be smaller than ex vivo ablations made using the same device.

13.3 Clinical Considerations of Ablative HIFU for Kidney Tumours

Given the wide range of clinical applications for HIFU, there are currently a variety of optimised clinical HIFU devices on the market for extracorporeal,[41, 42, 61–63] interstitial[64] or intracavitary use,[65] the first being the only truly non-invasive approach. Interstitial applications include an intravascular approach for cardiac ablation,[66] whilst intracavitary applications include the trans-rectal approach for the prostate.[67]

Specifically designed laparoscopic devices have fairly recently been used for laparoscopic ablation of small renal tumours including the Sonatherm device (Misonix, Inc., NY, USA). One 10-patient study demonstrated complete ablation of 4 of 7 excised tumours of around 10 cm^3 volume without complication[68] and a 12-patient UK case series has demonstrated safety and feasibility of the laparoscopic technique following optimisation of the ablation protocol.[69] However, whilst laparoscopic devices may have a useful role in particular clinical settings for the treatment of small renal cancers, one of HIFU's most attractive capabilities, that is non-invasive yet highly specific tissue targeting (shared only with external radiotherapy, photodynamic therapy, molecular targeted chemotherapeutics and radionuclide therapies), is lost in laparoscopic surgery.

Promising clinical outcomes for extracorporeal renal ablations have been demonstrated using a variety of device designs: handheld or non-portable, US- or MR-guided, single element or phased array, concave or cylindrical transducers with parabolic reflectors. Transducers built for delivering ablation at short distances, for use in interstitial or intracavitary devices, tend to operate at the higher frequencies of 3–4MHz,[70] producing smaller, well-defined lesions. Whilst such devices have been used to perform ex vivo[49] or laparoscopic[59] kidney ablations in animal studies, they are not suitable for extracorporeal kidney ablations in human subjects due to their smaller transducer diameters and higher frequencies, with consequent inadequate depth of penetration.

For successful extracorporeal kidney HIFU ablation, in order to create ablative lesions with clear demarcation, clinical devices must employ higher powers, and transducers with lower curvature in order to achieve the required increased depth of penetration of 5–15 cm.[71] Devices must be capable of generating in situ focal intensities in the region of 1.5 kW/cm^2.[72] As the attenuation coefficient of most tissues is directly related to the ultrasound frequency,[73] clinical extracorporeal devices[70] require lower operating frequencies (of 0.8–1.6 MHz) to facilitate this increased depth of penetration.[74]

A major obstacle in extracorporeal HIFU ablation of the liver, kidney and heart is that the incident focused ultrasound must cross the protective rib cage in order to reach the target organ. Ribs obstructing the ultrasound path undergo very high levels of absorption and reflection of the transmitted energy, and thus begin to heat up, with consequent unwanted thermal effects of the overlying tissues and skin, a major side effect of ablative treatments across the ribs.[74] As the rib position becomes closer to the focal point, the off-target temperature rises are greater and the focal intensity decreases,[75] both being undesirable results, as consequently higher powers are required to achieve ablation, thus pushing the rib temperature up further.

Due to physical limitations, at the cost of device portability, clinical extracorporeal devices employ either single or multiple-element transducers with a large diameter, upwards of 10 cm. With increasing transducer diameter the larger surface area reduces the energy density crossing the skin, fat, muscle and ribs, thus minimising off target-effects for the same focal intensity compared with a smaller transducer. In addition, a larger transducer will naturally reduce the potential impact of rib shielding due to a larger area of incident wave transmission. This is because larger-diameter transducers transmit energy through several intercostal spaces simultaneously, whilst a small-diameter transducer will typically transmit through a single intercostal space and thus, for some target positions, may undergo a significantly greater shielding effect from a single rib lying within the transmitted ultrasound field.

In addition to reducing the energy density transmitted across the costal wall, minimising rib heating, larger-diameter transducers have greater curvature consequent with increased depth of penetration, making them ideal for extracorporeal use. Since their introduction by McGough et al.[76] and Botros et al.[77, 78] in the late 1990s, phased array HIFU devices have been under investigation[55, 75, 79–88] for their ability to steer the focus through the intercostal spaces, thus minimising unwanted effects such as rib overheating or reflections. Phased array devices have typically been designed for non-portable extracorporeal applications using large-diameter multiple-element transducers; however, portable phased array devices are now emerging.[89] HIFU devices with this so-called 'beam-steering' technology are now in clinical use. These include the Sonalleve MRgHIFU device (Philips Healthcare),[62] although this is not yet a clinically established technique for transcostal kidney ablations.

The Model-JC and JC200 Tumour Therapy Systems (Chongqing HAIFU Company) are extracorporeal clinical devices approved by China's State Food and Drug Administration (SFDA). The devices indicated for use in solid tumours including primary and metastatic liver cancer, kidney cancer, pancreatic cancer, breast cancer, primary and metastatic malignant bone tumours, soft tissue sarcomas and benign tumours such as uterine fibroids and breast fibroadenomas. In 2005 and 2009 respectively, the Model-JC and JC200 devices gained European Conformity (CE) marking for treatment of the liver, breast, pancreas, uterus, bone and soft tissues, subsequently superseded by UK Conformity Assessed (UKCA) marking. They have since been used to treat a large number of patients worldwide, including in China, Japan, Korea, United Kingdom, Italy, Spain, Russia, Romania, Ukraine and Saudi Arabia.[90] An interchangeable therapeutic transducer lies in the centre of the treatment table immersed in a reservoir of degassed water, and can be moved with millimetric precision in orthogonal axes via a computer console. The Model-JC has operating frequencies of 0.8–1.6 MHz and generates free field focal intensities of 5–15 kW/cm^2 at focal lengths of 9–15 cm.[91] The Model JC200 has operating frequencies of 0.8–2.4 MHz with a maximum free field focal intensity of 25 kW/cm^2 for similar focal depths. Both devices have a co-axially aligned 3.5-MHz diagnostic ultrasound probe, which lies in a central aperture of the therapy transducer. These diagnostic probes can be used to provide on-line targeting and feedback based on the presence or absence of hyperechoic signal following attempted ablation. By controlled translational movements of the transducer along Cartesian axes, driven from the operating interface, the device offers a conventional dot-by-dot approach to forming rows, planes and volumes, and a linear mode, which provides lines of continuous sonication for more rapid dose 'painting' of the target volume.

Depending on the target organ, ablative HIFU can be performed with the patient fully conscious, under light sedation or under regional or general anaesthetic (GA).[92] Whilst light sedation allows the patient to provide verbal feedback based on their sensations, such as pain from nerve stimulation, it offers no respiratory control. Despite being retroperitoneal, respiratory-related movement of the kidney, with 16–17 mm movements in the cranio-caudal direction,[93] has long been an important consideration for targeted therapy of the upper abdominal organs.[94] For HIFU ablation of intra-abdominal tumours, although one clinical study proceeded without,[72] GA is usually required in order for the patient to remain immobile throughout the treatment.[92] Furthermore, accurate placement of one lesion next to another in order to form rows and volumes requires a stable target organ, and relatively long treatment times, make breath holding impractical. Under GA, increased control over ventilation using respiratory gating,[92] lung separation techniques, such as bronchial blocking and double-lumen intubation for single lung ventilation,[95–97] have proved to be of great value for stabilisation of upper abdominal target organs in HIFU ablations. High-frequency jet ventilation, which has a role in percutaneous ablation of (microwave, radiofrequency and cryoablation) of intrathoracic and intra-abdominal organs including the liver,[98] kidneys and heart[99–101] and has shown benefit in microwave lung ablation,[102] also offers a less-invasive alternative for HIFU anaesthesia (see Chapter 24) (TARDOX Trial, Oxford, UK).[103] Another group has developed a sophisticated motion tracking platform integrated within an MRgFUS device, for ablation of abdominal targets such as the liver.[104]

13.4 Expert Commentary

The mechanisms for the effects induced by HIFU on neoplastic tissues are likely to comprise both direct and indirect destructive effects.[105–107] Evidence from pre-clinical studies has shown that HIFU can induce thermal damage in small vessels, depriving cancer cells of vital nutrients and oxygen.[108–111] This mechanism is likely to contribute to the instantaneous and irreversible cell death insults from the direct and instantaneous thermal and cavitation effects of HIFU.[112] Between 1997 and 1999, Wu et al. examined vessel destruction in 164 patients receiving extracorporeal HIFU for solid malignancies histologically, the majority being liver tumours.[113] Comprehensive radiological follow-up was performed, including contrast-enhanced MRI, colour Doppler US imaging, digital subtraction angiography (DSA) and dynamic radionuclide scanning. All modalities revealed a reduction, or absence, of blood supply in the treated region, indicating successful ablation. Thirty patients went on to have conventional surgery 1–2 weeks post-HIFU and histopathology revealed homogenous coagulation necrosis of tumour tissue and severe destruction of small blood vessels including arteries and veins in the treated region. It is known that the neoplastic microvasculature is more sensitive to hyperthermia-induced injury than that of normal tissue due to key histological differences, thus potentiating secondary tumour cell death.[114–116] This study concluded that HIFU induces neoplastic tumour vessel damage and this mechanism likely to contribute to coagulative necrosis by secondary tumour death.

Since the early pre-clinical histological studies of HIFU lesions in tissue,[107, 109, 112, 117, 118] several clinical studies involving surgical resection post-HIFU have been undertaken that have employed histological analysis to confirm the presence, and extent, of ablation in tissue sections,[108, 119, 120] and, more specifically, renal tumours.[42, 121] Haematoxylin and eosin (H&E) stain (Figure 13.1) can be used to demonstrate coagulative necrosis and irreversible cell death, by identifying the histological features of nuclear pyknosis, erythrocyte disruption, loss of cell membrane detail, granular protein deposits on vessel walls, endothelial damage and homogenisation of vascular smooth muscle.[120, 121] In particular, lesions in tissue harvested shortly after HIFU have classically been described as demonstrating an 'island and moat' appearance, where some regions of the central 'island' of tissue may look normal due to instantaneous heat fixation.[122] The central area is surrounded by a penumbra or 'moat' of clear cellular debris, and at its outer edge there is a very sharp demarcation from unaffected tissue, with a transition zone as narrow as six cells wide.[107, 109, 120] Over days, the irreversibly damaged cells at the centre of the lesions will disaggregate

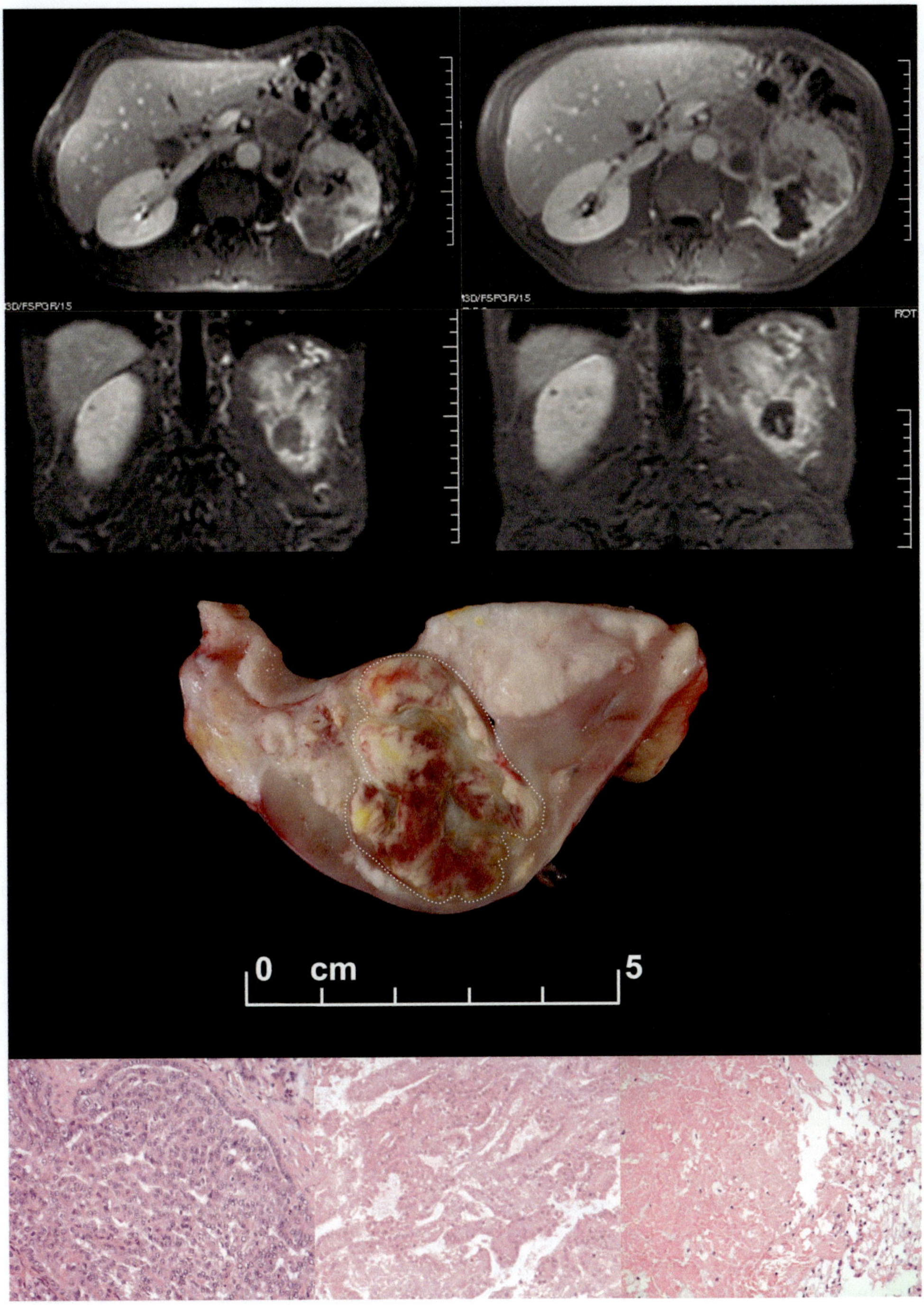

FIGURE 13.1 1: TOP – Axial (above) and coronal (below) contrast-enhanced MRI images taken prior (left) and 12 days post HIFU ablation (right), demonstrating a sharply demarcated region of reduced perfusion in the treated left kidney lesion. MIDDLE – Macroscopic view of the same large renal tumour treated with HIFU and subsequently surgically excised. The white dotted region represents the macroscopic borders of the tumour and ablated region. Several haemorrhagic regions are visible within. BOTTOM – Haematoxylin and eosin (H&E) stained sections of the same tumour, resected days later, showing viable solid variant papillary carcinoma in untreated tumour (left), marginal area of ablation zone of treated tumour showing liquefactive necrosis with inflammatory response with macrophage infiltration on the right of the image (middle) and heat-fixed ablation zone retaining architecture and nuclear outline in treated tumour (right). Images obtained courtesy of James Kennedy, Oxford, UK 113.

and demonstrate the absence of distinct nuclei or cytoplasm.[123] In the boundary between treated and untreated cells, granulation tissue appears around 7 days and there is infiltration by fibroblasts, which are involved in scarring and repair processes.[120, 124] Typically, small blood vessels of the target region less than 0.5–2 mm in diameter, depending on flow rate, are significantly damaged and occluded, with irreversible destruction of endothelial cells,[109, 125] resulting in a delayed secondary response due to reduced blood supply to the tumour.[113, 118, 126] NADH-diaphorase is a standard histochemical vitality stain, which has been utilised for electron microscopy of snap-frozen sections of HIFU-ablated tumour tissue, having the advantage over H&E in its ability to differentiate non-viable heat-fixed cells.[123, 127–129] Several other vitality stains have also been used for histological analysis post-ablation including cytokeratins and triphenyl tetrazolium chloride (TTC). Cytokeratin immunohistochemistry, for example CK8/18, are epithelial specific, and have utility in histological subtyping of carcinomas. In addition cytokeratins can offer information on cell vitality and have an advantage over NADH-diaphorase in that the stain works in paraffin sections and may demonstrate improved morphology.[129] Cytokeratins have been used in the identification of ablation of various tumour types by a variety of devices, including HIFU.[129–133]

Whilst histology will remain the gold standard for assessing the presence and margins of HIFU ablation, outside early phase studies, obtaining clinical tissue is rarely possible. Contrast-enhanced cross-sectional imaging, in the form of MR or CT, provides a convenient and reliable alternative.[41] In the early weeks following HIFU treatment, CE-MRI demonstrates a lack of central enhancement in the 'ablation zone', consistent with coagulative necrosis and destruction of tumour vasculature so that contrast cannot penetrate the region. The associated surrounding thin peripheral rim of enhancement is known as benign peri-ablational enhancement[134] and corresponds to an early inflammatory reaction.[113] CE-MRI has now become the imaging modality of choice in the assessment of response following HIFU ablation for most tumour types, including renal tumours (Figure 13.1). To ensure the full extent of tumour ablation, timely radiological evaluation by CE-MRI, or other suitable imaging modality, is critical in oncology patients. However as microscopic foci of tumour cells cannot be visualised radiologically,[134] early radiological evaluation is only a surrogate marker of treatment success, and consequently there is a need for further clinical studies with long-term follow-up and survival data.

In the treatment of renal tumours by extracorporeal HIFU ablation, whilst safety and feasibility has been demonstrated clinically, the reproducibility of ablation volumes is notably less reliable here than for its application in other solid organs, such as the liver.[42] Clinical studies have demonstrated successful ablation in only approximately two-thirds of attempted treatments[97] and, whilst promising, a higher success rate is sought before the modality becomes adopted as a readily acceptable alternative treatment to surgical excision, for example in co-morbid patients.

The delicate balance between avoidance of off-target effects, including skin burns due to rib reflections and pre-focal heating, and achievement of effective ablation, has been apparent across the breadth of pre-clinical and clinical studies. One study has compared ablation zones formed using identical HIFU parameters and focal depths, and found smaller volumes of coagulative necrosis in the kidney compared to those in liver and muscle tissue.[135] There are several possible mechanisms that may result in these smaller, and indeed less predictable, ablation zones seen in extracorporeal HIFU of the kidneys. When considering the ultrasound propagation path to the kidney, beyond subcutaneous fat, ribs overlying tumours in the upper poles have the effect of absorbing and/or reflecting a significant amount of energy, which can only pass effectively through intercostal spaces, significantly reducing the peak intensity relative to lower pole targets. Deeper still, the abdominal musculature and peri-nephric fat are also highly attenuating, and the greater depth of some renal tumours serves to further reduce the peak intensity. In addition, the kidneys are highly perfused organs and, at rest, receive approximately a quarter of cardiac output. In well-perfused organs such as the kidney, there is a consequent high level of conductive cooling.[52] To compensate for these characteristics, higher pressures are likely to be required before successful ablation, with transient echogenic changes, is achieved. With increased power there is increased the risk of pre-focal heating[136] and skin toxicity.[42]

Of all these limitations, perhaps the most important characteristic that distinguishes ultrasound propagation to the kidneys from that to the liver, is the presence of perinephric fat. This is a protective layer of fat which surrounds the kidney and is typically 2–4 cm thick. Not only is it highly attenuating, thus reducing the intensity at the focal region, but it also has a deleterious effect on the accuracy of focusing and targeting of the HIFU field. One study has determined that fresh perinephric fat obtained from nephrectomy patients attenuated the intensity of a clinical HIFU device at 0.8 MHz from 58% at 2 cm to 26% at 5 cm thickness.[136] Furthermore, the study showed that a 10-cm-thick layer of fat in front of the focus induced defocusing by 1 mm in both transverse directions, providing mistargeting by a full HIFU beam width. It may be that there is a correlation between increasing body mass index with a declining success rate in kidney ablations, but this is a currently unpublished hypothesis.

Micro-bubbles are systemically administered US contrast agents, whose enhancing effects on HIFU ablation are being investigated in pre-clinical models.[137–144] With low inertial cavitation thresholds, micro-bubbles serve to nucleate cavitation, ultimately increasing both cavitation effects and ultrasonic absorption in the target tissue. Such a combined therapy can potentially achieve a larger ablation zone in a faster time, using less total energy.[145, 146] This appears highly applicable to the problem of kidney HIFU ablations, and indeed improved efficacy of ablation has been demonstrated pre-clinically.[57] However micro-bubbles have a short half-life in vivo with rapid clearance from the circulation within minutes.[147] Furthermore they are not targeted specifically to tumour tissue and remain confined to the perivascular space due to their size, thus not penetrating the target tumour.[148] For these reasons, whilst micro-bubbles offer a promising avenue for exploration, further research and early phase clinical studies are warranted before combination therapies like this are seen in routine clinical practice as ablation-enhancing agents.

Despite promising results from early phase prospective studies in the West, there is a paucity of much-needed later phase randomised studies, which compare outcomes in cancer patients treated with HIFU with the many competing minimally invasive treatment modalities available, and this is, in part, attributable to ethical considerations. The ethics involved in randomising cancer patients to different treatments arms is a well-debated subject; when an established treatment option already exists, is it ethical to clinically explore a novel (and potentially better) treatment? The stakes are high in cancer patients, and there is a concern that for participants to consent to a randomised study, they must hold altruism above their own best interests, for the benefit of future patients.[149] This is true of any novel cancer therapy, but in favour of continued HIFU research is the large and ever-increasing body of evidence demonstrating the excellent safety profile of HIFU for oncological treatment, its clinical efficacy and repeatability. This has made it an attractive area for continued pre-clinical and clinical studies across the globe and progress continues to be made year on year.

13.5 Summary

The truly noninvasive nature of HIFU coupled with its flexibility, repeatability and favourable safety profile makes it a very attractive treatment modality for solid tumours. The absence of any increased risk of metastasis and evidence of enhancement of the immune response following ablative therapies further strengthens its case. However, as with other competing therapies, HIFU ablation of solid organ tumours has its limitations, including the relatively lengthy treatment times compared with RFA, and the obstruction of the propagation path to some target regions by the presence of bone or air-filled structures.

The safety, feasibility and efficacy of extracorporeal HIFU for treatment of kidney tumours in both curative and palliative settings has been discussed. The lack of associated morbidities such as urinary leakage, haemorrhage or infection[97] provides a clear advantage over surgical management. However, achieving consistent extracorporeal ablation in kidney tumours is particularly challenging for ultrasound-guided HIFU devices for the reasons discussed, namely:

i) The acoustic blocking effects of the rib cage
ii) The respiratory motion of the kidney
iii) Highly attenuating perinephric fat which serves to defocus the HIFU beam

Despite the challenges and the relative infancy of HIFU technology, preliminary clinical studies for renal cancers have demonstrated response and tumour stability in two-thirds of patients treated, with minimal morbidity.

Despite limitations in the expense of development and deployment, the paradigm shift 'from knife to needle to nothing'[150] in the non-invasive treatment of solid organ malignancies is taking ever closer steps to becoming a reality. Further advances in clinical HIFU devices and/or combination therapy such as the use of intra-procedural micro-bubbles[59] or pre-procedural trans-arterial embolisation[151] to lower the intensity threshold for ablation, and improve targeting accuracy, may serve to further progress this rapidly emerging and promising treatment modality. Targeted drug delivery studies using HIFU with or without microbubbles are also under clinical investigation for other cancer types.[152, 153] The advent of immunotherapy approvals for renal cancer, including sunitinib, offer opportunity for new research avenues of combined device trials.

For the future it is hoped that future improvements in device technology can lead to reproducible extracorporeal HIFU renal ablation, or that HIFU combined with intravenous agents and/or chemotherapies will achieve reliable (chemo-)ablation. Such clinical advancement would preserve the great advantage of extracorporeal HIFU over other competing minimally invasive therapies, namely, its ability to provide non-invasive and repeatable treatments. Such an opportunity would serve a great number of renal cancer patients who are under active imaging surveillance due to being high risk for surgery due to co-morbidities.

NOTE

1 Focus Surgery, Inc., Fremont, CA. Single 30-mm-diameter, curved, ceramic piezoelectric, 4-MHz element of 30 mm diameter with a 30-mm fixed focus, capable of producing temperatures of up to 90 °C at the focal zone and used for both imaging and therapy. Device prototype later became commercialised as Sonablate by SonaCare Medical.

REFERENCES

1. Luciani LG, Cestari R, Tallarigo C. Incidental renal cell carcinoma-age and stage characterization and clinical implications: Study of 1092 patients (1982–1997). Urology. 2000;56(1):58–62.
2. Chow WH, Devesa SS, Warren JL, Fraumeni JF, Jr. Rising incidence of renal cell cancer in the United States. JAMA. 1999;281(17):1628–31.
3. Jayson M, Sanders H. Increased incidence of serendipitously discovered renal cell carcinoma. Urology. 1998;51(2):203–5.
4. Chen DY, Uzzo RG. Evaluation and management of the renal mass. The Medical Clinics of North America. 2011;95(1):179–89.
5. Chow WH, Dong LM, Devesa SS. Epidemiology and risk factors for kidney cancer. Nat Rev Urol. 2010;7(5):245–57.
6. Ferlay J, Shin HR, Bray F, Forman D, Mathers C, Parkin DM. Estimates of worldwide burden of cancer in 2008: GLOBOCAN 2008. Int J Cancer. 2010;127(12):2893–917.
7. NCI. SEER Cancer Statistics Fact Sheets: Kidney and Renal Pelvis Cancer. National Cancer Institute; 2015. A vailable from: http://seer.cancer.gov/statfacts/html/kidrp.html.
8. Birnbaum BA, Bosniak MA, Megibow AJ, Lubat E, Gordon RB. Observations on the growth of renal neoplasms. Radiology. 1990;176(3):695–701.
9. Bosniak MA. Observation of small incidentally detected renal masses. Seminars in Urologic Oncology. 1995;13(4):267–72.
10. Kunkle DA, Crispen PL, Li T, Uzzo RG. Tumor size predicts synchronous metastatic renal cell carcinoma: Implications for surveillance of small renal masses. The Journal of Urology. 2007;177(5):1692–6; discussion 7.
11. Mickisch GH. Rational selection of a control arm for randomised trials in metastatic renal cell carcinoma. Eur Urol. 2003;43(6):670–9.
12. McDermott DF, Atkins MB. Interleukin-2 therapy of metastatic renal cell carcinoma-predictors of response. Semin Oncol. 2006;33(5):583–7.
13. Motzer RJ, Hutson TE, Tomczak P, Michaelson MD, Bukowski RM, Oudard S, et al. Overall survival and updated results for sunitinib compared with interferon alfa in patients with metastatic renal cell carcinoma. Journal of Clinical Oncology. 2009;27(22):3584.

14. D'Armiento M, Damiano R, Feleppa B, Perdona S, Oriani G, De Sio M. Elective conservative surgery for renal carcinoma versus radical nephrectomy: A prospective study. British Journal of Urology. 1997;79(1):15–9.
15. Clark AT, Breau RH, Morash C, Fergusson D, Doucette S, Cagiannos I. Preservation of renal function following partial or radical nephrectomy using 24-hour creatinine clearance. Eur Urol. 2008;54(1):143–49.
16. McKiernan J, Simmons R, Katz J, Russo P. Natural history of chronic renal insufficiency after partial and radical nephrectomy. Urology. 2002;59(6):816–20.
17. Stephenson AJ, Hakimi AA, Snyder ME, Russo P. Complications of radical and partial nephrectomy in a large contemporary cohort. The Journal of Urology. 2004;171(1):130–4.
18. Van Poppel H, Da Pozzo L, Albrecht W, Matveev V, Bono A, Borkowski A, et al. A prospective, randomised EORTC intergroup phase 3 study comparing the oncologic outcome of elective nephron-sparing surgery and radical nephrectomy for low-stage renal cell carcinoma. European urology. 2011;59(4):543–52 %@ 0302–2838.
19. Porpiglia F, Volpe A, Billia M, Scarpa RM. Laparoscopic versus open partial nephrectomy: Analysis of the current literature. Eur Urol. 2008;53(4):732–42; discussion 42–3.
20. Cohen HT, McGovern FJ. Renal-cell carcinoma. The New England Journal of Medicine. 2005;353(23):2477–90.
21. Solbiati L, Ahmed M, Cova L, Ierace T, Brioschi M, Goldberg SN. Small liver colorectal metastases treated with percutaneous radiofrequency ablation: Local response rate and long-term survival with up to 10-year follow-up. Radiology. 2012;265(3):958–68.
22. Hamada A, Yamakado K, Nakatsuka A, Uraki J, Kashima M, Takaki H, et al. Radiofrequency ablation for colorectal liver metastases: Prognostic factors in non-surgical candidates. Jpn J Radiol. 2012;30(7):567–74.
23. Shady W, Petre EN, Gonen M, Erinjeri JP, Brown KT, Covey AM, et al. Percutaneous radiofrequency ablation of colorectal cancer liver metastases: Factors affecting outcomes-a 10-year experience at a single center. Radiology. 2016;278(2):601–11.
24. Gillams AR, Lees WR. Five-year survival in 309 patients with colorectal liver metastases treated with radiofrequency ablation. Eur Radiol. 2009;19(5):1206–13.
25. Van Tilborg AA, Meijerink MR, Sietses C, Van Waesberghe JH, Mackintosh MO, Meijer S, et al. Long-term results of radiofrequency ablation for unresectable colorectal liver metastases: A potentially curative intervention. The British Journal of Radiology. 2011;84(1002):556–65.
26. Kunkle DA, Uzzo RG. Cryoablation or radiofrequency ablation of the small renal mass: A meta-analysis. Cancer. 2008;113(10):2671–80.
27. Burov AK. High-intensity ultrasonic vibrations for action on animal and human malignant tumours. Dokl Akad Nauk SSSR. 1956;106:239–41.
28. Madersbacher S, Marberger M. Therapeutic applications of ultrasound in urology. Application of Newer Forms of Therapeutic Energy in Urology. Marberger M. ed. ISIS; 1995. p. 115–36.
29. Fry FJ, Johnson LK. Tumor irradiation with intense ultrasound. Ultrasound Med Biol. 1978;4(4):337–41.
30. Yang R, Reilly CR, Rescorla FJ, Faught PR, Sanghvi NT, Fry FJ, et al. High-intensity focused ultrasound in the treatment of experimental liver cancer. Archives of Surgery. 1991;126(8):1002–9; discussion 9–10.
31. Chapelon JY, Margonari J, Vernier F, Gorry F, Ecochard R, Gelet A. In vivo effects of high-intensity ultrasound on prostatic adenocarcinoma Dunning R3327. Cancer Research. 1992;52(22):6353–7.
32. Goss S, Fry FJ. The effect of high intensity ultrasonic irradiation on tumor growth. Sonics and Ultrasonics, IEEE Transactions on. 1984;31(5):491–6 %@ 0018–9537.
33. Oosterhof GO, Cornel EB, Smits GA, Debruyne FM, Schalken JA. Influence of high-intensity focused ultrasound on the development of metastases. Eur Urol. 1997;32(1):91–5.
34. Gelet A, Chapelon J. Effects of high-intensity focused ultrasound on malignant cells and tissues. Application of Newer Forms of Therapeutic Energy in Urology. Marberger M. ed. ISIS; 1995. p. 107–14.
35. den Brok MH, Sutmuller RPM, van der Voort R, Bennink EJ, Figdor CG, Ruers TJM, et al. In situ tumor ablation creates an antigen source for the generation of antitumor immunity. Cancer Research. 2004;64(11):4024–9 %@ 0008–5472.
36. Hu Z, Yang XY, Liu Y, Morse MA, Lyerly HK, Clay TM, et al. Release of endogenous danger signals from HIFU-treated tumor cells and their stimulatory effects on APCs. Biochemical and Biophysical Research Communications. 2005;335(1):124–31.

37. Hu Z, Yang XY, Liu Y, Sankin GN, Pua EC, Morse MA, et al. Investigation of HIFU-induced anti-tumor immunity in a murine tumor model. Journal of Translational Medicine. 2007;5:34.
38. Wu F, Wang ZB, Lu P, Xu ZL, Chen WZ, Zhu H, et al. Activated anti-tumor immunity in cancer patients after high intensity focused ultrasound ablation. Ultrasound Med Biol. 2004;30(9):1217–22.
39. Xu ZL, Zhu XQ, Lu P, Zhou Q, Zhang J, Wu F. Activation of tumor-infiltrating antigen presenting cells by high intensity focused ultrasound ablation of human breast cancer. Ultrasound Med Biol. 2009;35(1):50–7.
40. Cranston D. A review of high intensity focused ultrasound in relation to the treatment of renal tumours and other malignancies. Ultrasonics Sonochemistry. 2015;27:654–8.
41. Wu F, Wang ZB, Chen WZ, Wang W, Gui Y, Zhang M, et al. Extracorporeal high intensity focused ultrasound ablation in the treatment of 1038 patients with solid carcinomas in China: An overview. Ultrasonics Sonochemistry. 2004;11(3–4):149–54.
42. Illing RO, Kennedy JE, Wu F, ter Haar GR, Protheroe AS, Friend PJ, et al. The safety and feasibility of extracorporeal high-intensity focused ultrasound (HIFU) for the treatment of liver and kidney tumours in a Western population. British Journal of Cancer. 2005;93(8):890–5.
43. Frizzell LA, Linke CA, Carstensen EL, Fridd CW. Thresholds for focal ultrasonic lesions in rabbit kidney, liver, and testicle. Biomedical Engineering, IEEE Transactions on. 1977(4):393–6 %@ 0018-9294.
44. Carstensen EL, Miller MW, Linke CA. Biological effects of ultrasound. Journal of Biological Physics. 1974;2(4):173–92.
45. Vallancien G, Chopin D, Davila C, Guiillonneau B, Perreira E, Veillon B, et al. [Focused extracorporeal pyrotherapy. Initial experimental results]. Progres en urologie: Journal de l'Association francaise d'urologie et de la Societe francaise d'urologie. 1991;1(1):149–53.
46. Vallancien G, Harouni M, Veillon B, Mombet A, Prapotnich D, Brisset JM, et al. Focused extracorporeal pyrotherapy: Feasibility study in man. Journal of Endourology. 1992;6(2):173–81 %@ 0892-7790.
47. Chapelon JY, Margonari J, Theillere Y, Gorry F, Vernier F, Blanc E, et al. Effects of high-energy focused ultrasound on kidney tissue in the rat and the dog. European Urology. 1991;22(2):147–52.
48. Hynynen K, Damianou CA, Colucci V, Unger E, Cline HH, Jolesz FA. MR monitoring of focused ultrasonic surgery of renal cortex: Experimental and simulation studies. Journal of magnetic resonance imaging: JMRI. 1995;5(3):259–66.
49. Adams JB, Moore RG, Anderson JH, Strandberg JD, Marshall FF, Davoussi LR. High-intensity focused ultrasound ablation of rabbit kidney tumors. Journal of Endourology/Endourological Society. 1996;10(1):71–5.
50. Watkin NA, Morris SB, Rivens IH, ter Haar GR. High-intensity focused ultrasound ablation of the kidney in a large animal model. Journal of Endourology/Endourological Society. 1997;11(3):191–6.
51. Billard BE, Hynynen K, Roemer RB. Effects of physical parameters on high temperature ultrasound hyperthermia. Ultrasound in medicine & biology. 1990;16(4):409–20 %@ 0301-5629.
52. Chen L, ter Haar G, Hill CR, Dworkin M, Carnochan P, Young H, et al. Effect of blood perfusion on the ablation of liver parenchyma with high-intensity focused ultrasound. Physics in Medicine and Biology. 1993;38(11):1661–73.
53. Watkin NA, ter Haar GR, Rivens I. The intensity dependence of the site of maximal energy deposition in focused ultrasound surgery. Ultrasound Med Biol. 1996;22(4):483–91.
54. Daum DR, Smith NB, King R, Hynynen K. In vivo demonstration of noninvasive thermal surgery of the liver and kidney using an ultrasonic phased array. Ultrasound Med Biol. 1999;25(7):1087–98.
55. Daum DR, Buchanan MT, Fjield T, Hynynen K. Design and evaluation of a feedback based phased array system for ultrasound surgery. IEEE Transactions on Ultrasonics, Ferroelectrics, and Frequency Control. 1998;45(2):431–8.
56. Tu G, Qiao TY, He S. An experimental study on high-intensity focused ultrasound in the treatment of VX-2 rabbit kidney tumours. Chin J Urol. 1999;20(8):456–8.
57. Yu T, Wang G, Hu K, Ma P, Bai J, Wang Z. A microbubble agent improves the therapeutic efficiency of high intensity focused ultrasound: A rabbit kidney study. Urological Research. 2004;32(1):14–9.
58. Blomley MJ, Cooke JC, Unger EC, Monaghan MJ, Cosgrove DO. Microbubble contrast agents: A new era in ultrasound. BMJ. 2001;322(7296):1222–5.
59. Paterson RF, Barret E, Siqueira TM, Jr., Gardner TA, Tavakkoli J, Rao VV, et al. Laparoscopic partial kidney ablation with high intensity focused ultrasound. The Journal of Urology. 2003;169(1):347–51.

60. Damianou C. In vitro and in vivo ablation of porcine renal tissues using high-intensity focused ultrasound. Ultrasound Med Biol. 2003;29(9):1321–30.
61. Ellis S, Rieke V, Kohi M, Westphalen AC. Clinical applications for magnetic resonance guided high intensity focused ultrasound (MRgHIFU): Present and future. J Med Imaging Radiat Oncol. 2013;57(4):391–9.
62. Köhler M, Enholm J, Mougenot C, Andreae T. Philips MR-guided High Intensity Focused Ultrasound (White Paper). Philips Healthcare; 2012.
63. Elias WJ, Huss D, Voss T, Loomba J, Khaled M, Zadicario E, et al. A pilot study of focused ultrasound thalamotomy for essential tremor. The New England Journal of Medicine. 2013;369(7):640–8.
64. Lafon C, Melodelima D, Salomir R, Chapelon JY. Interstitial devices for minimally invasive thermal ablation by high-intensity ultrasound. International Journal of Hyperthermia: The Official Journal of European Society for Hyperthermic Oncology, North American Hyperthermia Group. 2007;23(2):153–63.
65. Abel M, Ahmed H, Leen E, Park E, Chen M, Wasan H, et al. Ultrasound-guided trans-rectal high-intensity focused ultrasound (HIFU) for advanced cervical cancer ablation is feasible: A case report. J Ther Ultrasound. 2015;3:21.
66. Meininger GR, Calkins H, Lickfett L, Lopath P, Fjield T, Pacheco R, et al. Initial experience with a novel focused ultrasound ablation system for ring ablation outside the pulmonary vein. Journal of Interventional Cardiac Electrophysiology: An International Journal of Arrhythmias and Pacing. 2003;8(2):141–8.
67. Mearini L, Porena M. Transrectal high-intensity focused ultrasound for the treatment of prostate cancer: Past, present, and future. Indian Journal of Urology: IJU: Journal of the Urological Society of India. 2010;26(1):4–11.
68. Haar GT, Coussios C. High intensity focused ultrasound: Physical principles and devices. International Journal of Hyperthermia: The Official Journal of European Society for Hyperthermic Oncology, North American Hyperthermia Group. 2007;23(2):89–104.
69. Klingler HC, Susani M, Seip R, Mauermann J, Sanghvi N, Marberger MJ. A novel approach to energy ablative therapy of small renal tumours: Laparoscopic high-intensity focused ultrasound. European Urology. 2008;53:810–6. discussion 817-8
70. Ritchie RW, Leslie TA, Turner GD, Roberts IS, D'Urso L, Collura D, Demarchi A, Muto G, Sullivan ME. Laparoscopic high-intensity focused ultrasound for renal tumours: a proof of concept study. BJU International. 2011 Apr;107(8):1290–6. doi: 10.1111/j.1464-410X.2010.09620.x. Epub 2010 Sep 21. PMID: 21929519
71. Köhrmann KU, Michel MS, Gaa J, Marlinghaus E, Alken P. High intensity focused ultrasound as noninvasive therapy for multilocal renal cell carcinoma: Case study and review of the literature. The Journal of Urology. 2002;167(6):2397–403 %@ 0022–5347.
72. Visioli AG, Rivens IH, ter Haar GR, Horwich A, Huddart RA, Moskovic E, et al. Preliminary results of a phase I dose escalation clinical trial using focused ultrasound in the treatment of localised tumours. European Journal of Ultrasound. 1999;9(1):11–8 %@ 0929–8266.
73. Hill CR, Bamber JC, ter Haar G. Physical Principles of Medical Ultrasonics. Wiley Online Library; 2004.
74. Li F, Gong X, Hu K, Li C, Wang Z. Effect of ribs in HIFU beam path on formation of coagulative necrosis in goat liver. AIP Conference Proceedings. 2006;829(1):477–80.
75. Civale J, Clarke R, Rivens I, ter Haar G. The use of a segmented transducer for rib sparing in HIFU treatments. Ultrasound in Medicine & Biology. 2006;32(11):1753–61.
76. McGough RJ, Kessler ML, Ebbini ES, Cain C. Treatment planning for hyperthermia with ultrasound phased arrays. Ultrasonics, Ferroelectrics, and Frequency Control, IEEE Transactions on. 1996;43(6):1074–84.
77. Botros YY, Volakis JL, VanBaren P, Ebbini ES. A hybrid computational model for ultrasound phased-array heating in presence of strongly scattering obstacles. Biomedical Engineering, IEEE Transactions on. 1997;44(11):1039–50 %@ 0018–9294.
78. Botros YY, Ebbini ES, Volakis JL. Two-step hybrid virtual array ray (VAR) technique for focusing through the rib cage. Ultrasonics, Ferroelectrics, and Frequency Control, IEEE Transactions on. 1998;45(4):989–1000 %@ 0885–3010.

79. Qiao S, Shen G, Bai J, Chen Y. Transcostal high-intensity focused ultrasound treatment using phased array with geometric correction. J Acoust Soc Am. 2013;134(2):1503–14.
80. Ji X, Bai JF, Shen GF, Chen YZ. High-intensity focused ultrasound with large scale spherical phased array for the ablation of deep tumors. J Zhejiang Univ Sci B. 2009;10(9):639–47.
81. Chapelon JY, Cathignol D, Cain C, Ebbini E, Kluiwstra JU, Sapozhnikov OA, et al. New piezoelectric transducers for therapeutic ultrasound. Ultrasound Med Biol. 2000;26(1):153–9.
82. Pernot M, Aubry JF, Tanter M, Thomas JL, Fink M. High power transcranial beam steering for ultrasonic brain therapy. Physics in Medicine and Biology. 2003;48(16):2577–89.
83. Ebbini ES, Yao H, Shrestha A. Dual-mode ultrasound phased arrays for image-guided surgery. Ultrason Imaging. 2006;28(2):65–82.
84. Tanter M, Pernot M, Aubry JF, Montaldo G, Marquet F, Fink M. Compensating for bone interfaces and respiratory motion in high-intensity focused ultrasound. International Journal of Hyperthermia. 2007;23(2):141–51 %@ 0265-6736.
85. Hand JW, Shaw A, Sadhoo N, Rajagopal S, Dickinson RJ, Gavrilov LR. A random phased array device for delivery of high intensity focused ultrasound. Physics in Medicine and Biology. 2009;54(19):5675–93.
86. Cochard E, Aubry JF, Tanter M, Prada C. Adaptive projection method applied to three-dimensional ultrasonic focusing and steering through the ribs. J Acoust Soc Am. 2011;130(2):716–23.
87. Cochard E, Prada C, Aubry JF, Fink M. Ultrasonic focusing through the ribs using the DORT method. Med Phys. 2009;36(8):3495–503.
88. Daum DR, Hynynen K. A 256-element ultrasonic phased array system for the treatment of large volumes of deep seated tissue. IEEE Transactions on Ultrasonics, Ferroelectrics, and Frequency Control. 1999;46(5):1254–68.
89. Choi JW, Lee JY, Hwang EJ, Hwang I, Woo S, Lee CJ, et al. Portable high-intensity focused ultrasound system with 3D electronic steering, real-time cavitation monitoring, and 3D image reconstruction algorithms: A preclinical study in pigs. Ultrasonography. 2014;33(3):191–9.
90. Moros E. Physics of Thermal Therapy: Fundamentals and Clinical Applications. CRC Press; 2012.
91. Kennedy JE, Wu F, ter Haar GR, Gleeson FV, Phillips RR, Middleton MR, et al. High-intensity focused ultrasound for the treatment of liver tumours. Ultrasonics. 2004;42(1–9):931–5.
92. Yao CL, Trinh T, Wong GT, Irwin MG. Anaesthesia for high intensity focused ultrasound (HIFU) therapy. Anaesthesia. 2008;63(8):865–72.
93. Bussels B, Goethals L, Feron M, Bielen D, Dymarkowski S, Suetens P, et al. Respiration-induced movement of the upper abdominal organs: A pitfall for the three-dimensional conformal radiation treatment of pancreatic cancer. Radiotherapy and Oncology: Journal of the European Society for Therapeutic Radiology and Oncology. 2003;68(1):69–74.
94. Schwartz LH, Richaud J, Buffat L, Touboul E, Schlienger M. Kidney mobility during respiration. Radiotherapy and Oncology: Journal of the European Society for Therapeutic Radiology and Oncology. 1994;32(1):84–6.
95. Campos JH. An update on bronchial blockers during lung separation techniques in adults. Anesthesia and Analgesia. 2003;97(5):1266–74.
96. Brodsky JB. Lung separation and the difficult airway. British Journal of Anaesthesia. 2009;103 Suppl 1:i66–75.
97. Ritchie RW, Leslie T, Phillips R, Wu F, Illing R, ter Haar G, et al. Extracorporeal high intensity focused ultrasound for renal tumours: A 3-year follow-up. BJU International. 2010;106(7):1004–9.
98. Biro P, Spahn DR, Pfammatter T. High-frequency jet ventilation for minimizing breathing-related liver motion during percutaneous radiofrequency ablation of multiple hepatic tumours. British Journal of Anaesthesia. 2009;102(5):650–3.
99. Perkins PE. High-frequency jet ventilation during radiofrequency ablation: A case report. AANA Journal. 2008;76(3):209–12.
100. Goode JS, Jr., Ranier RL, Buffington CW, Klain MM, Schwartzman D. To the editor-on the safety and efficacy of high-frequency jet ventilation during posterior left atrial ablation. Heart Rhythm. 2011;8(8):e1; author reply e-2.
101. Goode JS, Jr., Taylor RL, Buffington CW, Klain MM, Schwartzman D. High-frequency jet ventilation: Utility in posterior left atrial catheter ablation. Heart Rhythm. 2006;3(1):13–9.

102. Chung DY, Tse DM, Boardman P, Gleeson FV, Little MW, Scott SH, et al. High-frequency jet ventilation under general anesthesia facilitates CT-guided lung tumor thermal ablation compared with normal respiration under conscious analgesic sedation. Journal of Vascular and Interventional Radiology: JVIR. 2014;25(9):1463–9.
103. Lyon PC, Griffiths LF, Lee J, Chung D, Carlisle R, Wu F, et al. Clinical trial protocol for TARDOX: A phase I study to investigate the feasibility of targeted release of lyso-thermosensitive liposomal doxorubicin (ThermoDox®) using focused ultrasound in patients with liver tumours. Journal of Therapeutic Ultrasound. 2017;5(1):1–8.
104. Mihcin, S, Strehlow J, Demedts D, Schwenke M, Levy Y, Melzer A. Evidence-based cross validation for acoustic power transmission for a novel treatment system. Minimally Invasive Therapy & Allied Technologies. 2017;26(3):151–61.
105. Fry FJ. Intense focused ultrasound in medicine. Some practical guiding physical principles from sound source to focal site in tissue. Eur Urol. 1993;23 Suppl 1:2–7.
106. Hill CR, ter Haar GR. Review article: High intensity focused ultrasound-potential for cancer treatment. The British Journal of Radiology. 1995;68(816):1296–303.
107. ter Haar GR, Robertson D. Tissue destruction with focused ultrasound in vivo. Eur Urol. 1993;23 Suppl 1:8–11.
108. Susani M, Madersbacher S, Kratzik C, Vingers L, Marberger M. Morphology of tissue destruction induced by focused ultrasound. European Urology. 1993;23 Suppl 1:34–8.
109. Chen L, Rivens I, ter Haar G, Riddler S, Hill CR, Bensted JP. Histological changes in rat liver tumours treated with high-intensity focused ultrasound. Ultrasound Med Biol. 1993;19(1):67–74.
110. Fowlkes JB, Ivey JA, Gardner EA, Rubin JM, Carson PL. New acoustical approaches to perfusion and other vascular dynamics. The Journal of the Acoustical Society of America. 1994;95(5):2855- %@ 0001–4966.
111. Vaezy S, Martin R, Kaczkowski P, Keilman G, Goldman B, Yaziji H, et al. Use of high-intensity focused ultrasound to control bleeding. Journal of Vascular Surgery. 1999;29(3):533–42 %@ 0741–5214.
112. ter Haar G. Ultrasound focal beam surgery. Ultrasound Med Biol. 1995;21(9):1089–100.
113. Wu F, Chen WZ, Bai J, Zou JZ, Wang ZL, Zhu H, et al. Tumor vessel destruction resulting from high-intensity focused ultrasound in patients with solid malignancies. Ultrasound Med Biol. 2002;28(4):535–42.
114. Denekamp J. Inadequate vasculature in solid tumours: Consequences for cancer research strategies. BJR Supplement/BIR. 1992;24:111–7.
115. Sweetland HM, Wyman A, Rogers K. Evaluation of the effect of interstitial laser hyperthermia on experimental subcutaneous tumours. Lasers in Medical Science. 1993;8(2):107–12 %@ 0268–8921.
116. Liu DL, Andersson-Engels S, Sturesson C, Svanberg K, Håkansson CH, Svanberg S. Tumour vessel damage resulting from laser-induced hyperthermia alone and in combination with photodynamic therapy. Cancer Letters. 1997;111(1):157–65.
117. Warwick R, Pond J. Trackless lesions in nervous tissues produced by high intensity focused ultrasound (high-frequency mechanical waves). J Anat. 1968;102(Pt 3):387–405.
118. Linke CA, Carstensen EL, Frizzell LA, Elbadawi A, Fridd CW. Localized tissue destruction by high-intensity focused ultrasound. Archives of Surgery. 1973;107(6):887–91.
119. Walter B, Weiss T, Hofstadter F, Gaumann A, Hartmann A, Rogenhofer S, et al. Utility of immunohistochemistry markers in the interpretation of post-high-intensive focussed ultrasound prostate biopsy cores. World J Urol. 2013;31(5):1129–33.
120. Wu F, Chen WZ, Bai J, Zou JZ, Wang ZL, Zhu H, et al. Pathological changes in human malignant carcinoma treated with high-intensity focused ultrasound. Ultrasound Med Biol. 2001;27(8):1099–106.
121. Ritchie RW, Leslie TA, Turner GD, Roberts IS, D'Urso L, Collura D, et al. Laparoscopic high-intensity focused ultrasound for renal tumours: A proof of concept study. BJU international. 2011;107(8):1290–6.
122. Wu F, Wang ZB, Cao YD, Xu ZL, Zhou Q, Zhu H, et al. Heat fixation of cancer cells ablated with high-intensity-focused ultrasound in patients with breast cancer. Am J Surg. 2006;192(2):179–84.
123. Mueller PR, Adam AU. Interventional Oncology: A Practical Guide for the Interventional Radiologist. Springer; 2011.
124. Jiang L, Hu B, Guo Q, Chen L. Sonographic and histological development of high-intensity focused ultrasound in rabbit muscle. Exp Ther Med. 2013;5(1):33–8.

125. Ichihara M, Sasaki K, Umemura S, Kushima M, Okai T. Blood flow occlusion via ultrasound image-guided high-intensity focused ultrasound and its effect on tissue perfusion. Ultrasound Med Biol. 2007;33(3):452–9.
126. Rowland IJ, Rivens I, Chen L, Lebozer CH, Collins DJ, ter Haar GR, et al. MRI study of hepatic tumours following high intensity focused ultrasound surgery. The British Journal of Radiology. 1997;70:144–53.
127. Neumann RA, Knobler RM, Pieczkowski F, Gebhart W. Enzyme histochemical analysis of cell viability after argon laser-induced coagulation necrosis of the skin. J Am Acad Dermatol. 1991;25(6 Pt 1):991–8.
128. Anderson JK, Baker M, Jaffers O, Pearle MS, Lindberg GL, Cadeddu JA. Time course of nicotinamide adenine dinucleotide diaphorase staining after renal radiofrequency ablation influences viability assessment. Journal of Endourology/Endourological Society. 2007;21(2):223–7.
129. Wang YN, Khokhlova T, Bailey M, Hwang JH, Khokhlova V. Histological and biochemical analysis of mechanical and thermal bioeffects in boiling histotripsy lesions induced by high intensity focused ultrasound. Ultrasound Med Biol. 2013;39(3):424–38.
130. Kreb DL, Bosscha K, Ernst MF, Rutten MJ, Jager GJ, van Diest PJ, et al. Use of cytokeratin 8 immunohistochemistry for assessing cell death after radiofrequency ablation of breast cancers. Biotech Histochem. 2011;86(6):404–12.
131. Lindner U, Lawrentschuk N, Weersink RA, Davidson SR, Raz O, Hlasny E, et al. Focal laser ablation for prostate cancer followed by radical prostatectomy: Validation of focal therapy and imaging accuracy. Eur Urol. 2010;57(6):1111–4.
132. Van Leenders GJ, Beerlage HP, Ruijter ET, de la Rosette JJ, van de Kaa CA. Histopathological changes associated with high intensity focused ultrasound (HIFU) treatment for localised adenocarcinoma of the prostate. J Clin Pathol. 2000;53(5):391–4.
133. Schassburger KU, Lofgren L, Lagerstedt U, Leifland K, Thorneman K, Sandstedt B, et al. Minimally-invasive treatment of early stage breast cancer: A feasibility study using radiofrequency ablation under local anesthesia. Breast. 2014;23(2):152–8.
134. Goldberg SN, Grassi CJ, Cardella JF, Charboneau JW, Dodd GD, 3rd, Dupuy DE, et al. Image-guided tumor ablation: Standardization of terminology and reporting criteria. Journal of Vascular and Interventional Radiology: JVIR. 2009;20(7 Suppl):S377–90.
135. Wang Z, Bai J, Li F, Du Y, Wen S, Hu K, et al. Study of a "biological focal region" of high-intensity focused ultrasound. Ultrasound in Medicine & Biology. 2003;29(5):749–54 %@ 0301–5629.
136. Ritchie R, Collin J, Coussios C, Leslie T. Attenuation and de-focusing during high-intensity focused ultrasound therapy through peri-nephric fat. Ultrasound Med Biol. 2013;39(10):1785–93.
137. Luo W, Zhou X, Ren X, Zheng M, Zhang J, He G. Enhancing effects of SonoVue, a microbubble sonographic contrast agent, on high-intensity focused ultrasound ablation in rabbit livers in vivo. Journal of Ultrasound in Medicine: Official Journal of the American Institute of Ultrasound in Medicine. 2007;26(4):469–76.
138. Kaneko Y, Maruyama T, Takegami K, Watanabe T, Mitsui H, Hanajiri K, et al. Use of a microbubble agent to increase the effects of high intensity focused ultrasound on liver tissue. European Radiology. 2005;15(7):1415–20 %@ 0938–7994.
139. Razansky D, Einziger PD, Adam DR. Enhanced heat deposition using ultrasound contrast agent-modeling and experimental observations. IEEE Transactions on Ultrasonics, Ferroelectrics, and Frequency Control. 2006;53(1):137–47.
140. Tung YS, Liu HL, Wu CC, Ju KC, Chen WS, Lin WL. Contrast-agent-enhanced ultrasound thermal ablation. Ultrasound Med Biol. 2006;32(7):1103–10.
141. Yu T, Xu C. Hyperecho as the indicator of tissue necrosis during microbubble-assisted high intensity focused ultrasound: Sensitivity, specificity and predictive value. Ultrasound Med Biol. 2008;34(8):1343–7.
142. He W, Wang W, Zhou P, Wang YX, Zhou P, Li RZ, et al. Enhanced ablation of high intensity focused ultrasound with microbubbles: An experimental study on rabbit hepatic VX2 tumors. Cardiovascular and Interventional Radiology. 2011;34(5):1050–7.
143. Elbes D, Denost Q, Laurent C, Trillaud H, Rullier A, Quesson B. Pre-clinical study of in vivo magnetic resonance-guided bubble-enhanced heating in pig liver. Ultrasound Med Biol. 2013;39(8):1388–97.
144. Chung DJ, Cho SH, Lee JM, Hahn ST. Effect of microbubble contrast agent during high intensity focused ultrasound ablation on rabbit liver in vivo. Eur J Radiol. 2012;81(4):e519–23.

145. Farny CH, Glynn Holt R, Roy RA. The correlation between bubble-enhanced HIFU heating and cavitation power. IEEE Transactions on Bio-medical Engineering. 2010;57(1):175–84.
146. Okita K, Sugiyama K, Takagi S, Matsumto Y. Microbubble behavior in an ultrasound field for high intensity focused ultrasound therapy enhancement. J Acoust Soc Am. 2013;134(2):1576–85.
147. Mullin L, Gessner R, Kwan J, Kaya M, Borden MA, Dayton PA. Effect of anesthesia carrier gas on in vivo circulation times of ultrasound microbubble contrast agents in rats. Contrast Media & Molecular Imaging. 2011;6(3):126–31.
148. Ferrara K, Pollard R, Borden M. Ultrasound microbubble contrast agents: Fundamentals and application to gene and drug delivery. Annual Review of Biomedical Engineering. 2007;9:415–47.
149. Edwards SJ, Lilford RJ, Hewison J. The ethics of randomised controlled trials from the perspectives of patients, the public, and healthcare professionals. BMJ. 1998;317(7167):1209–12.
150. Clayman RV. From knife to needle to nothing: The waning of the wound. Braz J Urol. 2001;27:209–14.
151. Wu F, Wang ZB, Chen WZ, Zou JZ, Bai J, Zhu H, et al. Advanced hepatocellular carcinoma: Treatment with high-intensity focused ultrasound ablation combined with transcatheter arterial embolization. Radiology. 2005;235(2):659–67.
152. Lyon PC, Gray MD, Mannaris C, Folkes LK, Stratford M, Campo L, et al. Safety and feasibility of ultrasound-triggered targeted drug delivery of doxorubicin from thermosensitive liposomes in liver tumours (TARDOX): A single-centre, open-label, phase 1 trial. The Lancet Oncology. 2018;19(8):1027–39.
153. Dimcevski G, Kotopoulis S, Bjånes T, Hoem D, Schjøtt J, Gjertsen BT, Biermann M, Molven A, Sorbye H, McCormack E, et al. A human clinical trial using ultrasound and microbubbles to enhance gemcitabine treatment of inoperable pancreatic cancer. Journal of Controlled Release. 2016;243:172–81.

14

Clinical Application of Ultrasound-Guided Focused Ultrasound Ablation for Pancreatic Cancer

Joan Vidal-Jové

14.1 Background

14.1.1 Pancreas Cancer Statistics: Stages and Percentages

Cancer is the second most common cause of death in the Western world. The American Cancer Society estimated that 48,960 Americans would be diagnosed with pancreatic cancer in 2015, and that 40,560 would die from the disease.[1, 2] Despite decades of effort, the 5-year survival rate remains at only 7%. There are no early detection tests, and most patients with localised disease have no recognizable symptoms or signs. As a result, most patients are not diagnosed until late in their disease, after their cancer has become unresectable or has metastasised to other organs. The stage distribution at diagnosis is 9% for localised tumours (stage I and II, the ones that are clearly surgically resectable), 28% for regional disease (stage III) and 53% for distant disease (stage IV).

Despite these poor statistics, we believe that there is real hope on the horizon.

14.1.2 Survival in Stage III and Stage IV Pancreas Cancer Patients with Chemotherapy Today

The median survival for patients with locally advanced pancreatic cancer (stage III) is around 6–12 months, and this falls to 3–6 months for patients with metastatic stage IVdisease.[1, 2] These times have increased with recent chemotherapy regimes.[3–5]

Ghosn et al.[3] reported a median time to progression and median survival of 4 and 7.5 months, respectively. They employed a combination called FOLFOX (fluorouracil and oxaliplatin). This combination was the gold standard for metastatic pancreatic cancer patients until the appearance of the gemcitabine combinations. Von Hoff reported a median time to progression and median survival of 5.5 and 8.5 months, respectively, but only for patients with metastatic pancreatic adenocarcinoma. Nab-paclitaxel plus gemcitabine significantly improved overall survival, progression-free survival, and response rate, but rates of peripheral neuropathy and myelosuppression were increased. Trouilloud[5] has shown a successful strategy employing fluorouracil and irinotecan combined with gemcitabine with an overall survival of 11 months.

In summary, we are dealing with a group of patients who in the best-case scenario and with the best chemotherapy options present a median expected survival of about 1.5 years. Those are the numbers we face when considering ablative options to add to chemotherapy treatments.

14.2 Clinical Use

14.2.1 Ablation Techniques for the Pancreas: Interventional Oncology Concepts

Interventional oncology claims its position in the multicentric place in which all oncological specialities converge. Interventional oncology is not surgery, nor chemotherapy nor radiotherapy. It involves a

 DOI: 10.1201/9780429162671-14

different group of treatments with direct impacts on the tumour itself that may provide local control, and with indirect impact on systemic disease through the immunological consequences of the application of the treatment. It is carried out by physicians with different backgrounds, mostly interventional radiologists, radiation oncologists or surgeons.

The concept of interventional oncology has been recently developed and includes all techniques which are aimed at local control of neoplastic disease.[6] By using these therapies, isolated lesions in different organs can be eliminated, and complete or partial responses which result in an increased progression-free interval, and even overall survival, of these patients can be elicited.[7–9] These therapies are effective in relatively easily accessible organs such as liver, lung or kidney. The pancreas, however, presents the difficulties of location and its anatomical relationships, with the added complexity of surrounding vessels. Treatment may be feasible, but it is very unusual for such treatment to produce high response rates. The problem is not only the access to the pancreas, but also getting an ablation that is clinically significant.

For all techniques that require a needle for access to the malignant lesion, it will be difficult not to damage neighbouring structures. Radiofrequency, electroporation and microwave techniques do not have easy access to the pancreas. High intensity focused ultrasound (HIFU) with real-time ultrasound guidance allows good visualisation and access, either directly to the tumour (Figure 14.1) or through the gastric window (Figure 14.2), since the thickness of the stomach wall allows HIFU ablation treatment through it.

14.2.2 HIFU Ablation for Malignant Tumours

HIFU or focused ultrasound surgery (FUS) are acronyms for a therapy that destroys tumours selectively, with no skin puncture or perforation, and with simultaneous direct control of the therapy that is being performed.[10–12] Several authors have studied and discussed the principles of this treatment, and it is not the purpose of this chapter to go deeply into this, since they are explained in more detail in other chapters of this book.[13–15]

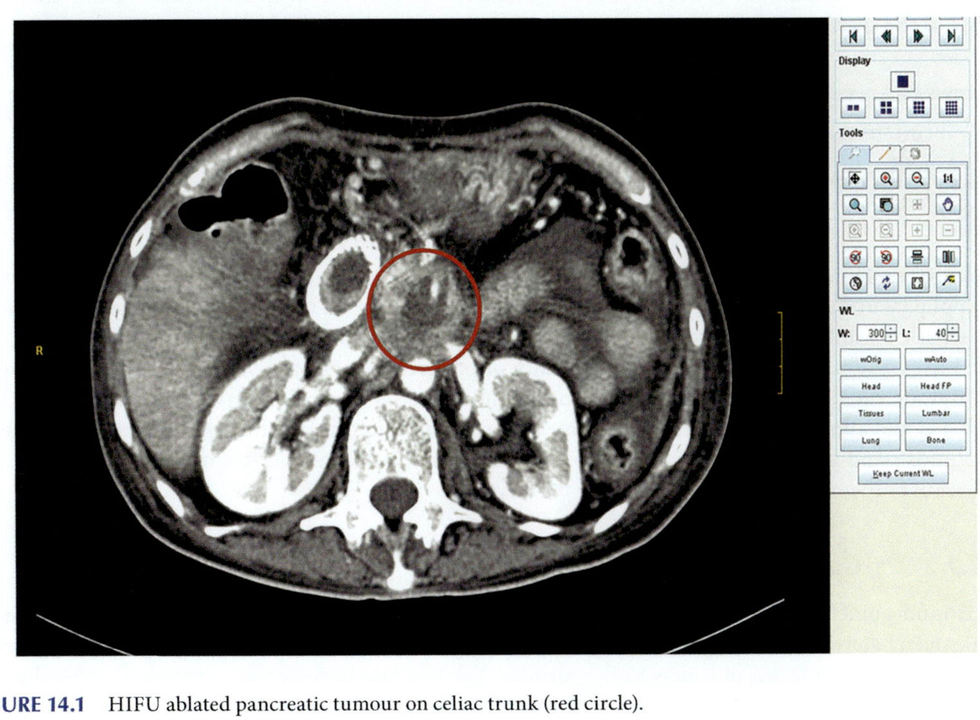

FIGURE 14.1 HIFU ablated pancreatic tumour on celiac trunk (red circle).

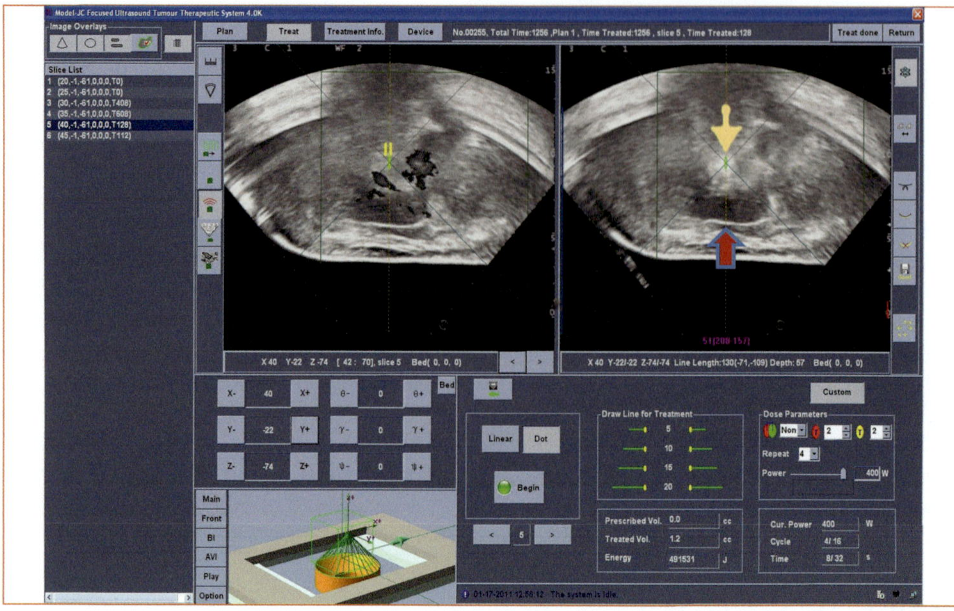

FIGURE 14.2 Treatment with HIFU from below. Patient is in a prone position. Red arrow, stomach. Yellow arrow, response to treatment.

HIFU has been used to treat primary or metastatic tumours in the liver, pancreas, kidney, prostate, retroperitoneal or pelvic malignancies, soft tissue tumours, bone metastases, breast, and thyroid nodules or even lung metastases. Its efficacy is proportional to the completeness of the ablation as well as to the bulk of the tumour treated.[16–19] Relevant issues are access to the tumours, the direct control of the ablation, and the evaluation of the response immediately after the treatment. Control of this affects the quality of the therapy and its long-term efficacy.[20–24]

14.3 Treatment Outcomes

14.3.1 HIFU for Pancreatic Tumours

14.3.1.1 MRI-Guided FUS

Magnetic resonance image–guided high intensity focused ultrasound (MRgHIFU) has been studied and applied with success in selected cases of pancreatic cancer.[25–27] It needs careful evaluation and selection of patients suitable for the procedure due to the characteristics of the device. It cannot be controlled in real time and needs to deal with the difficulty of pancreatic motion resulting from patient respiration. But, on the other hand, MRgHIFU provides much better control in terms of image quality than USgHIFU and allows temperature measurement of the tumour and skin during the ablation. This helps avoid injury and gives relevant information on thermal ablation at the tumour site, allowing better evaluation of the response of the procedure performed.

14.3.1.2 US-Guided FUS

Ultrasound-guided high-intensity focused ultrasound (USgHIFU) was developed to ablate benign uterine fibroids. Lately, it has been proposed for malignant tumours due to the characteristics of the ablation and its suitability in terms of access to the tumour. For the case of pancreatic tumours, control in real time, as well as efficacy of the ablation without side effects has become the outstanding measure for success. HIFU should be considered to be the gold standard for ablation in pancreatic tumours. Several authors have demonstrated that HIFU for pancreatic tumours is feasible with very low morbidity and no mortality.[28–38] Others consider this to be the main option along with chemotherapy for stage III tumours and stage IV that have responded to chemotherapy. Unresectable, locally advanced, late stage or similar malignant pancreatic tumours seem to benefit either from symptom control or from survival increase. The difficulties in the procedure arise from the experience of the operator, position of the tumour relative to structures that may be harmed (bowel, etc.), difficulties with the biliary stent placement and cooling of the ablation due to the nearby presence of vessels with high flow.

14.3.1.3 Palliative Intent

At present, stage III and IV pancreatic tumours are considered incurable. In this context, HIFU has been advocated as being a good option for inclusion as one of the treatment options for the provision of best supportive care. The main complications expected during the progression of pancreatic tumours are pain, due to either nerve involvement or bowel obstruction, or complications due to the involvement of gastrointestinal structures close to the tumour. In either case, local control of the tumour by means of ablation may prevent or delay the onset of these complications.[39, 40]

14.3.1.4 Curative Intent

HIFU alone cannot be considered as a potentially curable strategy for pancreatic cancer in any circumstance. At this point, the evidence does not support HIFU as a therapy that can manage cancer on its own. All options should at this point be considered as a part of a multispeciality strategy to obtain better results. In stage I and II cases, surgery is the main treatment and adjuvant chemotherapy should be considered in all cases. In stage III and IV cases, chemotherapy is the main option with radiotherapy being considered in some cases. In these cases, HIFU has demonstrated that it may be of a great help in controlling local disease and improving survival.[41–44]

In our own experience, we compared FUS-HIFU plus standard chemotherapy regimes with a cohort of patients treated at the same institution in the same period with standard chemotherapy regimens only. This was a 7-year observational retrospective comparative cohort study. Malignant advanced non resectable stage III and IV pancreatic tumours treated with FUS-HIFU + chemotherapy: 57 cases. We only included stage IV patients that had previously responded to chemotherapy. As a control group, we had a cohort of 58 patients treated at the same institution at the same time. Those patients underwent systemic chemotherapy with similar standard combinations. Mean survival was 23.5 months (6 months to 4.3 years) and overall percent survival was 18% at 5-year follow-up. Survival analysis between the two cohorts of patients showed a statistically significant benefit for the group of patients treated with FUS-HIFU plus chemotherapy ($p = 0.0025$). On multivariate analysis the hazard ratio was 0.45. Patients treated with the combination of chemotherapy plus FUS-HIFU had a 45% lower probability of dying during this follow-up period, independently from other variables (Figure 14.3).

14.3.1.5 HIFU Toxicity

Several studies have addressed safety issues arising from HIFU treatments of pancreatic tumours.[45–51] Complications reported include skin burn, abdominal wall burn, gastric or bowel perforations, pancreatitis with several degrees of severity, gastrointestinal vessel bleeding, pseudocyst formation and vertebral periosteum injury. In most cases, the severity of these complications was minimal, with percentages between 5% and 10%. The reported mortality is very low, with few cases related to the previous conditions of the patients treated.

14.3.1.6 Stent Role

An important number of pancreatic tumour cases are diagnosed from the onset of jaundice. Some series report 45% incidence of jaundice. On these cases, the placement of a biliary stent is mandatory. The usual

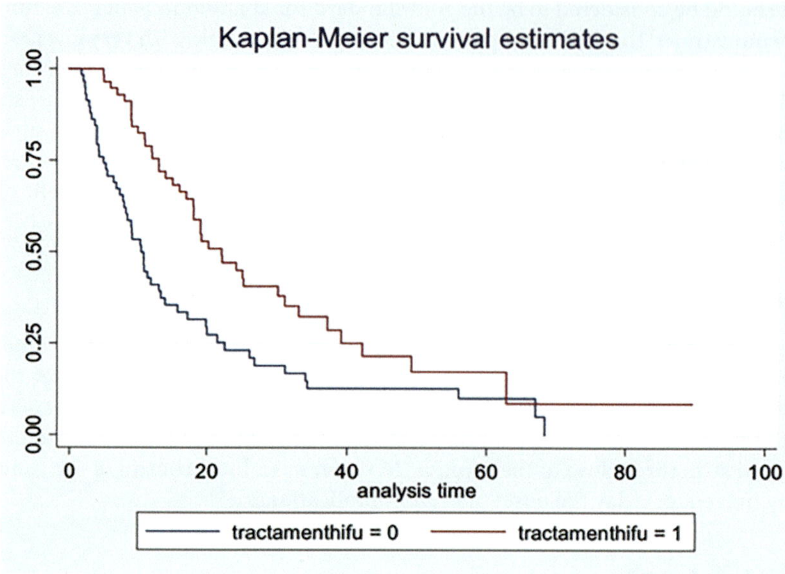

FIGURE 14.3 Survival curves of two cohorts of patients treated at the same institution with HIFU plus chemotherapy versus chemotherapy alone. There is a statistically significant benefit for the group of patients treated with FUS-HIFU plus chemotherapy ($p = 0.0025$). See text.

choice of this device is between metallic or plastic materials. Most remain permanently and become an issue to be dealt with when ablation becomes an option. In these cases, it presents an additional difficulty.[52, 53] A biliary stent will act as a barrier to complete ablation of the tumour located behind the stent. On the other hand, it will concentrate the thermal effect and may act as a mirror, reflecting the heat to tissues in front and giving the risk of thermal injury to surrounding tissues.

14.3.1.7 HIFU Response Evaluation

When considering a HIFU ablation, the issue of knowing when the ablation is completed remains unsolved when a clear image it is not seen during the procedure. Response can sometimes be seen as a "white" (hyperechoic) image at the tumour site reflecting the coagulative necrosis produced. In others, no "white" response can be seen, probably due to tumour texture characteristics or to major vessels occurring near the tumour that have a cooling effect (Figure 14.4), and we remain blinded in terms of response evaluation.[54]

Evaluation of the response once the procedure has been performed remains an issue too. Radiologists unfamiliar with this type of ablation may confuse the immediate swelling that is usual with ablation, with progression of the disease. Careful evaluation of the grey scale where a CT scan is performed needs to be considered. If MRI is employed, we suggest perfusion evaluation image sequences to evaluate tumour activity response. If a positron emission tomography (PET) scan is used, it will be difficult to distinguish between low-level inflammation and tumour activity with standardised uptake values (SUVs) between 2 and 3.

14.3.1.8 HIFU Plus Surgery, Radiotherapy or Chemotherapy

There is little experience in the use of HIFU as a neoadjuvant treatment to downgrade pancreatic tumours and to render them resectable. Wang and colleagues show a 93% resectability rate in their series of 30 borderline resectable cases.[55] In our experience, these cases would not be considered as surgical candidates and are addressed with neoadjuvant chemotherapy.

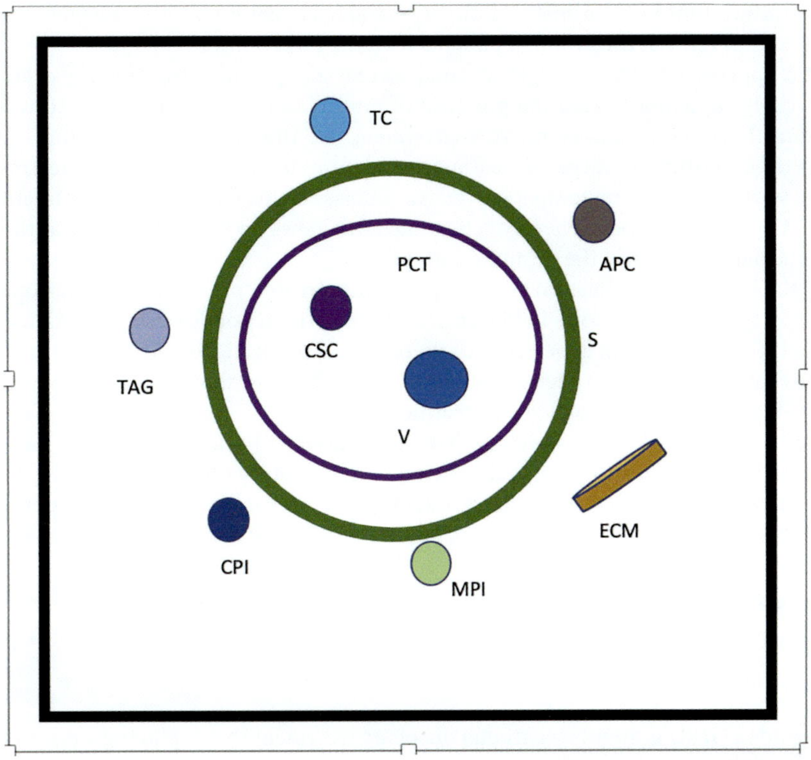

FIGURE 14.4 Constituents of the pancreatic tumour microenvironment: PCT pancreatic cancer tumour, CSC cancer stem cell, V vessel, S stromal tissue, T lymphocyte T cell, APC antigen presenting cell, ECM extracellular matrix, MPI membrane protein immunogenic, CPI checkpoint inhibitor, TAG tumour antigen.

Combination strategies that employ HIFU and radiotherapy have been reported with good success.[56] Careful patient evaluation and dosimetry analysis should be performed to avoid excessive exposure of the patient. In these cases, HIFU as an hyperthermic treatment may be considered, despite also being an ablative option.

The same strategy may apply to the combined use of HIFU plus chemotherapy. Reports are more common here.[57–63] The concurrent use of HIFU as a hyperthermic treatment is a recent trend and added to immuno-therapeutic considerations, its effect to provide enhanced delivery to the tumour may play an interesting role. Enhanced delivery of chemotherapy drugs, either standard, or with liposomes, need to be evolved, employing HIFU as a hyperthermic device. These studies are underway by the Oxford group, and we are eager to see their results.[64]

14.3.1.9 Tumour Microenvironment and Immunotherapy

In recent years, several authors have emphasised the role of the tumour microenvironment as a key factor in protecting the pancreatic tumour either from the immune system of the patient or from the chemotherapy treatments.[65, 66] If this is the case, disrupting this tumour protection may be a suitable way of increasing survival in selected patients. The advantages of this approach emphasise the effect of the liberation of tumour antigens that may be recognised by antigen-presenting cells and liberate the immune effect. A correlation with immunotherapy trials available at present indicate a positive way to dedicate research in that direction.

A study published by a group in the University of Bergen[67] shows an interesting approach. They use a combination of microbubbles (Sonovue contrast) as a sonoporation agent, activated by a common diagnostic ultrasound probe administered during standard chemotherapy treatment. This application shows prolonged survival in the group of patients with the intervention.

Therapeutic approaches which target stromal tissue, along with strategies to overcome specific immune targets have demonstrated the presence of multiple immunoregulatory pathways within the pancreatic ductal adenocarcinoma microenvironment. In this setting, combining complementary stromal-targeted and immune-targeted treatment modalities offer a more rational treatment approach. There are two very interesting review papers that summarise all available options for treating pancreatic cancer with FUS.[68, 69] Their comprehensive effort includes views on how to enhance antitumour effects by invoking the participation of the immune system.

Following the leadership in Eastern Asia on pancreatic treatments with HIFU, Europe has recently leveraged this subject.[70–73] The efforts in Pleven, Barcelona, Milan, London and Oxford have been clearly reinforced with the outstanding experience of Bonn University leaded by Milka Marinova and Holger Strunk. More than 100 cases have been successfully treated by now, showing the efficacy of a model that integrates HIFU with standard oncological treatments.

Recently, a new type of FUS, histotripsy, has been developed and tested in clinical trials in liver tumours.[74] This technique employs a "bubble cloud" that destroys tumour tissue by cavitation, and avoids thermal effects. Its potential to better interact and activate the immune responses generating abscopal effects seems greater than the other ablation methods used until now.[75]

14.4 Expert Commentary

14.4.1 Future Prospects

Ultrasound-guided HIFU is an interventional oncology treatment that is playing a role in the treatment of localised solid tumours, specially pancreatic tumours, where other options are scarce. It has proven its efficacy in terms of projected survival with low morbidity and mortality rates. Technical improvements of the device need to appear to gain momentum before the technology becomes obsolete. There are several issues to be addressed, with evaluation of response being the most important. Combination strategies between HIFU, chemotherapy and radiotherapy need to be considered to improve results.

Multicentric trials are also needed to confirm the results seen in single centre reports. We have not been successful in engaging institutions from East and West to include enough patients to test the many clinical questions that remain unanswered.

Combining therapies appears to be the most successful way of obtaining better results with the tools available today.

The role of immunotherapy seems pre-eminent as more information is being obtained about the characteristics of the pancreatic tumour microenvironment. HIFU ablation seems indicated to generate favourable immune effects.

Histotripsy is a recently developed FUS modality that does not use thermal energy. Available research shows that it may favour superior immune effects, but this needs to be confirmed in clinical trials.

REFERENCES

1. Siegel R, Miller K, Jemal A. Cancer statistics, 2015. CA Cancer J Clin 2015;65:5–29.
2. Wolfgang C, Herman J, Laheru D, Klein A, Erdek M, Fishman E, Hruban R. Recent progress in pancreatic cancer. CA Cancer J Clin 2013;63:318–348.
3. Ghosn M, Farhat F, Kattan J, Younes F, Moukadem W, Nasr F, Chahine G. FOLFOX-6 combination as the first-line treatment of locally advanced and/or metastatic pancreatic cancer. Am J Clin Oncol. 2007 Feb;30(1):15–20.
4. Von Hoff DD, Ervin T, Arena FP, Chiorean EG, Infante J, Moore M, Seay T, Tjulandin SA, Ma WW, Saleh MN, et al. Increased survival in pancreatic cancer with nab-paclitaxel plus gemcitabine. N Engl J Med. 2013 Oct 31;369(18):1691–703.

5. Trouilloud I, Dupont-Gossard AC, Malka D, Artru P, Gauthier M, Lecomte T, Aparicio T, Thirot-Bidault A, Lobry C, Asnacios A, et al. Fixed-dose rate gemcitabine alone or alternating with FOLFIRI.3 (irinotecan, leucovorin and fluorouracil) in the first-line treatment of patients with metastatic pancreatic adenocarcinoma: An AGEO randomised phase II study (FIRGEM). Eur J Cancer. 2014 Dec;50(18):3116–24.
6. Salgado S, Sharaiha R, Gaidhane M, Kahaleh. Ablation therapies for pancreatic cancer: An updated review. M. Minerva Gastroenterol Dietol. 2014 Dec;60(4):215–25. Epub 2014 Sep 12. Review.
7. Ierardi AM, Lucchina N, Petrillo M, Floridi C, Piacentino F, Bacuzzi A, Fonio P, Fontana F, Fugazzola C, Brunese L, Carrafiello G. Systematic review of minimally invasive ablation treatment for locally advanced pancreatic cancer. Radiol Med. 2014 Jul;119(7):483–98.
8. Rombouts SJ, Vogel JA, van Santvoort HC, van Lienden KP, van Hillegersberg R, Busch OR, Besselink MG, Molenaar IQ. Systematic review of innovative ablative therapies for the treatment of locally advanced pancreatic cancer. Br J Surg. 2015 Feb;102(3):182–93.
9. Keane MG, Bramis K, Pereira SP, Fusai GK. Systematic review of novel ablative methods in locally advanced pancreatic cancer. World J Gastroenterol. 2014 Mar 7;20(9):2267–78.
10. Copelan A, Hartman J, Chehab M, Venkatesan AM. High-intensity focused ultrasound: Current status for image-guided therapy. Semin Intervent Radiol. 2015 Dec;32(4):398–415.
11. ter Haar G. HIFU tissue ablation: Concept and devices. Adv Exp Med Biol. 2016;880:3–20. doi:10.1007/978-3-319-22536-4_1.
12. Maloney E, Hwang JH. Emerging HIFU applications in cancer therapy. Int J Hyperthermia. 2015 May;31(3):302–9.
13. Al-Bataineh O, Jenne J, Huber P. Clinical and future applications of high intensity focused ultrasound in cancer. Cancer Treat Rev. 2012 Aug;38(5):346–53.
14. Zhou YF. High intensity focused ultrasound in clinical tumour ablation. World J Clin Oncol. 2011 Jan 10;2(1):8–27.
15. Orsi F, Arnone P, Chen W, Zhang L. High intensity focused ultrasound ablation: A new therapeutic option for solid tumours. J Cancer Res Ther. 2010 Oct-Dec;6(4):414–20.
16. Orgera G, Monfardini L, Della Vigna P, Zhang L, Bonomo G, Arnone P, Padrenostro M, Orsi F. High-intensity focused ultrasound (HIFU) in patients with solid malignancies: Evaluation of feasibility, local tumour response and clinical results. Radiol Med. 2011 Aug;116(5):734–48.
17. Zhang L, Wang ZB. High-intensity focused ultrasound tumour ablation: Review of ten years of clinical experience. Front Med China. 2010 Sep;4(3):294–302.
18. Orsi F, Zhang L, Arnone P, Orgera G, Bonomo G, Vigna PD, Monfardini L, Zhou K, Chen W, Wang Z, et al. High-intensity focused ultrasound ablation: Effective and safe therapy for solid tumours in difficult locations. AJR Am J Roentgenol. 2010 Sep;195(3):W245–52.
19. Dubinsky TJ, Cuevas C, Dighe MK, Kolokythas O, Hwang JH. High-intensity focused ultrasound: Current potential and oncologic applications. AJR Am J Roentgenol. 2008 Jan;190(1):191–9. Review.
20. Leslie TA, Kennedy JE. High intensity focused ultrasound in the treatment of abdominal and gynaecological diseases. Int J Hyperthermia. 2007 Mar;23(2):173–82. Review.
21. ter Haar G, Coussios C. High intensity focused ultrasound: Physical principles and devices. Int J Hyperthermia. 2007 Mar;23(2):89–104. Review.
22. Wu F. Extracorporeal high intensity focused ultrasound in the treatment of patients with solid malignancy. Minim Invasive Ther Allied Technol. 2006;15(1):26–35. Review.
23. Kennedy JE, ter Haar GR, Cranston D. High intensity focused ultrasound: Surgery of the future? Br J Radiol. 2003 Sep;76(909):590–9. Review.
24. Bhutani MS. Endoscopic ultrasound guided antitumour therapy. Endoscopy. 2003 Aug;35(8): S54–6. Review.
25. Anzidei M, Marincola BC, Bezzi M, Brachetti G, Nudo F, Cortesi E, Berloco P, Catalano C, Napoli A. Magnetic resonance-guided high-intensity focused ultrasound treatment of locally advanced pancreatic adenocarcinoma: Preliminary experience for pain palliation and local tumour control. Invest Radiol. 2014 Dec;49(12):759–65.
26. Anzidei M, Napoli A, Sandolo F, Marincola BC, Di Martino M, Berloco P, Bosco S, Bezzi M, Catalano C. Magnetic resonance-guided focused ultrasound ablation in abdominal moving organs: A feasibility study in selected cases of pancreatic and liver cancer. Cardiovasc Intervent Radiol. 2014 Dec;37(6):1611–7.

27. Napoli A, Anzidei M, Ciolina F, Marotta E, Cavallo Marincola B, Brachetti G, Di Mare L, Cartocci G, Boni F, Noce V, Bertaccini L, et al. MR-guided high-intensity focused ultrasound: Current status of an emerging technology. Cardiovasc Intervent Radiol. 2013 Oct;36(5):1190–203.
28. Wu F. High intensity focused ultrasound: A noninvasive therapy for locally advanced pancreatic cancer. World J Gastroenterol. 2014 Nov 28;20(44):16480–8.
29. Zhou Y. High-intensity focused ultrasound treatment for advanced pancreatic cancer. Gastroenterol Res Pract. 2014;205325.
30. Chen Q, Zhu X, Chen Q, Wang K, Meng Z. Unresectable giant pancreatic neuroendocrine tumour effectively treated by high-intensity focused ultrasound: A case report and review of the literature. Pancreatology. 2013 Nov-Dec;13(6):634–8.
31. Xiaoping L, Leizhen Z. Advances of high intensity focused ultrasound (HIFU) for pancreatic cancer. Int J Hyperthermia. 2013 Nov;29(7):678–82.
32. Gao HF, Wang K, Meng ZQ, Chen Z, Lin JH, Zhou ZH, Wang P, Shi WD, Sheng YH. High intensity focused ultrasound treatment for patients with local advanced pancreatic cancer. Hepatogastroenterology. 2013 Nov-Dec;60(128):1906–10.
33. Li PZ, Zhu SH, He W, Zhu LY, Liu SP, Liu Y, Wang GH, Ye F. High-intensity focused ultrasound treatment for patients with unresectable pancreatic cancer. Hepatobiliary Pancreat Dis Int. 2012 Dec 15;11(6):655–60.
34. Sofuni A, Moriyasu F, Sano T, Yamada K, Itokawa F, Tsuchiya T, Tsuji S, Kurihara T, Ishii K, Itoi T. The current potential of high-intensity focused ultrasound for pancreatic carcinoma. J Hepatobiliary Pancreat Sci. 2011 May;18(3):295–303. doi:10.1007/s00534-010-0355-4.
35. Jang HJ, Lee JY, Lee DH, Kim WH, Hwang JH. Current and future clinical applications of high-intensity focused ultrasound (HIFU) for pancreatic cancer. Gut Liver. 2010 Sep;4 Suppl 1:S57–61.
36. Orgera G, Krokidis M, Monfardini L, Bonomo G, Della Vigna P, Fazio N, Orsi F. High intensity focused ultrasound ablation of pancreatic neuroendocrine tumours: Report of two cases. Cardiovasc Intervent Radiol. 2011 Apr;34(2):419–23.
37. Wu F, Wang ZB, Zhu H, Chen WZ, Zou JZ, Bai J, Li KQ, Jin CB, Xie FL, Su HB. Feasibility of US-guided high-intensity focused ultrasound treatment in patients with advanced pancreatic cancer: Initial experience. Radiology. 2005 Sep;236(3):1034–40. Epub 2005 Jul 29.
38. Wang X, Sun J. High-intensity focused ultrasound in patients with late-stage pancreatic carcinoma. Chin Med J (Engl). 2002 Sep;115(9):1332–5.
39. Khokhlova TD, Hwang JH. HIFU for palliative treatment of pancreatic cancer. Adv Exp Med Biol. 2016;880:83–95. doi:10.1007/978-3-319-22536-4_5.
40. Wang K, Chen Z, Meng Z, Lin J, Zhou Z, Wang P, Chen L, Liu L. Analgesic effect of high intensity focused ultrasound therapy for unresectable pancreatic cancer. Int J Hyperthermia. 2011;27(2):101–7.
41. Vidal-Jove J, Perich E, del Castillo MA. Ultrasound guided high intensity focused ultrasound for malignant tumours: The Spanish experience of survival advantage in stage III and IV pancreatic cancer. Ultrason Sonochem. 2015 Nov;27:703–6. doi:10.1016/j.ultsonch.2015.05.026. Epub 2015 May 27.
42. Luo J, Ren X, Yu T. Efficacy of extracorporeal ultrasound-guided high intensity focused ultrasound: An evaluation based on controlled trials in China. Int J Radiat Biol. 2015 Jun;91(6):480–5. doi:10.3109/09553002.2015.1021962. Epub 2015 Mar 28. Review.
43. Li CC, Wang YQ, Li YP, Li XL. High-intensity focused ultrasound for treatment of pancreatic cancer: A systematic review. J Evid Based Med. 2014 Dec;7(4):270–81. doi:10.1111/jebm.12128. Review.
44. Sung HY, Jung SE, Cho SH, Zhou K, Han JY, Han ST, Kim JI, Kim JK, Choi JY, Yoon SK, et al. Long-term outcome of high-intensity focused ultrasound in advanced pancreatic cancer. Pancreas. 2011 Oct;40(7):1080–6.
45. Shi Y, Ying X, Hu X, Zhao J, Fang X, Wu M, Chen TZ, Shen H. Influence of high intensity focused ultrasound (HIFU) treatment to the pancreatic function in pancreatic cancer patients. Pak J Pharm Sci. 2015 May;28(3 Suppl):1097–100.
46. Sofuni A, Moriyasu F, Sano T, Itokawa F, Tsuchiya T, Kurihara T, Ishii K, Tsuji S, Ikeuchi N, et al. Safety trial of high-intensity focused ultrasound therapy for pancreatic cancer. World J Gastroenterol. 2014 Jul 28;20(28):9570–7.
47. Ge HY, Miao LY, Xiong LL, Yan F, Zheng CS, Wang JR, Jia JW, Cui LG, Chen W. High-intensity focused ultrasound treatment of late-stage pancreatic body carcinoma: Optimal tumour depth for safe ablation. Ultrasound Med Biol. 2014 May;40(5):947–55.

48. Wang K, Zhu H, Meng Z, Chen Z, Lin J, Shen Y, Gao H. Safety evaluation of high-intensity focused ultrasound in patients with pancreatic cancer. Onkologie. 2013;36(3):88–92. doi:10.1159/000348530. Epub 2013 Feb 25.
49. Shehata IA. High intensity focused ultrasound (HIFU): Call for careful patient selection! Abdom Imaging. 2013 Apr;38(2):419–20.
50. Wang K, Chen L, Meng Z, Lin J, Zhou Z, Wang P, Chen Z. High intensity focused ultrasound treatment for patients with advanced pancreatic cancer: A preliminary dosimetric analysis. Int J Hyperthermia. 2012;28(7):645–52.
51. Jung SE, Cho SH, Jang JH, Han JY. High-intensity focused ultrasound ablation in hepatic and pancreatic cancer: Complications. Abdom Imaging. 2011 Apr;36(2):185–95.
52. Kang KM, Lee JY, Kim H, Han JK, Choi BI. Gel phantom study with high-intensity focused ultrasound: Influence of metallic stent containing either air or fluid. Ultrasound Med Biol. 2014 Dec;40(12):2851–6.
53. Hassanuddin A, Choi JH, Seo DW, Ryu CH, Kim SH, Park do H, Lee SS, Lee SK, Kim MH. Factors affecting tumour ablation during high intensity focused ultrasound treatment. Gut Liver. 2014 Jul;8(4):433–7. doi:10.5009/gnl.2014.8.4.433. Epub 2013 Dec 24.
54. Ge HY, Miao LY, Wang JR, Xiong LL, Yan F, Zheng CS, Jia JW, Cui LG, Chen W. Correlation between ultrasound reflection intensity and tumour ablation ratio of late-stage pancreatic carcinoma in HIFU therapy: Dynamic observation on ultrasound reflection intensity. Sci World J. 2013 Dec 26;2013:852874.
55. Wang G, Zhou D. Preoperative ultrasound ablation for borderline resectable pancreatic cancer: A report of 30 cases. Ultrason Sonochem. 2015 Nov;27:694–702.
56. Liu CX, Gao XS, Xiong LL, Ge HY, He XY, Li T, Zhang HJ, Bai HZ, Lin Q, Zhang M, et al. A preclinical in vivo investigation of high-intensity focused ultrasound combined with radiotherapy. Ultrasound Med Biol. 2011 Jan;37(1):69–77.
57. Dimitrov D, Andreev T, Feradova H, Ignatov B, Zhou K, Johnson C, Delijski T, Gortchev G, Tomov S. Multimodality treatment by FOLFOX plus HIFU in a case of advanced pancreatic carcinoma. A case report. JOP. 2015 Jan 31;16(1):66–9.
58. Kim JH, Kim H, Kim YJ, Lee JY, Han JK, Choi BI. Dynamic contrast-enhanced ultrasonographic (DCE-US) assessment of the early response after combined gemcitabine and HIFU with low-power treatment for the mouse xenograft model of human pancreatic cancer. Eur Radiol. 2014 Sep;24(9):2059–68.
59. Lee ES, Lee JY, Kim H, Choi Y, Park J, Han JK, Choi BI. Pulsed high-intensity focused ultrasound enhances apoptosis of pancreatic cancer xenograft with gemcitabine. Ultrasound Med Biol. 2013 Nov;39(11):1991–2000.
60. Zhong GC, Zhang XY, Chen J, Sun Y, Zhang WH, Gui YZ, Long HX, Zhu B. Efficacy evaluation of high intensity focused ultrasound combined with intra-arterial infusion of gemcitabine in the treatment of pancreatic cancer. Zhonghua Zhong Liu Za Zhi. 2012 Jan;34(1):68–72. Chinese.
61. Lee JY, Choi BI, Ryu JK, Kim YT, Hwang JH, Kim SH, Han JK. Concurrent chemotherapy and pulsed high-intensity focused ultrasound therapy for the treatment of unresectable pancreatic cancer: Initial experiences. Korean J Radiol. 2011 Mar-Apr;12(2):176–86.
62. Yuan Y, Shen H, Hu XY, Gu FY, Li MD, Zhong X. Multidisciplinary treatment with chemotherapy, targeted drug, and high-intensity focused ultrasound in advanced pancreatic carcinoma. Med Oncol. 2012 Jun;29(2):957–61.
63. Zhao H, Yang G, Wang D, Yu X, Zhang Y, Zhu J, Ji Y, Zhong B, Zhao W, Yang Z, et al. Concurrent gemcitabine and high-intensity focused ultrasound therapy in patients with locally advanced pancreatic cancer. Anticancer Drugs. 2010 Apr;21(4):447–52.
64. Grundy M, Coussios C, Carlisle R. Advances in systemic delivery of anti-cancer agents for the treatment of metastatic cancer. Expert Opin Drug Deliv. 2016 Apr 15;1–15.
65. Won Jin Ho, Elizabeth M. Jaffee and Lei Zheng. The tumour microenvironment in pancreatic cancer, clinical challenges and opportunities. Nature reviews Clinical oncology. 2020 Sep;17(9):527–40. doi:10.1038/s41571-020-0363-5
66. Carpenter E, Nelson S, Bednar F, Cho C, Nathan H, Sahai V, di Magliano MP, Frankel TL. Immunotherapy for pancreatic ductal adenocarcinoma. J Surg Oncol. 202 1;123:751–759. https://doi.org/10.1002/jso.26312
67. Dimcevski G, Kotopoulis S, Bjånes T, Hoem D, Schjøtt J, Gjertsen BT, Biermann M, Molven A, Sorbye H, McCormack E, et al. A human clinical trial using ultrasound and microbubbles to enhance gemcitabine treatment of inoperable pancreatic cancer. J Control Release 2016;243:172–81.

68. Mouratidis, PXE, ter Haar G. Latest advances in the use of therapeutic focused ultrasound in the treatment of pancreatic cancer. Cancers. 2022;14:638. doi:10.3390/cancers14030638
69. Maloney E, Khokhlova T, Pillarisetty VG, Schade GR, Repasky EA, Wang Y-N, Giuliani L, Spring M, Hwang JH. Focused ultrasound for immuno-adjuvant treatment of pancreatic cancer: An emerging clinical paradigm in the era of personalized oncotherapy. International reviews of immunology. 2017 Nov 2;36(6):338–51. doi:10.1080/08830185.2017.1363199
70. Yamaguchi T, Kitahara S, Kusuda K, Okamoto J, Horise Y, Masamune K, Muragaki Y. Current landscape of sonodynamic therapy for treating cancer. Cancers. 2021;13:6184. doi:10.3390/cancers13246184
71. Marinova M, Wilhelm-Buchstab T, Strunk H. Advanced pancreatic cancer: High-intensity focused ultrasound (HIFU) and other local ablative therapies. RöFo-Fortschritte auf dem Gebiet der Röntgenstrahlen und der bildgebenden Verfahren 2019 Mar (Vol. 191, No. 03, pp. 216–227). © Georg Thieme Verlag KG. doi:10.1055/a-0820-5564
72. Sofuni A, Asai Y, Tsuchiya T, Ishii K, Tanaka R, Tonozuka R, Honjo M, Mukai S, Nagai K, Yamamoto K, et al. Novel therapeutic method for unresectable pancreatic cancer – the impact of the long-term research in therapeutic effect of high-intensity focused ultrasound (HIFU) therapy. Curr Oncol. 2021;28:4845–61. doi:10.3390/curroncol28060409
73. Bai L, Pfeifer T, Gross W, De La Torre C, Zhao S, Liu L, Schaefer M, Herr I. (2021) Establishment of tumor treating fields combined with mild hyperthermia as novel supporting therapy for pancreatic cancer. Front. Oncol. 11:738801. doi:10.3389/fonc.2021.738801
74. Hendricks-Wenger A, Hutchison R, Vlaisavljevich E, Allen IC. Immunological effects of histotripsy for cancer therapy. Front Oncol. 2021;11:681629. doi:10.3389/fonc.2021.681629
75. Qu S, Worlikar T, Felsted AE, Ganguly A, Beems MV, Hubbard R, Pepple Al, Kevelin AA, Garavaglia H, Dib J, et al. Non-thermal histotripsy tumor ablation promotes abscopal immune responses that enhance cancer immunotherapy. J Immuno Ther Cancer 2020;8:e000200. doi:10.1136/jitc-2019-000200

15

Clinical Application of Ultrasound-Guided Focused Ultrasound Ablation for Breast Tumours

Mirjam C.L. Peek, M. Ahmed, and M. Douek

15.1 Background

Breast tumours are very common and can cause anxiety and fear in women, young or old. The vast majority of breast tumours are benign.[1] The most common benign breast tumours are fibroadenomata (FAD) which occur in about 10% of all women and are the primary finding in approximately 50% of all breast biopsies.[2] Breast cancer is much less common, but is the most common malignant tumour in the United Kingdom with over 55,920 women diagnosed with invasive breast cancer in 2018 and over 11,500 deaths in 2021.[3]

Patients usually present symptomatically with a palpable lesion detected either during self-examination, or incidentally following radiographic investigations. Furthermore, breast tumours are identified at an increasingly earlier stage, due to the wider use of mammographic screening in patients >50 years old.[4–6] A diagnosis is made using triple assessment, involving a physical examination, imaging (mostly mammography or ultrasound [US]) and a core needle biopsy (CNB).[4,7,8] In patients >40 years, breast cancer is more common, and the priority should therefore be the exclusion of breast cancer in these patients.[1]

The management of palpable and impalpable FAD is conservative. Excision should be considered in breast tumours with diagnostic uncertainty. For symptomatic and anxious patients there are two main treatment options available: vacuum-assisted mammotomy (VAM) or surgical excision; however, VAM is not licensed for the treatment of FAD.[8] In other patients, surgery might involve unnecessary excisions of benign lesions and compromised cosmesis.[7] High intensity focused ultrasound (HIFU) ablation is therefore ideal for the treatment of breast FAD, conferring advantages such as avoidance of scarring, improved cosmesis and the possibility of treating patients under local anaesthesia in an outpatient setting.

For breast cancer, breast-conserving surgery (BCS) has proven to be effective and well accepted by patients. However, BCS can be associated with changes in the size and symmetry of the treated breast, and this can lead to a detrimental effect on patient quality of life.[9] This is especially the case with larger tumours, which require large volume excisions of greater than 10%.[10] Successful treatment with BCS is furthermore dependent upon clear margins. However, since it is not possible to visualise the tumour intra-operatively to aid in determining clear margins, there are high re-excision rates of 20%.[11] Over 95% of all non-palpable breast cancers are visible on US. For the small proportion that are not, US visible markers can be positioned to identify them. This makes HIFU ideal for the treatment of non-palpable breast cancers.[12] Furthermore, with HIFU, breast tissue can be conserved rather than displaced or replaced as is performed in surgery. There is a clinical need to develop alternative techniques which further reduce re-operation rates by defining the target and the tumour margins intra-operatively. Minimally invasive ablative techniques not only provide potential benefit from the absence of general anaesthesia, but also from reduced recovery times, absence of scarring and consequent possible economic benefits.[13]

DOI: 10.1201/9780429162671-15

15.2 Established Clinical Trials

Several clinical trials have been performed over the last few years using US-guided-HIFU (USgHIFU) for the treatment of both breast FAD and cancer. In general, clinical research on a new technique usually starts with feasibility phase 1 and 2 trials on benign lesions, followed by phase I and II trials on malignant lesions, before being implemented in clinical practice. However, the first trials using HIFU were performed on breast cancer and the most recent on benign breast FAD. A systematic review of the use of HIFU in breast tumours by Peek et al.[14] noted the paucity of HIFU trials for FAD. Furthermore, it was concluded that before HIFU can be evaluated within larger prospective trials, consistent tumour and margin necrosis with reliable follow-up imaging is required.

Between April 1998 and December 2006, three trials[15–17] were conducted using HIFU for the treatment of breast cancer (Table 15.1). All trials used the JC-HIFU therapeutic system (Chongqing HAIFU Technology Company, People's Republic of China; Figure 15.1). In two studies by Wu et al.[15, 16], the therapeutic US beam was produced by a 12.0-cm-diameter, 1.6-MHz transducer with a focal length of 9.0 cm and a 3.5–5.0 MHz imaging transducer. The focal region was 0.33 by 0.11 cm and the target tissue was exposed at free field acoustic focal peak intensities from 5000 to 15000 W/cm^2 (maximum 25000 W/cm^2), using an acoustic focusing efficacy of 28000 and a maximum acoustic power of 400 W_{AC}.[18] In the study by Kim et al.,[17] the transducer had a diameter of 15.5 cm, a focal length of 13.5 cm, a central hole of

TABLE 15.1

Characteristics of Cancer Studies

Study	N (Breast Tumours)	Study Type	Anaesthesia	Margin	Follow-up
Wu et al. 2003[15]	23	RCT	IV and GA	1.5–2.0 cm	Up to 2 wk post-op when mastectomy is performed
Wu et al. 2005[16]	22	Feasibility	IV and GA	1.5–2.0 cm	2wk, 3M, 6M and 12M with US-guided biopsy
Kim et al. 2010[17]	6	Feasibility	GA	1.0 cm	2M, 4M, every 4–6M in the first year and every 5–8M thereafter.

** RCT = randomised controlled trial, IV = intravenous, GA = general anaesthesia, wk = weeks, M = months.*

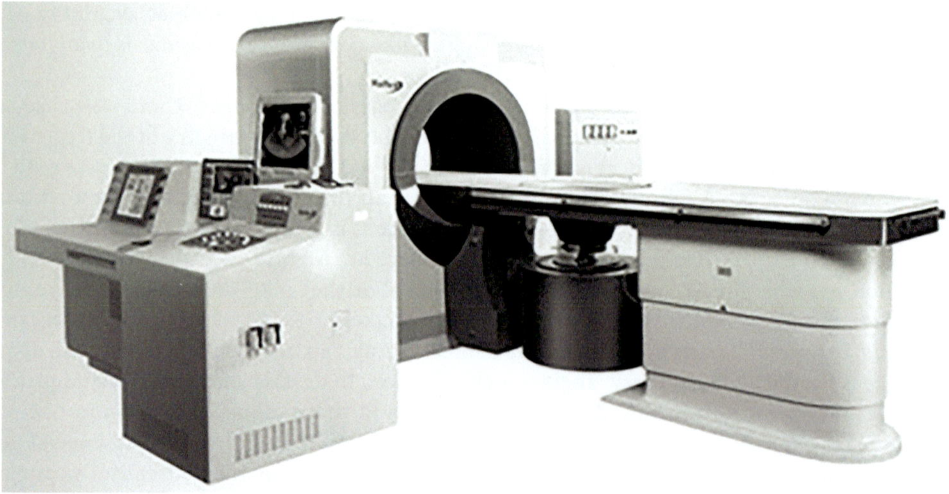

FIGURE 15.1 Chongqing HAIFU Technology (China).

6.0 cm and a frequency of 0.8 MHz. The mean focal field region was 0.11 by 0.98 cm with a focal distance of 13.5 cm. The therapy power used was between 80 and 240 W_{AC} (maximum 350 W_{AC}) and total sonication times were between 1942 and 3831 seconds. The inclusion criteria allowed patients of 18 years or older with histologically proven invasive breast cancer, single palpable tumours at least 0.5–1.0 cm from the skin and chest wall and 2.0 cm from the nipple.

Wu et al.[15] included 48 patients in a randomised control trial (RCT) to investigate the efficacy, safety and feasibility of HIFU ablation. Patients were eligible if the lesion was ≤6.0 cm in diameter and the boundaries were visible on colour Doppler US imaging. Patients with breast implants, lack of stable haematological parameters and a history of active myocardial infarction within the last 6 months were excluded. Patients were randomised to two groups; a control group (n = 25), in which modified radical mastectomy was performed, and a HIFU group (n = 23), in which HIFU was performed, followed by mastectomy within 2 weeks. HIFU was performed under intravenous sedation (n = 4) or general anaesthesia (n = 19), and a margin of 1.5–2.0 cm of normal tissue was ablated. Patient response was assessed prior to and after surgical excision using magnetic resonance imaging (MRI) in three patients and with histopathology.

Wu et al.[16] reported on 22 patients between April 1998 and April 2001 in a non-randomised prospective trial to determine patient acceptance, tumour regression, pathological changes, cosmesis, local recurrence and survival post-treatment. Patients were eligible if the lesion was ≤5.0 cm, the patient was not suitable for or had refused modified radical mastectomy or surgical excision, the lesion was visible on US and the patient had a Karnofsky performance status score of 70% or higher. Patients with three or more lesions, or with metastases visible on bone scan or radiography were excluded. Treatment was performed under intravenous sedation (n = 8) or general anaesthesia (n = 14), and a margin of 1.5–2.0 cm of normal tissue was ablated. Follow-up was performed after 2 weeks and 3, 6 and 12 months, with a physical examination and US-guided CNB.

Kim et al.[17] included six patients with small or intermediate sized (≤5.0 cm) invasive tumours to evaluate MRI features after HIFU ablation between March and December 2006. The lesion boundary needed to be visible on US, and there could be no distant metastases. In patients with large tumours (≥5.0 cm) chemotherapy was first performed for three cycles to shrink the lesion. Patients were treated under general anaesthesia and follow-up was performed at 2 and 4 months and then at intervals of 4–6 and 5–8 months, using MRI.

In 2010, Orgera et al.[19] published a case report in which USgHIFU was performed in a non-resectable retroperitoneal lymph node of a women with invasive mixed ductal and lobular carcinoma of the breast. The patient underwent wide local surgical excision and sentinel lymph node biopsy, followed by radiotherapy and adjuvant hormonal therapy for 2 years. A month after the last treatment, US showed a single 3.0 cm hypo-echoic solid mass considered to be a metastatic lymph node which was confirmed by US-guided core biopsy. The patient was not suitable for resection, and a month later the lesion had grown by 1.0 cm. The patient was enrolled into a phase I study for HIFU treatment of solid tumours under general anaesthesia using the JC-HAIFU system with a 0.8 MHz therapeutic probe and a 1.0–8.0 MHz imaging probe. She was followed up after 5 and 8 months.

Since 2011, four phase I feasibility studies[20–24] have been reported or are currently being performed (Table 15.2). All but one [25] used the Echopulse device (Theraclion, Malakoff, France; Figure 15.2) which has received European Conformity (CE) marking for treating breast FAD and thyroid nodules. The other study[25] used the JC-HAIFU therapeutic system. The Echopulse device consists of a 3.0 MHz piezoelectric treatment transducer with a diameter of 5.6 cm and a focal length of 3.8 cm, and a 7.5–12.0 MHz imaging transducer with a diameter of 3.8 cm. The maximum acoustic power during treatment is 125 W_{AC}. In general, patients were eligible for participation in the study if they were 18 years or older, with a palpable FAD diagnosed by triple assessment (and a mammogram if the patient is 35 years or older) and which was visible on US. Exclusion criteria were pregnancy or lactation, breast implants, history of breast cancer, laser or radiation therapy to the ipsilateral breast and participation in other trials using drugs or devices.

Kovatcheva and Boulanger et al.[24, 26] evaluated the efficacy and safety of US-guided HIFU in patients with breast FAD. Between May 2011 and February 2013, 42 patients were included, of whom five underwent treatment of multiple FAD. Patients were included if they were ≥18 years with a palpable FAD

TABLE 15.2

Characteristics of Fibroadenoma Studies

Study	N (FAD)	Study Type	Anaesthesia	Follow-up
Kovatcheva et al. 2014[26]	42(51)	Feasibility	IV and conscious sedation	2M, 6M, 12M
Cavallo-Marincola et al. 2015[25]	10(12)	Feasibility	LA and conscious sedation	3M
Boulanger et al. 2015[24]	24	Feasibility	–	2M, 4M, 6M, 12M
Hahn et al. 2015[23]	27	Feasibility	–	>12M
Douek et al. 2015[21]	51(53)	Feasibility	LA	2wk, 3M, 6M, 12M
Brenin et al. 2015[20]	20		–	3M, 6M, 12M

* *FAD = fibroadenomata, IV = intravenous, LA = local anaesthesia, wk = weeks, M = months.*

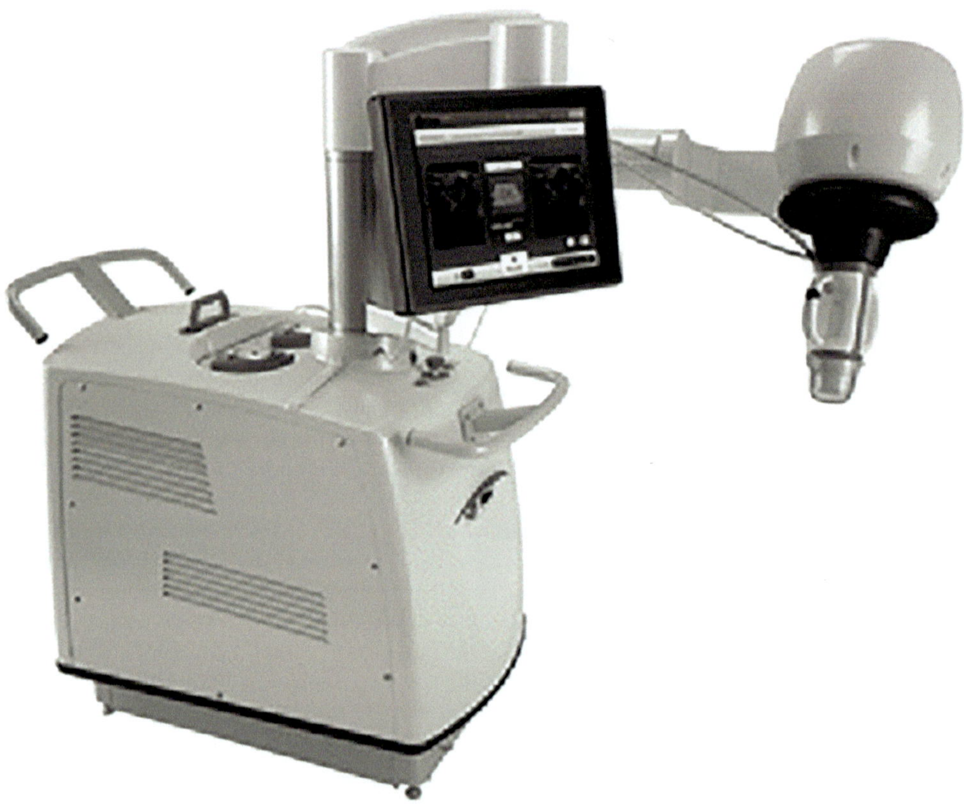

FIGURE 15.2 Echopulse device (Theraclion, France).

visible on US. For patients older than 35 years, the lesion had to be negative for micro-calcifications on mammography, and two independent readers had to confirm the FAD on biopsy. Technical inclusion criteria included a FAD size of ≥1.0 cm and distance between the focal point and the pectoralis major ≥1.0 cm. The distance between the skin and the FAD had to be between 0.5 and 2.3 cm to prevent burning of the skin or reaching the maximum depth of treatment. Post-treatment, patients were followed up by physical examination after one week and using US at 2, 6 and 12 months. Outcome measures were short-term complications, volume reduction as measured on US and pain score at the end of the treatment.

Cavallo-Marincola et al.[25] performed a small study in ten patients with 12 breast FAD between October 2013 and April 2014. Patients obtained cytological/histological confirmation of single or multiple FAD which were at least 1.5 cm in maximum diameter. Patients were treated on an outpatient basis under local anaesthesia with conscious sedation. Follow-up was performed at 3 months.

In the single-centre, prospective study described by Hahn et al.[23], 27 patients were to be recruited between December 2013 and January 2016 to evaluate the efficacy of HIFU in the treatment of breast FAD. The secondary outcome measure was the tolerability of HIFU. Inclusion was possible if the FAD was ≤2.5 cm in maximum diameter. Patients were excluded if they had interstitial laser therapy or cryoablation of a FAD within 1 year of inclusion. Follow-up was performed for 12 months.

Douek et al.[21] managed the HIFU-F trial, a feasibility study to assess circumferential HIFU treatment of FAD. Two circumferential rings around the FAD were treated by deselecting the centre of the FAD. Between January 2014 and October 2015, 50 patients were included. The primary outcome measure is the change in size of FAD volume as recorded on US imaging. Secondary outcome measures are post-treatment complications, patient outcome measures (pain prior, during and post HIFU treatment, measured using Visual Analog Scale (VAS) and palpability of the FAD determined during physical examination), mean treatment time and cost-effectiveness of the HIFU treatment compared to surgical excision of FAD. Patients were eligible if the local breast multi-disciplinary meeting confirmed the diagnosis of FAD. FAD with atypia or suspicion of phyllodes are excluded from the study. Follow-up was set at 2 weeks, 3, 6 and 12 months with physical examination and imaging US to determine the decrease in FAD volume.

Brenin et al.[20] performed a feasibility study to determine the safety and efficacy of HIFU treatment. The aim was to include 20 patients between April 2014 and May 2016. Primary outcome measures included the change in FAD volume, as measured by US, size of FAD on physical examination, patient outcomes by determining patient rated pain and patient response using satisfaction questionnaires. The secondary outcome measure was the incidence of adverse events. Patients were eligible if they had an FAD smaller than 1.0 cm, with a volume between 2 and 10 cc. An additional exclusion criterion was the presence of a cyst within the FAD. Patients were followed up at 3, 6 and 12 months.

15.3 Clinical Trial Treatment Outcomes

In the treatment of breast cancer, all three studies[15–17] have reported the outcomes of the trials (Table 15.3). The Wu et al. trial[15] included 23 patients with a median age of 46.5 ± 1.7 years. Tumours were 3.1 ± 0.79 cm (range 2.0–4.7 cm) in size and mean treatment time was 78 minutes (45–210 minutes). At 2-week follow-up, oedema surrounding the tumour was noticed, but this disappeared within 7–10 days. One patient had a minimal skin burn, and 14 patients experienced mild local pain, warmth and

TABLE 15.3

Outcomes of Cancer Studies

Study	Age (years)	Tumour Size	Treatment Time (median)	Volume	Complications
Wu et al. 2003[15]	46.5	3.1 ± 0.79 cm^3 (2.0–4.7)	78 min (45–210 min)†	Complete necrosis 100%	Oedema (all) Skin burn (1) Mild pain (14)
Wu et al. 2005[16]	48.6	3.4 cm (2.0–4.8)	132 min (60–180 min)†	Complete necrosis 100% Volume reduction: 26.7 ± 12.2% (6M) 45.2 ± 22.1% (12M) 90.4 ± 4.9% (60M)	Oedema (all) Pain (14)
Kim et al. 2010[17]	62.1	2.56 cm (1.2–3.7)	171 min (80–285 min)	Complete ablation in 67% (4/6)	Oedema (all) Pectoralis major injury (all)

* *Min = minutes, M = months; †Median, all mean ± standard deviation (range).*

sensation of heaviness in the treated breast. Macroscopic and histological examination showed complete homogenous coagulative necrosis of the target tissue, which included a margin of 1.80 ± 0.58 cm in all patients. At the margin between treated and untreated tissue, a rim of congestion was present. This represented an inflammatory reaction to thermal ablation. Using histochemical staining (Victoria bleu and ponceau's) vascular elasticity and collagen fibrin were found to be significantly collapsed and disturbed,. MRI showed a thin rim of enhancement at the periphery and an absence of enhancement at the index tumour and 1.5–2.0 cm of normal tissue. Immunohistological staining post-treatment showed no expression of PCNA, CD44v6 and MMP-9 within the tumour cells, suggesting a loss of ability to proliferate, invade and metastasise.

The results from the same patient population have been discussed further.[27–29] The first article[27] reported the use of immuno-histochemical staining, messenger RNA in-situ hybridisation and telomere repeat amplification protocol-enzyme-linked immunosorbent assay techniques to detect tumour expression of PCNA, CD44v6, MMP-9, erbB2 mRNA and to measure telomerase activity. In patients undergoing HIFU, significant alterations in PCNA, CD44v6, MMP-9 and erbB2 mRNA expression were found, together with a decrease in telomerase activity. The second article[28] described the use of biotin-streptavidin-peroxidase immune-histochemical technology to stain a variety of cellular molecules expressed on breast cancer cells, including tumour antigens and HSP-70. After HIFU ablation, some tumour antigens remained in the tumour debris, thus providing a potential antigen source to stimulate anti-tumour immune response. The third study[29] looked at the therapeutic effects in the treated region by using terminal deoxy-nucleotidyl (TUNEL) methods. After HIFU treatment, no apoptotic cells were detected in either treated tumour or normal breast tissue, demonstrating cell-cycle stability after therapy.

The trial described by Wu et al.[16] included 22 patients with a median age of 48.6 years (36–68 years). Median tumour size was 3.4 cm (2.0–4.8 cm) and the mean treatment time was 132 minutes (60–180 minutes). The median follow-up was 54.8 months. Colour Doppler US imaging was repeated every 3–6 months postoperatively and showed a heterogeneous increase in grey-scale within the treated lesions in 15 patients and an absence of blood flow in 19 patients. The tumour had disappeared on US imaging in eight patients, whilst in 14 patients the tumour had decreased in size. In two women, an increase in tumour size was seen after an initial reduction due to local recurrence. A decrease in volume of 26.7 ± 12.2% was measured after 6 months, 45.2 ± 22.1% after 12 months and 90.4 ± 4.9% after 60 months. MRI showed an absence of contrast enhancement in the treated region and a thin peripheral rim of enhancement surrounding the coagulative necrosis, indicating an inflammatory reaction to thermal ablation. Single photon emission computed tomography (SPECT) results showed a disappearance of uptake after HIFU treatment. Mild local pain was felt in 14 patients, and oedema noticed immediately after treatment disappeared within 2 weeks. Haematoxylin and eosin staining of a core needle biopsy, taken at 1 weeks, revealed no viable cells in any patient. Coagulative necrosis of the treated tumour and the normal tissue margin was seen. At 3 months, partial fibrosis was visible, and complete fibrosis could be seen at six and 12 months. Two patients opted for surgical excision due to anxiety, and local recurrence was found in another two patients. Cosmesis was good to excellent in 16 patients and acceptable in 1 patient.

The trial reported by Kim et al.[17] included six patients with a median age of 62.1 years (46–68 years). Median tumour size was 2.56 cm (1.2–3.7 cm) and a maximum acoustic power of 35 W_{AC} was used. The mean treatment time was 171 minutes (80–285 minutes). Complete ablation was seen in patients with no enhancement of the index tumour and thin rim enhancement on subtracted MR imaging. After the first session, three patients had complete ablation (50%) and after a second session performed in two patients, one more patient (17%) had a complete ablation. The other two patients underwent surgery after the first treatment due to oedema and nipple depression. Two patients with complete ablation also underwent surgery, and coagulative necrosis was found within the treated volume. The thin rim of enhancement visible on MRI corresponded to fibrosis with foreign body reaction. Injury to the pectoralis major muscle and oedema was found in all patients.

For the treatment of FAD with USgHIFU only two studies have published results; the other trials have not published thus far (Table 15.4).

TABLE 15.4

Outcomes of Fibroadenoma Studies

Study	Age (years)	Tumour Size	Treatment Time	Volume	Complications
Kovatcheva et al. 2014 [26]	32 (16–52)	3.89 ml (0.34–19.66)	118 min (60–255)	33.2 ± 19.1% (3M) 59.2 ± 18.2% (6M) 72.5 ± 16.7% (12M)	Skin blister (3) Induration (1) Hyperpigmentation (1)
Cavallo-Marincola et al. 2015 [25]	26 (18–24)	2.65 cm (1.9–4.4)	57.2 min (40–100)	50% reduction at 3M	Mild swelling and hardness of area (all)

** Min = minutes, M= months; mean (range).*

Kovatcheva et al.[26] presented the results of 41 symptomatic patients (mean age 32.0 years, 16–52 years) with 51 FAD treated under conscious sedation in an outpatient setting. Mean treatment time was 118 minutes (60–255 minutes). A second HIFU session was performed between months 3 and 9 in eight patients due to a reduction of less than 50% or an absolute volume value that exceeded 1.5 ml at 6 months. The mean FAD volume was 3.89 ml (0.34–19.66 ml). At 3 months, the mean reduction in volume was 33.2 ± 19.1%, at 6 months 59.2 ± 18.2% and at 12 months 72.5 ± 16.7%. No significant change in echogenicity was seen on US during follow-up. All patients were reported as tolerating the treatment well and no serious adverse events were documented. Short term complications were superficial skin blisters (n = 3), induration (n = 1) and hyperpigmentation (n = 1). The mean pain scale score at the end of treatment was 2.97 ± 2.75 cm (0–8.0 cm).

Cavallo Marincola et al.[25] performed a study with ten patients and 12 FAD with a median diameter of 2.65 cm (1.9–4.4 cm). The mean procedure time was 57.2 minutes (40–100 minutes) and an average of 88 sonications (54–148) were applied. The mean total delivered energy was 115.9 J/site (102–199 J with a sonication time of 3–7 seconds). At three month follow-up, a reduction of 50% was seen. No adverse events were documented, apart from mild swelling and hardness of the treatment area.

15.4 Expert Commentary

Several studies have used USgHIFU for the treatment of breast tumours. The earliest studies were performed on patients with breast cancer. The first was a 'treat and resect' study, but the following two did not excise the treated tissues unless there was a suspicion of residual or recurrence of breast cancer. However, for both studies, tissue was obtained through post-treatment CNBs to determine the presence of residual tumour, using histopathology.

The first studies of HIFU treatment of breast cancer were performed using the JC-HIFU therapeutic system, and the most recent studies, which all involved FAD, used the JC-HIFU device or the Echopulse device. The JC-HIFU device was not first used for benign lesions in published trials, but was used directly on breast cancer. Recently, Cavallo Marincola[25] used this device for breast FAD. The second USgHIFU technique is currently being optimised within FAD trials before potential progression to clinical trials on breast cancer.

Since the study by Kim et al., no other studies have been reported using USgHIFU in the treatment of breast cancers. This raises questions about what halted further progression of the technique. Currently, there are ongoing trials using MR-guided HIFU (MRgHIFU) for the treatment of breast cancer, and therefore the HIFU technique is unlikely to be the limitation. A potential limitation may be the difficulty in accurately visualising breast cancers using US. However, with a strict selection process and US-visible markers, USgHIFU trials in the treatment of breast cancer should be feasible in the future.

All breast cancer studies, even though they have limited numbers of patients (23, 22 and 6), show promising results (23/23, 22/22 and 4/6 complete ablation, respectively). However, long-term follow-up is needed to determine the recurrence rates. Currently, only one study[16] has had a follow-up of 5 years and showed two recurrences.

The current limitation of HIFU is the treatment time. In the study by Peek et al.[30] this drawback is tackled by a circumferential ablation technique. This technique has demonstrated a significant reduction in treatment time, which would make it more amenable to patients. This would not, of course, be applicable to malignant disease. Therefore, the treatment time should be reduced further through technological improvements in the treatment head, to allow the targeting of a greater zone of ablation, or several targeted sites, simultaneously.

Another limitation is the influence of patient motion upon treatment. Respiratory movements result in a shift of the target treatment zone, compromising the precision of ablation, which is completely unacceptable in oncological management. Consequently, it is imperative to develop effective immobilisation methods and, potentially, software, which adjusts for target movement. Currently, research is being conducted on such software and hopefully will be available soon to provide a precise, targeted treatment. Such advances are essential when HIFU is applied to breast cancer. The correct target volume must be treated since tissue is not excised, and no histological tumour margin assessment can be conducted. It is therefore likely that window studies (treat and resect) will be the first step in the direction of modern breast cancer trials.

While MRgHIFU offers images with good resolution, and the possibility of monitoring the treatment with thermometry, USgHIFU offers convenient inexpensive real-time imaging.[31] The benefit of HIFU treatment of breast cancer would be the previously mentioned ability to visualise the tumour margins intra-operatively using US. However, not all tumours are visible on US and/or MRI and therefore strict guidelines regarding patient selection are required. A disadvantage of HIFU is that there is no histopathological specimen available after treatment. However, all important information regarding the type, grade and receptor status of the tumour can be assessed pre-operatively using core needle biopsies. An adjuvant treatment plan can be put in place prior to HIFU treatment. HIFU can be used in combination with adjuvant treatment options such as radiotherapy, chemotherapy and hormonal therapy; the technique simply replaces the surgical section of the patient pathway. Further assessment is required to determine whether HIFU may eliminate or reduce the need for such adjuvant therapies.

Post-treatment imaging is currently not sufficiently conclusive to determine the adequacy of treatment. Therefore, in the published HIFU literature, all patients underwent either core biopsies or surgical excision post-treatment. MRI has been used in all breast cancer studies to determine the presence of complete ablation – which was recognised by an absence of enhancement seen pre-treatment and a thin rim of enhancement at the periphery. This thin rim could, however, also represent residual disease and therefore histopathology was needed to confirm a complete treatment.

Common complications included local pain combined with a sensation of heat and pressure at the treatment site, oedema, pectoralis major injury and, rarely, skin burns. These are common complications for HIFU treatment guided with either US or MRI and are all short-term and self-limiting.

15.5 Summary

USgHIFU studies performed on FAD and breast cancer can induce coagulative necrosis. However, complete ablation has not been reported consistently on histology, and the percentage of complete ablation has not been confidently predicted using imaging modalities. Well-structured, adequately powered, prospective clinical trials are now crucially needed to rectify these deficiencies in order for USgHIFU treatment to progress into mainstream clinical practice.

REFERENCES

1. Njeze, G.E., *Breast lumps: A 21-year single-center clinical and histological analysis.* Nigerian J Surg, 2014. **20**(1): p. 38–41.
2. Dent, D.M. and P.J. Cant, *Fibroadenoma.* World J Surg, 1989. **13**(6): p. 706–10.
3. *Breast Cancer.* 2013 [cited 2014]; A vailable from: http://publications.cancerresearchuk.org/downloads/Product/CS_KF_BREAST.pdf.
4. *Breast Cancer Treatment.* 25/09/2014 [cited 2014/20/10]; A vailable from: www.cancer.gov/cancertopics/pdq/treatment/breast/healthprofessional.

5. Dooley, W.C., et al., *Focused microwave thermotherapy for preoperative treatment of invasive breast cancer: A review of clinical studies.* Ann Surg Oncol, 2010. **17**(4): p. 1076–93.
6. Gianfelice, D., et al., *MR imaging-guided focused US ablation of breast cancer: Histopathologic assessment of effectiveness-initial experience.* Radiology, 2003. **227**(3): p. 849–55.
7. Greenberg, R., Y. Skornick, and O. Kaplan, *Management of breast fibroadenomas.* J Gen Intern Med, 1998. **13**(9): p. 640–5.
8. Sperber, F., et al., *Diagnosis and treatment of breast fibroadenomas by ultrasound-guided vacuum-assisted biopsy.* Arch Surg, 2003. **138**(7): p. 796–800.
9. Yoshinaga, Y., et al., *Image and pathological changes after radiofrequency ablation of invasive breast cancer: A pilot study of nonsurgical therapy of early breast cancer.* World J Surg, 2013. **37**(2): p. 356–63.
10. Cochrane, R.A., et al., *Cosmesis and satisfaction after breast-conserving surgery correlates with the percentage of breast volume excised.* Br J Surg, 2003. **90**(12): p. 1505–1509.
11. Jeevan, R., et al., *Reoperation rates after breast conserving surgery for breast cancer among women in England: retrospective study of hospital episode statistics.* Br Med J, 2012. **345**: p. e4505.
12. Ahmed, M., et al., *Surgical treatment of nonpalpable primary invasive and in situ breast cancer.* Nature Reviews Clinical Oncology. 2015 Nov;12(11):645–63.
13. Furusawa, H., et al., *Magnetic resonance-guided focused ultrasound surgery of breast cancer: reliability and effectiveness.* J Am Coll Surg, 2006. **203**(1): p. 54–63.
14. Peek, M.C., et al., *Systematic review of high-intensity focused ultrasound ablation in the treatment of breast cancer.* Br J Surg, 2015. **102**(8): p. 873–82; discussion 882.
15. Wu, F., et al., *A randomised clinical trial of high-intensity focused ultrasound ablation for the treatment of patients with localised breast cancer.* Br J Cancer, 2003. **89**(12): p. 2227–33.
16. Wu, F., et al., *Extracorporeal high intensity focused ultrasound treatment for patients with breast cancer.* Breast Cancer Res Treat, 2005. **92**(1): p. 51–60.
17. Kim, S.H., et al., *The potential role of dynamic MRI in assessing the effectiveness of high-intensity focused ultrasound ablation of breast cancer.* Int J Hyperthermia, 2010. **26**(6): p. 594–603.
18. Ltd., C.H.M.T.C., *Model JC Focused Ultrasound Tumor Therapeutic System*, H.M. Technology, Editor. 2015: Chongqing, China. p. 2.
19. Orgera, G., et al., *High-intensity focused ultrasound effect in breast cancer nodal metastasis.* Cardiovasc Intervent Radiol, 2010. **33**(2): p. 447–449.
20. Brenin, R., *Treatment of Breast Fibroadenoma With High Intensity Focused Ultrasound.* Clinical Trials 2014 [cited 2014/18/11]; A vailable from: http://clinicaltrials.gov/show/NCT02078011.
21. Douek, M., *Feasibility Study Assessing the Treatment of Fibroadenomata with a Circumferential Sonication Treatment with HIFU.* Clinical Trials 2013 [cited 2014/18/11]; A vailable from: http://clinicaltrials.gov/show/NCT02139683.
22. Kovatcheva, R., *Treatment of Breast Fibroadenoma with High Intensity Focused Ultrasound (HIFU).* Clinical Trials 2011 [cited 2014/18/11]; A vailable from: http://clinicaltrials.gov/show/NCT01331954.
23. Hahn, M., *Treatment of Breast Fibroadenoma with High Intensity Focused Ultrasound (HIFU).* Clinical Trials 2013 [cited 2014/18/11]; A vailable from: http://clinicaltrials.gov/show/NCT02011919.
24. Boulanger, L., *High Intensity Focused Ultrasound (HIFU) to Treat Breast Fibroadenoma.* Clinical Trials 2011 [cited 2014/18/11]; A vailable from: http://clinicaltrials.gov/show/NCT01422629.
25. Cavallo Marincola, B., et al., *High-intensity focused ultrasound in breast pathology: non-invasive treatment of benign and malignant lesions.* Expert Rev Med Devices, 2015. **12**(2): p. 191–9.
26. Kovatcheva, R., et al., *Ultrasound-guided high-intensity focused ultrasound treatment of breast fibroadenoma-a multicenter experience.* J Ther Ultrasound, 2015. **3**(1): p. 1.
27. Wu, F., et al., *Changes in biologic characteristics of breast cancer treated with high-intensity focused ultrasound.* Ultrasound Med Biol, 2003. **29**(10): p. 1487–92.
28. Wu, F., et al., *Expression of tumor antigens and heat-shock protein 70 in breast cancer cells after high-intensity focused ultrasound ablation.* Ann Surg Oncol, 2007. **14**(3): p. 1237–42.
29. Wu, F., et al., *"Wide local ablation" of localized breast cancer using high intensity focused ultrasound.* J Surg Oncol, 2007. **96**(2): p. 130–6.
30. Peek, M.C., M. Ahmed, and M. Douek, *High-intensity focused ultrasound for the treatment of fibroadenomata (HIFU-F) study.* J Ther Ultrasound, 2015. **3**: p. 6.
31. Li, S. and P.-H. Wu, *Magnetic resonance image-guided versus ultrasound-guided high-intensity focused ultrasound in the treatment of breast cancer.* Chin J Cancer, 2013. **32**(8): p. 441–452.

16

Clinical Application of Ultrasound-Guided High-Intensity Focused Ultrasound Treatment for Primary Bone Malignancies and Soft Tissue Sarcomas

Feng Wu

16.1 Introduction

Primary bone malignancies include osteosarcoma, chondrosarcoma, and Ewing sarcoma. Of these, osteosarcoma is the most common primary malignant tumour of the bone, representing 35% of total primary bone malignancies. It is an aggressive malignant tumour in children and adolescents, with an incidence of 3–4.5 cases per million population per year worldwide.[1] Osteosarcoma can present in any bone in the body, but the most common sites are around the knee (the femur and tibia) and the proximal humerus,[2] where the bone is growing quickly.

Typically, clinical presentation includes the onset of localised pain and swelling in the affected bone. These are usually attributed to "growing pains" and commonly last for weeks to months prior to presentation. Approximately 10%–20% of patients present with macroscopic evidence of detectable metastases at diagnosis, and approximately 80% of patients present with microscopic metastatic disease, which is subclinical or undetectable using current diagnostic imaging modalities.[3] The most common site of metastasis is the lung, with bone being the second most common site of distant disease. Five-year survival rate ranges from 65% to 75% in children and adolescents with localised disease.[4] Patients with metastasis have the worst prognosis, with the 3-year survival rate being less than 30%.[5]

16.2 Diagnosis and Staging

Persistent pain in an extremity is a major symptom in patients with osteosarcoma. It is sufficiently intense to wake the patient from sleep at night. The pain is usually accompanied by swelling at the same site. For any suspected bone lesion, a diagnostic imaging protocol is carried out immediately. This includes plain-film radiography, magnetic resonance imaging (MRI), computed tomography (CT) and bone scintigraphy or positron emission tomography (PET).[6]

A bone tissue sample is essential for the diagnosis of osteosarcoma. It can be obtained using either a minimally invasive core needle biopsy approach or an open surgical biopsy. The pathological diagnosis of osteosarcoma depends on the identification of malignant mesenchymal cells producing osteoid and irregularly woven bone within the regions of tumour cells.[7] The tumour cells usually exhibit marked atypia with a high degree of pleiotropism, and multiple morphologies may exist within the same tumour, such as spindle, epithelioid, small round, and giant cells. Based on the predominant matrix being produced, osteosarcoma can be subdivided into chondroblastic, fibroblastic, osteoblastic, and telangiectatic types.[8]

The staging classification used in osteosarcoma is the Musculoskeletal Tumour Society staging scheme (known as the Enneking system), originally developed and described by Enneking.[9] This system defines tumours as being either low or high grade (I or II), intra-compartmental or extra-compartmental (A or B), and metastatic (III). For instance, stage IA represents a low-grade tumour that is intra-cortical,

 DOI: 10.1201/9780429162671-16

and IIB represents a high-grade tumour that is extra-cortical. A patient with metastatic disease is in stage III. Most commonly, patients with osteosarcoma are diagnosed at stage IIB.

16.3 Treatment

The general principle for treating osteosarcoma is based on its histological grade. It requires an expert multidisciplinary team that includes surgeons, medical and radiation oncologists, pathologists, radiologists, and specialist nurses. A combination of chemotherapy and complete surgical resection is essential for cure in patients with either localised disease or metastasis. The current management strategy for newly diagnosed high-grade osteosarcoma includes neoadjuvant chemotherapy, surgical removal of the primary tumour along with all clinically known metastases, plus the addition of adjuvant chemotherapy postoperation.[10] The goal of surgery is complete resection of disease by wide excision of the tumour. It involves limb salvage or amputation. Limb salvage surgery includes two essential steps: resection and reconstruction. It provides a safe treatment for 85–90% of patients with osteosarcoma.[11]

Surgery plays an important role in the management of patients with low-grade osteosarcoma, including central and peri-osteal lesions. These patients are typically treated by surgical resection alone, whereas chemotherapy can be avoided if final pathology confirms a low grade. For intermediate-grade osteosarcoma, surgery is also important for resection of the tumour. But the role of chemotherapy is controversial and may be associated with the same risk-to-benefit relationship as high-grade osteosarcoma.

Although osteosarcoma is a radio-resistant tumour, radiotherapy can be considered as a local control option for unresectable osteosarcoma or for challenging sites such as in pelvic, trunk, and craniofacial primary disease, where complete surgical resection may cause unacceptable morbidities.[12] Radiotherapy used for osteosarcoma includes heavy particles, proton beam therapy, and carbon ion radiotherapy. Clinical results are encouraging, and 5-year local control rates range from 62% to 67% in patients with inoperable pelvic and trunk sarcomas.[13, 14]

The treatment of osteosarcoma has evolved greatly during the last 4 decades. Unfortunately, since the mid-1980s, clinical outcomes in the survival of patients with osteosarcoma have barely improved. According to National Cancer Institute SEER program data, 5-year survival rates in patients with newly diagnosed, resectable osteosarcoma were 60.6% between 1987 and 1990, 68.1% between 1991 and 1994, 61.7% between 1995 and 1998, and 66.4% between 1999 and 2002.[15] On the other hand, intensive chemotherapy regimens used for osteosarcoma are associated with severe acute and long-term toxic effects and have considerable impact on quality of life. Patients with unresectable a primary tumour or metastasis, and those with disease relapse have extremely poor outcomes.[16] Novel therapies are therefore urgently required for the management of osteosarcoma.

16.4 HIFU for Primary Bone Malignancies

16.4.1 Technique and Principles

The amplitude and intensity of an ultrasound beam decreases when it travels through tissue; this process is known as attenuation. Each tissue has a characteristic attenuation coefficient, with bone having the second highest amplitude attenuation coefficients,[17] ranging from 150 to 350 Npm^{-1} MHz^{-1}(see Chapter 2). Attenuation derives from the energy losses from absorption, scattering, and reflection between the bone and soft tissue interfaces. Absorption determines that portion of ultrasonic wave that is converted into heat. The propagation of ultrasonic waves through bone is more complex than in soft tissue. In cortical bone such as in the femur, only a small part of the attenuation is due to absorption and most is due to reflection, scattering, and mode conversion.[17]

Due to its high attenuation, it is difficult for a focused ultrasound beam to propagate through intact bone. However, osteosarcoma typically appears as a mixed radiodense and lytic lesion arising in an eccentric manner from the metaphyseal region of the long bone. Most osteosarcoma is lytic, and cortical destruction with periosteal reaction is common.[6] There is frequently mass extension into the

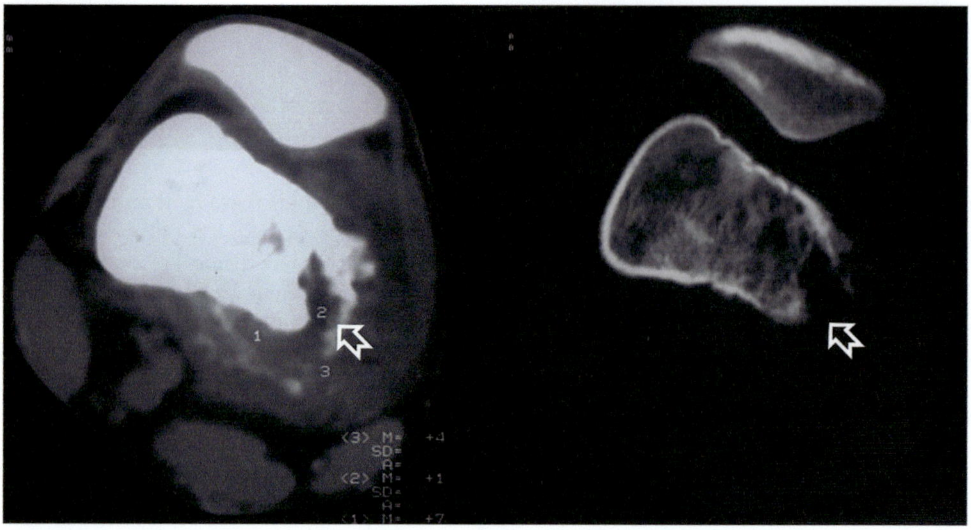

FIGURE 16.1 Transverse computed tomography (CT) images in a patient with distal femoral osteosarcoma. The image on CT soft tissue window (left) shows extensive cortical destruction (arrow), soft tissue mass extension, and periosteal reaction. The image on CT bone window (right) shows complete cortical destruction (arrow), creating an acoustic window for HIFU treatment.

adjacent tissue. Osteosarcoma patients are most often diagnosed at stage IIB (extra-cortical), where the tumour has already penetrated the cortex of the bone with slight to complete cortical destruction (Figure 16.1). This creates an acoustic window on the diseased bone that allows the focused ultrasound beam to propagate through the damaged cortex into the medullary cavity, from where the tumour cells initially originate. HIFU can thus be used as a non-invasive approach to treat osteosarcoma through the tumour-damaged cortex of the bone. In addition, because of the low thermal conductivity and high ultrasound attenuation in the periosteum and bone cortex, acoustic powers used for treating osteosarcoma are much lower than those for soft tissue tumours. This can significantly reduce thermal damage to normal tissues surrounding the treated bone, resulting in improved safety of HIFU treatment.

16.4.2 Post-HIFU Imaging Assessment

Medical imaging modalities have been widely used for disease detection, diagnosis, staging, post-treatment assessment, and follow-up in patients with osteosarcoma. Of these, MRI plays an important role in assessment of therapeutic effects because it provides high-resolution imaging for musculoskeletal systems. Although a wide variety of MRI sequences are available for post-ablation assessment, the most common for assessing HIFU ablation is gadolinium contrast-enhanced T1-weighted imaging.[18] Figure 16.2 shows MR images before and after HIFU in a patient with proximal tibial osteosarcoma. Compared to the pre-HIFU image, an absence of contrast enhancement in the treated region is seen on contrast-enhanced T1-weighted image after HIFU. This ablation zone is surrounded by a smooth, continuous rim of peripheral hyper-enhancement, which is the result of local inflammation and hyperaemia at the interface between the ablation zone and normal muscles. However, the hyper-vascular rim is differentiated from residual unablated tumour, which usually presents with nodular, thickened, and irregular enhancement around the periphery of the ablation zone.

Additionally, single photon emission computed tomography (SPECT) and PET have high sensitivity and specificity for the assessment of tumour response after ablation. They use radiolabelled compounds to provide physiological information about the metabolism and function of tumours. Interpretation of both imaging methods is based on observed intensity relative to expected normal activity. It can either be increased (often called a "hot spot") or decreased (termed "photopenic"). Figure 16.3 shows ^{99m}technetium

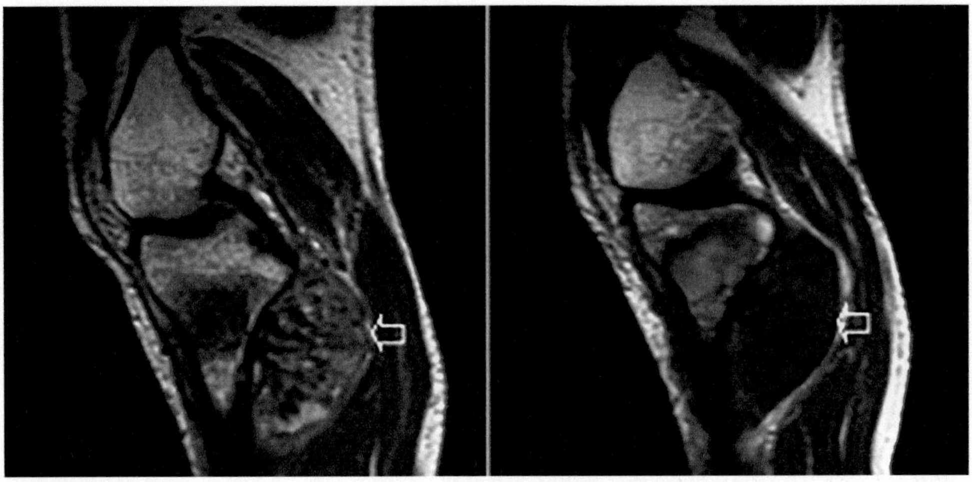

FIGURE 16.2 Sagittal contrast-enhanced T1-weighted MR images before and after USgHIFU treatment in a patient with proximal tibia osteosarcoma. Before HIFU (left), there is contrast enhancement in the target tumour (arrow). Two weeks after HIFU (right), no evidence of contrast enhancement is seen in the treated tumour (arrow) with smooth peripheral hyperenhancement rim, indicative of complete ablation in the osteosarcoma. (From Wu F, et al. Ultrasound Med Bio 2002; 28:535–542.)[19]

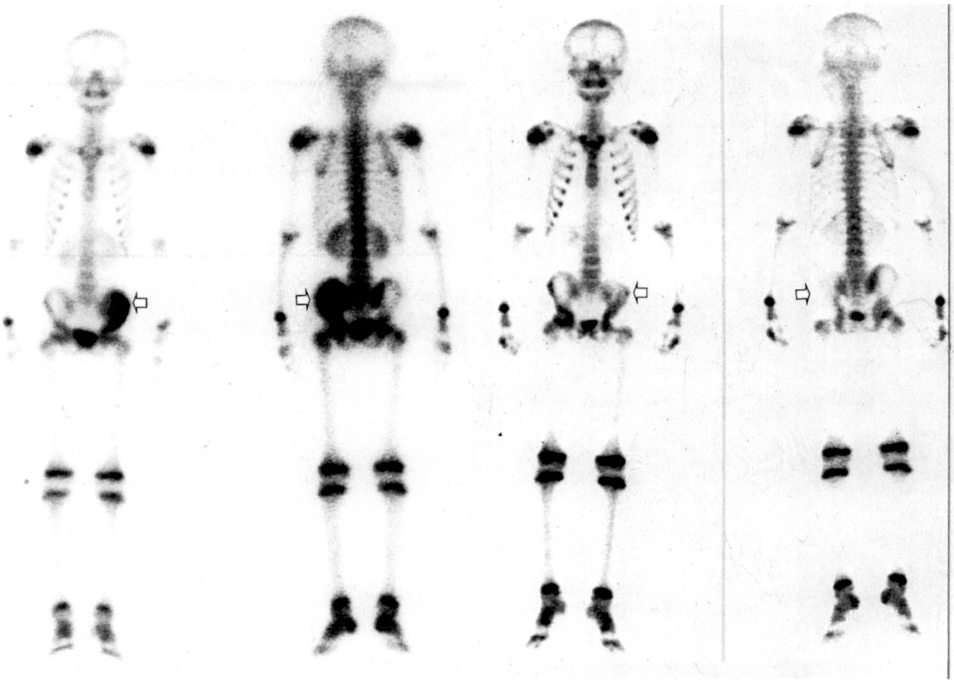

FIGURE 16.3 ^{99m}Technetium methylene diphosphonate SPECT images before and after USgHIFU treatment in a patient with left pelvic osteosarcoma. Before HIFU (left), an increased uptake of the radioisotope is detected in local abnormality (arrow). One week after HIFU (right), the tracer uptake disappears completely in the treated tumour (arrow), indicating a radioactive photopenic area.

methylene diphosphate (^{99m}Tc-MDP) SPECT images pre- and post-HIFU in a patient with left pelvic osteosarcoma. One week after treatment, no abnormal ^{99m}Tc-MDP signal was detected in the treated region, indicating a positive therapeutic response with an absence of residual viable tumour.

16.4.3 Clinical Outcomes

The first USgHIFU trial for the treatment of patients with primary bone malignancy was reported in 2002. A total of 44 patients were treated with HIFU plus chemotherapy (n = 40) or HIFU alone (n = 4), with a mean follow-up of 17.6 months. The results showed that HIFU combined with chemotherapy for primary malignant bone tumour in the extremity was safe and effective with good function preservation in the limbs, suggesting that HIFU could provide a limb-salvaging treatment.[20]

In 2010, this team published their long-term follow-up results. This is the largest clinical trial for primary bone malignancy to date, wherein 80 patients received HIFU treatment, including 60 in stage IIb and 20 in stage III disease.[21] Of them, HIFU combined with chemotherapy was performed in 66 patients (osteosarcoma 62; Ewing's sarcoma 3; periosteal osteosarcoma 1), and the remaining 14 patients underwent HIFU treatment alone, including chondrosarcoma, malignant giant cell tumour of bone, and sarcoma of the periosteum. CT, MRI, and SPECT (^{99m}Tc-MDP) scans were performed to assess tumour response after ablation. The results showed complete tumour ablation in 69 patients (86%) and partial ablation (>50% tumour ablation) in the remaining 11. Figure 16.4 shows contrast-enhanced T1-weighted MR images before and after HIFU in a patient with proximal tibia osteosarcoma. Compared to the image pre-treatment, no contrast enhancement is observed in the target tumour post-treatment, indicative of positive response with complete ablation. During 36-month follow-up, the innovation of the ablation zone occured over time, with no evidence of local recurrence. The overall 5-year survival rate

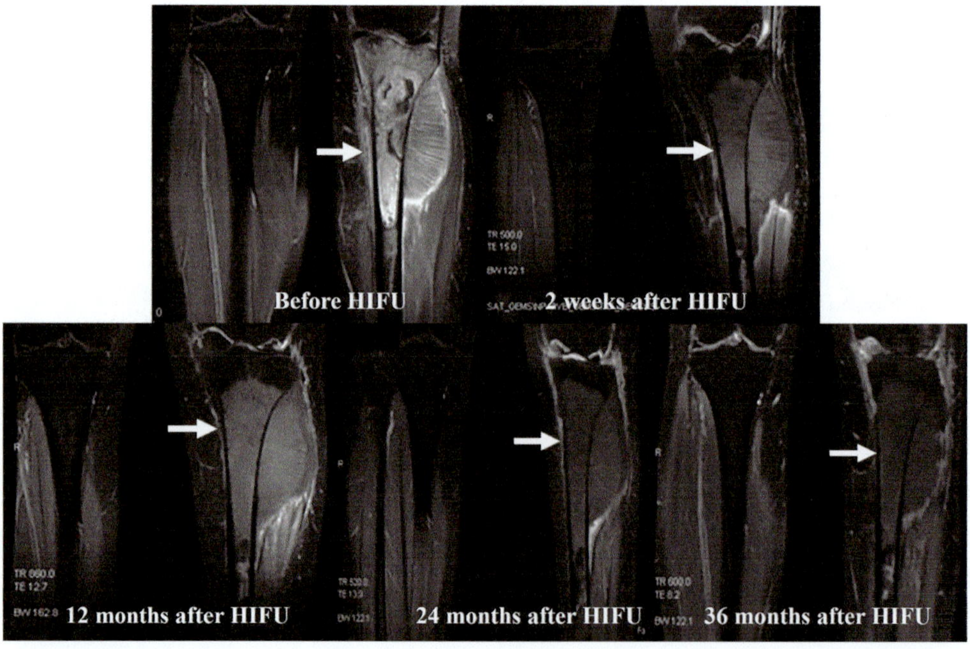

FIGURE 16.4 Coronary contrast-enhanced T1-weighted MR images before and after USgHIFU treatment in a patient with proximal tibia osteosarcoma. Before HIFU treatment, there is contrast enhancement in the target tumour (arrow). Two weeks after HIFU (right), an absence of contrast enhancement is observed in the treated tumour (arrow) with smooth peripheral hyperenhancement rim, indicative of positive tumour response with complete ablation. The ablation zone decreases in size during 36-month follow-up without any evidence of recurrence in the treated region. (From Chen W, et al. Radiology 2010; 255:967–978.)[20]

was 51%, with 64% in stage IIb and 16% in stage III. However, this study found that in the stage IIb patients, 30 patients who completed the treatment schedule (complete tumour ablation plus all cycles of chemotherapy) had a significantly longer 5-year survival (86%), in comparison with 36% in patients with either incomplete chemotherapy cycles (n = 24) or partial ablation only (n = 6). Only 5 (7%) of the 69 patients with complete tumour ablation had local recurrence during the follow-up period. Bone healing occurred post-treatment to restore the diseased bone to its normal state. Figure 16.5 shows the

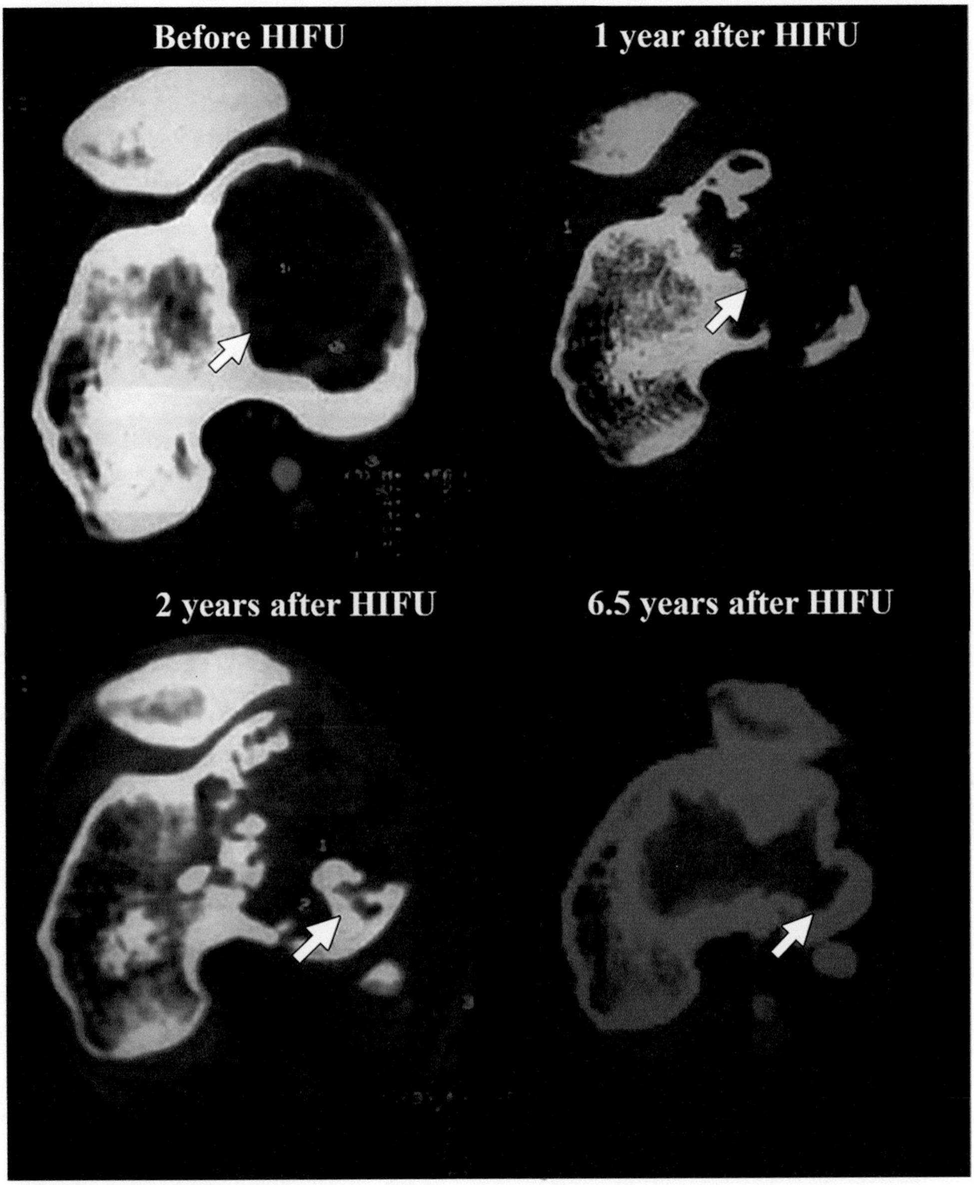

FIGURE 16.5 Transverse unenhanced CT images before and after USgHIFU treatment in a 40-year-old patient with malignant giant cell tumour of the distal femur. Before HIFU, it shows single lesion (arrow) in the femur with cortical destruction. After HIFU, a repair process of the diseased bone develops with remineralisation in the treated tumour (arrow) until almost complete restoration of normal cortical structure occurs during follow-up period. (From Chen W, et al. Radiology 2010; 255:967–978.)[20]

repair process in cortical bone on unenhanced CT images in a patient with malignant giant cell tumour of the distal femur. The repair process in diseased bone develops with remineralisation posttreatment and progresses with time. Almost complete restoration of normal cortical structure is observed during the follow-up period.

USgHIFU can also be used to treat bone metastasis. Li and colleagues[22] reported their experience of using HIFU treatment for primary and metastatic bone malignancy. All patients experienced significant pain relief immediately after treatment, including 21 (87.5%) patients with complete relief of pain. Follow-up MRI/PET-CT showed that complete ablation was achieved in 6 (46.2%) of 13 patients with primary bone malignancy, and 5 (41.7%) of 12 patients with bone metastasis. 5-year survival rate was 39% in patients with primary bone malignancy, but no patients with bone metastasis survived for 3 years. Subsequently, Wang and colleagues performed a retrospective analysis of HIFU-treated 11 patients with primary malignant tumours of the pelvic bone. Of these, 4 patients received HIFU treatment with curative intent, and the remaining 7 patients underwent HIFU as a palliative option for pain control. Follow-up MRI showed 100% tumour ablation in 4 patients treated with curative intent, and these were alive at the time of publication, ranging from 11 to 154 months. In the remaining patients treated for palliation, partial ablation was achieved with pain relief in all patients. In addition, HIFU was used to treat locally unresectable recurrence of osteosarcoma in 27 patients.[23] Posttreatment MRI showed that the tumour response rate was 51.8% and the local disease control rate was 85.2%. The median local disease progression-free time was 14 months, the median progression-free time was 13 months, and the median overall survival time was 21 months. Patients with no lung metastasis had better local disease control rate than patients with lung metastasis.

In 2019, Wang reported a randomised clinical trial, which compared chemotherapy (Adriamycin) plus HIFU (n = 36) with chemotherapy alone (n = 36) for the treatment of patients with stage III osteosarcoma.[24] Using the Response Evaluation Criteria in Solid Tumours (RECIST), therapeutic efficacy was classified as complete response, partial response, stable disease, or progressive disease. In the combined group the overall response (88.9%) and disease control rate (94.4%) were significantly higher than in the chemotherapy group (66.7% and 75.0%, respectively). The 2- and 3-year survival rates were significantly higher in the combined group than in the control group (2y: 69.4% vs 52.8%; 3y: 38.9% vs 22.2%), indicative that HIFU combined with chemotherapy could provide better survival benefit in patients with advanced-stage osteosarcoma. In addition, this study found that after thermal ablation, the serum levels of tumour necrosis factor-alpha, interleukin-2, and interleukin-8 were significantly higher in the combined group, suggesting that HIFU combined with chemotherapy may enhance antitumour effects of the immune system via activation of these cytokines.

Besides typical HIFU-related side effects that are usually transient and resolved without any additional medication two weeks post-treatment. Serious complications vary depending on the location and size of primary bone malignancy. It has been reported that in a total of 80 HIFU-treated patients, peripheral nerve damage is observed in 10 patients (12%), bone fracture in 6 (8%), ligamentous laxity in 3 (4%), epiphysiolysis in 2 (2%), and local infection in 2 (2%).[20]

16.5 HIFU for Soft Tissue Sarcoma

Soft tissue sarcomas (STS) are rare and heterogeneous mesenchymal neoplasms, which develop in connective tissues such as the muscle, nerve, tendon, blood vessel, fat, and fibrous tissues. These are diverse tumours with more than 70 histological subtypes. STS can be found in any part of the body but mostly in the arms, legs, and trunk. Their symptoms vary depending on the size and location of the tumour. The overall 5-year survival rate is only 50–60% in STS patients.[25] Most patients die of metastatic disease, and the overall median survival for patients with lung metastases was 15 months.[26]

Conservative surgery combined with pre- and post-operative radiotherapy is standard treatment for localised STS in the limb and trunk, with the aim of achieving high rates of local control whilst maintaining optimal function.[27] Radiotherapy may be avoided in patients with low grade STS or small high-grade tumours post-operation. The role of adjuvant chemotherapy for most STS remains unproven. But neoadjuvant chemotherapy may be considered as a treatment option for patients, whose surgical resection is difficult due to tumour size or position. In addition, treatment for patients with locally recurrent STS after initial wide resection is challenging, because further surgery and radiotherapy are extremely difficult to deliver appropriately.[28, 29] Therefore, non-ionising ablative therapies are of great interest in treating patients with local recurrence, particularly with oligometastatic disease.

The first clinical experience of using USgHIFU treatment for STS was reported in 2004. This was a clinical overview of patient data collected from 10 Chinese hospitals, and HIFU was used as a palliative option for treating local recurrence of STS after surgical resection.[30] Ultrasonography, CT, and MRI were performed to assess tumour response after ablation. Figure 16.6 shows a significant decrease of blood flow signals within the treated STS lesion on colour Doppler ultrasonography, indicative of positive tumour response. An absence of contrast enhancement is also observed within the treated tumour on contrast-enhanced MRI scan after the treatment (Figure 16.7).

To date, most clinical HIFU results have been published in the form of case reports, and treated STS include chordoma,[32] leiomyosarcoma,[33] gastric leiomyosarcoma,[34] malignant fibrous histiocytoma,[35] and synovial sarcoma.[36] Yu and colleagues[37] reported a retrospective analysis of USgHIFU treatment for 36 patients with locally unresectable recurrent STS, including lipoblastoma in 8 patients, undifferentiated pleomorphic sarcoma in 7, leiomyosarcoma in 3, fibrosarcoma in 6, chondrosarcoma in 4, synovial sarcoma in 3, aggressive fibromatosis in 2, and alveolar rhabdomyosarcoma, and clear cell sarcoma and primitive neurotodermal tumour in 1, respectively. Pain score, tumour response, progression-free survival, overall survival, and adverse events were used to assess clinical outcomes. Following RECIST v1.1, follow-up MRI/CT scan showed that 17 (47.3%) patients had partial response at 3 months and 14 (38.9%) at 12 months. No patients showed a complete response. The overall survival, median local disease progression-free survival and progression-free survival time were 20 months, 13 months, and 10 months, respectively. Pain relief was achieved in 25 (75.8%) of 33 patients at 1 month and remained stable 3 months after HIFU treatment. This study concluded that HIFU is a tolerated treatment modality with promising activity and safety in STS patients with local unresectable recurrence. Although there are only limited data on survival benefit, current clinical results show that HIFU can improve local control of recurrent STS and play an important role in control of oligometastatic disease in sarcoma patients who cannot tolerate surgery and radiotherapy.

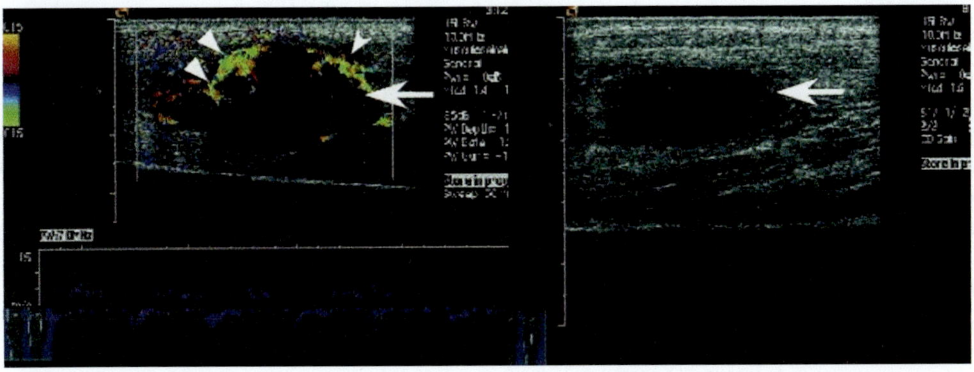

FIGURE 16.6 Longitudinal colour Doppler ultrasonography images before and after USgHIFU treatment in a 29-year-old patient with superficial soft tissue sarcoma in the thigh. Before HIFU (left), it shows hypoechoic mass with numerous blood flow signals (arrowhead) within the tumour (arrow); 2 weeks after HIFU (right), no flow signals are seen within the treated tumour (arrow). (From Wu F, et al. Ultrasound Med Bio 2002; 28:535–542.)[19]

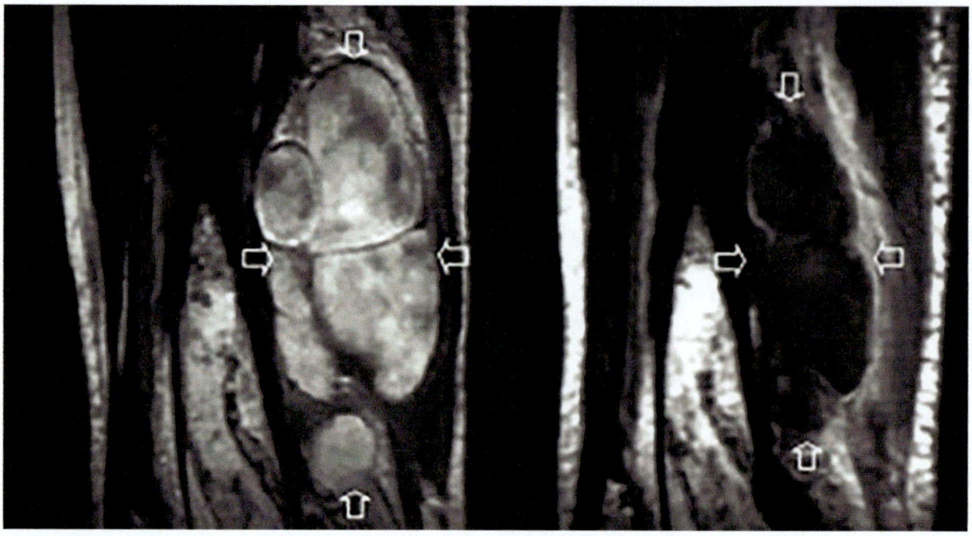

FIGURE 16.7 Coronary contrast-enhanced T1-weighted MR images before and after USgHIFU treatment in a patient with soft tissue sarcoma of the leg. Before HIFU (left), there is contrast enhancement in the tumour (arrows). Two weeks after HIFU (right), an absence of contrast enhancement is observed within the treated tumour (arrows), indicating a positive tumour response with complete ablation. (From Wu F, et al. Ultrasound Med Bio 2004; 30:245–260.)[31]

16.6 Summary

The current management strategy for patients with high-grade osteosarcoma includes neoadjuvant chemotherapy, surgery, and adjuvant chemotherapy, plus radiation therapy if appropriate. Of these, neoadjuvant chemotherapy is extremely important since approximately 80% of patients present with microscopic metastatic disease at diagnosis.[38, 39] It is routinely used as a standard treatment with high-dose methotrexate, doxorubicin and cisplatin (MAP regimen) and has significantly improved long-term survival in patients with osteosarcoma.[40] In addition, there seems to be a big difference between the good and poor responders in survival. Patients with more than 90% necrosis after neoadjuvant chemotherapy have a greater than 90% 5-year event-free survival, whereas those with less than 90% necrosis have only 50–60% 5-year survival.[41, 42] However, this claim has not been repeated by other investigators.[43, 44]

Clinical results have shown that HIFU therapy is technically and clinically safe, feasible, and effective for the local treatment of osteosarcoma. It can be offered as a curative option that destroys an entire tumour for limb salvage, or as a debulking option in advanced-stage patients. For patients with femoral and tibial osteosarcoma, it is important to use either a plaster or splint support to fix the treated bone and adjacent joints immediately after HIFU treatment. This fixation should last 3–6 months to allow the treated bone to repair and fuse. During the follow-up period, patients can walk with the aid of weight-bearing support, which should continue until remineralisation of the new-growth normal bone visible in CT scan is strong enough to support free ambulation.

Compared to current treatment options for primary bone malignancy, such as radiotherapy, surgery, radiofrequency and microwave ablation, the noninvasive nature of HIFU has already made it more desirable to patients and clinicians. HIFU has shown its value in many clinical studies and has emerged as a competitive option for radiation therapy and other thermal ablation modalities. Where clinically appropriate, HIFU should give at least the same result as surgery. It has become clear that HIFU will take its place in the multidisciplinary management of patients with primary bone malignancy in the future. However, multicentral, randomised clinical trials are needed to provide evidence-based results for HIFU as a first-line treatment option in the management of primary bone malignancies.

REFERENCES

1. Mirabello, L., Troisi, R. J., and Savage, S. A. 2009. International osteosarcoma incidence patterns in children and adolescents, middle ages and elderly persons. *Int J Cancer* 125:229–234.
2. Jafari, F., Javdansirat, S., Sanaie, S., et al. 2020. Osteosarcoma: A comprehensive review of management and treatment strategies. *Ann Diagn Pathol* 49:151654.
3. Bielack, S. S., Kempf-Bielack, B., Delling, G., et al. 2002. Prognostic factors in high-grade osteosarcoma of the extremities or trunk: An analysis of 1,702 patients treated on neoadjuvant cooperative osteosarcoma study group protocols. *J Clin Oncol* 20:776–790.
4. Gorlick, R., Janeway, K., Lessnick, S., Randall, R. L., and Marina, N. 2013. Children's Oncology Group's 2013 blueprint for research: Bone tumors. *Pediatr Blood Cancer* 60:1009–1015.
5. Aljubran, A. H., Griffin, A., Pintilie, M., and Blackstein, M. 2009. Osteosarcoma in adolescents and adults: Survival analysis with and without lung metastases. *Ann Oncol* 20:1136–1141.
6. Geller, D. S., and Gorlick, R. 2010. Osteosarcoma: A review of diagnosis, management, and treatment strategies. *Clin Adv Hematol Oncol* 8:705–718.
7. Choi, J. H., and Ro, J. Y. 2021. The 2020 WHO classification of tumors of bone: An updated review. *Adv Anat Pathol* 28:119–138.
8. Klein, M. J., and Siegal, G. P. 2006. Osteosarcoma: Anatomic and histologic variants. *Am J Clin Pathol* 125:555–581.
9. Enneking, W. F. 1986. A system of staging musculoskeletal neoplasms. *Clin Orthop Relat Res* 204:9–24.
10. Beird, H. C., Bielack, S. S., Flanagan, A. M., et al. 2022. Osteosarcoma. *Nat Rev Dis Primers* 2022 8:77.
11. Isakoff, M. S., Bielack, S. S., Meltzer, P., and Gorlick, R. 2015. Osteosarcoma: Current treatment and a collaborative pathway to success. *J Clin Oncol* 33:3029–3035.
12. Strauss, S. J., Frezza, A. M., Abecassis, N., et al. 2021. Bone sarcomas: ESMO-EURACAN-GENTURIS-ERN PaedCan clinical practice guideline for diagnosis, treatment and follow-up. *Ann Oncol* 32:1520–1536.
13. Ciernik, I. F., Niemierko, A., Harmon, D. C., et al. 2011. Proton-based radiotherapy for unresectable or incompletely resected osteosarcoma. *Cancer* 117:4522–4530.
14. Matsunobu, A., Imai, R., Kamada, T, et al. 2012. Impact of carbon ion radiotherapy for unresectable osteosarcoma of the trunk. *Cancer* 118:4555–4563.
15. Smith, M. A., Seibel, N. L., Altekruse, S. F., et al. 2010. Outcomes for children and adolescents with cancer: Challenges for the twenty-first century. *J Clin Oncol* 28:2625–2634.
16. Kempf-Bielack, B., Bielack, S. S., Jürgens, H., et al. 2005. Osteosarcoma relapse after combined modality therapy: An analysis of unselected patients in the Cooperative Osteosarcoma Study Group (COSS). *J Clin Oncol* 23:559–568.
17. Pinton, G., Aubry, J. F., Bossy, E., Muller, M., Pernot, M., and Tanter, M. 2012. Attenuation, scattering, and absorption of ultrasound in the skull bone. *Med Phys* 39:299–307.
18. Fite, B. Z., Wang, J., Ghanouni, P., and Ferrara, K. W. 2022. A review of imaging methods to assess ultrasound-mediated ablation. *BME Front* 2022:9758652.
19. Wu, F., Chen, W. Z., Bai, J., et al. 2002. Tumor vessel destruction resulting from high-intensity focused ultrasound in patients with solid malignancies. *Ultrasound Med Biol* 28:535–542.
20. Chen, W., Wang, Z., Wu, F., et al. 2002. High intensity focused ultrasound in the treatment of primary malignant bone tumor. *Zhonghua Zhong Liu Za Zhi* 24:612–615.
21. Chen, W., Zhu, H., Zhang, L., et al. 2010. Primary bone malignancy: Effective treatment with high intensity focused ultrasound ablation. *Radiology* 255:968–78.
22. Li, C., Zhang, W., Fan, W., Huang, J., Zhang, F., and Wu, P. 2010. Noninvasive treatment of malignant bone tumors using high-intensity focused ultrasound. *Cancer* 116:3934–3942.
23. Yu, W., Tang, L., Lin, F., Yao, Y., Shen, Z., and Zhou, X. 2015. High-intensity focused ultrasound: Noninvasive treatment for local unresectable recurrence of osteosarcoma. *Surg Oncol* 24:9–15.
24. Wang, C. 2019. Therapeutic effects of adriamycin combined with high-intensity focused ultrasound on osteosarcoma. *J Balk Union Oncol* 24:826–831.
25. Howlader, N., Noone, A. M., Krapcho, M. et al. (eds). SEER Cancer Statistics Review, 1975–2017, National Cancer Institute. 2020.
26. Bourcier, K., Le Cesne, A., Tselikas, L., et al. 2019. Basic knowledge in soft tissue sarcoma. *Cardiovasc Intervent Radiol* 42:1255–1261.

27. Dangoor, A., Seddon, B., Gerrand, C., Grimer, R., Whelan, J., and Judson, I. 2016. UK guidelines for the management of soft tissue sarcomas. *Clin Sarcoma Res* 6:20.
28. Cormier, J. N., and Pollock, R. E. 2004. Soft tissue sarcomas. *CA Cancer J Clin* 54:94–109.
29. Sugiura, H., Tsukushi, S., Yoshida, M., and Nishida, Y. 2018. What is the success of repeat surgical treatment of a local recurrence after initial wide resection of soft tissue sarcomas? *Clin Orthop Relat Res* 476:1791–1800.
30. Wu, F., Wang, Z. B., Chen, W. Z., et al. 2004. Extracorporeal high intensity focused ultrasound ablation in the treatment of 1038 patients with solid carcinomas in China: An overview. *Ultrason Sonochem* 11:149–154.
31. Wu, F., Wang, Z. B., Chen, W. Z., et al. 2004. Extracorporeal focused ultrasound surgery for treatment of human solid carcinomas: Early Chinese clinical experience. *Ultrasound Med Biol* 30:245–260.
32. Gillies, M. J., Lyon, P. C., Wu, F., et al. 2017. High-intensity focused ultrasonic ablation of sacral chordoma is feasible: A series of four cases and details of a national clinical trial. *Br J Neurosurg* 31:446–451.
33. Li, J., Chen, X., and Hu, X. 2020. High-intensity focused ultrasound for treatment of recurrent uterine leiomyosarcoma: A case report and literature review. *J Int Med Res* 48:300060520942107.
34. Cheng, C. S., Chen, L., Xie, J., and Chen, Z. 2019. Multimodality palliative treatment with transarterial chemoembolization and high-intensity focused ultrasound for gastric leiomyosarcoma multiple liver metastasis pain: A case report. *Med (United States)* 98: e17328.
35. Zhou, M., Hu, X., He, H., Chen, J., Chen, L., and Deng, Y. 2012. Neoadjuvant HIFU treatment for malignant fibrous histiocytoma: Report of a case. *J Med Ultrason* 39:259–264.
36. Hu, X., Cai, H., Zhou, M., et al. 2013. New clinical application of high-intensity focused ultrasound: Local control of synovial sarcoma. *World J Surg Oncol* 11:265.
37. Yu, W., Tang, L., Lin, F., Jiang, L., and Shen, Z. 2019. Significance of HIFU in local unresectable recurrence of soft tissue sarcoma, a single-center, respective, case series in China. *Surg Oncol* 30:117–121
38. Eilber, B. y. F., Giuliano, A., Eckardt, J., Patterson, K., Moseley, S., and Goodnight, J. 1987. Adjuvant chemotherapy for osteosarcoma: A randomized prospective trial. *J Clin Oncol* 5:21–26.
39. O'Kane, G. M., Cadoo, K. A., Walsh, E. M., et al. 2015. Perioperative chemotherapy in the treatment of osteosarcoma: A 26-year single institution review. *Clin Sarcoma Res* 5:1–8.
40. Marina, N. M. Smeland, S., Bielack, S. S., et al. 2016. Comparison of MAPIE versus MAP in patients with a poor response to preoperative chemotherapy for newly diagnosed high-grade osteosarcoma (EURAMOS-1): An open-label, international, randomised controlled trial. *Lancet Oncol* 17:1396–1408.
41. Meyers, P. A., Schwartz, C. L., Krailo, M., et al. 2005. Osteosarcoma: A randomized, prospective trial of the addition of ifosfamide and/or muramyl tripeptide to cisplatin, doxorubicin, and high-dose methotrexate. *J Clin Oncol* 23:2004–2011.
42. Provisor, A. J., Ettinger, L. J., Nachman, J. B., et al. 1997. Treatment of nonmetastatic osteosarcoma of the extremity with preoperative and postoperative chemotherapy: A report from the children's Cancer Group. *J Clin Oncol* 15:76–84.
43. Meyers, P. A., Gorlick, R., Heller, G., et al. 1998. Intensification of preoperative chemotherapy for osteogenic sarcoma: Results of the Memorial Sloan-Kettering (T12) protocol. *J Clin Oncol* 16:2452–2458.
44. Lewis, I. J., Nooij, M. A., Whelan, J., et al. 2007. Improvement in histologic response but not survival in osteosarcoma patients treated with intensified chemotherapy: A randomized phase III trial of the European Osteosarcoma Intergroup. *J Natl Cancer Inst* 99:112–128.

17

Clinical Extracorporeal MR-Guided Focused Ultrasound Systems: Treatment Planning, Therapy Delivery, and Online Monitoring via Thermometry and Thermal Dose Mapping

Ryan M. Jones, Yuexi Huang, and Kullervo Hynynen

17.1 Introduction

It has been known for many years that ultrasound is capable of inducing biological effects in vivo when appropriate acoustic parameters are employed.[1, 2] Acoustic energy can be focused within small volumes (with millimetric dimensions) deep inside the body (with up to several centimeters penetration depth), depending on the operating frequency and nature of the ultrasound applicator employed.[3] This localised energy deposition can be exploited to produce a range of mechanical and/or thermal bioeffects on the vasculature and in tissue. These have been reviewed extensively in the literature.[4–7]

The potential of focused ultrasound (FUS) as a tool for non-invasive, localised tissue ablation in humans for medical therapy was first demonstrated more than 60 years ago, when it was used to treat patients suffering from a variety of neurological disorders of the brain.[8] Yet, FUS therapy failed to gain widespread clinical acceptance for many years after these promising initial human trials, due largely to limitations in the available methods for treatment guidance (i.e., targeting, monitoring, and evaluation) at that time. These initial procedures[8] used a complex FUS delivery system consisting of four separate quartz transducers, each coupled to a polystyrene lens, which were co-aligned to further confine and amplify the acoustic focus. Therapy targeting was performed using X-ray imaging of nearby bony landmarks, and the ultrasound exposures were delivered through an open skin and bone flap, which at the time was thought to be required for successful application of FUS therapy in the brain due to the aberrating nature of the skull bone.[2]

Later, diagnostic ultrasound imaging was proposed for guiding FUS therapy in soft tissues.[9, 10] This approach has since led to the development of several clinical ultrasound-guided FUS (USgFUS) systems; for example, extracorporeal USgFUS devices have been used to treat patients with a variety of solid tumours, including those located in the liver, kidney, breast, pancreas, uterus, and in bone,[11–18] primarily in China and the United Kingdom. However, the majority of thermal USgFUS treatments currently rely on open-loop energy delivery with fixed exposure settings, meaning that the acoustic parameters (e.g., applied acoustic power, exposure duration) chosen are based on theoretical and experimental models, as well as prior clinical experience. This is due largely to the fact that ultrasound is currently unable to provide reliable and precise thermometry information over a clinically relevant temperature range. Hyperechoic backscatter resulting from bubble formation is used as an indicator of treatment efficacy during some clinical USgFUS procedures[19]; however, this is known to correlate poorly with the spatial extent of lesion formation and tends to underestimate the true amount of tissue damage.[20]

Magnetic resonance imaging (MRI) allows high-resolution 3D imaging (over millimeter length scales) with exceptional soft tissue contrast, making it particularly well suited for FUS treatment planning. This involves determining the required number, location, and power of individual ultrasound

DOI: 10.1201/9780429162671-17

exposures and their associated beam paths, as well as the identification of critical structures that should be avoided (e.g., bone, nerves, gas). These features motivated the first experimental integration of a FUS thermal ablation system with an MRI scanner.[21] Furthermore, MRI can detect and map temperature changes spatially within the body[22] in a quantitative manner,[23] as will be discussed in more detail later (see Section 17.5). This unique ability allows MR-guided FUS (MRgFUS) system operators to confirm targeting, monitor the induced temperature elevations in near real time, and predict the treated (e.g., ablated) volume through calculation of the cumulative thermal dose.[24, 25] Finally, MRI can be employed for post-treatment evaluation (see Section 17.8); in breast, uterine fibroid, and bone applications the ablated volume is commonly mapped using contrast-enhanced T_1-weighted (T_1w) imaging,[26–30] which can identify perfusion-deficient regions indicative of tissue coagulation, whereas during brain treatments T_2-weighted (T_2w) sequences are often used to detect edema[30] and to estimate the size of the induced lesion.[31, 32] It is therefore evident that MRI offers many beneficial features as a modality for guiding FUS therapy, particularly thermally based applications such as those involving hyperthermia or tissue ablation.

This chapter concentrates on clinical extracorporeal MRgFUS devices and will begin with a brief history of the existing systems. Their principle system components will be described, followed by an illustration of how MRI is used for treatment planning, as well as for online thermometry and thermal dose mapping during FUS therapy. Methods for MRgFUS system calibration and quality assurance will then be discussed. Finally, an overview of the outcomes from the clinical treatments carried out to date with these devices will be presented.

17.2 History of Existing Extracorporeal MRgFUS Systems

Although the potential of using MRI for FUS therapy guidance was recognised in the early 1980s, it wasn't until roughly ten years later that the two modalities were combined successfully.[21, 33] The encouraging results from the first animal experiments using MRgFUS for thermal ablation[21] spurred extensive collaboration with General Electric Medical Systems (GEMS), ultimately resulting in the development of the first clinical prototype (Figure 17.1C). This device consisted of an MRI-compatible spherically focused transducer (10 cm diameter, 8 cm radius of curvature, 1.5 MHz operating frequency) mounted on a mechanical translation stage and was used in the first clinical tests of MRgFUS technology, which investigated the feasibility of treating malignant breast tumours and benign fibroadenomas.[26, 28, 34] The results from these initial clinical trials were promising; however, the FUS systems employed in these studies were limited by the small focal volume afforded by a mechanically scanned single-element transducer. Similarly, the therapy systems were limited from a treatment monitoring perspective; although they were capable of displaying MR-thermometry maps at an acceptable rate, the thermal dose distribution was not tracked during exposures.[28]

Based on the clinical experience gained from this first-generation prototype system, as well as concurrent simulation and pre-clinical studies that demonstrated the benefits of ultrasound phased array technology[36–38] and thermal dose mapping for therapy guidance,[24, 39] the first commercial MRgFUS system was developed (ExAblate Body, formerly: ExAblate 2000; InSightec, Inc., Tirat Carmel, Israel) by InSightec in collaboration with GEMS and researchers from Brigham and Women's Hospital (BWH) in Boston (Figure 17.1D). The device is contained within a specialised MRI bed and consists of a fully populated, hybrid sector-vortex and concentric ring phased array design (12 cm spherically curved circular aperture, 16 cm radius of curvature, 208 elements, 0.96–1.14 MHz operating frequency), which allows electronic focusing primarily in the depth direction with a small steering range laterally. The array is positioned mechanically to aim the acoustic focus, and the device can also be rotated in two angular directions to provide further control over the beam orientation so that near- or far-field structures can be avoided. MR-thermometry is carried out during the ultrasound exposures and the associated thermal dose buildup is monitored online during the procedures,[40, 41] a strategy that is now commonplace amongst MRgFUS devices (see Sections 17.5 and 17.6). The ExAblate Body system received U.S. Food and Drug Administration (FDA) approval for treating uterine fibroids[29] and for pain palliation from bone metastases[42] in 2004 and 2012, respectively. Subsequent technological advancements to this

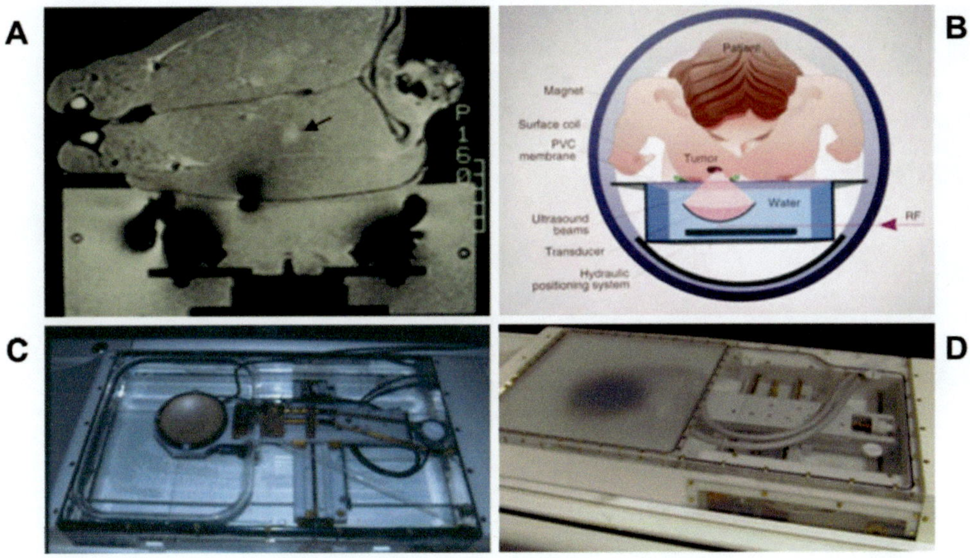

FIGURE 17.1 First MRgFUS systems used clinically (figure reproduced with permission from[35]). (A) A proton density-weighted MR image showing a small volume of thermally coagulated tissue (arrow) *in vivo* in dog thigh muscle. This was the first in vivo thermal ablation using FUS under MRI guidance. The dark hole on the skin is a large susceptibility artifact caused by a small air bubble. (B) A diagram of the first clinical hydraulic prototype system used in the first clinical treatments of breast fibroadenoma. The system transmitted the mechanical motion of master cylinders via water lines to the slave cylinders in the tank on the scanner table. The slave cylinders moved the transducer in three dimensions. (C) The second-generation prototype system manufactured by GEMS that was used during a part of the fibroadenoma study. (D) The ultrasound array and positioning system mounted in an MRI scanner table of the first commercial MRgFUS system (ExAblate 2000; InSightec, Inc., Tirat Carmel, Israel).

MRgFUS device have resulted in improvements in both treatment efficacy and patient safety, as demonstrated in a recently reported single-centre, retrospective study.[43] Because many patients have difficulty lying on their painful bone tumours, InSightec has developed an MRI-guided phased array system dedicated for bone applications (ExAblate 2100 Conformal Bone System; 76 mm flat square aperture, 1000 elements, 550 kHz operating frequency) that can be strapped to the patient, on top of the tumour.[44]

The very first animal experiments demonstrated the difficulties imposed by the presence of the skull bone when applying FUS in the brain.[2] Indeed, it was assumed for a long time that the use of FUS in the brain required a craniotomy.[8, 45] However, based on experiments with ex vivo human skulls[46] and subsequent simulation studies,[47, 48] researchers at BWH demonstrated that it was feasible to deliver sufficient ultrasound energy through the human cranium to achieve focal thermal coagulation of tissue. By using a large hemispherical array design[49, 50] together with phase corrections derived from high-resolution CT scans of the head[51] and measurements of human skull bone's acoustic properties,[52] methods were developed that enabled in vivo demonstration of non-invasive trans-skull ablation.[53] Based on these findings, InSightec has developed two clinical transcranial MRgFUS devices (ExAblate Neuro, formerly: ExAblate 3000/4000; 30 cm diameter hemispherical dome, 1024 elements) for brain applications, one operating at 220–230 kHz and the other at 650–720 kHz. Both of these systems consist of a hemispherical transducer helmet built on to a specialised MRI bed (Figure 17.2); the patient lies supine with their head fixed in place relative to the array using a stereotactic frame. The high frequency ExAblate Neuro system has been employed predominantly for thermal ablation of brain tissue (see Section 17.8.4), and was granted U.S. FDA clearance for treating patients with essential tremor (ET) in 2016,[54] tremor-dominant Parkinson's disease (PD) in 2018,[55] and most recently, advanced PD (i.e., including mobility, rigidity, or dyskinesia symptoms) in 2021.[56] Researchers in France have developed a higher-frequency prototype MRgFUS brain system (23 cm aperture, 15 cm radius of curvature, 512 elements, 1 MHz operating frequency.[57]) This device has been shown to provide good targeting ability

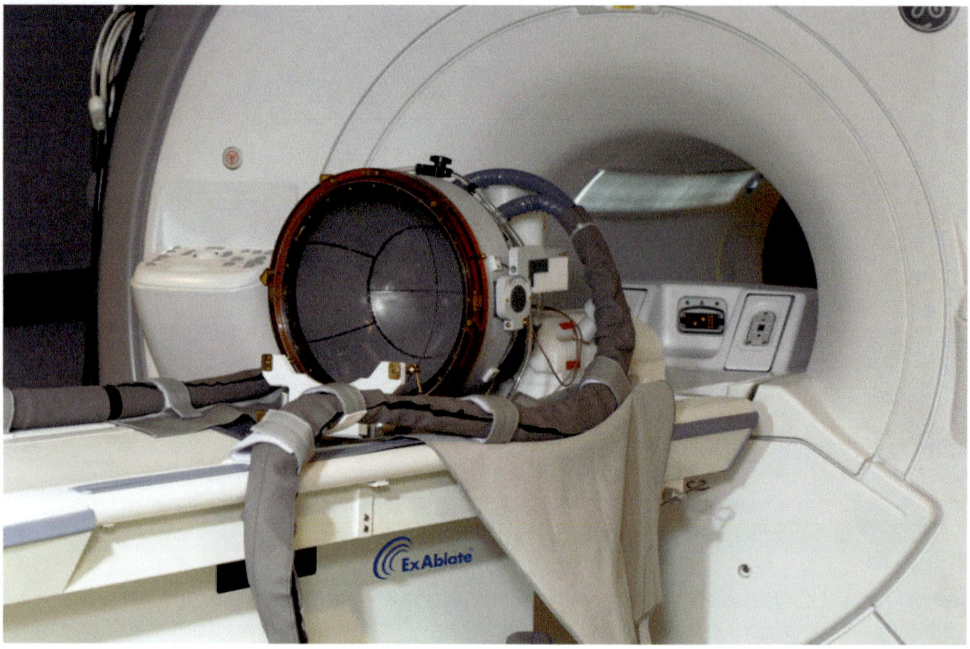

FIGURE 17.2 InSightec's high-frequency MRgFUS hemispherical transducer helmet on an MRI table. The hose to the helmet carries cooled, degassed water that is used to both couple the patient's head acoustically to the transducer and cool the scalp to avoid overheating during the treatment.

during experiments performed on ex vivo human cadaver heads; however, the induced temperature elevations reported thus far have been insufficient to achieve brain tissue ablation in this model.[58, 59] The low-frequency ExAblate Neuro system was developed originally for cavitation-based applications, used initially for pre-clinical work[60–63] and has since entered clinical testing to assess the feasibility and safety of transcranial FUS-mediated blood-brain barrier (BBB) opening for treating various diseases of the central nervous system (see Section 17.8.4). An MRgFUS system consisting of a single-element spherically focused transducer (6 cm diameter, 8 cm focal length, 650 kHz operating frequency) has been developed (BX Pulsar 1002; BrainSonix, Corp., Sherman Oaks, CA, USA) and is being used to investigate neuromodulation applications.[64] Both neuronavigation-guided[65–67] and patient-specific skull-conformal phased arrays[68, 69] represent alternate extracorporeal device designs for image-guided microbubble-mediated FUS brain treatments.

Several other companies have developed external MRgFUS devices; Chongqing Haifu developed an MRgFUS applicator (JM series; Chongqing Haifu Medical Technology Co., Ltd., Chongqing, China) in collaboration with Siemens Healthcare[70] based on prior experience with their ultrasound-guided platforms.[11] This device is similar in design to InSightec's first prototype system, consisting of a mechanically positioned single-element transducer (18 cm diameter, 15 cm radius of curvature, 0.7–1.2 MHz operating frequency), and has been used to treat patients with uterine fibroids in China.[71] Philips Healthcare developed an MRgFUS system (Sonalleve, Philips Healthcare, Inc., Vantaa, Finland) built within a custom MRI bed, which exploits a random sparse array design (12–14 cm spherically curved aperture, 12–14 cm radius of curvature, 256 elements, 0.8–1.45 MHz operating frequency) and employs volumetric ultrasound exposures controlled by feedback from MR-thermometry and thermal dose mapping.[72, 73] The Sonalleve MRgFUS system was acquired by Profound Medical (Mississauga, Canada) in 2017. Having received the European Conformity (CE) mark of approval for fibroid ablation and palliation of pain from bone metastases treatment in 2010 and 2011, respectively, this device obtained FDA approval for treating osteoid osteoma in the extremities in 2017, and is currently being investigated for several additional clinical applications.[74–76] All of the aforementioned extracorporeal

MRgFUS systems designed for abdominal applications carry out exposures with patients placed in the prone position. A recently described MRgFUS system developed in Taiwan (ArcBlate 100 M; EpiSonica, Corp., Hsinchu, Taiwan) performs sonications with supine patient positioning.[77] Lastly, two MRgFUS systems dedicated to breast applications have been developed, one by Philips Healthcare[78] and the other by researchers at the University of Utah[79]) in collaboration with Siemens Healthcare and Image Guided Therapy (Image Guided Therapy, Inc., Pressac, France). Both of these systems employ a phased array transducer mounted laterally, a design that minimises the potential for far-field heating on the thoracic cage and may also allow a wider variety of locations within the breast to be treated successfully.

17.3 Main System Components

The basic components of a typical ultrasound generation system are illustrated in Figure 17.3. The radiofrequency (RF)-drive line contains a computer-controlled signal source that generates a sinusoidal RF signal near the transducer's resonance frequency. This signal is amplified and split into a power meter, for monitoring the transmitted and reflected power, as well as a tuning network that matches the transducer's impedance to the output impedance of the amplifier at the driving frequency. Due to the reverse piezoelectric effect, the transducer material expands and contracts in proportion to the applied time-varying voltage and generates a mechanical disturbance, at the frequency of the RF signal, in the medium in contact with the front surface. For multi-element phased array systems, each of the array elements is driven independently with its own signal line.

It is worth noting that for MRI-guided systems all of the aforementioned drive system components, as well as the transducer itself, must be made of materials that are compatible with the high magnetic fields present within the scanner environment. The existing clinical external MRgFUS systems are integrated with standard 1.5 or 3.0 tesla MRI scanners and use either body (3.0 tesla brain systems) or custom built-in coils (bone/fibroid systems, dedicated breast systems, 1.5 tesla brain systems) for MR imaging purposes. Recently, a dual-channel RF receive-only head coil designed specifically for use with InSightec's 3.0 tesla brain device was shown to augment imaging performance relative to the body coil[80] and may become a standard component of this MRgFUS system in the future. The FUS transducers in the Sonalleve and ExAblate Body systems are built into customised MRI beds and are submerged in mineral oil and degassed deionised water, respectively, to enable acoustic coupling to the patient's skin via gel pads.[81] With the InSightec brain systems, a circular rubber membrane with a central opening is stretched to fit tightly around the patient's head and is mounted on the hemispherical array to allow cooled, degassed water to be circulated over the patient's scalp to keep the absolute skull temperatures within an acceptable range.[82] The latest version of the Sonalleve system is equipped with a temperature controlled water coupling system, which aims to maintain the patient's skin over the ultrasound window at ~20°C to help avoid skin burns.[83]

Several safety measures are in place during MRgFUS procedures. Patients are given a button that can stop the sonications immediately at any time if they experience discomfort during the treatment. Many clinical MRgFUS systems are also equipped with passive detectors to monitor for inertial cavitation, the

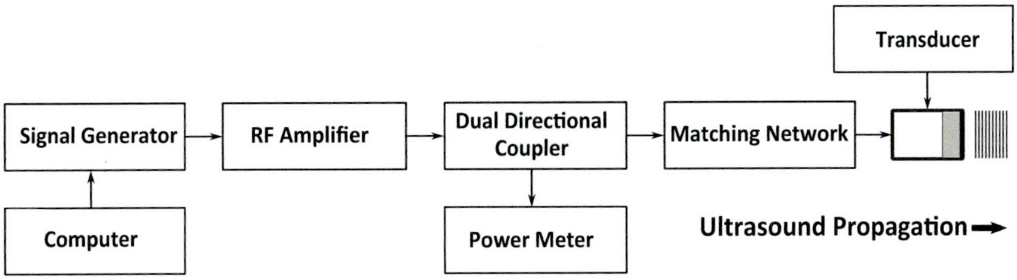

FIGURE 17.3 Block diagram of the basic components of an ultrasound generation system.

growth and subsequent collapse of bubbles generated from the absorbed gases present in vivo,[84] to avoid potential hemorrhage and other unwanted bioeffects associated with this type of activity.[85] For example, sonications with InSightec's ExAblate Neuro systems are terminated automatically if the energy in a spectral band centred about the subharmonic frequency exceeds a calibrated threshold level[63] since a marked increase in subharmonic emissions accompanied by a rise in broadband signals is indicative of inertial cavitation activity.[86–88] The latest version of the high-frequency brain system allows sonications to be delivered in power modulation mode. This modulates the applied acoustic power over the course of each exposure to deliver the prescribed acoustic energy while minimising excessive cavitation signals. Similarly, the latest version of the low-frequency brain system enables closed-loop feedback control of the FUS exposures during microbubble-mediated BBB opening procedures based on the detected cavitation signals.[89]

17.4 Patient Screening and Treatment Planning

Once a patient has been deemed to be an appropriate candidate for MRgFUS based on their current medical symptoms and prior clinical history, a medical imaging-based screening process is carried out. This involves a series of standard MRI scans (e.g., T_2w, T_1w with and/or without the injection of intravenous contrast) that are used to characterise the target volume and confirm that it is acoustically accessible, and treatable by FUS.[28, 29] In the case of brain treatments, pre-treatment computed tomography (CT) scans are also acquired at this time.[90]

On the day of the treatment the patient is prepared for the procedure, which may involve shaving any hair within the beam path for both bone and brain treatments.[91] The patient is then positioned on the MRgFUS platform, to which they are coupled acoustically using a gel pad and/or degassed deionised water, and T_2w MR images are acquired in three orthogonal planes (axial, sagittal, and coronal) allowing the system operator to determine the required orientation of the transducer with respect to the patient. Corresponding 3D T_1w datasets are also acquired at this time during bone treatments with the Sonalleve device, to help with target visualisation.[92] Once adequate positioning of the transducer with respect to the patient is obtained, the MRgFUS operator will define the target volume to be treated and delineate "no-pass" zones within the beam path (e.g., scar tissue, air bubbles, nerves, sinuses, bowel, bladder) using the available MRI data. Based on this information, the MRgFUS system software determines the individual array element apodisation to be used during the sonications and estimates the initial power required using look up tables. For uterine fibroid treatments with InSightec's device, the MRgFUS user also outlines the outer skin layer boundary,[93] which is taken into account during these calculations. The MR-thermometry slices that are to be viewed over the course of the treatment are then prescribed; for example, during uterine fibroid treatments with the Sonalleve system, a near field thermometry slice is positioned in the muscle behind the subcutaneous fat layer and a far field thermometry slice is positioned in front of the spine for monitoring unwanted heating (see Section 17.5).

For brain treatments, the pre-procedural CT data is fused with the treatment planning MR images to determine the relative orientation of the patient's skull and the transducer array. The registered skull geometry and density maps allow calculation of the element driving signals (i.e., phase and amplitude) needed to focus through the cranial bone.[51, 94] The human skull is a strongly aberrating structure at ultrasonic frequencies.[95, 96] The high-frequency InSightec brain system modulates the amplitude of each element such that a uniform acoustic intensity is achieved on the outer skull surface[97] to avoid the generation of local hot spots.[52] Array elements with an angle of incidence above 45° at the outer skull surface are assumed to undergo total reflection[98] and are disabled by the system.[90] The pre-treatment CT data is also examined for the presence of intracranial calcifications,[99] which, due to their high acoustic absorption, must be avoided by turning off beams passing through calcified tissues. Recently, contrast agent microbubble imaging-based aberration correction has been shown to improve trans-skull focal quality relative to traditional CT-based focusing during MRgFUS thalamotomy.[100] This may help expand the treatment envelope of MRgFUS thermoablation in the brain.

17.5 MR Thermometry

As the magnetic properties of water (which makes up a substantial proportion of most human tissues) are temperature-dependent,[101] MRI can be used to image temperature elevations in tissue within the body non-invasively. Temperatures in fat and bone cannot be measured easily due to their relatively low water content. Although several MR parameters are temperature dependent, MR-thermometry based on the water proton resonance frequency (PRF) shift[23] is the most commonly employed method for monitoring FUS therapy. The physical mechanism behind the PRF shift is that a local elevation in temperature acts to weaken hydrogen bonds that, in turn, leads in an increase of the shielding of protons and, as a result, their resonance frequency. Using this method, the change in temperature between a set of consecutive images (ΔT) is estimated using the equation:

$$\Delta T = \frac{\nabla \phi}{\gamma \mathrm{TE} \alpha B_0} \qquad \text{(Eq.17.1)}$$

where $\Delta\phi$ is the phase difference between the two images, γ is the gyromagnetic ratio of water protons, TE is the prescribed echo time, α is the PRF shift coefficient, and B_0 is the strength of the main magnetic field. Spatial maps of temperature elevation are most commonly obtained by subtracting baseline images acquired prior to heating at normal body temperature. The PRF coefficient α is relatively constant over a wide range of temperatures (0–100 °C) and insensitive to tissue type (–0.0096 to –0.0113 ppm/°C.[102, 103]) Importantly, the PRF shift thermometry technique is adequately sensitive for detection of temperature elevations on the order of a few degrees Celsius in most soft tissues. This allows low-power sonications to be delivered to confirm targeting prior to inducing irreversible effects on the tissue. An example of the application of PRF shift thermometry during a clinical uterine fibroid treatment is given in Figure 17.4.

MR-thermometry implementations differ among the existing clinical MRgFUS systems, based on tradeoffs for specific applications. During brain treatments with InSightec's high frequency device, a single plane intersecting the acoustic focus is imaged with a gradient echo sequence (echo time: 13 ms; in-plane resolution: 1 mm × 2 mm, zero-padded to 1 mm × 1 mm; slice thickness: 3 mm; temporal resolution: 3.5 s[32, 104]) and it was recently discovered that the associated phase data contains anatomic

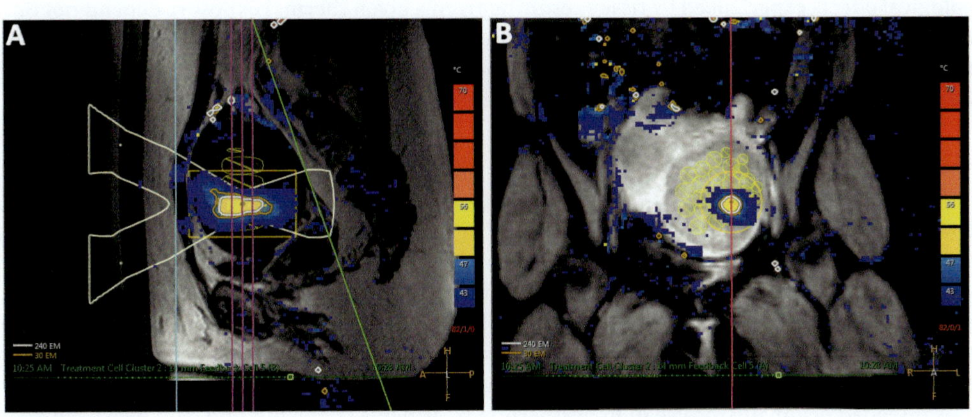

FIGURE 17.4 Six planes used for online MR-thermometry monitoring during uterine fibroid patient treatments with the Sonalleve MRgFUS system. (A) Sagittal localizer image illustrating the near-field (cyan), far-field (green), and three coronal (pink) planes monitored during MRgFUS treatment. (B) Coronal magnitude thermometry image [middle of the three coronal planes shown in (A)] illustrating the sagittal plane (rose) monitored during MRgFUS treatment. Both the temperature and thermal dose (30 CEM_{43} and 240 CEM_{43}) distributions are overlaid in colour (orange and white, respectively).

information that can be useful in guiding the procedures.[105] A similar prescription is carried out by InSightec's Body system (echo time: 20 ms; in-plane resolution: 1 mm × 2 mm, slice thickness: 3 mm; temporal resolution: 5 s[40]). For uterine fibroid treatments with the Sonalleve system, six separate planes (Figure 17.4) are monitored using a fat-saturated echo planar imaging (EPI) sequence: four slices (three coronal and one sagittal) are used to monitor the focal region, and two oblique slices monitor for heating in the near- and far-fields (echo time: 19 ms; in-plane resolution: 2.5 mm × 2.5 mm; slice thickness: 7.0 mm; temporal resolution: 2.9 s[106]). One clinical study with this device applied T_2-based thermometry to check the temperature of the subcutaneous fat layer periodically.[107] For bone treatments with the Sonalleve device, four separate planes (one coronal, one sagittal, two oblique) are monitored using a fat-saturated EPI sequence (echo time: 16 ms; in-plane resolution: 1.5 mm × 1.5 mm; slice thickness: 5.3 mm; temporal resolution: 4.1 s[92]). The initial clinical trial with Philips' dedicated breast system employed fat-suppressed EPI thermometry (echo time: 30 ms; in-plane resolution: 1.7 mm × 1.7 mm; slice thickness: 5.0 mm; temporal resolution: 2.3 s[108]), together with a look up table-based correction method to account for errors in the temperature maps caused by respiration-induced magnetic field disturbances.[109] Similarly to sonications performed with the Sonalleve system, multiple slices are monitored throughout the exposures: two in the focal region (one coronal and one sagittal) and one in both the near- and far-fields. Since most breast tumours are at least partially surrounded by adipose tissue, the authors suggested that T_1- and/or T_2-based thermometry methods[107, 110] be incorporated into this system in the future. Unfortunately, the PRF shift technique cannot measure temperature elevations in bone reliably, due to the high fat concentration in bone marrow and the short T_2 of cortical bone, the latter of which leads to low signal levels when conventional MR sequences are employed. Therefore, during palliative bone pain treatments the adjacent muscle tissue is monitored to provide an indirect measure of heating in the targeted bone region,[42] though several methods to obtain a more direct measurement are currently being investigated.[111] In the first patient treatments with the dedicated breast system developed in Utah, a 3D segmented EPI gradient recalled echo pulse sequence was employed with fat saturation (echo time: 15 ms; voxel size: 1.5 mm × 1.5 mm × 4.0 mm; temporal resolution: 5.7 s), and the utility of performing MR acoustic radiation force imaging[112] for targeting verification in scenarios when MR-thermometry monitoring failed due to high fat content was demonstrated.[113]

17.6 Thermal Dose Delivery and Mapping

The biological effects experienced by tissue resulting from a given thermal exposure depend not only on the absolute temperature attained but also on the duration of the exposure. For this reason, a thermal dose metric was developed to give an indication of the tissue effects resulting from thermal exposures.[114] The thermal dose distribution, $D(\boldsymbol{r})$, is calculated as follows:

$$D(\boldsymbol{r}) = \int R^{(43-T(\boldsymbol{r};t))} dt \qquad \text{(Eq.17.2)}$$

where R is a piecewise constant ($R[T > 43\ °C] = 0.5$; $R[T \leq 43\ °C] = 0.25$) and the integration is carried out over the duration of heating as well as a portion of the cooling period. The values for R were determined empirically based on in vitro experiments that examined the temperature-time dependence of thermally induced cell necrosis in various human and animal cell lines.[115] For an arbitrary thermal exposure, the thermal dose D can be interpreted as the number of cumulative minutes at 43 °C that would be required to achieve an equivalent biological effect (CEM_{43}). Although the concept of thermal dose was intended originally for use in hyperthermia treatments,[116] the method has since been adopted widely for assessing thermal ablation therapy.

Each tissue type has a different sensitivity to thermal dose; however, existing data suggests a dose of 240 CEM_{43} is sufficient to induce necrosis in the vast majority of normal tissue types.[117, 118] For this reason, 240 CEM_{43} is often used as a conservative treatment goal in FUS-mediated ablation therapies to ensure that thermal coagulation is achieved.[93] Although spatial maps of 240 CEM_{43} correlate well with the size

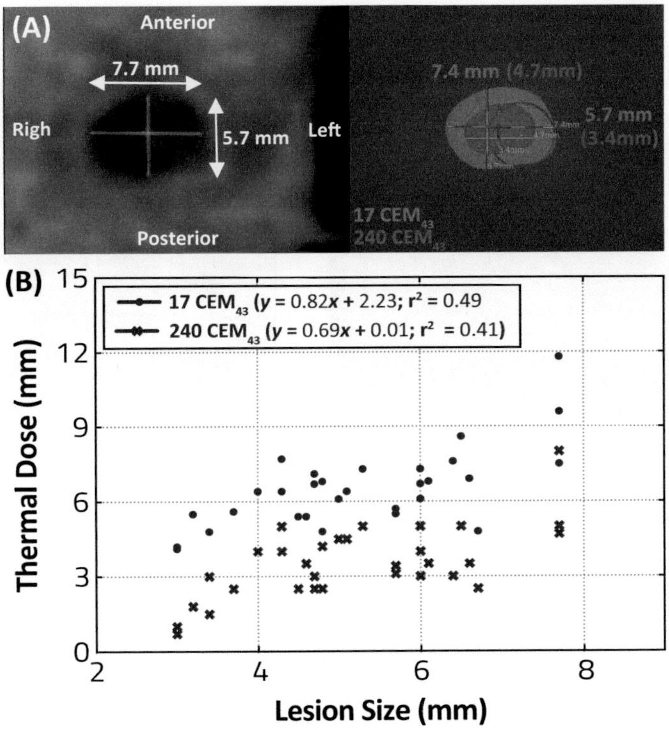

FIGURE 17.5 (A) Representative example of an MRgFUS-induced brain lesion on T_1w imaging one day post-treatment (left) together with the corresponding 17 CEM_{43} (yellow) and 240 CEM_{43} (green) thermal dose maps (right) obtained using MR-thermometry during the procedure. (B) Correlation of lesion size (measured via T_1w imaging) and thermal dose (17 CEM_{43} and 240 CEM_{43}) size for 16 patients treated with MRgFUS thalamotomy for ET at our institution (early subset of patients reported in Huang et al. 2018). Distance measurements along the right-left and anterior-posterior directions are plotted for each patient. The lines of best fit demonstrate that dose sizes based on 240 CEM_{43} and 17 CEM_{43} tend to under- and over-estimate the corresponding lesion size measured via T_2w MRI, respectively.

of thermal lesions generated in muscle tissue,[119, 120] they tend to underestimate the size of brain lesions both in animal models[121] and clinical treatments (Figure 17.5). Indeed, a study of ultrasound-induced thermal bioeffects in rabbit brain found that a dose of 17.5 CEM_{43} corresponded to a 50% probability of inducing tissue damage.[121] Additionally, in some uterine fibroid ablation procedures the immediate non-perfused volume, an important indicator of treatment success,[122] can extend far beyond the ablation region predicted from thermal dosimetry due to the occlusion or spasm of large blood vessels in the treated zone.[93] More precise dose thresholds for various clinical applications have yet to be established.

With the existing clinical MRgFUS systems, thermal dose distributions can be accumulated over multiple sonications in 2D if the imaging planes remain unchanged, with appropriate corrections to compensate for off-resonance-induced spatial shifting artifacts induced along the frequency-encoding direction.[32, 123, 124] During uterine fibroid treatments with the Sonalleve system, both temperature maps and thermal dose volumes are used for real-time feedback to control the timing on the steering of the acoustic beam.[72, 73] An example of FUS uterine fibroid ablation with the Sonalleve system is shown in Figure 17.6. With this system, volumetric sonications are performed by steering the acoustic focus electronically along concentric circular trajectories of 4, 8, 12, and 16 mm in diameter. These treatment cells are divided up into 8, 16, 24, and 32 evenly spaced points, respectively, and the order in which they are sonicated individually is chosen to promote a uniform temperature elevation by maximising the spatial distance between successive points [Figure 17.6(A)]. Starting from the innermost prescribed circle, sonications are performed until either all voxels within that circle receive a thermal dose of 240 CEM_{43}

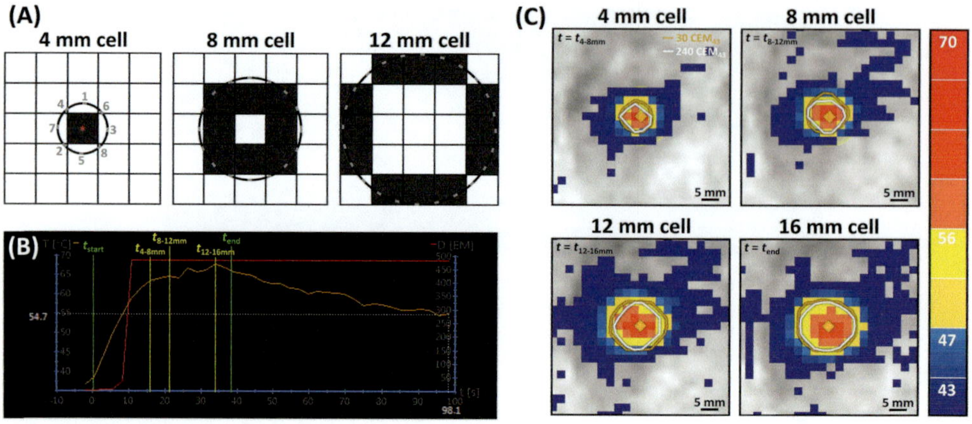

FIGURE 17.6 Illustration of MR thermometry feedback-controlled volumetric sonications using the Sonalleve MRgFUS system. (A) Circular trajectories are divided up into a series of evenly spaced points (light gray). The order in which these control points are sonicated is specified for the 4 mm treatment cell case. The voxels (2.5 mm × 2.5 mm in size) used for feedback control for a given cell size are filled in (dark gray). (B) Temperature and thermal dose accumulation (CEM_{43}) in the middle of the treatment cell [red asterisk in (A)] as a function of time during a uterine fibroid treatment conducted at our institution with the Sonalleve system. The time points at which the sonications transition between the various treatment cell sizes are specified (yellow), along with the start and stop points of sonication (green). (C) Coronal magnitude thermometry images at four different time points along the temperature and dose curves in (B) corresponding to 4, 8, 12, and 16 mm treatment cell sonications. Both the temperature and thermal dose (30 CEM_{43} and 240 CEM_{43}) distributions are overlaid in colour (orange and white, respectively).

or until the mean temperature level exceeds a predetermined threshold, at which point either sonications around a larger treatment circle are carried out or the procedure is terminated.[72, 73] The Sonalleve system also allows volumetric sonications to be carried out without feedback control, and this strategy is employed during current bone treatments[92, 125]; the ultrasound exposures are truncated if the peak temperature is assessed to have exceeded 80 °C. Figure 17.6(B) demonstrates the calculation of thermal dose for a single voxel given its temperature as a function of time (via Eq. 17.2). Figure 17.6(C) shows an example of a spatial thermal dose map; the thermal dose is calculated independently for each voxel and the white (orange) contours denote regions that have reached at least 240 (30) CEM_{43}.

17.7 System Calibration and Quality Assurance

Several methods exist for calibrating clinical MRgFUS systems (see review): bulk measurements of the total acoustic power output for a given electrical input can be performed using a radiation force balance,[126, 127] and local measurements of the acoustic field can be obtained via hydrophone scans.[128, 129] If the device is positioned outside the MRI suite, the oscillation pattern at the surface of the transducer can be characterised using laser vibrometry[130] or hydrophone measurements of a pre-focal 2D planar field combined with back-projection techniques.[49, 131, 132] This latter combined measurement and modelling approach has several uses as a quality assurance (QA) tool: for example, it can be used to identify defective elements or to test whether any significant phase or amplitude variations exist from element-to-element within a phased array, which could be compensated for to improve the overall acoustic field generated by the device.

On the treatment day, a QA protocol that consists of a series of test sonications within a re-useable tissue-mimicking gel phantom is carried out to verify the overall functionality of the MRgFUS system.[41, 133, 134] Several low-power thermal exposures are carried out and the corresponding MR-thermometry images are examined to ensure that quantities such as the peak temperature rise, targeting accuracy, shape of the heated zone, and image noise level are within acceptable tolerance levels. With InSightec's brain systems, a high power sonication designed to nucleate cavitation activity within the gel phantom is carried out, to confirm the system's ability to halt sonications automatically based on the acoustic signals received by the passive cavitation detectors.

The specific pulsing scheme (i.e., applied acoustic power, pulse duration, pulse repetition frequency) employed during clinical MRgFUS treatments depends on the nature of the desired biological effect. As will be seen later, the majority of clinical MRgFUS procedures performed to date have intended to induce thermal coagulative necrosis (see Section 17.8). During these ablative treatments, continuous wave (CW) ultrasound exposures are applied for tens of seconds, with in situ spatial-peak time-averaged intensities that are typically within the range of 10^3-10^4 W/cm^2, to raise the absolute temperature of the target tissue to 55–60 °C. Dwell times of the order of 1–100 s allow the overlying tissue to cool between successive sonications. MRgFUS mild hyperthermia employs CW ultrasound at reduced exposure levels (10^2-10^3 W/cm^2 spatial-peak time-averaged intensity) over tens of minutes with the aim of maintaining the target tissue volume between 40–43 °C. To date, six patients have been treated with MRgFUS mild hyperthermia using the Sonalleve device in a phase I trial investigating its use for the sensitisation of radiation and chemotherapy for recurrent rectal cancer.[74] In contrast, during FUS-mediated BBB opening low power pulsed ultrasound exposures (e.g., pulse length = 2 ms, duty cycle <1%, exposure duration = 50 s[63] during initial clinical testing[135, 136] are applied in combination with an intravenous injection of contrast agent microbubbles, resulting in a temporary and localised increase in cerebral microvascular permeability (see Section 17.8.4). At frequencies suitable for trans-skull sonications (0.2–1.5 MHz), the spatial-peak time-averaged acoustic intensities required for BBB opening are approximately two orders of magnitude lower than the threshold for inducing thermal effects in the brain.[63, 137]

17.8 Clinical Applications of Extracorporeal MRgFUS

17.8.1 Breast

Breast tumours were chosen as the first clinical target for MRgFUS technology, as they are easily accessible with therapeutic ultrasound anatomically and since, given the choice, many patients would prefer a non-invasive treatment option that preserves cosmetic integrity.[138] In their seminal work, Hynynen et al. targeted benign focal breast fibroadenomas with a mechanically scanned single-element transducer, and 73% (8/11) of the treated lesions showed partial or complete lack of gadolinium-based contrast material uptake on post-treatment MRI.[28] Later that same year, a case study in which MRgFUS was used to ablate a malignant breast tumour prior to breast conserving surgery was reported.[34] Since these initial feasibility studies, several trials investigating MRgFUS ablation for breast cancer have been carried out using follow up surgical resection to evaluate the extent of tumour coagulation.[26, 139] Although the MRgFUS breast tumour treatments performed to date have been able to ablate the majority of malignant tissue successfully, the proportion of reported cases that have resulted in complete tumour necrosis has been relatively low (e.g., 54% in one study[139]). Several technical obstacles need to be addressed before MRgFUS is employed routinely in the clinic for breast treatments, including the development of methods for accurate MR-thermometry in fatty tissues, and strategies for reducing the currently lengthy procedure times. The two dedicated phased array MRgFUS breast systems currently under development[78, 79] aim to overcome some of these limitations.

17.8.2 Uterus

Thermal ablation using FUS is a relatively new treatment approach for uterine fibroids (leiomyomas or myomas). These are extremely prevalent, noncancerous neoplasms of the uterus.[109, 140] The ExAblate Body,[29, 43] JM,[70, 71] and Sonalleve[106] systems have all been shown to be safe and effective in treating these myomas. For example, one study reported that 73% (40/55) of patients with uterine fibroids treated with MRgFUS had significant symptom improvement one year post-treatment. This proportion increased to 90% (19/21) once less conservative treatment protocols were adopted.[141] FUS ablation has several advantages compared to traditional surgical-based approaches for treating fibroids: it has a short recovery time (primarily this is recovery from sedation) and can thus be performed as an outpatient procedure,[142] the treatments are well tolerated and are associated with comparatively low complication rates, and several recent retrospective studies suggest that MRgFUS has no negative impact on fertility.[143] Indeed, in a recent literature review, MRgFUS was deemed to be a "safe and effective non-invasive uterine-preserving treatment from which they [patients] can rapidly recover" by a Canadian government agency,[144] and a compatriot economic analysis concluded that the technology could result in a saving of over 4 million Canadian dollars annually in the province of Ontario alone.[145] However, despite the excellent clinical success achieved worldwide in treating uterine fibroids using MRgFUS, the procedure times for large fibroids are currently lengthy (typically over 3 h[146, 147]), and many patients do not pass the inclusion criteria for the existing clinical systems (e.g., lack of scarring, surgical clips, and bowel loops within the FUS beam path, target depth from skin surface ≤8 cm.[76]) Recent computer simulations[148, 149] have suggested that some of these limitations may be overcome by employing an improved phased array design.[150] Based on these studies, a fully electronically steerable MRgFUS phased array system (17 cm flat aperture, 6144 elements, 0.5 MHz operating frequency) has been developed (Arrayus Technologies, Inc., Burlington, Canada) and is currently undergoing clinical testing at our institution for the treatment of uterine fibroids.

17.8.3 Bone

Common malignant cancers, including those of breast, gastrointestinal tract, and lung, usually metastasise to bone and can result in pain that is not only extremely difficult to control but also has an associated reduction in the quality of life of many patients. Both the ExAblate Body[151–153] and Sonalleve[44, 92, 125, 154, 155] systems have been used successfully in the clinic to treat pain from bone metastases. The results from a multicentre phase III trial demonstrated the effectiveness of MRgFUS both in rapid pain palliation and in improved quality of life in patients with bone metastases.[152] Furthermore, the time until response of MRgFUS ablation is typically a few days.[152] This compares favourably to external beam radiotherapy (on the order of weeks), which is the current standard of care for painful bone metastases that do not respond to opioid pain relief.[156] Similar clinical success has been found in treating pain from lumbar facet joints[125, 157] and benign bone tumours[158–160] with these MRgFUS devices. In a multicentre clinical trial, 90% (26/29) of osteoid osteoma patients that underwent MRgFUS ablation reported complete pain relief 1 year post-treatment.[158] To the best of the authors' knowledge, there are only two published reports concerning the clinical use of InSightec's dedicated bone system, one in which two of the five patients treated with bone metastases had complete pain reduction at the 1-year follow-up point[44] and another in which 74% (14/19) of patients treated with medial knee osteoarthritis reported a partial treatment response (i.e., ≥50% decrease in numerical rating scale pain score) at 12 months post-treatment.[161] Further clinical testing is therefore required to assess this MRgFUS device.

Since bone has a very high acoustic absorption coefficient,[162] these tumours and periosteal nerves, which are the desired target for pain palliation applications, can generally be heated sufficiently to achieve ablation with relatively low-level ultrasound exposures. However, in cases where the bone has been infiltrated by malignant soft tissue, higher power levels can be required. Nevertheless, in practice it is difficult to monitor the heating accurately during MRgFUS bone treatments. Because the temperature maps are obtained by subtraction of a baseline reference (see Eq. 17.1), they are extremely sensitive to motion during heating, which can occur as a result of patient pain during the exposures. To help minimise motion-induced MR-thermometry artifacts, patients are sedated continuously during palliation of pain from metastatic bone lesions[92], and in some benign tumour cases general anaesthesia is applied.[159]

17.8.4 Brain

Non-invasive approaches to the treatment of neurological disorders are particularly attractive, since invasive interventions in the brain can be associated with detrimental complications and side effects due to damage to overlying tissue. The first clinical test of MRgFUS in the brain was a trial that investigated the feasibility of ultrasound-induced thermal ablation for treating glioblastoma (GBM) in three patients at BWH.[90] The early-stage device employed in this study was limited in that it was unable to deliver sufficient acoustic power to achieve coagulation, nonetheless it was demonstrated that acoustic waves could be focused transcranially into the brain, and that the induced heating distribution could be visualised using MR-thermometry.[90] Several improvements were subsequently made to InSightec's high-frequency system, and it has since been shown capable of producing thermal lesions within the brain for the treatment of a variety of neurological disorders, as will be discussed later. A phase I clinical trial of the safety and efficacy of MRgFUS ablation for GBM, using this updated system, is ongoing in Switzerland. A case study, which reports partial tumour ablation in a single patient with a centrally located GBM without any observable neurological deficits or other adverse events, has been published from this cohort.[163] A separate MRgFUS approach for brain tumour therapy is to harness the interactions of ultrasound with contrast agent microbubbles for non-invasive, targeted drug delivery to the brain by temporary opening of the BBB.[63, 137, 164, 165] InSightec's low-frequency system has been employed in early phase clinical trials aiming to enhance the delivery of chemotherapy in patients with glioma[89, 136] and Her2-positive brain metastases,[166] as well as several studies investigating the feasibility and safety of FUS-induced BBB opening for different neurological indications, including Alzheimer's disease,[135, 167] amyotrophic lateral sclerosis,[168] and PD.[169]

Based on the clinical experience gained from the first GBM trial, MRgFUS thalamotomy was tested in nine patients for the treatment of chronic neuropathic pain in Zurich.[170] Thermal lesions were generated in the posterior part of the central lateral thalamic nucleus, resulting in a mean pain relief of 68% 2 days post-treatment.[170] In a follow-up study, it was observed that the pain relief was temporally varying within this patient population, with mean values of 49% and 57% reported at 3 and 12 months post-treatment, respectively.[171] One of the additional patient treatments reported in this follow-up study resulted in a permanent neurological complication due to bleeding at the focal target and associated ischemia that extended into the motor thalamus.[171] This complication led to the incorporation of passive detectors within the MRgFUS system to monitor for unwanted cavitation activity.[171]

To date, most of the clinical experience employing transcranial MRgFUS has been obtained in treating ET, one of the most prevalent movement disorders worldwide. Following previously developed RF ablation and deep brain stimulation approaches,[172, 173] several groups have shown that precise unilateral lesioning in the central intermediate nucleus of the thalamus using MRgFUS can lead to reduced contralateral hand tremor in patients suffering from ET.[54, 104, 174, 175] These studies paved the way for a multi-centre, randomised controlled trial, which demonstrated that patients treated with MRgFUS for ET had significantly improved tremor scores compared to sham controls, and that the improvement was maintained at the 1-year follow-up point.[54] A follow-up study reported that tremor suppression in this patient population was maintained stably at the 2-year time point.[175] Ongoing trials are investigating the safety profile of staged, bilateral MRgFUS thalamotomy to address ipsilateral symptoms.[176] Apart from ET, several brain targets have been investigated for MRgFUS thermal ablation treatment in patients with tremor-dominant PD,[55] advanced PD,[56] and behavioural and psychiatric disorders such as obsessive-compulsive disorder and major depressive disorder.[177, 178]

The use of ultrasound therapies in the brain is also discussed in Chapters 20 and 26.

17.9 Summary

FUS can be used to deliver energy that can be harnessed to induce localised therapeutic effects, and it can be performed deep into the body in a completely non-invasive manner using extracorporeal devices. MRI's unrivalled soft tissue contrast and ability to measure temperature elevations quantitatively make it the modality of choice for thermal FUS therapy guidance, as it allows precise treatment planning, online monitoring using MR-thermometry and thermal dose mapping, as well as post-treatment evaluation. Clinical investigations with external MRgFUS devices to date have, for the most part, involved treatments that have aimed to induce cell death via thermal ablation (e.g., in malignant and benign breast tumours, benign uterine fibroids, periosteal nerves, as well as brain malignancies or targets for functional/psychiatric neurosurgery). Some promising non-thermal applications (e.g., FUS-induced BBB opening) are now also in the early stages of human testing. Further improvements in both ultrasound phased array and image guidance technology[179] will improve the speed, safety, and efficacy of the existing FUS therapies, as well as increase the number of clinical indications for which it is a viable and effective treatment option, ultimately resulting in therapeutic ultrasound being used more routinely to enhance patient well-being worldwide.

REFERENCES

1. Lynn JG, Zwemer RL, Chick AJ, Miller AE. A new method for the generation and use of focused ultrasound in experimental biology. The Journal of General Physiology. 1942;26(2):179.
2. Lynn JG, Putnam TJ. Histology of cerebral lesions produced by focused ultrasound. The American Journal of Pathology. 1944;20(3):637.
3. O'Neil H. Theory of focusing radiators. The Journal of the Acoustical Society of America. 1949;21(5):516–26.
4. Baker KG, Robertson VJ, Duck FA. A review of therapeutic ultrasound: Biophysical effects. Physical Therapy. 2001;81(7):1351–8.
5. Coussios C, Farny C, ter Haar G, Roy R. Role of acoustic cavitation in the delivery and monitoring of cancer treatment by high-intensity focused ultrasound (HIFU). International Journal of Hyperthermia. 2007;23(2):105–20.
6. Goertz DE. An overview of the influence of therapeutic ultrasound exposures on the vasculature: High intensity ultrasound and microbubble-mediated bioeffects. International Journal of Hyperthermia. 2015;31(2):134–44.
7. O'Brien Jr WD. Ultrasound–biophysics mechanisms. Progress in Biophysics and Molecular Biology. 2007;93(1–3):212–55.
8. Fry W, Fry F. Fundamental neurological research and human neurosurgery using intense ultrasound. IRE Transactions on Medical Electronics. 1960(3):166–81.
9. Okuyama D, Fry WJ, Fry FJ, Leichner GH, Kelly E. Acoustic visualization of transient inhomogeneities induced by intense focused ultrasound in lucite. The Journal of the Acoustical Society of America. 1966;39(6_Supplement):1236.
10. Fry F, Sanghvi N, Eggleton R, Erdmann W, editors. Ultrasonic visualization and therapeutic computer controlled system. Ultrasound in Medicine: Volume 2 Proceedings of the 20th Annual Meeting of the American Institute of Ultrasound in Medicine. Springer; 1976.
11. Wu F, Chen W-Z, Bai J, Zou J-Z, Wang Z-L, Zhu H, et al. Pathological changes in human malignant carcinoma treated with high-intensity focused ultrasound. Ultrasound in Medicine & Biology. 2001;27(8):1099–106.
12. Wu F, Wang Z-B, Chen W-Z, Wang W, Gui Y, Zhang M, et al. Extracorporeal high intensity focused ultrasound ablation in the treatment of 1038 patients with solid carcinomas in China: An overview. Ultrasonics Sonochemistry. 2004;11(3–4):149–54.
13. Kennedy J, Wu F, ter Haar G, Gleeson F, Phillips R, Middleton M, et al. High-intensity focused ultrasound for the treatment of liver tumours. Ultrasonics. 2004;42(1–9):931–5.
14. Peek M, Ahmed M, Scudder J, Baker R, Pinder S, Douek M, et al. High intensity focused ultrasound in the treatment of breast fibroadenomata: Results of the HIFU-F trial. International Journal of Hyperthermia. 2016;32(8):881–8.
15. Gray MD, Lyon PC, Mannaris C, Folkes LK, Stratford M, Campo L, et al. Focused ultrasound hyperthermia for targeted drug release from thermosensitive liposomes: Results from a phase I trial. Radiology. 2019;291(1):232–8.
16. Lyon PC, Gray MD, Mannaris C, Folkes LK, Stratford M, Campo L, et al. Safety and feasibility of ultrasound-triggered targeted drug delivery of doxorubicin from thermosensitive liposomes in liver tumours (TARDOX): A single-centre, open-label, phase 1 trial. The Lancet Oncology. 2018;19(8):1027–39.
17. Vidal-Jové J, Serres-Créixams X, Ziemlewicz TJ, Cannata JM. Liver histotripsy mediated abscopal effect – Case report. IEEE Transactions on Ultrasonics, Ferroelectrics, and Frequency Control. 2021;68(9):3001–5.

18. Drost L, Hynynen K, Huang Y, Lucht B, Wong E, Czarnota G, et al. Ultrasound-guided focused ultrasound treatment for painful bone metastases: A pilot study. Ultrasound in Medicine & Biology. 2020;46(6):1455–63.
19. Illing R, Kennedy J, Wu F, ter Haar G, Protheroe A, Friend P, et al. The safety and feasibility of extracorporeal high-intensity focused ultrasound (HIFU) for the treatment of liver and kidney tumours in a Western population. British Journal of Cancer. 2005;93(8):890–5.
20. Rivens I, Shaw A, Civale J, Morris H. Treatment monitoring and thermometry for therapeutic focused ultrasound. International Journal of Hyperthermia. 2007;23(2):121–39.
21. Hynynen K, Darkazanli A, Unger E, Schenck J. MRI-guided noninvasive ultrasound surgery. Medical Physics. 1993;20(1):107–15.
22. Parker DL. Applications of NMR imaging in hyperthermia: An evaluation of the potential for localized tissue heating and noninvasive temperature monitoring. IEEE Transactions on Biomedical Engineering. 1984(1):161–7.
23. Ishihara Y, Calderon A, Watanabe H, Okamoto K, Suzuki Y, Kuroda K, et al. A precise and fast temperature mapping using water proton chemical shift. Magnetic Resonance in Medicine. 1995;34(6):814–23.
24. Chung AH, Jolesz FA, Hynynen K. Thermal dosimetry of a focused ultrasound beam in vivo by magnetic resonance imaging. Medical Physics. 1999;26(9):2017–26.
25. Graham S, Chen L, Leitch M, Peters R, Bronskill M, Foster F, et al. Quantifying tissue damage due to focused ultrasound heating observed by MRI. Magnetic Resonance in Medicine: An Official Journal of the International Society for Magnetic Resonance in Medicine. 1999;41(2):321–8.
26. Gianfelice D, Khiat A, Amara M, Belblidia A, Boulanger Y. MR imaging-guided focused ultrasound surgery of breast cancer: Correlation of dynamic contrast-enhanced MRI with histopathologic findings. Breast Cancer Research and Treatment. 2003;82:93–101.
27. Hynynen K, Darkazanli A, Damianou CA, Unger E, Schenck JF. The usefulness of a contrast agent and gradient-recalled acquisition in a steady-state imaging sequence for magnetic resonance imaging-guided noninvasive ultrasound surgery. Investigative Radiology. 1994;29(10):897–903.
28. Hynynen K, Pomeroy O, Smith DN, Huber PE, McDannold NJ, Kettenbach J, et al. MR imaging-guided focused ultrasound surgery of fibroadenomas in the breast: A feasibility study. Radiology. 2001;219(1):176–85.
29. Tempany CM, Stewart EA, McDannold N, Quade BJ, Jolesz FA, Hynynen K. MR imaging–guided focused ultrasound surgery of uterine leiomyomas: A feasibility study. Radiology. 2003;226(3):897–905.
30. Mörocz IÁ, Hynynen K, Gudbjartsson H, Peled S, Colucci V, Jólesz FA. Brain edema development after MRI-guided focused ultrasound treatment. Journal of Magnetic Resonance Imaging. 1998;8(1):136–42.
31. Wintermark M, Druzgal J, Huss D, Khaled M, Monteith S, Raghavan P, et al. Imaging findings in MR imaging–guided focused ultrasound treatment for patients with essential tremor. American Journal of Neuroradiology. 2014;35(5):891–6.
32. Huang Y, Lipsman N, Schwartz ML, Krishna V, Sammartino F, Lozano AM, et al. Predicting lesion size by accumulated thermal dose in MR-guided focused ultrasound for essential tremor. Medical Physics. 2018;45(10):4704–10.
33. Cline HE, Schenck JF, Hynynen K, Watkins RD, Souza SP, Jolesz FA. MR-guided focused ultrasound surgery. Journal of Computer Assisted Tomography. 1992;16(6):956–65.
34. Huber PE, Jenne JW, Rastert R, Simiantonakis I, Sinn H-P, Strittmatter H-J, et al. A new noninvasive approach in breast cancer therapy using magnetic resonance imaging-guided focused ultrasound surgery. Cancer Research. 2001;61(23):8441–7.
35. Hynynen K. MRIgHIFU: A tool for image-guided therapeutics. Journal of Magnetic Resonance Imaging. 2011;34(3):482–93.
36. Fjield T, Hynynen K. The combined concentric-ring and sector-vortex phased array for MRI guided ultrasound surgery. IEEE Transactions on Ultrasonics, Ferroelectrics, and Frequency Control. 1997;44(5):1157–67.
37. Daum DR, Hynynen K. A 256-element ultrasonic phased array system for the treatment of large volumes of deep seated tissue. IEEE Transactions on Ultrasonics, Ferroelectrics, and Frequency Control. 1999;46(5):1254–68.
38. Daum DR, Smith NB, King R, Hynynen K. In vivo demonstration of noninvasive thermal surgery of the liver and kidney using an ultrasonic phased array. Ultrasound in Medicine & Biology. 1999;25(7):1087–98.

39. Cline HE, Hynynen K, Hardy CJ, Watkins RD, Schenck JF, Jolesz FA. MR temperature mapping of focused ultrasound surgery. Magnetic Resonance in Medicine. 1994;31(6):628–36.
40. Pilatou MC, Stewart EA, Maier SE, Fennessy FM, Hynynen K, Tempany CM, et al. MRI-based thermal dosimetry and diffusion-weighted imaging of MRI-guided focused ultrasound thermal ablation of uterine fibroids. Journal of Magnetic Resonance Imaging: An Official Journal of the International Society for Magnetic Resonance in Medicine. 2009;29(2):404–11.
41. McDannold N, Hynynen K. Quality assurance and system stability of a clinical MRI-guided focused ultrasound system: Four-year experience. Medical Physics. 2006;33(11):4307–13.
42. Catane R, Beck A, Inbar Y, Rabin T, Shabshin N, Hengst S, et al. MR-guided focused ultrasound surgery (MRgFUS) for the palliation of pain in patients with bone metastases – preliminary clinical experience. Annals of Oncology. 2007;18(1):163–7.
43. Browne JE, Gorny KR, Hangiandreou NJ, Edmonson HA, Long Z, Brandt KR, et al. Comparison of clinical performance between two generations of magnetic resonance-guided focused ultrasound systems in treatments of uterine leiomyomas. Academic Radiology. 2021;28(10):1361–7.
44. Joo B, Park M-S, Lee SH, Choi HJ, Lim ST, Rha SY, et al. Pain palliation in patients with bone metastases using magnetic resonance-guided focused ultrasound with conformal bone system: A preliminary report. Yonsei Medical Journal. 2015;56(2):503–9.
45. Guthkelch A, Carter L, Cassady J, Hynynen K, Iacono R, Johnson P, et al. Treatment of malignant brain tumors with focused ultrasound hyperthermia and radiation: Results of a phase I trial. Journal of Neuro-Oncology. 1991;10:271–84.
46. Hynynen K, Jolesz FA. Demonstration of potential noninvasive ultrasound brain therapy through an intact skull. Ultrasound in Medicine & Biology. 1998;24(2):275–83.
47. Sun J, Hynynen K. Focusing of therapeutic ultrasound through a human skull: A numerical study. The Journal of the Acoustical Society of America. 1998;104(3):1705–15.
48. Sun J, Hynynen K. The potential of transskull ultrasound therapy and surgery using the maximum available skull surface area. The Journal of the Acoustical Society of America. 1999;105(4):2519–27.
49. Clement G, Hynynen K. Field characterization of therapeutic ultrasound phased arrays through forward and backward planar projection. The Journal of the Acoustical Society of America. 2000;108(1):441–6.
50. Clement GT, Sun J, Giesecke T, Hynynen K. A hemisphere array for non-invasive ultrasound brain therapy and surgery. Physics in Medicine & Biology. 2000;45(12):3707.
51. Clement GT, Hynynen K. A non-invasive method for focusing ultrasound through the human skull. Physics in Medicine & Biology. 2002;47(8):1219.
52. Connor CW, Clement GT, Hynynen K. A unified model for the speed of sound in cranial bone based on genetic algorithm optimization. Physics in Medicine & Biology. 2002;47(22):3925.
53. Hynynen K, Clement GT, McDannold N, Vykhodtseva N, King R, White PJ, et al. 500-element ultrasound phased array system for noninvasive focal surgery of the brain: A preliminary rabbit study with ex vivo human skulls. Magnetic Resonance in Medicine: An Official Journal of the International Society for Magnetic Resonance in Medicine. 2004;52(1):100–7.
54. Elias WJ, Lipsman N, Ondo WG, Ghanouni P, Kim YG, Lee W, et al. A randomized trial of focused ultrasound thalamotomy for essential tremor. New England Journal of Medicine. 2016;375(8):730–9.
55. Bond AE, Shah BB, Huss DS, Dallapiazza RF, Warren A, Harrison MB, et al. Safety and efficacy of focused ultrasound thalamotomy for patients with medication-refractory, tremor-dominant Parkinson disease: A randomized clinical trial. JAMA Neurology. 2017;74(12):1412–8.
56. Eisenberg HM, Krishna V, Elias WJ, Cosgrove GR, Gandhi D, Aldrich CE, et al. MR-guided focused ultrasound pallidotomy for Parkinson's disease: Safety and feasibility. Journal of Neurosurgery. 2020;135(3):792–8.
57. Marsac L, Chauvet D, Larrat B, Pernot M, Robert B, Fink M, et al. MR-guided adaptive focusing of therapeutic ultrasound beams in the human head. Medical Physics. 2012;39(2):1141–9.
58. Aubry J-F, Marsac L, Pernot M, Robert B, Boch A-L, Chauvet D, et al. Ultrasons focalisés de forte intensité pour la thérapie transcrânienne du cerveau. IRBM. 2010;31(2):87–91.
59. Chauvet D, Marsac L, Pernot M, Boch A-L, Guillevin R, Salameh N, et al. Targeting accuracy of transcranial magnetic resonance–guided high-intensity focused ultrasound brain therapy: A fresh cadaver model. Journal of neurosurgery. 2013;118(5):1046–52.

60. Alkins R, Huang Y, Pajek D, Hynynen K. Cavitation-based third ventriculostomy using MRI-guided focused ultrasound. Journal of neurosurgery. 2013;119(6):1520–9.
61. Monteith SJ, Harnof S, Medel R, Popp B, Wintermark M, Lopes MBS, et al. Minimally invasive treatment of intracerebral hemorrhage with magnetic resonance–guided focused ultrasound. Journal of Neurosurgery. 2013;118(5):1035–45.
62. Arvanitis CD, Vykhodtseva N, Jolesz F, Livingstone M, McDannold N. Cavitation-enhanced non-thermal ablation in deep brain targets: Feasibility in a large animal model. Journal of Neurosurgery. 2016;124(5):1450–9.
63. Huang Y, Alkins R, Schwartz ML, Hynynen K. Opening the blood-brain barrier with MR imaging–guided focused ultrasound: Preclinical testing on a trans–human skull porcine model. Radiology. 2017;282(1):123–30.
64. Badran BW, Caulfield KA, Stomberg-Firestein S, Summers PM, Dowdle LT, Savoca M, et al. Sonication of the anterior thalamus with MRI-Guided transcranial focused ultrasound (tFUS) alters pain thresholds in healthy adults: A double-blind, sham-controlled study. Brain Stimulation. 2020;13(6):1805–12.
65. Chen K-T, Chai W-Y, Lin Y-J, Lin C-J, Chen P-Y, Tsai H-C, et al. Neuronavigation-guided focused ultrasound for transcranial blood-brain barrier opening and immunostimulation in brain tumors. Science Advances. 2021;7(6):eabd0772.
66. Wei K-C, Tsai H-C, Lu Y-J, Yang H-W, Hua M-Y, Wu M-F, et al. Neuronavigation-guided focused ultrasound-induced blood-brain barrier opening: A preliminary study in swine. American Journal of Neuroradiology. 2013;34(1):115–20.
67. Pouliopoulos AN, Wu S-Y, Burgess MT, Karakatsani ME, Kamimura HA, Konofagou EE. A clinical system for non-invasive blood–brain barrier opening using a neuronavigation-guided single-element focused ultrasound transducer. Ultrasound in Medicine & Biology. 2020;46(1):73–89.
68. Hughes A, Hynynen K. Design of patient-specific focused ultrasound arrays for non-invasive brain therapy with increased trans-skull transmission and steering range. Physics in Medicine & Biology. 2017;62(17):L9.
69. Adams C, Jones RM, Yang SD, Kan WM, Leung K, Zhou Y, et al. Implementation of a skull-conformal phased array for transcranial focused ultrasound therapy. IEEE Transactions on Biomedical Engineering. 2021;68(11):3457–68.
70. Wang Y, Wang Z-B, Xu Y-H. Efficacy, efficiency, and safety of magnetic resonance-guided high-intensity focused ultrasound for ablation of uterine fibroids: Comparison with ultrasound-guided method. Korean Journal of Radiology. 2018;19(4):724–32.
71. Zhang L, Chen W-Z, Liu Y-J, Hu X, Zhou K, Chen L, et al. Feasibility of magnetic resonance imaging-guided high intensity focused ultrasound therapy for ablating uterine fibroids in patients with bowel lies anterior to uterus. European Journal of Radiology. 2010;73(2):396–403.
72. Köhler MO, Mougenot C, Quesson B, Enholm J, Le Bail B, Laurent C, et al. Volumetric HIFU ablation under 3D guidance of rapid MRI thermometry. Medical Physics. 2009;36(8):3521–35.
73. Enholm JK, Kohler MO, Quesson B, Mougenot C, Moonen CT, Sokka SD. Improved volumetric MR-HIFU ablation by robust binary feedback control. IEEE Transactions on Biomedical Engineering. 2009;57(1):103–13.
74. Chu W, Staruch RM, Pichardo S, Tillander M, Köhler MO, Huang Y, et al. Magnetic Resonance–Guided high-intensity focused ultrasound hyperthermia for recurrent rectal cancer: Mr thermometry evaluation and preclinical validation. International Journal of Radiation Oncology* Biology* Physics. 2016;95(4):1259–67.
75. Lee J, Farha G, Poon I, Karam I, Higgins K, Pichardo S, et al. Magnetic resonance-guided high-intensity focused ultrasound combined with radiotherapy for palliation of head and neck cancer – a pilot study. Journal of Therapeutic Ultrasound. 2016;4:1–7.
76. Shim J, Staruch R, Koral K, Xie X-J, Chopra R, Laetsch TW. Anatomical distribution and radiological characteristics of pediatric sarcoma and neuroblastoma: Eligibility for treatment with non-invasive ablative therapies. Pediatric Blood & Cancer. 2016;63(10):1753.
77. Wang C-J, Lin G, Huang Y-T, Weng CH, Wu K-Y, Su Y-Y, et al. A feasibility analysis of the ArcBlate MR-guided high-intensity focused ultrasound system for the ablation of uterine fibroids. Abdominal Radiology. 2021;46:5307–15.

78. Merckel LG, Bartels LW, Köhler MO, van den Bongard HD, Deckers R, Mali WPTM, et al. MR-guided high-intensity focused ultrasound ablation of breast cancer with a dedicated breast platform. Cardiovascular and Interventional Radiology. 2013;36:292–301.
79. Payne A, Merrill R, Minalga E, Vyas U, Bever Jd, Todd N, et al. Design and characterization of a laterally mounted phased-array transducer breast-specific MRgHIFU device with integrated 11-channel receiver array. Medical Physics. 2012;39(3):1552–60.
80. Bitton RR, Sheingaouz E, Assif B, Kelm N, Dayan M, Butts Pauly K, et al. Evaluation of an MRI receive head coil for use in transcranial MR guided focused ultrasound for functional neurosurgery. International Journal of Hyperthermia. 2021;38(1):22–9.
81. Gorny K, Hangiandreou N, Hesley G, Felmlee J. Evaluation of mineral oil as an acoustic coupling medium in clinical MRgFUS. Physics in Medicine & Biology. 2006;52(1):N13.
82. Hynynen K, McDannold N, Vykhodtseva N, Raymond S, Weissleder R, Jolesz FA, et al. Focal disruption of the blood–brain barrier due to 260-kHz ultrasound bursts: A method for molecular imaging and targeted drug delivery. Journal of Neurosurgery. 2006;105(3):445–54.
83. Ikink ME, van Breugel JM, Schubert G, Nijenhuis RJ, Bartels LW, Moonen CT, et al. Volumetric MR-guided high-intensity focused ultrasound with direct skin cooling for the treatment of symptomatic uterine fibroids: Proof-of-concept study. BioMed Research International. 2015;2015.
84. Leighton T. The Acoustic Bubble. Academic Press; 2012.
85. Hynynen K, Chung AH, Colucci V, Jolesz FA. Potential adverse effects of high-intensity focused ultrasound exposure on blood vessels in vivo. Ultrasound in Medicine & Biology. 1996;22(2):193–201.
86. Lele PP. Effects of ultrasound on "solid" mammalian tissues and tumors in vivo. Ultrasound: Medical Applications, Biological Effects, and Hazard Potential. Springer; 1987. p. 275–306.
87. Lele PP, editor Thresholds and mechanisms of ultrasonic damage to "organized" animal tissues. Symposium on Biological Effects and Characterizations of Ultrasound Sources. Vol 1977 Jun 2 (Vol. 78, p. 8048).
88. Eller A, Flynn H. Generation of subharmonics of order one-half by bubbles in a sound field. The Journal of the Acoustical Society of America. 1969;46(3B):722–7.
89. Anastasiadis P, Gandhi D, Guo Y, Ahmed A-K, Bentzen SM, Arvanitis C, et al. Localized blood–brain barrier opening in infiltrating gliomas with MRI-guided acoustic emissions–controlled focused ultrasound. Proceedings of the National Academy of Sciences. 2021;118(37):e2103280118.
90. McDannold N, Clement GT, Black P, Jolesz F, Hynynen K. Transcranial magnetic resonance imaging–guided focused ultrasound surgery of brain tumors: Initial findings in 3 patients. Neurosurgery. 2010;66(2):323–32.
91. Raymond SB, Hynynen K. Acoustic transmission losses and field alterations due to human scalp hair. IEEE Transactions on Ultrasonics, Ferroelectrics, and Frequency Control. 2005;52(8):1415–9.
92. Chan M, Dennis K, Huang Y, Mougenot C, Chow E, DeAngelis C, et al. Magnetic resonance–guided high-intensity-focused ultrasound for palliation of painful skeletal metastases: A pilot study. Technology in Cancer Research & Treatment. 2017;16(5):570–6.
93. McDannold N, Tempany CM, Fennessy FM, So MJ, Rybicki FJ, Stewart EA, et al. Uterine leiomyomas: MR imaging–based thermometry and thermal dosimetry during focused ultrasound thermal ablation. Radiology. 2006;240(1):263–72.
94. Aubry J-F, Tanter M, Pernot M, Thomas J-L, Fink M. Experimental demonstration of noninvasive transskull adaptive focusing based on prior computed tomography scans. The Journal of the Acoustical Society of America. 2003;113(1):84–93.
95. Fry FJ, Barger JE. Acoustical properties of the human skull. The Journal of the Acoustical Society of America. 1978;63(5):1576–90.
96. Pichardo S, Sin VW, Hynynen K. Multi-frequency characterization of the speed of sound and attenuation coefficient for longitudinal transmission of freshly excised human skulls. Physics in Medicine & Biology. 2010;56(1):219.
97. Hynynen K, McDannold N, Clement G, Jolesz FA, Zadicario E, Killiany R, et al. Pre-clinical testing of a phased array ultrasound system for MRI-guided noninvasive surgery of the brain – a primate study. European Journal of Radiology. 2006;59(2):149–56.
98. Clement GT, White PJ, Hynynen K. Enhanced ultrasound transmission through the human skull using shear mode conversion. The Journal of the Acoustical Society of America. 2004;115(3):1356–64.
99. Makariou E, Patsalides AD. Intracranial calcifications. Applied Radiology. 2009;38(11).

100. Jones RM, Huang Y, Meng Y, Scantlebury N, Schwartz ML, Lipsman N, et al. Echo-focusing in transcranial focused ultrasound thalamotomy for essential tremor: A feasibility study. Movement Disorders. 2020;35(12):2327–33.
101. Hindman J. Proton resonance shift of water in the gas and liquid states. The Journal of Chemical Physics. 1966;44(12):4582–92.
102. Chung AH, Hynynen K, Colucci V, Oshio K, Cline HE, Jolesz FA. Optimization of spoiled gradient-echo phase imaging for in vivo localization of a focused ultrasound beam. Magnetic Resonance in Medicine. 1996;36(5):745–52.
103. Peters RT, Hinks RS, Henkelman RM. Ex vivo tissue-type independence in proton-resonance frequency shift MR thermometry. Magnetic Resonance in Medicine. 1998;40(3):454–9.
104. Lipsman N, Schwartz ML, Huang Y, Lee L, Sankar T, Chapman M, et al. MR-guided focused ultrasound thalamotomy for essential tremor: A proof-of-concept study. The Lancet Neurology. 2013;12(5):462–8.
105. McDannold N, White PJ, Cosgrove GR. Using phase data from MR temperature imaging to visualize anatomy during MRI-guided focused ultrasound neurosurgery. IEEE Transactions on Medical Imaging. 2020;39(12):3821–30.
106. Kim Y-s, Keserci B, Partanen A, Rhim H, Lim HK, Park MJ, et al. Volumetric MR-HIFU ablation of uterine fibroids: Role of treatment cell size in the improvement of energy efficiency. European Journal of Radiology. 2012;81(11):3652–9.
107. Baron P, Ries M, de Greef M, Deckers R, Kohler M, Tanttu J, et al., editors. In Vivo Validation of T2-based MR Thermometry in Adipose Tissue Layers for HIFU Near-field Monitoring. International Society Magnetic Resonance in Medicine; 2014.
108. Merckel LG, Knuttel FM, Deckers R, van Dalen T, Schubert G, Peters NH, et al. First clinical experience with a dedicated MRI-guided high-intensity focused ultrasound system for breast cancer ablation. European Radiology. 2016;26:4037–46.
109. Deckers R, Merckel L, De Senneville BD, Schubert G, Köhler M, Knuttel F, et al. Performance analysis of a dedicated breast MR-HIFU system for tumor ablation in breast cancer patients. Physics in Medicine & Biology. 2015;60(14):5527.
110. Bohris C, Schreiber WG, Jenne Ju, Simiantonakis I, Rastert R, Zabel HJ, et al. Quantitative MR temperature monitoring of high-intensity focused ultrasound therapy. Magnetic Resonance Imaging. 1999;17(4):603–10.
111. Ramsay E, Mougenot C, Kazem M, Laetsch TW, Chopra R. Temperature-dependent MR signals in cortical bone: Potential for monitoring temperature changes during high-intensity focused ultrasound treatment in bone. Magnetic Resonance in Medicine. 2015;74(4):1095–102.
112. McDannold N, Maier SE. Magnetic resonance acoustic radiation force imaging. Medical Physics. 2008;35(8):3748–58.
113. Payne A, Merrill R, Minalga E, Hadley JR, Odéen H, Hofstetter LW, et al. A breast-specific MR guided focused ultrasound platform and treatment protocol: First-in-human technical evaluation. IEEE Transactions on Biomedical Engineering. 2020;68(3):893–904.
114. Sapareto SA, Dewey WC. Thermal dose determination in cancer therapy. International Journal of Radiation Oncology* Biology* Physics. 1984;10(6):787–800.
115. Roizin-Towle L, Pirro JP. The response of human and rodent cells to hyperthermia. International Journal of Radiation Oncology* Biology* Physics. 1991;20(4):751–6.
116. Oleson JR, Samulski TV, Leopold KA, Clegg ST, Dewhirst MW, Dodge RK, et al. Sensitivity of hyperthermia trial outcomes to temperature and time: Implications for thermal goals of treatment. International Journal of Radiation Oncology* Biology* Physics. 1993;25(2):289–97.
117. Dewhirst MW, Viglianti B, Lora-Michiels M, Hanson M, Hoopes P. Basic principles of thermal dosimetry and thermal thresholds for tissue damage from hyperthermia. International Journal of Hyperthermia. 2003;19(3):267–94.
118. Yarmolenko PS, Moon EJ, Landon C, Manzoor A, Hochman DW, Viglianti BL, et al. Thresholds for thermal damage to normal tissues: An update. International Journal of Hyperthermia. 2011;27(4):320–43.
119. Damianou CA, Hynynen K, Fan X. Evaluation of accuracy of a theoretical model for predicting the necrosed tissue volume during focused ultrasound surgery. IEEE Transactions on Ultrasonics, Ferroelectrics, and Frequency Control. 1995;42(2):182–7.

120. McDannold NJ, King RL, Jolesz FA, Hynynen KH. Usefulness of MR imaging-derived thermometry and dosimetry in determining the threshold for tissue damage induced by thermal surgery in rabbits. Radiology. 2000;216(2):517–23.
121. McDannold N, Vykhodtseva N, Jolesz FA, Hynynen K. MRI investigation of the threshold for thermally induced blood–brain barrier disruption and brain tissue damage in the rabbit brain. Magnetic Resonance in Medicine: An Official Journal of the International Society for Magnetic Resonance in Medicine. 2004;51(5):913–23.
122. Lénárd ZM, McDannold NJ, Fennessy FM, Stewart EA, Jolesz FA, Hynynen K, et al. Uterine leiomyomas: MR imaging–guided focused ultrasound surgery – imaging predictors of success. Radiology. 2008;249(1):187–94.
123. Gaur P, Partanen A, Werner B, Ghanouni P, Bitton R, Butts Pauly K, et al. Correcting heat-induced chemical shift distortions in proton resonance frequency-shift thermometry. Magnetic Resonance in Medicine. 2016;76(1):172–82.
124. Jones RM, Kamps S, Huang Y, Scantlebury N, Lipsman N, Schwartz ML, et al. Accumulated thermal dose in MRI-guided focused ultrasound for essential tremor: Repeated sonications with low focal temperatures. Journal of Neurosurgery. 2019;132(6):1802–9.
125. Huisman M, Lam MK, Bartels LW, Nijenhuis RJ, Moonen CT, Knuttel FM, et al. Feasibility of volumetric MRI-guided high intensity focused ultrasound (MR-HIFU) for painful bone metastases. Journal of Therapeutic Ultrasound. 2014;2(1):1–10.
126. Wells P, Bullen M, Follett D, Freundlich H, James JA. The dosimetry of small ultrasonic beams. Ultrasonics. 1963;1(2):106–10.
127. Hynynen K. Acoustic power calibrations of cylindrical intracavitary ultrasound hyperthermia applicators. Medical Physics. 1993;20(1):129–34.
128. Staudenraus J, Eisenmenger W. Fibre-optic probe hydrophone for ultrasonic and shock-wave measurements in water. Ultrasonics. 1993;31(4):267–73.
129. Beard P, Mills T. Extrinsic optical-fiber ultrasound sensor using a thin polymer film as a low-finesse Fabry–Perot interferometer. Applied Optics. 1996;35(4):663–75.
130. Song J, Hynynen K. Feasibility of using lateral mode coupling method for a large scale ultrasound phased array for noninvasive transcranial therapy. IEEE Transactions on Biomedical Engineering. 2009;57(1):124–33.
131. Schafer ME, Lewin PA. Transducer characterization using the angular spectrum method. The Journal of the Acoustical Society of America. 1989;85(5):2202–14.
132. Kreider W, Yuldashev PV, Sapozhnikov OA, Farr N, Partanen A, Bailey MR, et al. Characterization of a multi-element clinical HIFU system using acoustic holography and nonlinear modeling. IEEE Transactions on Ultrasonics, Ferroelectrics, and Frequency Control. 2013;60(8):1683–98.
133. Wu T, Felmlee JP. A quality control program for MR-guided focused ultrasound ablation therapy. Journal of Applied Clinical Medical Physics. 2002;3(2):162–7.
134. Gorny K, Hangiandreou N, Hesley G, Gostout B, McGee K, Felmlee J. MR guided focused ultrasound: Technical acceptance measures for a clinical system. Physics in Medicine & Biology. 2006;51(12):3155.
135. Lipsman N, Meng Y, Bethune AJ, Huang Y, Lam B, Masellis M, et al. Blood–brain barrier opening in Alzheimer's disease using MR-guided focused ultrasound. Nature Communications. 2018;9(1):2336.
136. Mainprize T, Lipsman N, Huang Y, Meng Y, Bethune A, Ironside S, et al. Blood-brain barrier opening in primary brain tumors with non-invasive MR-guided focused ultrasound: A clinical safety and feasibility study. Scientific Reports. 2019;9(1):321.
137. Hynynen K, McDannold N, Vykhodtseva N, Jolesz FA. Noninvasive MR imaging–guided focal opening of the blood-brain barrier in rabbits. Radiology. 2001;220(3):640–6.
138. Cavallo Marincola B, Pediconi F, Anzidei M, Miglio E, Di Mare L, Telesca M, et al. High-intensity focused ultrasound in breast pathology: Non-invasive treatment of benign and malignant lesions. Expert Review of Medical Devices. 2015;12(2):191–9.
139. Furusawa H, Namba K, Thomsen S, Akiyama F, Bendet A, Tanaka C, et al. Magnetic resonance–guided focused ultrasound surgery of breast cancer: Reliability and effectiveness. Journal of the American College of Surgeons. 2006;203(1):54–63.
140. Stewart EA. Uterine fibroids. The Lancet. 2001;357(9252):293–8.
141. Fennessy FM, Tempany CM, McDannold NJ, So MJ, Hesley G, Gostout B, et al. Uterine leiomyomas: MR imaging–guided focused ultrasound surgery – results of different treatment protocols. Radiology. 2007;243(3):885–93.

142. Stewart EA, Rabinovici J, Tempany CM, Inbar Y, Regan L, Gastout B, et al. Clinical outcomes of focused ultrasound surgery for the treatment of uterine fibroids. Fertility and Sterility. 2006;85(1):22–9.
143. Bohlmann M, Hoellen F, Hunold P, David M. High-intensity focused ultrasound ablation of uterine fibroids–potential impact on fertility and pregnancy outcome. Geburtshilfe und Frauenheilkunde. 2014;74(02):139–45.
144. Pron G. Magnetic resonance–guided high-intensity focused ultrasound (MRgHIFU) treatment of symptomatic uterine fibroids: An evidence-based analysis. Ontario Health Technology Assessment Series. 2015;15(4):1.
145. Babashov V, Palimaka S, Blackhouse G, O'Reilly D. Magnetic resonance-guided high-intensity focused ultrasound (MRgHIFU) for treatment of symptomatic uterine fibroids: An economic analysis. Ontario Health Technology Assessment Series. 2015;15(5):1.
146. Fennessy FM, Tempany CM. An update on magnetic resonance guided focused ultrasound surgery (MRgFUS) of uterine fibroids. Current Radiology Reports. 2013;1:136–46.
147. Park MJ, Kim Y-s, Keserci B, Rhim H, Lim HK. Volumetric MR-guided high-intensity focused ultrasound ablation of uterine fibroids: Treatment speed and factors influencing speed. European Radiology. 2013;23:943–50.
148. Ellens N, Hynynen K. Simulation study of the effects of near-and far-field heating during focused ultrasound uterine fibroid ablation using an electronically focused phased array: A theoretical analysis of patient safety. Medical Physics. 2014;41(7):072902.
149. Ellens N, Hynynen K. Frequency considerations for deep ablation with high-intensity focused ultrasound: A simulation study. Medical Physics. 2015;42(8):4896–910.
150. Ellens NP, Lucht BB, Gunaseelan ST, Hudson JM, Hynynen KH. A novel, flat, electronically-steered phased array transducer for tissue ablation: Preliminary results. Physics in Medicine & Biology. 2015;60(6):2195.
151. Gianfelice D, Gupta C, Kucharczyk W, Bret P, Havill D, Clemons M. Palliative treatment of painful bone metastases with MR imaging–guided focused ultrasound. Radiology. 2008;249(1):355–63.
152. Hurwitz MD, Ghanouni P, Kanaev SV, Iozeffi D, Gianfelice D, Fennessy FM, et al. Magnetic resonance–guided focused ultrasound for patients with painful bone metastases: Phase III trial results. Journal of the National Cancer Institute. 2014;106(5):dju082.
153. Liberman B, Gianfelice D, Inbar Y, Beck A, Rabin T, Shabshin N, et al. Pain palliation in patients with bone metastases using MR-guided focused ultrasound surgery: A multicenter study. Annals of Surgical Oncology. 2009;16:140–6.
154. Simões Corrêa Galendi J, Yeo SY, Simic D, Grüll H, Stock S, Müller D. A time-driven activity-based costing approach of magnetic resonance-guided high-intensity focused ultrasound for cancer-induced bone pain. International Journal of Hyperthermia. 2022;39(1):173–80.
155. Yeo SY, Bratke G, Grüll H. High intensity focused ultrasound for treatment of bone malignancies – 20 years of history. Cancers. 2022;15(1):108.
156. Huisman M, van den Bosch MA, Wijlemans JW, van Vulpen M, van der Linden YM, Verkooijen HM. Effectiveness of reirradiation for painful bone metastases: A systematic review and meta-analysis. International Journal of Radiation Oncology* Biology* Physics. 2012;84(1):8–14.
157. Weeks EM, Platt MW, Gedroyc W. MRI-guided focused ultrasound (MRgFUS) to treat facet joint osteoarthritis low back pain – case series of an innovative new technique. European Radiology. 2012;22:2822–35.
158. Geiger D, Napoli A, Conchiglia A, Gregori L, Arrigoni F, Bazzocchi A, et al. MR-guided focused ultrasound (MRgFUS) ablation for the treatment of nonspinal osteoid osteoma: A prospective multicenter evaluation. JBJS. 2014;96(9):743–51.
159. Napoli A, Mastantuono M, Cavallo Marincola B, Anzidei M, Zaccagna F, Moreschini O, et al. Osteoid osteoma: MR-guided focused ultrasound for entirely noninvasive treatment. Radiology. 2013;267(2):514–21.
160. Rovella MS, Martins GL, Cavalcanti CF, Bor-Seng-Shu E, Camargo OP, Cerri GG, et al. Magnetic resonance-guided high-intensity focused ultrasound ablation of osteoid osteoma: A case series report. Ultrasound in Medicine & Biology. 2016;42(4):919–23.
161. Kawasaki M, Muramatsu S, Namba H, Izumi M, Ikeuchi M, Yaogawa S, et al. Efficacy and safety of magnetic resonance-guided focused ultrasound treatment for refractory chronic pain of medial knee osteoarthritis. International Journal of Hyperthermia. 2021;38(2):46–55.

162. Hynynen K, DeYoung D. Temperature elevation at muscle-bone interface during scanned, focused ultrasound hyperthermia. International Journal of Hyperthermia. 1988;4(3):267–79.
163. Coluccia D, Fandino J, Schwyzer L, O'Gorman R, Remonda L, Anon J, et al. First noninvasive thermal ablation of a brain tumor with MR-guided focusedultrasound. Journal of Therapeutic Ultrasound. 2014;2(1):1–7.
164. Choi J, Pernot M, Brown T, Small S, Konofagou E. Spatio-temporal analysis of molecular delivery through the blood–brain barrier using focused ultrasound. Physics in Medicine & Biology. 2007;52(18):5509.
165. McDannold N, Arvanitis CD, Vykhodtseva N, Livingstone MS. Temporary disruption of the blood–brain barrier by use of ultrasound and microbubbles: Safety and efficacy evaluation in rhesus macaques. Cancer Research. 2012;72(14):3652–63.
166. Meng Y, Reilly RM, Pezo RC, Trudeau M, Sahgal A, Singnurkar A, et al. MR-guided focused ultrasound enhances delivery of trastuzumab to Her2-positive brain metastases. Science Translational Medicine. 2021;13(615):eabj4011.
167. Rezai AR, Ranjan M, D'Haese P-F, Haut MW, Carpenter J, Najib U, et al. Noninvasive hippocampal blood– brain barrier opening in Alzheimer's disease with focused ultrasound. Proceedings of the National Academy of Sciences. 2020;117(17):9180–2.
168. Abrahao A, Meng Y, Llinas M, Huang Y, Hamani C, Mainprize T, et al. First-in-human trial of blood–brain barrier opening in amyotrophic lateral sclerosis using MR-guided focused ultrasound. Nature Communications. 2019;10(1):4373.
169. Gasca-Salas C, Fernández-Rodríguez B, Pineda-Pardo JA, Rodríguez-Rojas R, Obeso I, Hernández-Fernández F, et al. Blood-brain barrier opening with focused ultrasound in Parkinson's disease dementia. Nature Communications. 2021;12(1):779.
170. Martin E, Jeanmonod D, Morel A, Zadicario E, Werner B. High-intensity focused ultrasound for noninvasive functional neurosurgery. Annals of Neurology: Official Journal of the American Neurological Association and the Child Neurology Society. 2009;66(6):858–61.
171. Jeanmonod D, Werner B, Morel A, Michels L, Zadicario E, Schiff G, et al. Transcranial magnetic resonance imaging–guided focused ultrasound: Noninvasive central lateral thalamotomy for chronic neuropathic pain. Neurosurgical Focus. 2012;32(1):E1.
172. Ondo W, Jankovic J, Schwartz K, Almaguer M, Simpson R. Unilateral thalamic deep brain stimulation for refractory essential tremor and Parkinson's disease tremor. Neurology. 1998;51(4):1063–9.
173. Pahwa R, Lyons KE, Wilkinson SB, Tröster AI, Overman J, Kieltyka J, et al. Comparison of thalamotomy to deep brain stimulation of the thalamus in essential tremor. Movement Disorders: Official Journal of the Movement Disorder Society. 2001;16(1):140–3.
174. Elias WJ, Huss D, Voss T, Loomba J, Khaled M, Zadicario E, et al. A pilot study of focused ultrasound thalamotomy for essential tremor. New England Journal of Medicine. 2013;369(7):640–8.
175. Chang JW, Park CK, Lipsman N, Schwartz ML, Ghanouni P, Henderson JM, et al. A prospective trial of magnetic resonance–guided focused ultrasound thalamotomy for essential tremor: Results at the 2-year follow-up. Annals of Neurology. 2018;83(1):107–14.
176. Iorio-Morin C, Yamamoto K, Sarica C, Zemmar A, Levesque M, Brisebois S, et al. Bilateral focused ultrasound thalamotomy for essential tremor (BEST-FUS phase 2 trial). Movement Disorders. 2021;36(11):2653–62.
177. Jung H, Kim S, Roh D, Chang J, Chang W, Kweon E, et al. Bilateral thermal capsulotomy with MR-guided focused ultrasound for patients with treatment-refractory obsessive-compulsive disorder: A proof-of-concept study. Molecular Psychiatry. 2015;20(10):1205–11.
178. Davidson B, Hamani C, Meng Y, Baskaran A, Sharma S, Abrahao A, et al. Examining cognitive change in magnetic resonance-guided focused ultrasound capsulotomy for psychiatric illness. Translational Psychiatry. 2020;10(1):397.
179. Hynynen K, Jones RM. Image-guided ultrasound phased arrays are a disruptive technology for non-invasive therapy. Physics in Medicine & Biology. 2016;61(17):R206.

18

Clinical Application of MR-Guided Focused Ultrasound Ablation for Uterine Fibroids

Stephen Derek Quinn and Wladyslaw M. Gedroyc

18.1 Background

Uterine fibroids (also known as leiomyomas or myomas) are the most common benign tumour found in women, with epidemiological studies indicating that up to 74% of pre-menopausal women will have histological evidence of uterine fibroids.[1] Although these are benign tumours, uterine fibroids may have a significant impact on the quality of life of women,[2] with a range of clinical manifestations related to the size and position of the fibroids. Heavy menstrual bleeding and painful periods are the most commonly encountered clinical problem. Bladder symptoms, such as urinary frequency and nocturia, and bowel symptoms such as constipation may also be experienced when the fibroids are of a significant volume. Fertility may also be adversely affected with increased rates of infertility, miscarriage and other pregnancy problems being more common in women with uterine fibroids.[3]

At present fibroids may be treated medically by using treatments to reduce bleeding such as antifibrinolytics (e.g. tranexamic acid), non-steroidal anti-inflammatory drugs (e.g. mefenamic acid) or hormonal preparations such as progestogens (e.g. norethisterone or the levonorgestrel releasing intrauterine system; Mirena coil). When these are insufficient to adequately alleviate symptoms, other more invasive methods are used. These include removal of the fibroid tissue surgically by hysteroscopic, laparoscopic or open myomectomy and hysterectomy, or by causing ischaemic infarction of the fibroid using uterine fibroid embolisation (UFE). In addition to these well-established treatments for uterine fibroids thermally ablative approaches have been developed.

The destruction of tumour tissue by thermal injury can be achieved by using radiofrequency energy, focused ultrasound or microwave energy. Increasing the temperature of tissue to 50–52°C for four to six minutes is sufficient to produce irreversible cellular damage.[4] When temperatures reach 60–100°C, rapid, irreversible damage caused by protein coagulation leads ultimately to coagulative necrosis.[5, 6] When temperatures exceed 105°C, resultant tissue vaporisation and carbonisation can worsen further ablation within the tissue due to the reduction in energy transmission.[4, 6] High-intensity ultrasound can be focused into a small volume to produce a rise in tissue temperature sufficient to cause irreparable cell damage in the target at depth within the body.[7] Therapeutic focused ultrasound can be guided by both MRI and diagnostic ultrasound to direct the energy to the targeted tissue. In 1992 the first report of the use of MR imaging to direct focused ultrasound in the targeting of deep lying tumour tissue was published.[8]

High-intensity focused ultrasound (HIFU) uses ultrasonic waves to create thermal damage within tissues. These ultrasound waves are generated by a transducer, a device that converts electrical pulses into pressure pulses. Most commonly, the transducer uses a piezoelectric plate that generates an ultrasound pulse. Piezoelectric materials expand or contract when a charge is applied.[9] It is this expansion and contraction that results in longitudinal ultrasound pressure waves. When an ultrasound wave passes through a medium, the molecules of that medium oscillate back and forth along the direction of propagation of the wave. The resulting friction transforms acoustic energy into heat and contributes

DOI: 10.1201/9780429162671-18

to the attenuation of the ultrasonic beam. The intensity of the ultrasound beam is a measure of energy flowing through an area of the beam, which is quoted in Wcm^2. The intensities used for typical diagnostic ultrasound scanning (B-mode, pulsed or continuous Doppler) can be up to 720 $mWcm^2$. In contrast, the intensity of focused ultrasound in the focal region is in the range of 100–10 000 Wcm^2.[10]

Ultrasound waves can be focused into a small volume either by a lens, a curved transducer, or a phased array, in a manner similar to that for light being focused through a magnifying glass onto a single point. The phased array transducer is constructed using multiple parallel transducer units.[9] The signal from each transducer is emitted at a different phase from that preceding it. Appropriate timing of these signals allows the ultrasound beam to be focused. By using ultrasound with energies of up to 7000 joules focused into an ellipsoidal focal spot of size in the range 2 × 2 × 4 mm to 10 × 10 × 70 mm, the tissues within the focal point are heated to temperatures greater than 56°C for a period of 1 second or longer. Each focal exposure is commonly referred to as a sonication. The temperature of 56°C has been established as the minimum temperature at the edges of a 2-second sonication for the ablated volume.[11] Temperatures at the centre of the sonication may be greater than 90°C, resulting in coagulative necrosis and apoptotic cell death of the targeted tissue.[12] Sonications within tissue can create 'lesions' that vary in size from one to seven centimetres in length. The absorption coefficients of tissues vary significantly: bone absorbs most ultrasound energy, while fluids such as blood absorb very little, with soft tissues such as myometrium falling in between.[9] When ultrasound is applied in a linear pressure regimen (for biological tissues this is typically below 5MPa), the energy is absorbed at a rate that is directly proportional to the local intensity, meaning that the highest rise in temperature will be at the focus of the beam. The temperature continues to rise as more energy is absorbed, although some heat is lost by the process of conduction to surrounding cooler areas.

18.2 Clinical Use

Since its introduction, increasing experience of MRgFUS in the treatment of uterine fibroids has led to a refinement of patient selection, with a tendency towards treating women with fewer fibroids and smaller uteri, while avoiding those with high signal intensity fibroids (on T2-weighted MR imaging).[13] As the reduction in fibroid volume is variable (13.5%–39.5%)[14, 15] the use of MRgFUS has tended to be avoided in those women with predominantly pressure-related symptoms arising from the size of their fibroids, as their symptoms are likely to persist in these cases. Menstrual related symptoms are much more likely to respond favourably to MRgFUS and these, along with other general fibroid-related symptoms are quantified using a standardised fibroid quality of life symptom severity score (UFS-QoL).[16] This allows objective assessment of fibroid-related symptom severity and provides a useful tool for studies investigating the effect of a treatment on fibroid symptoms.

Many studies have reported diminished results in symptom severity score improvement and volume reduction in patients with fibroids of high signal intensity on T2-weighted MR images.[13, 14] The signal intensity of uterine fibroids may be described as i. hypointense, or of low intensity, when compared with the myometrium or skeletal muscle on T2 images (type 1); ii. lower or equal to the myometrium but higher than skeletal muscle (type 2); or iii. a signal intensity higher that of skeletal muscle or myometrium (type 3).[17]

HIFU has been used to treat uterine fibroids under the guidance of both ultrasound and MRI. Sonographically guided focused ultrasound uses changes in echogenicity to determine the area of fibroid ablation.[18] The HIFUNIT 9000 tumour therapy system (Shanghai Aishen Technology, Shanghai, China) comprises six self-focusing acoustic therapeutic transducers which focus the ultrasound beam, and a diagnostic transducer located in the centre of the therapeutic transducers.[19] This allows tissues in the path of therapeutic ultrasound waves to be viewed in diagnostic ultrasound images. Initial results with this system were encouraging, with 85.5% of patients undergoing this treatment experiencing an improvement in their symptoms at one year, 59.3% having total relief from their symptoms at 1 year, and a 9.7% re-intervention rate at 1 year (n = 145).[20] An alternative system has been used with a similar arrangement of a central 3.5- to 5.0-MHz convex diagnostic ultrasound probe and a 20-cm-diameter therapeutic transducer with a focal length of 150 mm operating at a frequency of 0.9 MHz (Model JC; Chongqing Haifu Technology, Chongqing, China).[21] This system has been used to treat submucosal uterine fibroids achieving a mean non-perfused volume of 80%, a mean reduction in fibroid volume of 90.1% at 24 months and vaginal expulsion of necrosed fibroid material in 58%.[21] The reduction in fibroid volumes following sonographically guided focused ultrasound have been notable, with reductions of between 50.3% and 78.9% at 12 months.[20, 21] These studies are, however, small, and, compared with magnetic resonance-guided focused ultrasound (MRgFUS), long-term data is limited. Sonographically guided focused ultrasound may have advantages over MRgFUS, including the cost of treatment and potentially shorter treatment times. A recent study used a modified treatment protocol consisting of repeated and shortened (less than 25 minutes) treatment sessions of high intensity (1000–1500 Wcm-^{2}), and repeated sonication pulses (1500–2000) at each spot.[22] This modified protocol was associated with a third-degree skin burn in one of the 20 subjects, two cases of skin blisters and eight patients experiencing pain after the treatment. However, ultrasound monitoring does not provide accurate real-time mapping of the thermal doses, unlike MR-guided treatments.

MRI enables assessment of the pelvic anatomy in three dimensions, allowing accurate targeting of the uterine fibroids. By using MRI the ultrasound beam path can be visualised, allowing the operator to avoid structures such as the bowel (Figure 18.1).

Passage through bowel and gas can result in perforation by reflection at gas/soft tissue interfaces. Prior to treatments, patients are catheterised, ensuring a static bladder volume during the treatment. Initial detailed MR imaging of the pelvis allows treatments to be carefully planned prior to the first sonication, and the position of surrounding bowel and far field bone are noted.

MRI allows near-real-time thermometry of the tissue to achieve the planned outcome (Figure 18.2).

MR thermometry relies on the temperature dependence of the proton-resonance phase shift of water molecules.[23, 24] This effect results in a phase shift of the gradient recalled MR-images: an effect which is both linear with observed temperature change, and independent of the type of tissue. MR thermometry allows the operator to titrate the focused ultrasound energy and spot-type against the result visualised in the tissues so that maximum results can be achieved in each individual patient.

MRI also enables the post-treatment assessment of the volume of fibroid ablated. Following the completed sonications, an intravascular contrast agent is given and T1-fat saturated images of the pelvis are obtained. From these, the degree of non-perfusion of the fibroid volume can be assessed (Figure 18.3).

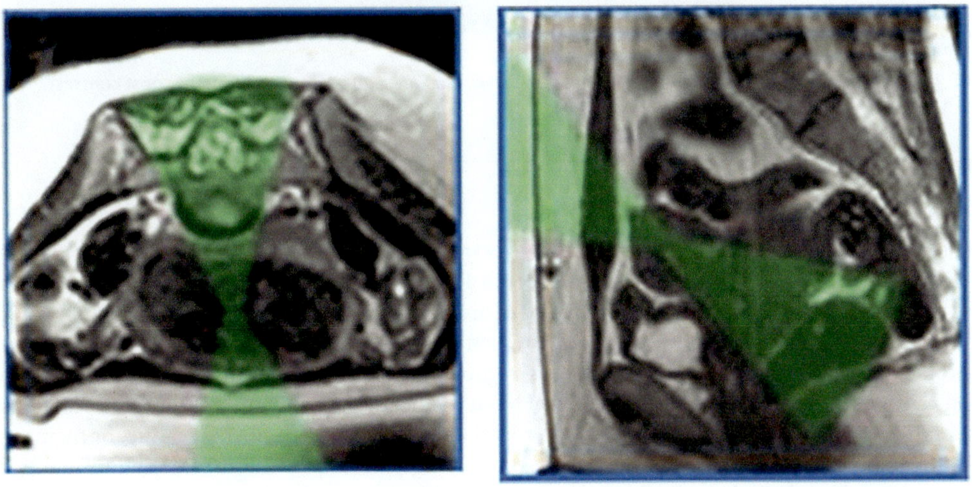

FIGURE 18.1 Visualising the ultrasound beam path using MRI.

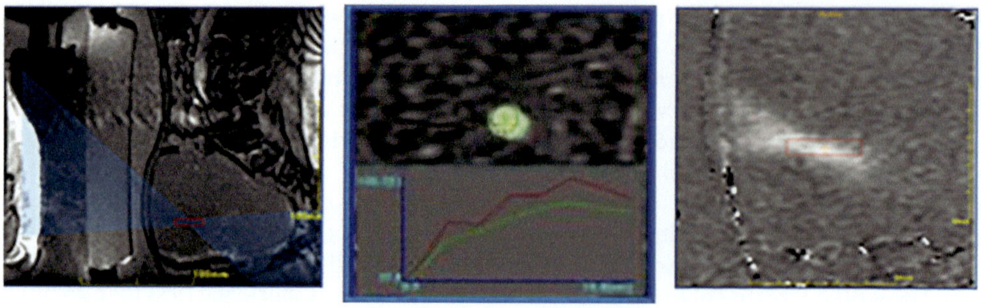

FIGURE 18.2 Real-time thermometry employed during MRgFUS.

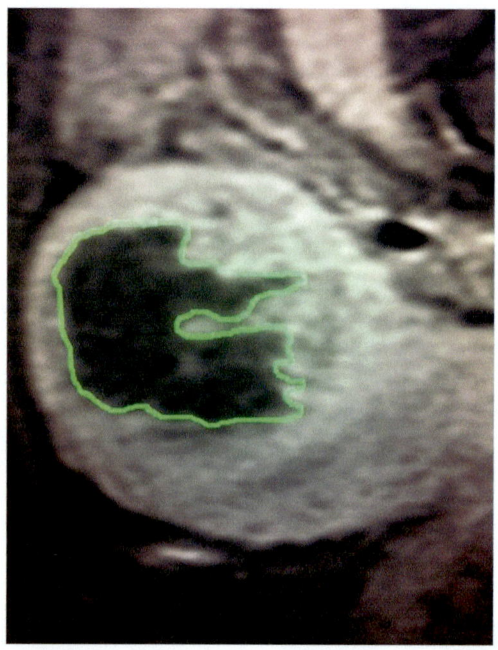

FIGURE 18.3 Non-perfused volume post treatment (marked area) on sagittal T1 weight images post contrast.

18.3 Treatment Outcomes

Since its introduction, increasing experience of this treatment has led to a refinement of patient selection, with a tendency towards treating women with fewer fibroids and smaller uteri.[25] In addition to patient selection, several clinical tactics have been used to treat fibroids, where treatments would be otherwise limited. The passage of the focused ultrasound beam through bowel in the treatment of uterine fibroids is contraindicated due to concerns regarding this organ's absorption of energy. Various methods have been used to move loops of bowel from the beam path including filling the bladder with normal saline, or by rectal filling using either a rectal balloon filled with normal saline, or by inserting rectal ultrasound gel.[26] One group has described applying pressure to the central abdominal wall in order to displace bowel via the use of a convex gel pad.[27] It is known that the signal intensity of fibroids can correspond to their cellular density, fibre content and vascularity[28, 29] and that this is a known predictor of the success of HIFU.[30] A study of 91 women undergoing MRgFUS in Japan found a 2-year re-intervention rate of 14.0% in women with hypointense or iso-intense fibroids.[14] These women had a mean non-perfused volume (NPV) of 54.7% and a mean tumour volume of 129.0 ml (SD 145.2 ml).[14]

A systematic review of the literature regarding HIFU found 38 prospective and retrospective studies, no randomised control trials and studies of limited quality overall.[31] The available data on long-term outcomes is currently very limited. Funaki et al. found a 2-year re-intervention rate of 21.6% for hyper-intense uterine fibroids (with a mean NPV of 36.2%) and 14.0% at 2 years for normo-intense fibroids (with a mean NPV of 54.35%).[14] This was the first study to examine how the overall percentage of fibroid tissue treated successfully (as defined by the post-contrast NPV appearance of the MR image) related to subsequent symptomatic response over a longer follow-up period. A more recent prospective study found a two year re-intervention rate of 24%, with an overall NPV of 40.9%.[32] This study also stratified outcome by signal intensity and NPV and found that women with hyper-intense fibroids had a higher risk of requiring further treatment after two years, compared with women with hypo-intense fibroids, although on multivariate analysis this failed to reach significance (OR 2.87 [0.64–14.4]). Treatment resulting in greater than 45% NPV had a 15% risk of re-intervention by 2 years, whereas treatments resulting in a 10–20% NPV had a 40% risk of re-intervention at 2 years (OR 5.22 [1.1–26.0]).[32] A recent retrospective study of women undergoing UAE and MRgFUS found a 5 year re-intervention rate of 66.7% following a mean NPV of 36.4%.[33] In this study, however, the less accurate ellipsoid formula method was used to calculate the NPV, no mention of fibroid signal intensity was made and 37% of their patients were lost to follow-up. A cohort study of 280 women undergoing MRgFUS found that the overall re-intervention rate at 5 years was 58.64%, but in those treatments with greater than 50% NPV the re-intervention rate was 50%.[13] Further improvement of the 5-year re-intervention rate was also found when 3 months pre-treatment of gonadotropin releasing hormone agonist (GnRHa) had been used.[34] It is the tissue effects of the GnRHa that are believed to improve the response of the fibroid tissue to thermal doses. GnRHa is also known to reduce the vascularity of uterine fibroids; this reduced vascularity may reduce the thermal conduction away from the fibroid during a focused ultrasound procedure. Overall, the trends in the studies have demonstrated that when larger NPVs are achieved, these lead to more successful, longer lasting treatment results.

In addition to the long-term outcomes, specific data regarding the safety of MRgFUS is encouraging. The initial multicentre prospective study by Stewart et al. (n = 155) found no deaths, life-threatening events or hysterectomies following MRgFUS.[31] There have been no recorded deaths, or hysterectomies following MRgFUS in any of the current literature. The most serious complication reported by that study was a sciatic nerve palsy in one woman, which had resolved by 1 year post treatment. This was believed to be a result of indirect injury of the nerve, caused by heating of the nearby bone following absorption of ultrasound energy in the far field of the treatment sonication. A cohort study of 280 women undergoing MRgFUS found a 1.4% risk of urinary tract infection (patients undergoing MRgFUS have a urinary catheter during the procedure), a 1.1% risk of minor skin burns requiring no repair and a 0.4% risk of major skin burn requiring secondary repair.[30] In this cohort there was, again, one woman who experienced persistent neuropathy following absorption of energy in the far-field bone. As a result of these cases, changes to the system and to treatment planning have been developed to reduce far field bone absorption by directing the beam with greater accuracy. Skin burns have greatly reduced due to the experience and reporting of adverse events. All reported cases of major skin burns have been in women with significant abdominal scarring, and avoidance of treating fibroids through significant abdominal scars, or the use of an energy-absorbing abdominal scar patch have reduced the incidents of further skin burns in recent years.[35]

Recent developments in MRgFUS have been aimed at improving the ablation volumes achieved, including the use of a three-dimensional treatment planner that automatically arranges sonication spots to cover a maximum targeted fibroid volume. By turning off elements in the transducer the beam of high intensity focused ultrasound may be shaped in such a way as to allow treatment in an area where otherwise bowel may have limited access. The transducer is able to get much closer to a patient's skin, resulting in reduced energy density in the beam path. The beam path will be wider at the skin and at the posterior bony structures leading to reduced energy absorption. This also allows there to be increased energy density safely at the focus without increased energy absorption in the skin and spine. Early results with this newer system suggest that it can produce a consistently larger area of fibroid destruction in most patients, with NPVs of 88% (range 38–100%) reported, which is likely to lead to improved treatment results.[36]

A cohort study of 36 women undergoing treatment for their uterine fibroids using the Sonalleve MRgFUS fibroid therapy system (Philips Healthcare, Vantaa, Finland) found 61.1% experienced a significant improvement in their quality of life score with a mean follow-up duration of 21.4 (95%CI: 16.3–26.5) months.[37] The main difference between the ExAblate system and the Sonalleve is the pattern and size of sonications produced. The ExAblate system performs point-by-point sonication using spots of variable length up to 76 mm, whereas the Sonalleve system produces volumetric heating, which utilises the heat diffusion within tissue by electronically moving the focal point between a number of predetermined locations.[38]

A small randomised controlled trial comparing MRgFUS with placebo in 20 women found an improvement in UFS-QoL score by 12 weeks post treatment compared with placebo, and a mean decrease in fibroid volume by 18%.[39] By 2 years post-MRgFUS 30% of the women had undergone another treatment procedure for their uterine fibroids. This study was small and the mean NPV ratios after treatment was 43%; however, this study did demonstrate the willingness of women to participate in an RCT involving this treatment, albeit not in direct comparison with an interventional or surgical treatment. Another RCT comparing outcomes with uterine artery embolisation is ongoing (the Fibroid Interventions: Reducing Symptoms Today and Tomorrow [FIRSTT]).[40]

18.4 Expert Commentary

MR-guided focused ultrasound of fibroids is accurate, safe and totally non-invasive. The image guidance that can be achieved using MRI thermometry and MR targeting provide high quality information about the site of temperature deposition and of the extent of power deposited which is quite unique in all aspects of image guidance currently available. This technique also has the added bonus that no ionising radiation is used at all in this procedure, and that it can easily be repeated. As the results in selected patients are very comparable to those for all other treatment modalities, why then is it not more widely adopted as a primary treatment modality for fibroids and what are the problems that we need to overcome to make this therapeutic modality more widely accepted and used?

One of the simplest problems that continually causes problems in trying to use this form of therapy is that the MR scanners in which these procedures are carried out are usually in continual demand for diagnostic imaging. To carry out MR-guided focused ultrasound requires one MR scanner to be solely devoted to one patient for a whole session, which, if only one scanner is available to an individual institution can be very problematic. Fortunately, most large institutions that want to carry out this type of procedure these days have more than one available MR scanner, and so the problem is not quite as acute as it was in the past and can be overcome with reasonable cooperation and planning.

MR-guided focused ultrasound of fibroids, and of other areas, can be problematic if carried out by one single specialty in isolation from other specialties. For focused ultrasound to be a successful process, it is clear that a multidisciplinary collaborative approach to implementing this type of complex clinical, imaging and technological process is required. To succeed effectively, all specialties involved in the care of each individual patient need to collaborate closely with each other, providing individual areas of expertise to achieve a single unified successful process. It is, sadly, surprisingly difficult to achieve such a unified multidisciplinary result in many instances.

It is important to understand that there is an immense variation in the nature of the fibroids that present with clinically symptomatic problems. The difference in volume between a symptomatic 3-cm-diameter, low-signal intensity fibroid and a 25-cm-diameter confluent fibroid mass that reaches almost to the liver are quite startling. Similarly, the range of MR signal changes that can be seen between different fibroids, reflecting the variations in tissue proportions within such leiomyomas (varying proportions of smooth muscle, vascular tissue, fibrous stroma and other connective tissue) is immense, often even within the same patient. Fibroids show a huge range in both size and nature of constituent tissue, and it is very unlikely that any one single treatment, short of removal of the whole uterus each time, will ever be able to provide comprehensive simple effective treatments for all the different variations that exist.

Currently focused ultrasound is most effective in treating smaller to medium-size fibroids which are not very numerous, and which can be easily accessed via a suitable acoustic window through the anterior abdominal wall. We know that the greater the NPV that is created in the target volume, the more effective and long-lasting the treatment result will be. Therefore, with current technology we tend to restrict our therapeutic procedures to those patients who fall into these most suitable categories. Patients with very large fibroids seem to be too difficult to treat effectively with focused ultrasound. It would theoretically be possible to do multiple procedures on individual patients, but this would require the devotion of an immense amount of time and the procedure would, as a result, become a very costly process. Furthermore, as a fibroid extends more superiorly it often lies very close to the lumbar spine, which lies immediately posteriorly, making propagated heat from bone absorption during focused ultrasound become a greater concern, as this may lead to damage to local neural structures in this area from bone heating. These are more susceptible to this type of heat damage than other soft tissues. Similarly, patients with multiple fibroids are also very difficult to treat effectively with our current technology. The frequently seen patient that presents with 10–30 fibroids is a very challenging problem for focused ultrasound since it is very problematic to treat multiple small, or even multiple large, fibroids scattered throughout the uterus. The acoustic window that is available, often just will not allow the treatment of so many peripheral fundal and inferior fibroids due to bowel obscuration and impingement on the spine, and again it is not usually possible to treat all of the fibroids in one or even two procedures in such patients, thus significantly reducing the chances long-term therapeutic success in these patients.

We currently estimate that only 25–30% of patients that present to our clinics with fibroid related problems are suitable for focused ultrasound using our current criteria. It is clear therefore that we need to find ways of improving our technology, and approach, to be able to treat more patients with fibroids, so that the very large fibroids that so commonly present, and the patients who have multiple fibroids can also be easily treated with this non-invasive technology.

How can we achieve such an improvement in the utilisation of this technology to encompass those patients who we currently exclude from treatment? We believe that there are two main principles that we need to explore to try and achieve these goals:

1) We need to be able to carry out FUS sonications much more quickly and to move from sonication site to subsequent sonication site much more speedily than we currently do, with almost no intervening time between sonications.
2) It would be highly desirable if we could find a way of enhancing the tissue effect of our focused ultrasound sonications in the targeted fibroids so that greater volumes of destruction could be produced per unit power application, whilst minimising changes in adjacent tissues.

Current MR-guided focused ultrasound machines for abdominal applications use approximately 220 ultrasound transducers in an electronic array and carry out sequential sonications. The manufacturers differ slightly in their application in this area with one manufacturer producing a volumetric area of destruction with a circular sonication pathway whilst another uses longer elongating spots, moving the focal spot anteriorly during a slightly longer individual sonication time. Could the technological future here hold out the possibility of greatly enlarging the number of transducers used from the current 220 or so to 5000–10,000, allowing the possibility of carrying out several sonications at different sites throughout the targeted fibroid at the same time. Are there other ways of using much higher transducer densities to increase power deposition into the targeted fibroids?

Methods of manipulating tissue response to ultrasound sonications and heat effects may also be able to increase the tissue response to focused ultrasound, producing greater results in much shorter times. There are a number of potential ways of producing such a response. GnRHa pre-treatment has been used for many years to shrink fibroids prior to surgery, or to focused ultrasound therapy, and it is well known that this is not only shrinks the fibroid itself but also decreases its vascularity, and both these effects are highly desirable in focused ultrasound. This method is already in significant use by practitioners in this field but is not a very comprehensive answer since it can only produce a certain amount of shrinkage and vascular improvement, and cannot bridge the gap that still remains in patients with very large fibroids and/or multiple fibroids to allow them to be treated.

Using a variety of pharmaceutical manipulations to reduce fibroid blood flow is an area that is currently being actively investigated by several practitioners around the world. The potential use of oxytocin or ergot derivatives to diminish uterine vascularity could have the effect of allowing fibroids with greater volumes to be more easily treated since they would be more responsive to thermal damage under these circumstances. Early studies utilising these preparations are underway and results are awaited. Another method currently being investigated to try to improve tissue response to focused ultrasound sonications is to use microbubbles such as are used in ultrasound contrast media. High energy focused ultrasound produces significant tissue cavitation when it impinges on volumes containing microbubbles, resulting in significant potentiation of local tissue damage. Some investigators use microbubble infusions during focused ultrasound administration to try and utilise this property to enlarge their results within the targeted fibroid. The theoretical concern, of course, is that not only will the microbubbles potentiate the results of focused ultrasound in the targeted fibroid but also to a lesser, but significant, level in the intervening tissues anterior to the fibroid through which the beam passes, particularly the skin, and also, potentially, in posterior sensitive tissues such as bone and neural structures. Such use could therefore potentially result in increased complications from this type of procedure and results are awaited again from small-scale implementations of this type of approach.

The fibroid response to heating is remarkably variable and it is well-known that fibroids that show T2 hyperintensity on MR respond relatively poorly to standard focused ultrasound. It is not completely clear why this happens. For many years people hypothesised that these were much more vascular fibroids, suggesting that there was a relative heat sink effect in these fibroids which meant they did not heat as well as the textbook-classic low-T2-signal fibroid. This may indeed partially be the case, but it also is becoming clear that the T2 hyperintense fibroids intrinsically contain much more cellular water, which appears to influence their response to heating. If we are to provide a comprehensive therapeutic solution for fibroids with focused ultrasound the problems of treating hyperintense T2 fibroids will also have to be addressed. To date none of the hormonal manipulations that have been attempted have effectively solved this problem and this still remains an area seeking further information and solutions.

18.5 Summary

It is clear that, in selected cases, using the inclusion and exclusion criteria we have described here, the results of focused ultrasound of fibroids can be extremely effective and long-lasting. Unfortunately, these current inclusion criteria mean that we can only apply therapy to about 25–30% of patients, and we undoubtedly need to find technological and medical solutions as discussed above to improve our ability to treat more patients with fibroids. Without these further refinements focused ultrasound will remain a treatment for the minority of patients.

A problem that has been experienced throughout this field is how to structure comparative trials using this type of technology. Regulators and funders demand category 1 evidence to recommend and reimburse treatments. The difficulty is that randomised controlled trials, often with placebo arms, which are conventionally used for drug therapy are expected to be employed in this type of medical device research. Medical devices, particularly large ones like those delivering focused ultrasound, however, are not simple tablets, and to equate the two in this manner can be quite erroneous. It is very difficult to assign patients to randomised groups which involve completely non-interventional therapy (focused ultrasound) and open invasive therapies such as surgery, and the ethical positions of this type of comparison can be quite problematic. Indeed many of the patients who potentially might be recruited for such trials flatly refuse to enter into such studies.

Currently a large registry with comparative myomectomy arm is being constructed to follow 1000 or more patients after focused ultrasound treatment and it may be that these types of registries are a much more acceptable method of collating information about medical devices research rather than the damaging overconcentration on randomised controlled trials which may not only be ethically problematic but are rather expensive, making them difficult to fund and complete.

REFERENCES

1. Cramer SF, Patel A. The frequency of uterine leiomyomas. Am J Clin Pathol. 1990;94(4):435–8.
2. Parker WH. Etiology, symptomatology, and diagnosis of uterine myomas. Fertil Steril. 2007;87(4):725–36.
3. Khaund A, Lumsden MA. Impact of fibroids on reproductive function. Best Pract Res Clin Obstet Gynaecol. 2008;22(4):749–60.
4. Goldberg SN, Gazelle GS, Halpern EF, Rittman WJ, Mueller PR, Rosenthal DI. Radiofrequency tissue ablation: Importance of local temperature along the electrode tip exposure in determining lesion shape and size. Acad Radiol. 1996;3(3):212–8.
5. Solbiati L, Ierace T, Goldberg SN, Sironi S, Livraghi T, Fiocca R, et al. Percutaneous US-guided radiofrequency tissue ablation of liver metastases: Treatment and follow-up in 16 patients. Radiology. 1997;202(1):195–203.
6. Goldberg SN, Gazelle GS, Mueller PR. Thermal ablation therapy for focal malignancy: A unified approach to underlying principles, techniques, and diagnostic imaging guidance. AJR Am J Roentgenol. 2000;174(2):323–31.
7. Lynn JG, Zwemer RL, Chick AJ, Miller AE. A new method for the generation and use of focused ultrasound in experimental biology. J Gen Physiol. 1942;26(2):179–93.
8. Cline HE, Schenck JF, Hynynen K, Watkins RD, Souza SP, Jolesz FA. MR-guided focused ultrasound surgery. J Comput Assist Tomogr. 1992;16(6):956–65.
9. Hoskins PR, Martin K, Thrush A. Diagnostic Ultrasound: Physics and Equipment. 2nd ed. ed. Cambridge: Cambridge University Press; 2010.
10. Zhou YF. High intensity focused ultrasound in clinical tumor ablation. World J Clin Oncol. 2011;2(1):8–27.
11. Hill CR, Rivens I, Vaughan MG, ter Haar GR. Lesion development in focused ultrasound surgery: A general model. Ultrasound Med Biol. 1994;20(3):259–69.
12. ter Haar G. Ultrasound focal beam surgery. Ultrasound Med Biol. 1995;21(9):1089–100.
13. Quinn SD, Vedelago J, Gedroyc W, Regan L. Safety and five-year re-intervention following magnetic resonance-guided focused ultrasound (MRgFUS) for uterine fibroids. Eur J Obstet Gynecol Reprod Biol. 2014;182:247–51.
14. Funaki K, Fukunishi H, Sawada K. Clinical outcomes of magnetic resonance-guided focused ultrasound surgery for uterine myomas: 24-month follow-up. Ultrasound Obstet Gynecol. 2009;34(5):584–9.
15. Stewart EA, Rabinovici J, Tempany CM, Inbar Y, Regan L, Gostout B, et al. Clinical outcomes of focused ultrasound surgery for the treatment of uterine fibroids. Fertil Steril. 2006;85(1):22–9.
16. Spies JB, Coyne K, Guaou Guaou N, Boyle D, Skyrnarz-Murphy K, Gonzalves SM. The UFS-QOL, a new disease-specific symptom and health-related quality of life questionnaire for leiomyomata. Obstet Gynecol. 2002;99(2):290–300.
17. Funaki K, Fukunishi H, Funaki T, Sawada K, Kaji Y, Maruo T. Magnetic resonance-guided focused ultrasound surgery for uterine fibroids: Relationship between the therapeutic effects and signal intensity of preexisting T2-weighted magnetic resonance images. Am J Obstet Gynecol. 2007;196(2):184.e1–6.
18. Cheung VY. Sonographically guided high-intensity focused ultrasound for the management of uterine fibroids. J Ultrasound Med. 2013;32(8):1353–8.
19. Ren XL, Zhou XD, Zhang J, He GB, Han ZH, Zheng MJ, et al. Extracorporeal ablation of uterine fibroids with high-intensity focused ultrasound: Imaging and histopathologic evaluation. J Ultrasound Med. 2007;26(2):201–12.
20. Ren XL, Zhou XD, Yan RL, Liu D, Zhang J, He GB, et al. Sonographically guided extracorporeal ablation of uterine fibroids with high-intensity focused ultrasound: Midterm results. J Ultrasound Med. 2009;28(1):100–3.
21. Wang W, Wang Y, Wang T, Wang J, Wang L, Tang J. Safety and efficacy of US-guided high-intensity focused ultrasound for treatment of submucosal fibroids. Eur Radiol. 2012;22(11):2553–8.
22. Leung JH, Yu SC, Cheung EC, Wong AS, Tong MM, Ho SS, et al. Safety and efficacy of sonographically guided high-intensity focused ultrasound for symptomatic uterine fibroids: Preliminary study of a modified protocol. J Ultrasound Med. 2014;33(10):1811–8.
23. McDannold N. Quantitative MRI-based temperature mapping based on the proton resonant frequency shift: Review of validation studies. Int J Hyperthermia. 2005;21(6):533–46.

24. Ishihara Y, Calderon A, Watanabe H, Okamoto K, Suzuki Y, Kuroda K. A precise and fast temperature mapping using water proton chemical shift. Magn Reson Med. 1995;34(6):814–23.
25. Zaher S, Gedroyc WM, Regan L. Patient suitability for magnetic resonance guided focused ultrasound surgery of uterine fibroids. Eur J Obstet Gynecol Reprod Biol. 2009;143(2):98–102.
26. Kim YS, Bae DS, Park MJ, Viitala A, Keserci B, Rhim H, et al. Techniques to expand patient selection for MRI-guided high-intensity focused ultrasound ablation of uterine fibroids. AJR Am J Roentgenol. 2014;202(2):443–51.
27. Hesley GK, Felmlee JP, Gebhart JB, Dunagan KT, Gorny KR, Kesler JB, et al. Noninvasive treatment of uterine fibroids: Early Mayo Clinic experience with magnetic resonance imaging-guided focused ultrasound. Mayo Clin Proc. 2006;81(7):936–42.
28. Yamashita Y, Torashima M, Takahashi M, Tanaka N, Katabuchi H, Miyazaki K, et al. Hyperintense uterine leiomyoma at T2-weighted MR imaging: Differentiation with dynamic enhanced MR imaging and clinical implications. Radiology. 1993;189(3):721–5.
29. Swe TT, Onitsuka H, Kawamoto K, Ueyama T, Tsuruchi N, Masuda K. Uterine leiomyoma: Correlation between signal intensity on magnetic resonance imaging and pathologic characteristics. Radiat Med. 1992;10(6):235–42.
30. Lénárd ZM, McDannold NJ, Fennessy FM, Stewart EA, Jolesz FA, Hynynen K, et al. Uterine leiomyomas: MR imaging-guided focused ultrasound surgery-imaging predictors of success. Radiology. 2008;249(1):187–94.
31. Gizzo S, Saccardi C, Patrelli TS, Ancona E, Noventa M, Fagherazzi S, et al. Magnetic resonance-guided focused ultrasound myomectomy: Safety, efficacy, subsequent fertility and quality-of-life improvements: A systematic review. Reproductive Sciences. 2014 Apr;21(4):465–76.
32. Machtinger R, Inbar Y, Cohen-Eylon S, Admon D, Alagem-Mizrachi A, Rabinovici J. MR-guided focus ultrasound (MRgFUS) for symptomatic uterine fibroids: Predictors of treatment success. Hum Reprod. 2012;27(12):3425–31.
33. Froeling V, Meckelburg K, Schreiter NF, Scheurig-Muenkler C, Kamp J, Maurer MH, et al. Outcome of uterine artery embolization versus MR-guided high-intensity focused ultrasound treatment for uterine fibroids: Long-term results. Eur J Radiol. 2013.
34. Smart OC, Hindley JT, Regan L, Gedroyc WM. Magnetic resonance guided focused ultrasound surgery of uterine fibroids-the tissue effects of GnRH agonist pre-treatment. Eur J Radiol. 2006;59(2):163–7.
35. Yoon SW, Seong SJ, Jung SG, Lee SY, Jun HS, Lee JT. Mitigation of abdominal scars during MR-guided focused ultrasound treatment of uterine leiomyomas with the use of an energy-blocking scar patch. J Vasc Interv Radiol. 2011;22(12):1747–50.
36. Trumm CG, Stahl R, Clevert DA, Herzog P, Mindjuk I, Kornprobst S, et al. Magnetic resonance imaging-guided focused ultrasound treatment of symptomatic uterine fibroids: Impact of technology advancement on ablation volumes in 115 patients. Invest Radiol. 2013;48(6):359–65.
37. Thiburce AC, Frulio N, Hocquelet A, Maire F, Salut C, Balageas P, et al. Magnetic resonance-guided high-intensity focused ultrasound for uterine fibroids: Mid-term outcomes of 36 patients treated with the Sonalleve system. Int J Hyperthermia. 2015;31(7):764–70.
38. Köhler MO, Mougenot C, Quesson B, Enholm J, Le Bail B, Laurent C, et al. Volumetric HIFU ablation under 3D guidance of rapid MRI thermometry. Med Phys. 2009;36(8):3521–35.
39. Jacoby VL, Kohi MP, Poder L, Jacoby A, Lager J, Schembri M, et al. The PROMISe trial: A pilot, randomized, placebo-controlled trial of magnetic resonance guided focused ultrasound for uterine fibroids. Fertility and sterility. 2016 Mar 1;105(3):773–80.
40. Bouwsma EV, Hesley GK, Woodrum DA, Weaver AL, Leppert PC, Peterson LG, et al. Comparing focused ultrasound and uterine artery embolization for uterine fibroids-rationale and design of the Fibroid Interventions: Reducing symptoms today and tomorrow (FIRSTT) trial. Fertil Steril. 2011;96(3):704–10.

19

Clinical Application of MR-Guided Focused Ultrasound Ablation for Tumours in the Breast

David Brenin

19.1 Background

Integration of technological advances and changes in our understanding of tumour biology results in the continuous evolution of breast cancer treatment. Radical mastectomy, although mutilating, was the most effective treatment in its time. Changes in our understanding of tumour metastasis led to modified radical mastectomy. Advances in radiation therapy, adjuvant systemic treatment, and the acceptance of multi-disciplinary care resulted in breast conserving surgery. Progress in gamma probe technology allowed sentinel lymph node biopsy to replace axillary dissection. Technological progress, and the evolution of our understanding of breast cancer biology has led to the less disabling and disfiguring breast tumour treatments that are now standard of care. Development of effective ablative therapies is a logical continuation of this trend.

The general concept underpinning the ablative treatment of breast tumours is that the in-situ destruction of a tumour should be similar to its surgical removal. Various energy forms can be utilised for in situ tumour ablation, but only focused ultrasound ablation (FUSA) is truly non-invasive, delivered, as it is, with no incision, and can result in near-perfect cosmesis (Figure 19.1). Gradient-echo magnetic resonance imaging (MRI) techniques for thermal monitoring, based on the temperature sensitivity of the proton chemical shift, can be used to monitor the temperature in the ablation zone in real time, requiring no incision or probe penetration into the breast.[1]

Lumpectomy is the current standard of care for the treatment of most women with early stage breast cancer. This can often be accomplished under local anaesthesia, provides excellent local control, results in good cosmesis, and can be done quickly, in less than 30 minutes. Focused ultrasound ablation can often be accomplished under local anaesthesia, provides excellent local control, and results in superior cosmesis. In contrast to lumpectomy, however, FUSA takes a long time to accomplish, often more than 120 minutes. While FUSA takes longer than lumpectomy it requires no incision, results in no scar, and, has a faster recovery. For the aforementioned reasons, if FUSA is found to be equivalent to surgery for local control, it is likely to become the treatment of choice. This chapter describes the clinical application of MR-guided focused ultrasound ablation (MRgFUSA) for the treatment of tumours of the breast. It should be noted that in this chapter, MRgFUSA and MRgHIFU (MR-guided high-intensity focused ultrasound) are both used to describe MR guided ablation using ultrasound. In general MRgFUSA is used when the ablation is achieved using the Insightec Exablate device, and MRgHIFU when it is performed using the Philips Sonalleve device. These are described in more detail later.

19.2 Clinical Use and Treatment Outcomes

Appropriate patient selection is essential. The tumour must be visible on MRI and clearly delineated from its surroundings. In order to prevent thermal injury to adjacent tissue, the anterior surface of the tumour must be at least 1 cm from the skin and not adjacent to the chest wall.

DOI: 10.1201/9780429162671-19

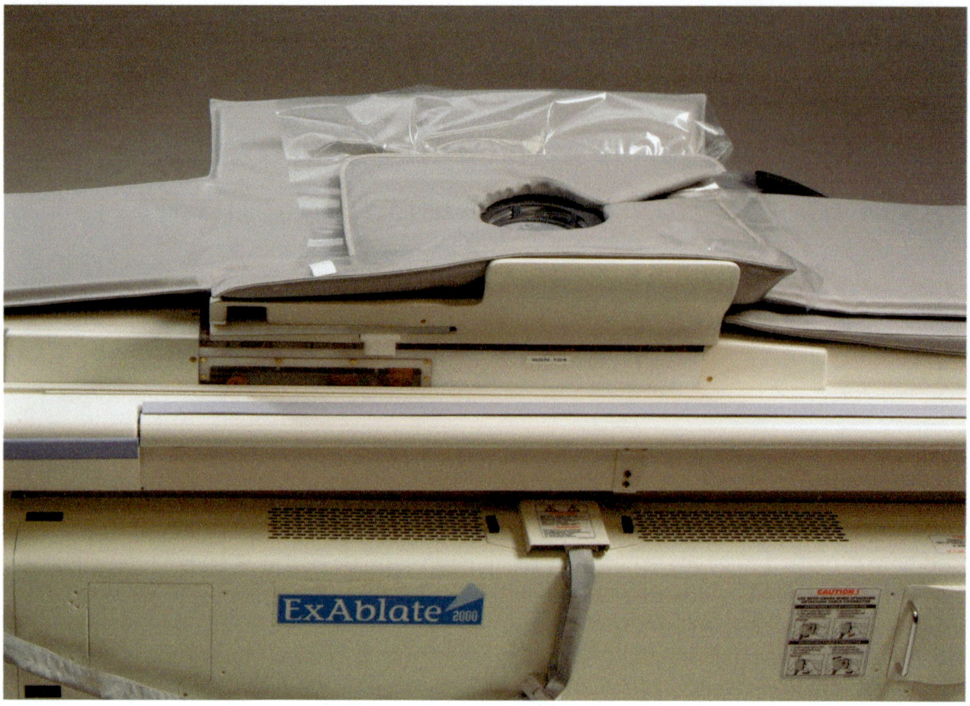

FIGURE 19.1 The MRgFUSA device embedded in the MRI table (ExAblate 2000, InSightec, Ltd, Haifa Israel). Insightec's first indications with FDA approved IDEs in 1999, 2000, and 2001 were for breast cancer and breast fibroadenoma using the pictured device.

The patient is positioned prone on a modified MRI table in which the treatment device is embedded (Figure 19.1). The breast is positioned in the centre of the MRgFUSA surface coil and an emergency stop button is placed in the patient's hand. The breast and surface coil are lowered into a tub containing the specialised ultrasound transducer. The tub is filled with degassed water to ensure acoustic coupling to the transducer. During the procedure, the degassed water is maintained at 20 degrees Celsius and circulated around the breast to provide active cooling of the skin. Conscious sedation is typically maintained with an intravenous anxiolytic/analgesic cocktail.

Contrast-enhanced MR images of the breast are obtained. The tumour is identified and the treatment volume is determined (Figure 19.2). The treatment is then delivered as a series of interlaced elliptical sonication zones delivered within the prescribed treatment area which comprises the tumour and a rim of surrounding normal tissue (Figure 19.3). Ideally, each sonication zone is individually exposed with near-real-time temperature monitoring. Total treatment duration is a function of the number of individual sonication zones required to cover the volume in the prescribed treatment region. Each sonication cycle (treatment and cooling) requires 18 to 74 seconds, with typical total treatment time ranging from 35 to 150 minutes.[2,3]

In 2001, Hynynen and co-workers[4] reported a feasibility study of MRI-guided HIFU using an MR imaging-compatible ultrasound surgery system (GE Medical Systems, Milwaukee, WI, USA) to treat 11 fibroadenomas in nine patients with a median age of 29 years (range 19–38 years). Mean tumour volume was 1.9 ± 1.5 cm^3 (range 0.7–6.5 cm^3). The treatment was provided in the prone position, with local anaesthesia and mild, oral sedation. Treatment plans were designed to ensure that "all intratumoural tissue was treated." Treatment times were reported to be approximately 2 hours for a 2-cm tumour and 45 minutes for a 1-cm tumour.

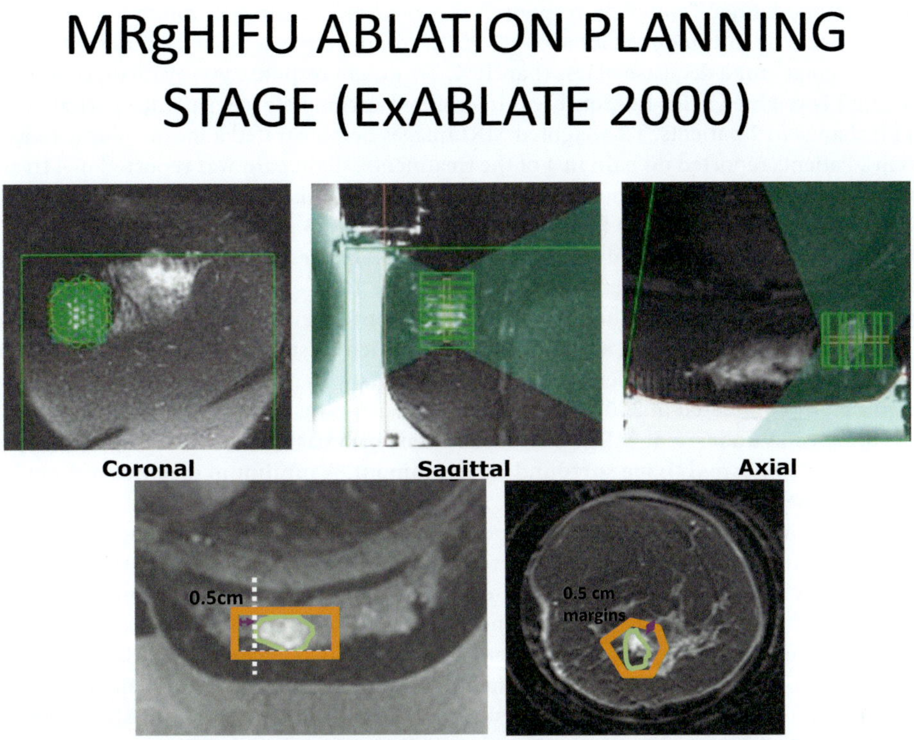

FIGURE 19.2 MRgFUSA breast treatment plan (ExAblate 2000, InSightec, Ltd, Haifa Israel). The treatment is provided as a series of interlaced elliptical sonication zones delivered within the prescribed treatment area comprising of the tumour and rim of surrounding tissue. Photos courtesy of Dr Furusawa at Breastopia, Namba Hospital, Miyazaki, Japan.

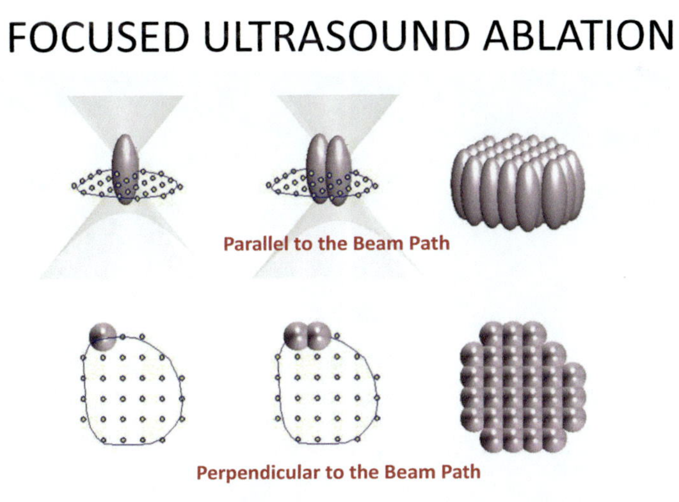

FIGURE 19.3 Depiction of "cigar"-shaped sonication zones arrayed side by side covering an entire tumour (blue circle) and small zone of surrounding tissue.

The investigators defined "complete response" as a decrease in tumour volume of >90%, "partial response" as a decrease in tumour volume of 50–90%, "minor response" as a decrease between 10 and 49%, and "no change" for a decrease of less than 10%. Treatment response was evaluated 6 months after ablation using T1-weighted MRI. Response was interpreted as complete in 6 patients, partial in 2, minor in 1, and no change in 2 patients. T2-weighted MRI images demonstrated a mean volume reduction of 1.3 ± 1.1 cm^3. Patients reported no pain in 4 of the treatments, slight pain was reported in 4 treatments, 2 patients experienced moderate pain, and one reported severe pain. Tenderness was the most common early toxicity, reported up to 10 days following the procedure. In 3 patients, additional bilateral mammograms were obtained and showed no treatment-related changes up to 4 years after therapy. MRI images, both before and after treatment, are shown in Figure 19.4.

To date, there have been 8 published papers relating to trials evaluating MRgFUSA for the treatment of breast cancer.[2,5–11] All but two can best be described as small feasibility studies. Gianfelice and co-workers were the first to describe a series of patients who underwent MRgFUSA followed by resection in a study completed in 2001.[5] Twelve patients with invasive breast cancers less than 3.5 cm in greatest dimension underwent MRgFUSA of a volume of breast tissue including the tumour and a margin of 0.5 cm of normal tissue surrounding the tumour. A minimum distance of 1 cm between the tumour and the skin or ribs was required. All patients underwent routine segmental resection within 24 days of MRgFUSA. The resected specimen was evaluated by mapping the tumour and treatment zone using three-dimensional macroscopic and microscopic histopathologic measurements combined with standard haematoxylin-eosin staining of 5 micron sections. At the time of excision, the first 3 patients treated were found to have a mean of 43.3% of the tumour ablated. Subsequent improvements in the targeting system used on the final 9 patients in this series resulted in 88.3% mean tumour volume necrosis. Two of the final 9 patients had no residual viable tumour. Two patients in this series suffered second-degree skin burns, both under 2.3 cm in size. Four patients reported slight discomfort, and 8 reported moderate discomfort on a 3-point scale (slight, moderate, intolerable). Based on their initial feasibility study, Gianfelice and co-workers concluded that MRgFUSA held significant promise in terms of patient tolerability, but that the observation of residual tumour at the margins of the treatment zone suggested that refinements in tumour imaging and targeting were required.

Zippel and Papa[8] reported the results of a phase 1 trial evaluating the use of MRgFUSA in 10 women with invasive breast cancer who ultimately underwent routine breast preserving surgery

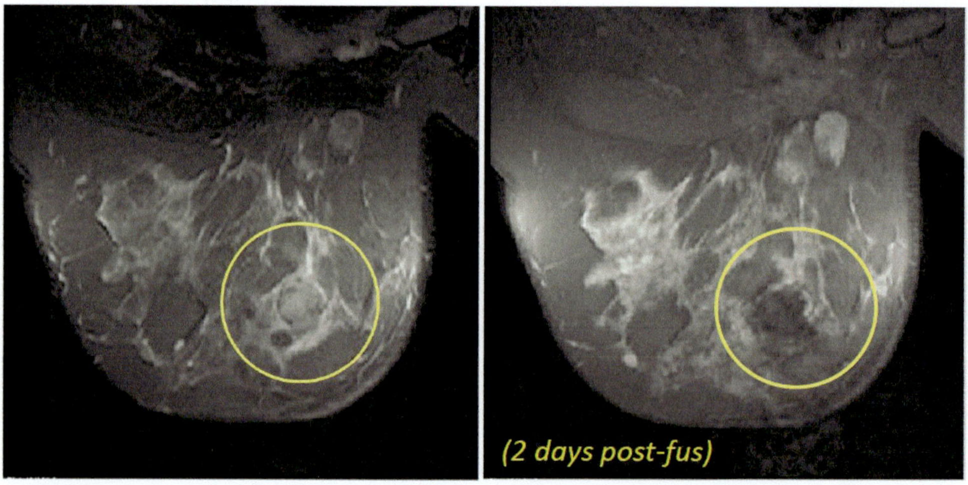

FIGURE 19.4 T1-weighted contrast enhanced MRI images of breast fibroadenoma are shown, both before and 48 h after MRI-guided focused ultrasound ablation. (Courtesy of K. Hynynen.)

between September 2002 and August 2004, using the ExAblate 2000 device (InSightec, Haifa Israel Ltd.) (Figure 19.1). Mean age was 56 years (range 45–72). All patients had tumours that were easily visible on non-enhanced MRI and were located more than 10 mm from the skin and chest wall. Tumour size was required to be less than 3 cm (mean 2.2 cm). Patients underwent standard lumpectomy and axillary sampling 7 to 10 days after the ablation procedure. On routine histopathologic evaluation of the excised specimens, 2 patients were found to have no residual tumour (Figure 19.5). Two patients had microscopic foci of residual carcinoma too small to quantify, 3 had 10% residual tumour, and 3 had 10–30% residual tumour. Procedure-related complications included pain requiring analgesia and sedation during the treatment, and 1 patient suffered a second degree skin burn over the area treated. The authors concluded that MRgFUSA had the potential to provide "non-invasive virtual surgery [that] can be safely and repeatedly done, with low morbidity to the patient."[8]

In 2006, Khiat and co-workers published the results of a study designed to determine the influence of post-treatment delay on the evaluation of the response to focused ultrasound ablation of breast cancer by dynamic contrast enhanced (DCE) MRI.[9] In this study, DCE-MRI data were collected immediately and several days after treatment for 25 patients (26 tumours), and these were then compared with the percentage of residual tumour as determined by histopathology of the excised treated mass. The mean age of patients treated was 61 years (range 45–87). All patients had invasive cancers less than 3.5 cm in diameter. One patient had 2 tumours treated. The MRgFUS treatments were performed by different versions of the ExAblate (2000 and 2100) system developed by InSightec, Inc. (Haifa, Israel and Dallas, TX). Dynamic contrast-enhanced MRI images used in this study were recorded both immediately and at a follow-up visit 3 to 14 days after the MRgFUS but before conventional surgery. A total of 26 treated tumours underwent ablation. On routine histopathologic analysis, 7 specimens had no detectable residual tumour at the site of MRgFUS, 11 specimens had less than 10% residual tumour volume, and 7 specimens were found to have a larger percentage of residual tumour, ranging between 20% and 90% of the originally measured volume on imaging. Based on their data, the authors concluded that "DCE-MRI parameters such as ISI and PEI are both useful in determining the effectiveness of MRgFUS in breast

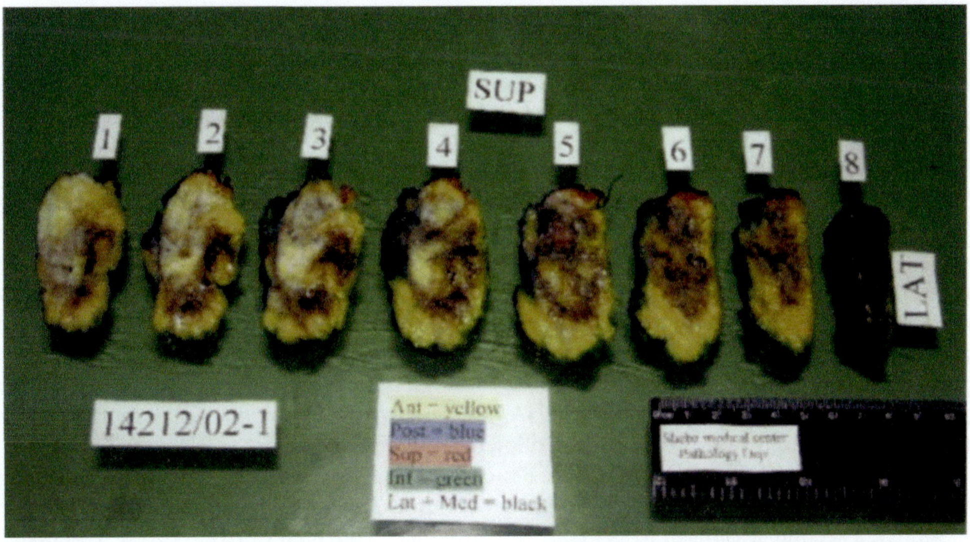

FIGURE 19.5 Breast lump pathology specimens showing haemorrhagic necrosis following FUS. (From Zippel DB, Papa MZ. The use of MR imaging guided focused ultrasound in breast cancer patients; a preliminary phase one study and review. Breast Cancer 2005;12:32–38.)

carcinomas, provided the measurements are performed sufficiently long after treatment, i.e. approximately 7 days or more after MRgFUS."[9]

Furusawa and colleagues reported on a study of 30 women with invasive breast cancer less than 3.5 cm in greatest diameter treated by MRgFUSA.[10] The tumour and "at least a 5-mm safety margin of normal tissue" were treated, followed 5 to 23 days later by routine breast conserving surgery or mastectomy. All tumours were greater than 1 cm from the skin or ribs. Histopathologic analysis of the specimens was conducted in a similar fashion to the previously mentioned study by Gianfelice and co-workers.[5] There were five protocol violations resulting in 25 evaluable patients. Mean tumour necrosis was 98% by volume (range 90–100%). One hundred percent necrosis was observed in 15 patients (60%), and only one patient had less than 95% necrosis of her tumour. One patient suffered a skin burn which was excised at the time of surgery. Two patients reported mild to moderate breast pain during sonication. Furusawa and co-workers concluded that MRgFUSA was well tolerated and effective, and that in well-selected patients, it had the potential to replace lumpectomy.[10]

Marincola and colleagues[11] reported on the treatment of 10 women with invasive breast cancer in a "treat and excise study" in which all patients underwent MRgFUSA followed by standard surgical excision at 10 to 21 days after ablation. The ExAblate 2100 device (InSightec, Haifa Israel Ltd.) was utilised. Tumours were required to be less than 2.0 cm in greatest dimension and located at least 15 mm from both skin and pectoral muscle. Mean tumour size of the patients treated was 1.2 cm. "Mild conscious sedation was performed in all cases."[11] Sonication planning incorporated 30% superimposition with complete coverage of the nodule and 5 mm-safety margin. Average treatment time was 2 h and 20 min (range: 1 h and 20 min to 3 h). No adverse events were recorded during or after the procedure. On routine histopathologic evaluation of the excised specimens, 6 patients were found to have no residual tumour and 4 patients had microscopic foci of residual carcinoma.

As of the writing of this chapter, Maurice A.A.J. van den Bosch and co-workers have an open trial evaluating a dedicated MR-HIFU breast platform specifically developed for ablation of breast tumours (Sonalleve, Philips Healthcare, Vantaa, Finland).[6] Similar in design to the ExAblate 2100 device (InSightec, Haifa Israel Ltd.), the platform consists of a water-filled table top with a breast cup positioned in the middle of an MRI table. The patient is positioned prone during the MR-HIFU treatment with the targeted breast inside the cup. The breast is surrounded by cooled water to enable ultrasound waves to target the breast. The Sonalleve device differs from previously evaluated units in that

> eight separate focused ultrasound modules with 32 transducer elements of 6.6 mm diameter each form a circular structure of 270 degrees surrounding the breast cup (Figures 19.6 and 19.7). The circular structure of the breast platform uses a mainly horizontal beam path orientation. Ultrasound beams target the breast from the lateral sides, hereby increasing the effective distance from focal point to rib cage, heart, and lungs. The larger distance reduces the heating of critical structures, because the far field, i.e. the area after the focal point, is mainly located inside the breast.[12]

The use of MRgFUSA as the primary treatment of breast cancer without excision was first reported by Gianfelice et al6, when he described a series of 24 patients with oestrogen receptor–positive, non-metastatic breast cancers. Mean tumour size was 1.5 cm (range 0.6–2.5 cm). All patients in the study had refused surgery or were considered to be "at too high a risk to undergo surgery." After consent was obtained, all patients underwent MRgFUSA followed by or concurrent with tamoxifen therapy. Patients did not undergo tumour excision. Following MRgFUSA, breast MRIs were obtained at 10 days, 1, 3, and 6 months. Following the MRI at 6 months, image-guided core biopsies (4–8 cores) were obtained from the area of the previously treated cancer. In the event that residual tumour was identified on biopsy, a second session of MRgFUSA was provided. Fourteen of twenty-four patients (58%) had no residual disease identified on core biopsy 6 months following MRgFUSA. Ten patients with positive post-ablation biopsies were re-treated with MRgFUSA, and five of the 10 were core biopsy

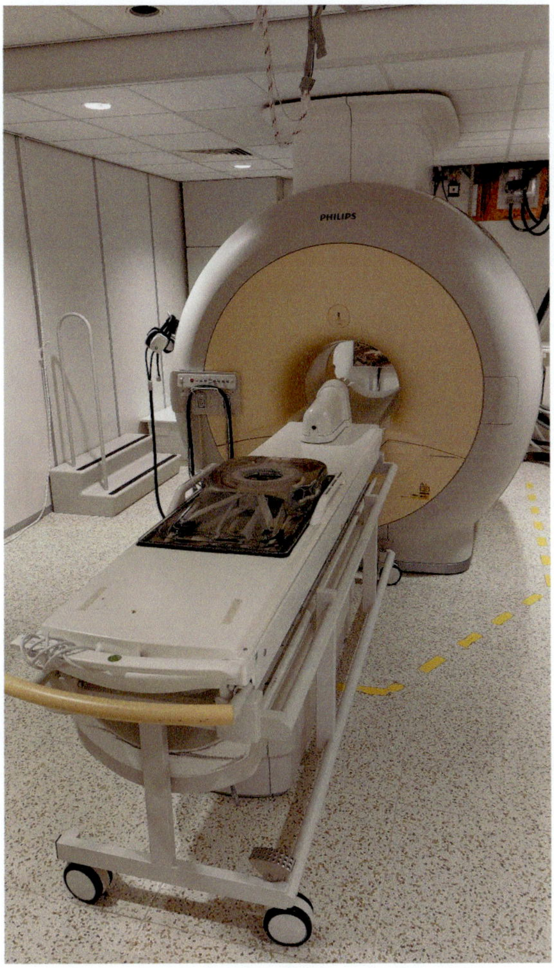

FIGURE 19.6

negative one month later. The final success rate, defined as core biopsy negative, 7 months after initial MRgFUSA treatment was 19 of 24 patients (79%). Mean follow-up was 20.2 months (range 12–39 months). One complication, in the form of a second-degree skin burn resolving with local wound care, was reported (4%). The treatment was well tolerated, with 10 patients reporting mild pain and 14 reporting moderate pain. Pain control was thought to be satisfactory with conscious intravenous sedation. The authors of the study concluded that MRgFUSA combined with adjuvant systemic treatment was well tolerated, had low-morbidity, and was an effective treatment for small breast cancers in selected patients.

In 2014, Dr Furusawa reported on the most recent experience in Japan with MRgFUSA for the treatment of patients with breast cancer at the 4th International Symposium on Focused Ultrasound.[7] At that time, Furusawa and colleagues had enrolled 74 patients in a prospective single arm trial of MRgFUSA followed by routine whole breast radiation therapy with no excision. All patients had a single well-demarcated tumour equal to or less than 1.5 cm in greatest dimension, well visualised on MRI, with a skin-to-tumour distance of 1.0 cm or greater. Prior to treatment, patients underwent definitive diagnosis by core biopsy and were found to be node negative by sentinel node biopsy.

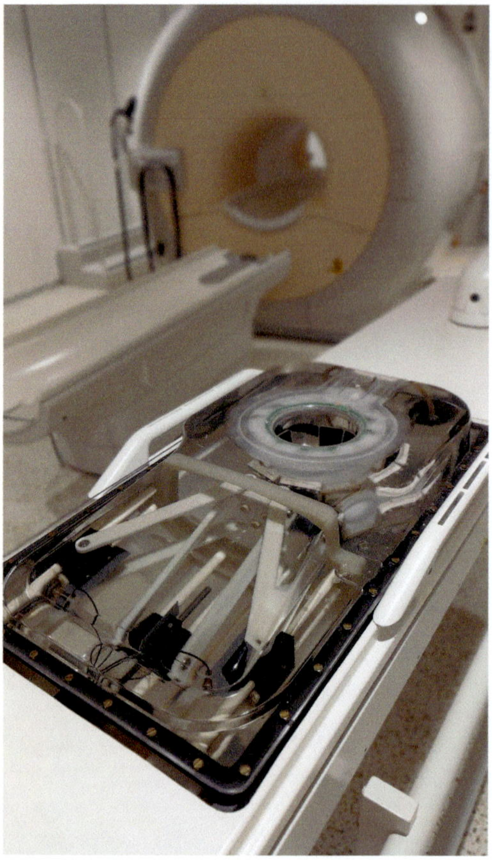

FIGURE 19.7

Patients underwent ultrasound guided core needle biopsy of the tumour site 3 weeks after completion of MRgFUSA. If no viable tumour was identified, patients received routine whole breast radiation therapy and were followed with mammography and breast MRI every 6 months (Figure 19.8). As of October 2014, 74 patients with mean tumour size of 1.1 cm (range 0.5–1.5cm) had been treated. The mean treatment duration was 120 minutes (range 41–246). Mean follow-up for all patients in the study was 77 months (range 11–126). Forty-eight patients had longer than 5-year follow-up. At the time of the presentation, there was 1 local recurrence (at 8 years post-ablation), and no significant adverse events and cosmesis was excellent (Figure 19.9). Dr Furusawa's treat and observe study remains open to accrual at this time in Japan.

19.3 Expert Commentary

Even if MRgFUSA is shown to be equivalent to breast-preserving surgery in the treatment of patients with small breast cancers, there are currently 3 significant obstacles to its clinical implementation: long duration of treatment, uncertainty of margin status, and the persistence of a breast mass after ablation in some patients. To date, these issues, along with a paucity of data, have prohibited the widespread adoption of ablative treatments of breast cancer.

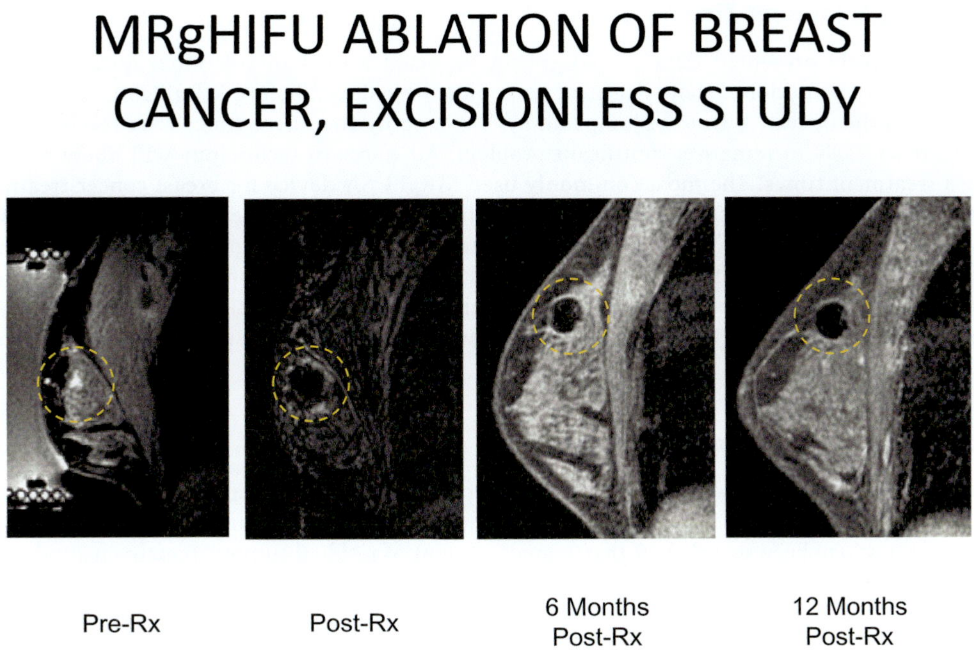

FIGURE 19.8 Serial breast MRIs of a breast cancer patient treated by MRgFUSA and no excision. The broken circle identifies the area where the treated tumour was present, not the treatment zone. Photos courtesy of Dr Furusawa at Breastopia, Namba Hospital, Miyazaki, Japan.

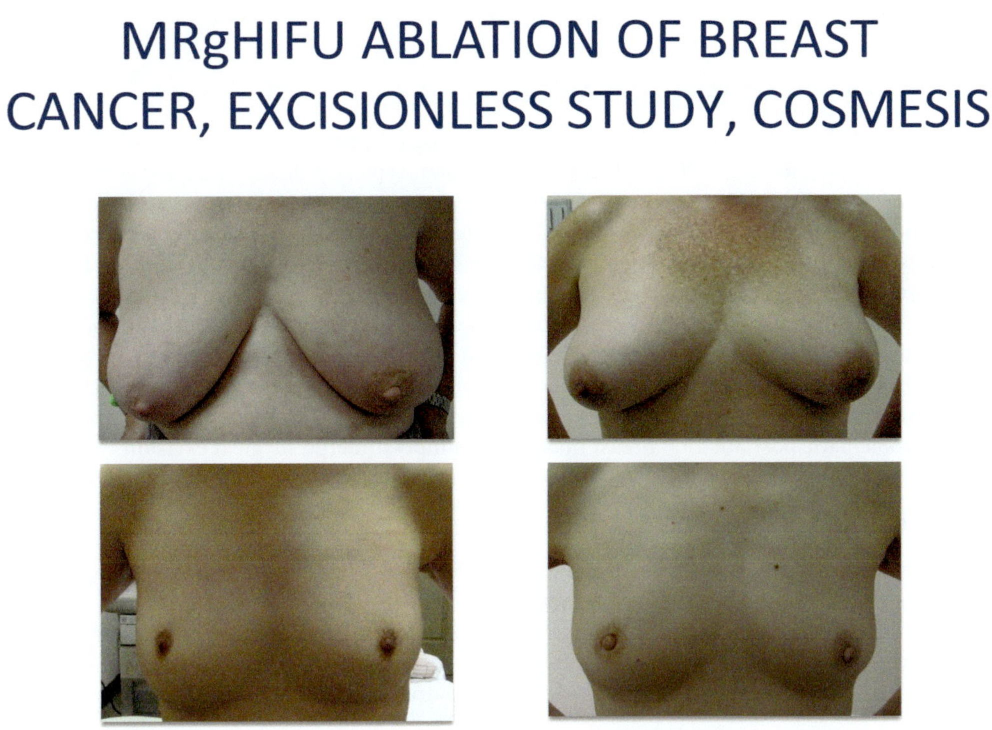

FIGURE 19.9 Four patients with T1, N0 breast cancers treated with MRgFUSA and no excision. Photos courtesy of Dr Furusawa at Breastopia, Namba Hospital, Miyazaki, Japan.

19.3.1 Long Treatment Time

The most recently presented data on MRgFUSA reported a median treatment duration of 120 minutes.[13] There is no doubt that treatment time must be reduced before MRgFUSA can compare favourably to the operative time of lumpectomy. The lengthy treatment times required by current devices are unlikely to remain a significant problem. Advances in technology will likely result in reduced treatment times. The most commonly used MRgFUSA device for breast cancer treatment and research, the ExAblate 2000 (InSightec, Ltd, Haifa Israel), is only somewhat specialised. Most of its components are utilised to treat a variety of organs including the uterus, breast, prostate, brain, and bone. If studies demonstrate that MRgFUSA is equivalent to breast-preserving surgery in the treatment of patients with small breast cancers, then it is likely that specialised, multi-transducer, breast specific treatment devices will be developed with the potential to substantially reduce treatment times.

19.3.2 Uncertainty of Margin Status

The idea that excellent margin control is vital to the prevention of local recurrence in cancer patients treated with standard breast preserving surgery is well-founded and should be closely adhered to. However, it has long been established that a small amount of residual tumour remains behind in the conserved breast in a substantial proportion of patients.[8] This residual tumour is typically undetectable on breast imaging, nor predictable by pathologic margin evaluation. Adjuvant radiation therapy is an integral component of breast preserving surgery, as it is intended to treat residual tumour assumed to remain in the breast.

The excellent local control observed to date in the limited number of patients enrolled in FUSA without excision studies is likely partially due to multi-modality care. Routine whole breast radiation therapy and adjuvant systemic treatment has been part of these protocols. Hopefully, these excellent results will prove durable on longer term follow-up and in future studies. If so, the uncertainty of margin status should not prove to be a significant obstacle to the clinical implementation of FUSA.

19.3.3 Persistent Breast Mass after Ablation

Fat necrosis, resulting in persistent palpable masses, can occur in a minority of patients following ablative therapy. Luckily, this is usually a self-limiting problem, typically slowly resolving over the course of a year.[9] A breast mass in a patient after breast preservation is problematic as it can be anxiety provoking to both the patient and her surgeon, and has the potential to obscure locally recurrent disease. Consistent use of various breast imaging modalities can minimise the likelihood of a missed local recurrence. However, there is little doubt that patients and surgeons will be intolerant of persistent palpable breast masses in cancer patients. Fat necrosis following ablative treatment of breast cancer may prove to be a significant challenge to the widespread adoption of the technique. However, the prevention and management of persistent palpable masses after ablation is an area that has yet to be investigated and may be amenable to systemic or local pharmacologic therapy. In the worst case, patients who develop a persistent, problematic post-ablation breast mass could simply undergo surgical excision.

19.3.3.1 Future of FUSA

Magnetic resonance–guided focused ultrasound ablation has been studied in several small trials. To date, these studies have proven it to be safe, but efficacy has ranged widely from 43% to 100% in the treat-and-excise trials. In Japan, the ongoing Furusawa "excisionless" MRgFUSA only trial has reported 1 recurrence in 74 carefully selected patients with mean follow-up of 77 months.[13] The results of this study have aided in the development of proper treatment guidelines and the standardisation of the procedure.

Focused ultrasound ablation has the potential to be a "disruptive technology," taking the primary treatment of patients with early stage breast cancer out of the hands of surgeons. However, surgeons should not feel imperilled. We already work closely with our breast imaging colleagues to provide outstanding multi-disciplinary breast cancer care. The same multi-disciplinary team will be required to develop and refine ablative techniques. There is no doubt that collaboration is the best way to assure that we continue to actively participate in the treatment of patients with early stage breast cancer

19.4 Summary

Breast conserving surgery combined with radiation therapy has been extensively studied and is the "gold standard" for the treatment of patients with small breast cancers.[10,11] Breast conserving surgery has been widely adopted because it is a brief outpatient procedure with low morbidity and exceedingly rare mortality that can be accomplished under local anaesthesia. It provides outstanding local control, and in experienced hands, most patients can expect good to excellent cosmesis. Breast conserving surgery requires minimal technology and can be successfully employed in almost any setting. In comparison, FUSA is a relatively new technique with minimal data, requiring complex technology with very limited availability. Much work remains to be completed before FUSA can be directly compared to breast preserving surgery. Studies of FUSA addressing local failure rates, cosmesis, cost effectiveness, and long-term patient satisfaction are ongoing.[13] There is little doubt that non-surgical ablative cancer therapies will become more commonplace in the future. Non-invasive ablative treatment of breast cancer has obvious advantages. Given equivalent results, few patients would choose surgery over no surgery. If ongoing studies find FUSA to be equivalent to breast conserving surgery, then FUSA will become the breast cancer treatment of choice for appropriately selected patients.

REFERENCES

1. Graham SJ, Chen L, Leitch M, Peters RD, Bronskill MJ, Foster FS, Henkelman RM, Plewes DB. Quantifying tissue damage due to focused ultrasound heating observed by MRI. Magnetic Resonance Medicine 1999;41:321–328.
2. Furusawa H, Namba K, Thomsen S, Akiyama F, Bendet A, Tanaka C, Yasuda Y, Nakahara H. Magnetic resonance-guided focused ultrasound surgery of breast cancer: Reliability and effectiveness. Journal of the American College of Surgeons 2006;203:54–63.
3. Gambos EC, Kacher DF, Furusawa H, Namba K. Breast focused ultrasound surgery with magnetic resonance guidance. Topics in Magnetic Resonance Imaging 2006;17:181–188.
4. Hynynen K, Pomeroy O, Smith DN, Huber PE, McDannold NJ, Kettenbach J, Baum J, Singer S, Jolesz F. MR imaging-guided focused ultrasound surgery of fibroadenomas in the breast: A feasibility study. Radiology. 2001;219(1):176–185.
5. Gianfelice D, Khiat A, Amara M, Belblidia A, Boulanger Y. MR imaging-guided focused US ablation of breast cancer: histopathologic assessment of effectiveness-initial experience. Radiology 2003;227:849–855.
6. Merckel L, Bartels L, Kohler M, van den Bongard H, Deckers R, Mali W, Binkert C, Moonen C, Gilhuijs K, van den and Bosch M. MR-Guided high-intensity focused ultrasound ablation of breast cancer with a dedicated breast platform. Cardiovascular Interventional Radiology 2013;36:292–301.
7. Furusawa H. Treatment of Breast Cancer. Plenary session presented at the 4th International Symposium on Focused Ultrasound, Bethesda, MD, 2004;10/15/14.
8. Holland R, Veling SHJ, Mravunac M, Hendriks JHCL. Histologic multifocality of Tis, T 1–2 breast carcinomas: implications for clinical trials of breast-conserving surgery. Cancer 1985;56:979–990.
9. Bland KL, Gass J, Klimberg VS. Radiofrequency, cryoablation, and other modalities for breast cancer ablation. Surgical Clinics of North America 2007;87:539–550.

10. Fisher B, Anderson S, Bryant J, Margolese RG, Deutsch M, Fisher ER, Jeong JH, Wolmark N. Twenty-year follow-up of a randomized trial comparing total mastectomy, lumpectomy, and lumpectomy plus irradiation for the treatment of invasive breast cancer. The New England Journal of Medicine 2002;347:1233–1241.
11. Veronesi U, Cascinelli N, Mariani L, Greco M, Saccozzi R, Luini A, Agular M, Marubini E. Twenty-year follow-up of a randomized study comparing breast-conserving surgery with radical mastectomy for early breast cancer. The New England Journal of Medicine 2002;347:1227–1232.

20

Clinical Application of MR-Guided Focused Ultrasound Ablation for Bone Metastasis

Alessandro Napoli, Luisa Di Mare, Giulia Alfieri, Monica Mattone, Alessandro De Maio, and Carlo Catalano

20.1 Background

Bone is the third most common organ involved in metastatic disease, coming behind lung and liver. Skeletal metastases occur in 20–30% of cancer patients. The tumours that most commonly metastasise to the bones include prostate, breast, kidney, thyroid, and lung. Breast, prostate, kidney, and lung primaries contribute 75% of all skeletal metastases. Prostate cancer contributes 60% of metastatic epithelial tumours in men, and breast cancer 75% of metastases in women.[1]

For breast cancer, bone is the second most common site of metastatic spread, and 90% of patients dying of breast cancer have bone metastasis. Breast and prostate cancer metastasise to bone most frequently, which reflects the high incidence of both these tumours, as well as their prolonged clinical courses.

The diagnosis of a metastatic lesion is usually straightforward in most cases. The lesions are quite amenable to diagnostic fine-needle aspiration cytology (this method is more difficult to use in primary bone lesions since sarcomas are heterogenous). In selected cases, a panel of antibodies can be helpful in establishing the diagnosis of metastatic carcinoma, and in locating the primary origin. Metastases occur via arterial transmission of cells into a distant intra-osseous artery. When lung metastases exist, bone metastases are considered to have spread from the lung lesion, but bone metastases often arise, even in the absence of lung metastases. Arterial metastases to the spine are typically located in the posterior aspect of the vertebral body, at the base of the pedicle, where many intraosseous arteries are present. As the tumour grows in this location, the radiographic contour of the pedicle is lost due to involvement at the junction between the vertebral body and the pedicle. Metastasis via a venous route occurs in the vertebra through the Batson venous plexus. This mechanism of metastasis arises mainly from tumours of abdomen and pelvis. These occur at a vertebral level close to the primary lesion. These lesions are typically in the centre of the vertebral body because of the distribution of the basi-vertebral vein.[2]

Bone metastases can severely impair mobility and significantly contribute to a general decrease in quality of life. Owing to progressively improved treatments for primary tumours, the incidence of distant metastases has increased, and the long-term management of their clinical effects has become important.[3] However, whereas systemic disease progression is managed with chemotherapy alone, bone metastases may often require additional, independent, local therapy to prevent concurrent skeletal complications and preserve quality of life.[4, 5] Pain is the most common symptom of bone metastases, with 50%–70% of patients suffering from severe pain.[6]

Current treatments for patients with bone metastases are primarily palliative and include analgesics (opioids and non-steroidal anti-inflammatory drugs), systemic therapies (chemotherapy, hormonal therapy, and bisphosphonates), and localised therapies (radiation therapy, percutaneous ablation, and surgical stabilisation) for local control.[7–12]

DOI: 10.1201/9780429162671-20

Recently, radiofrequency ablation has been tested as a treatment option for bone metastases. Moreover, the off-label use of cryoablation techniques is currently being tested as another alternative for bone metastasis palliation.[13]

At present, external beam radiation therapy (EBRT) is the current standard noninvasive treatment for palliation of local pain and the treatment of choice for clinically active bone metastases; however, this has proven ineffective in 20–30% of cases and is only temporarily effective in 27% of cases.[2, 12]

There is also an increased risk of pathological fracture in the peri-irradiation period, due to an induced hyperaemic response at the periphery of the tumour. The hyperaemic response weakens the adjacent bone and increases the risk of spontaneous fracture. Furthermore, patients who have recurrent pain at a site previously irradiated may not be eligible for further radiation therapy because of the limitations of normal tissue tolerance. Higher radiation doses also produce a greater risk of complications such as fibrosis of normal soft tissue, which can cause a decrease in the quality of life when life expectancy is longer than 6 months. High intensity focused ultrasound is a noninvasive technique that can facilitate coagulative necrosis at a precise focal point in the body. The location and extent of this treatment can be monitored accurately with real-time imaging, using either ultrasonography (US) or magnetic resonance (MR) techniques. Indeed, the advent of more sophisticated imaging techniques (especially MR thermometry) has led to a resurgence of interest in high intensity focused ultrasound. At the beginning, this technique was used to treat patients with hepatocellular carcinoma and breast cancer[14, 15] and, more recently, the treatment options have widely increased in clinical practice, and now include neurofunctional brain surgery.[16]

There has been a long-standing general consensus that ultrasound energy cannot enter bone at an intensity sufficient for therapeutic ablation. However, various groups have initially investigated whether high intensity focused ultrasound (HIFU) ablation therapy can be effectively applied to bone tumours. In particular, US-guided high intensity focused ultrasound ablation (USgHIFU) has been successfully applied in the treatment of 80 patients with primary bone malignancies (62 with osteosarcoma). Follow-up images demonstrated completely ablated malignant bone tumours in 69 patients and greater than 50% tumour ablation in the remaining 11 patients. Overall survival rates at 1, 2, 3, 4, and 5 years were 89.8%, 72.3%, 60.5%, 50.5%, and 50.5%, respectively. Survival rates at 1, 2, 3, 4, and 5 years were 93.3%, 82.4%, 75.0%, 63.7%, and 63.7%, respectively, in the patients with stage IIb cancer and 79.2%, 42.2%, 21.1%, 15.8%, and 15.8%, respectively, in those with stage III disease. The pain disappeared within 3–4 days of HIFU treatment. Local oedema was also observed in all patients immediately after the ultrasound ablation, reached its peak the day after the ablation and subsided within an average of 19 days.[17]

MR-guided focused ultrasound (MRgFUS) combines the ablative properties of high intensity focused ultrasound with MR imaging for target definition and real-time guidance and monitoring. It has been used to thermally ablate various types of soft tissue[18] and has the potential to achieve clinical goals in the treatment of bone tumours; in the management of bone metastasis. Clinically measured outcomes include pain relief, preservation and restoration of functional levels and local tumour control.[19]

20.2 Clinical Use

Clinical MRgFUS is already European Conformity (CE) marked and Food and Drug Administration (FDA) approved for treatment of uterine leiomyomas and palliative care of bone metastases and is currently under evaluation for the treatment of solid tumours in the brain, breast, prostate, liver, and pancreas.[20–24]

Although the success rate of combined treatment for bone tumours, ranging from surgery to chemoradiation and various forms of percutaneous ablation, is more than acceptable, a significant percentage of patients either do not benefit from symptom relief or face symptom recurrence in the short term.[5, 12] In these cases, MRgFUS can represent a safe and effective approach for both pain palliation and, potentially, tumour control. Hurwitz et al., in a multicentre phase III trial, demonstrated that MRgFUS was a safe and effective, noninvasive treatment for alleviating pain resulting from bone metastases in patients that had failed standard treatments Response to MRgFUS was typically rapid, with about two-thirds of responses seen within days after treatment. Additionally, 47% of the patients treated by MRgFUS reduced (21%) or completely stopped (26%) their morphine equivalent daily dose consumption.[25]

A study from the Radiological Department of University Medical Center of Utrecht demonstrated a significant pain score decrease, compared to baseline three days after treatment and pain scores significantly lower than at baseline at 1 month follow-up.[2].

In our experience, we have evaluated the efficacy of MRgFUS for pain management for the primary treatment of bone lesions accessible to the focused beam (after an imaging workup with computed tomography and MR to determine the size and the location of the lesions, as well as the feasibility of treatment and the lesion viability). Unlike previous studies, in which patients were enrolled for MRgFUS treatment because of the failure of other therapies, we treated patients who had not previously received other therapies. Although performed in a limited population, the absence of adverse events in our study suggests the use of this treatment option as a viable noninvasive alternative to standard pain palliation treatments. We noted a reduction of lesion viability after the MRgFUS procedure and a remineralisation of spongious bone in accordance with the MDA criteria. These parameters are important for evaluating the response of bone metastases to therapy; moreover, MR's ability to rapidly determine the response of a lesion to treatment might have great value in clinical practice. This is important, given the possibility of increased adverse effects and the greater patient morbidity associated with the persistent use of a potentially ineffective treatment if there is no possibility of immediately evaluating the response. Under MR guidance, treatment success or failure is rapidly addressed in terms of the amount of nonviable tissue in the target area.[3]

Patients should meet the following inclusion criteria for MRgFUS ablation of bone metastases: (a) treatable lesions must be located in the ribs, sternum, extremities, pelvis, shoulders, or posterior aspects of dorsal, lumbar, and sacral vertebra (S1–S5); (b) the lesion must be visible on MR images or computed tomographic (CT) images; (c) the lesion must be accessible to the focused ultrasound beam without being shielded by extensive scarring, hollow viscera, or non-targeted bone; and (d) the interface between the bone and targeted lesions should be deeper than 10 mm from the skin surface.[6]

The purpose of using MRgFUS is to treat a lesion in the region causing pain in order to achieve relief. Efficacy is determined by the level of pain relief (as measured by the Numerical Rating Scale [NRS]), decrease in analgesics/opiates, and improved quality of life. Initial studies have shown MRgFUS to be effective for pain control through thermal cell death and periosteal denervation induced by cortical heating as a result of acoustic energy absorption. Moreover, there is evidence that a high intensity focused ultrasound beam can penetrate through the cortical bone to the medullary space, producing thermal necrosis of malignant tissue. To understand the theoretical basis of these two different clinical approaches, it is important to realise that cortical bone has high acoustic absorption and low thermal conduction coefficients; hence, the focused US energy is absorbed by the cortical surface with little or no penetration into the medullary bone.[27] When pain palliation is the treatment aim, the interaction between focused US and intact cortical bone can be used to produce a temperature increase over the periosteal surface of the target area, causing thermal damage to the periosteal nerves (Figure 20.1), which are responsible for nociception.[28] On the other hand, when tumour control or tumour debulking is the primary clinical intent, focused US should be applied over a damaged (severely thinned or eroded) bony cortex, thus allowing thermal damage to lesions located deep into the medullary bone.

At our institution, all MRgFUS procedures, including pre-treatment imaging, are performed on a 3-T MR imaging scanner combined with the MRgFUS system. This system is approved for the ablation of bone lesions. Treatment takes place while the patient lies on the table inside the bore of the MR scanner. The transducer is embedded in the patient table and features a 208-element annular phased array (diameter, 120 mm; radius of curvature, 160 mm; focal distance, 60–200 mm; frequencies, 0.95–1.35 MHz; and energy range 500–7200 J). This transducer uses a wide-beam approach with the focal point placed behind the bone cortex and the ablation area located at the intersection of the ultrasound beam with the bone surface[3] (Figure 20.2).

Treatment begins by acquiring a series of MR images of the target organ. The physician then reviews the images on the system workstation, identifies a target volume on the MR images, delineates the treatment contours on the images, and reviews the treatment plan (Figures 20.3 and 20.4). Therapy planning software calculates the parameters required to treat the defined region effectively. During the treatment,

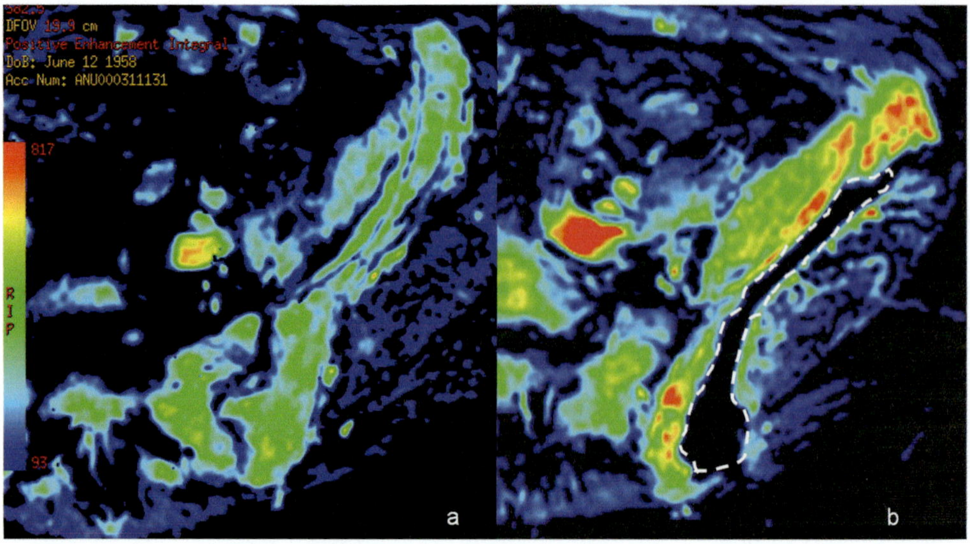

FIGURE 20.1 Periosteal neurolysis of iliac bone. Axial dynamic contrast-enhanced colour-coded T1-weighted image with fat saturation acquired before MR-guided focused ultrasound treatment (a) clearly shows diffuse metastatic involvement of iliac bone involving and also the medullar compartment. MR image obtained with the same parameters at 3 months follow-up (b) reveals that the pathologic tissue is entirely replaced by necrosis of the proximal cortex periostium, with a "black band" (dashed line), as demonstrated by absent perfusion. Despite residual tumour perfusion, the patient experienced pain relief within 3 days (VAS: from 8 [pre-treatment] to 1 [post-treatment]) of the periosteal neurolysis.

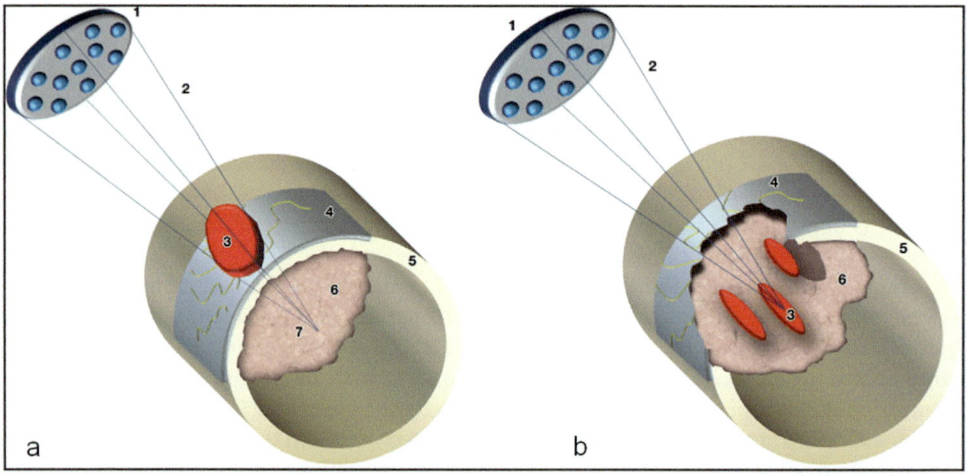

FIGURE 20.2 Wide-beam approach used for treating bone metastases. In a. Intact cortical bone (5): the ultrasound beam (2) is entirely absorbed by the cortical surface, even if the focus of the ultrasound beam is placed beyond the cortical line. The amount of energy at the intersection between the ultrasound beam and the bone is insufficient to cause ablation in any regular tissue; in bone, given its extraordinary acoustic absorption, the limited amount of energy is enough to create a wide area of increased temperature. In fact, temperature rises exponentially with energy increase; periosteal neurolysis is obtained with limited amount of focused ultrasound energy. In b: Transcortical growth of bone metastasis (4): when a discontinuity of the bone surface is seen, the solid component of the metastatic lesion (6) can be treated with focal spots, as in MR-guided focused ultrasound treatment of a regular solid lesion, for which the ablation area (3) corresponds to the acoustic focus (7).

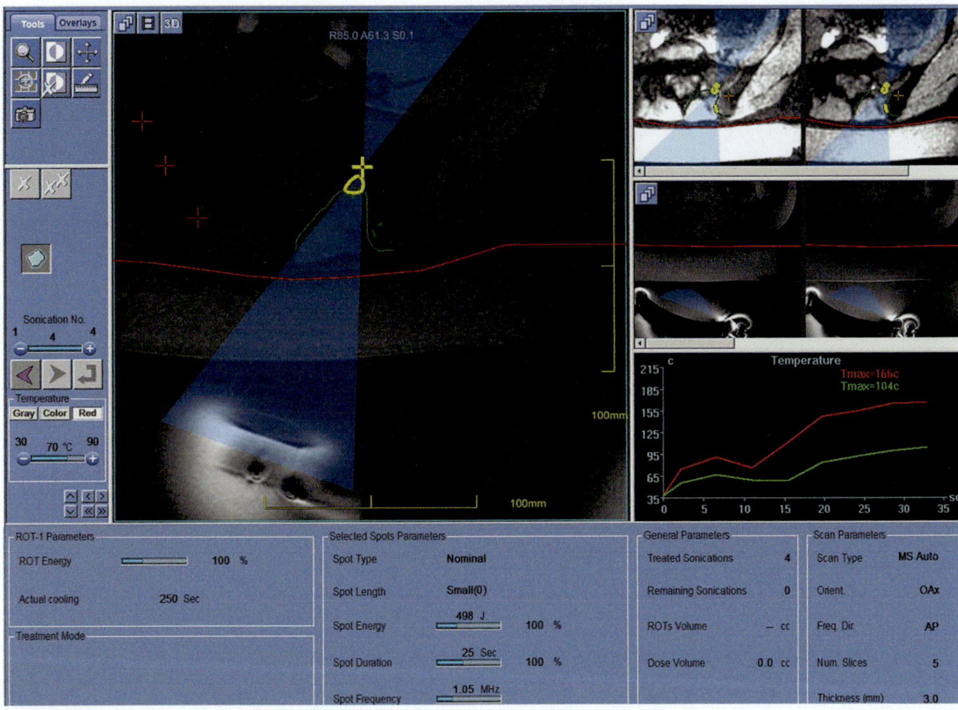

FIGURE 20.3 Pre-treatment MR images show the anatomical areas of interest that have been manually defined by the operator: the bone cortex surface (outlined with green), region of treatment (outlined with yellow) and skin line (outlined with red).

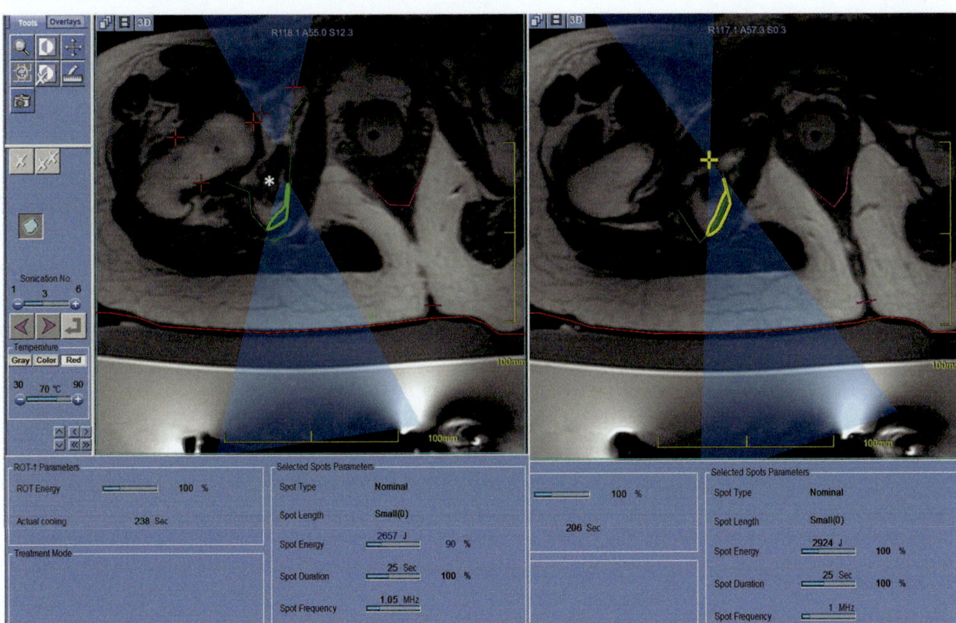

FIGURE 20.4 Pre-treatment stage in 58-year-old man with colon cancer. Axial planning image shows the presence of a lytic lesion (*) in a difficult to treat anatomical site, without damage to adjacent structures. The operator manually adjusts and defines the correct and safe angle of the beam to reach the target area. The small red crosses are the "fiducials" used to monitor any movement of the patient during energy delivery in real time, observed during thermometry acquisition. Highly fibrotic structures (such as the rectal canal and the anus) are spared with non-passing zone lines that prevent local energy deposition.

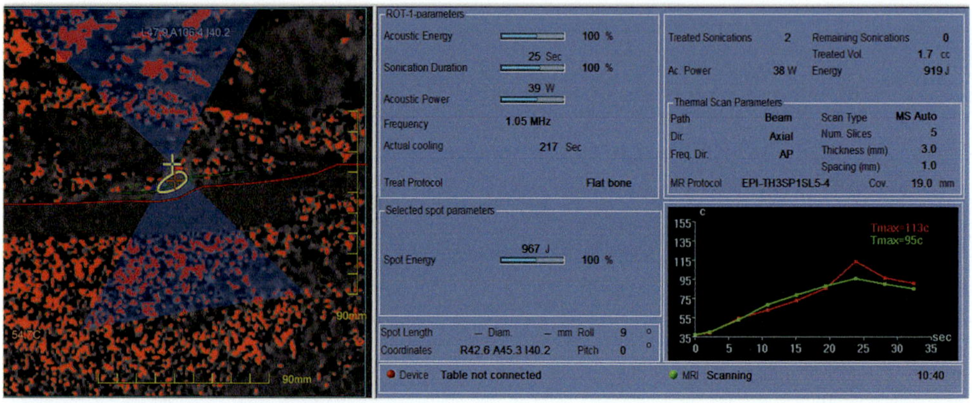

FIGURE 20.5 Verification stage. MR thermometry map image shows a low-energy sonication point (red cursor), that has been placed at the bone and soft-tissue interface (outlined with yellow). During the verification stage, a low-energy sonication test is performed to confirm the path and correct direction of the ultrasound beam into the target area (geometric verification). At the same time, the system automatically performs an energy test to confirm the equivalence between the planned energy dose and the effective dose deployed to the target lesion (dose verification).

an ultrasound transducer generates a burst of focused ultrasound energy, known as a *sonication*. The sonication raises the tissue temperature within a well-defined region, causing thermal coagulation. MR images acquired during sonication provide a quantitative, real-time temperature map (Figure 20.5) of the entire field-of-view around the target area, to confirm the location of the sonication and the size of the coagulated region. The sonication process is repeated at several adjacent points to cover the entire prescribed treatment volume. Patients are positioned according to tumour location, and general, epidural, or peripheral anaesthesia is chosen on the basis of a number of different parameters (lesion location, patient age, clinical condition). In all cases, pre-treatment planning is performed with T2-weighted MR sequences acquired in multiple planes with, and without, fat saturation pulses. Treatment is started after delivering low-energy sonications to verify the correct position of the focus; the ablation is therefore performed over the periosteal surface for osteoid osteoma (Figure 20.6) and bone metastases with an intact cortex, or through the eroded cortex in cases of lytic metastases. The effect of each sonication is measured on MRI using phase map imaging, with the proton resonance frequency (PRF) shift method reflecting the temperature-dependent change in resonance frequency. The PRF sequence allows thermal measurement within the target area because of the bone energy absorption and direct temperature increase of soft periskeletal structures. Moreover, PRF ensures proper targeting in the desired volume, thereby avoiding thermal damage to the surrounding anatomical structures.

Acoustic power is adjusted throughout the treatment, to achieve maximum tissue temperatures between 65°C and 85°C at the bone-tissue interface. Immediately after treatment, a series of MR scans are performed. The scanning includes T2-weighted and T1-weighted contrast-enhanced sequences to evaluate general anatomy and to assess treatment effect.[29] The number of sonications per single treatment can vary greatly, depending on lesion size and treatment protocol; usually, in the attempt to achieve tumour control, the sonication density is higher by a factor of three than that used for periosteal neurolysis.[3]

20.3 Treatment Outcomes

MR-guided high intensity focused US ablation is offered in our institution to patients with bone metastasis who have exhausted or refused other therapies and for primary pain palliation. When compared with other nonsurgical treatment options for both pain palliation and tumour control and, most of all, with radiotherapy, the relevant advantage of MRgFUS ablation is the fact that treatments can be

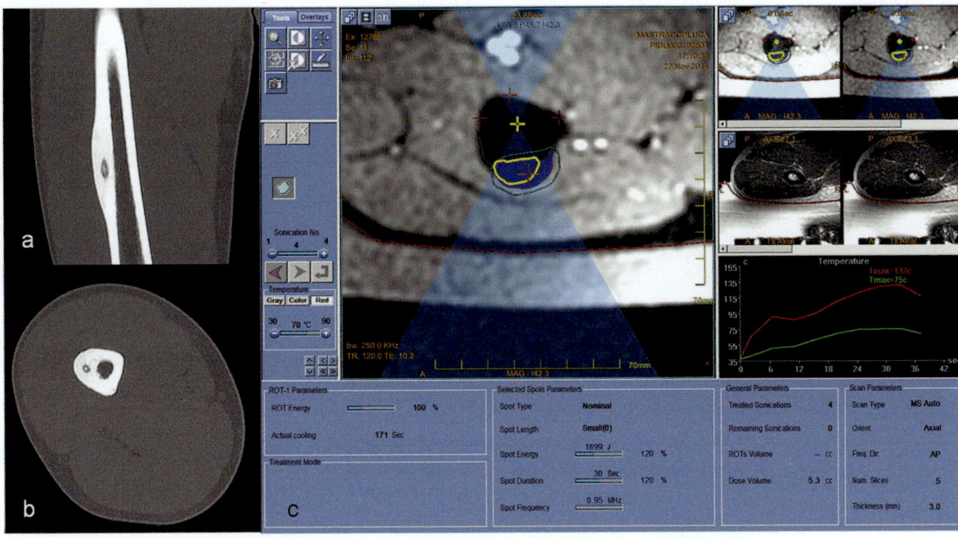

FIGURE 20.6 Treatment of subperiosteal osteoid osteoma. Coronal (a) and axial (b) CT images of a 18-years-old man with osteoid osteoma within the periosteum, in the femoral shaft. Pre-treatment MR planning (c): ablation is performed over the periosteal surface (yellow line). In order to obtain complete necrosis of the nidus, sonication duration can be increased to allow penetration into the exuberant sclerotic bone (almost invariably present in osteoid osteoma); MR thermometry eventually shows temperature rise into the nidus thus confirming technical success.

repeated indefinitely until the clinical aim is achieved, with no issues related to radiation absorption or other toxic effects.

Similar considerations to those that often present a clinical challenge for surgeons apply for the treatment of benign bone lesions. Nevertheless, most MRgFUS treatments are carried out in a single session, requiring further intervention in only an extremely limited population. Gianfelice et al. treated 11 patients with painful localised bone metastases. They evaluated symptom relief using a 0–10 pain score and reported progressive pain reduction in treated regions, with a decrease in pain medication use during a 3-month follow-up period.[30] Another multicentre study performed by Liberman et al. followed up 39 patients with painful bone metastases. They demonstrated significant reductions in pain scores during 3-month follow-up.[31]

In our department, we are evaluating the safety and efficacy of MRgFUS treatment for pain palliation in patients with both benign (osteoid osteoma, osteoblastoma, aneurismal bone cyst) and malignant (metastases, primary bone tumours) lesions.

No treatment related complications have been observed during or after any of the procedures. With regard to the treatment of painful bone metastases, we have so far performed 30 ablations of bone metastasis from different known primary tumours. Patients included in the study were all either receiving chemotherapy and could not undergo other pain palliation treatment, or they had exhausted or refused other therapy options. After the treatment, all patients were scheduled to undergo follow-up clinical examinations 1 and 3 days; 1 and 2 weeks; and 1, 2, and 3 months after the MRgFUS treatment. In addition, all patients underwent follow-up CT and MR imaging 1 and 3 months after the treatment. Follow-up MR imaging was performed using the same protocol as was used for the pre-procedural examination.

To evaluate treatment efficacy in terms of pain palliation, the Brief Pain Inventory – Quality of Life (BPIQOL) criteria were used to calculate the pain severity score. This scale consists of seven questions that ask respondents to indicate the extent to which pain interferes with general activity, mood, walking ability, normal work, relations with other people, sleep, and enjoyment of life using a 0–10 numerical rating scale, where 0 represents "Does not interfere" and 10 represents "Completely interferes". Responses to the 7 items are averaged to give the Pain Interference Scale score. To evaluate treatment

TABLE 20.1

MD Anderson (MDA) Criteria

Response Category	Criteria
Complete response	Complete sclerotic fill-in of lytic lesions on XR or CT Normalisation of bone density on XR or CT Normalisation of signal intensity on MRI Normalisation of tracer uptake on SS
Partial response	Development of a sclerotic rim or partial sclerotic fill-in of lytic lesions on XR or CT Osteoblastic flare: Interval visualisation of lesions with sclerotic rims or new sclerotic lesions in the setting of other signs of PR and absence of progressive bony disease Q50% decrease in measurable lesions on XR, CT, or MRI Q50% subjective decrease in the size of ill-defined lesions on XR, CT, or MRI Q50% subjective decrease in tracer uptake in SS
Progressive disease	Q25% increase in size of measurable lesions on XR, CT, or MRI Q25% subjective increase in the size of ill-defined lesions on XR, CT, or MRI Q25% subjective increase in tracer uptake in SS New bone metastases
Stable disease	No change G25% increase or G50%decrease in size of measurable lesions G25% subjective increase or G50% subjective decrease in size of ill-defined lesions No new bone metastases

XR, X-ray; CT, computed tomography; SS, skeletal scintigraphy; MRI, magnetic resonance imaging.

efficacy in terms of local tumour control, lesion changes were evaluated according to MD Anderson (MDA) criteria (Table 20.1). HIFU creates variable degrees of lesion necrosis, quantifiable in terms of non-perfused volume (NPV), defined as the volume of cancer tissue enhancing at baseline that shows no contrast uptake after treatment. The use of the NPV parameter can give added value in the evaluation of the treated region, and should be analysed in association with the MDA criteria. The use of NPV as an immediate predictor of tumour necrosis, and thus of the efficacy of the treatment, might play an important role in future patient management, avoiding continuation of a potentially ineffective treatment, and thus consequences such as toxic effects and morbidity, accelerated tumour growth, delay in delivery of other, potentially effective, treatment and unnecessary expense. Clinical data include an evaluation of a visual analogue pain score (VAS), changes in the drug schedule, and improvements in quality of life. The VAS is an 11-point pain scale that ranges between 0 and 10, where 0 is considered to be no pain at all and 10 is the worst pain.[32] The pain severity score in our patients has changed significantly from a baseline average of 7.1 ± 2.08 (4–10) to 1 ± 1.1 (0–3) at 3-month follow-up. In particular, at the end of the protocol 72.2% of patients have reported a zero score for pain severity without medication intake, consistent with a complete response to treatment. CT examinations performed at 3-month follow-up have revealed an increase of bone density with restoration of the cortical border in 27.7% of patients (Figure 20.7). According to MDA criteria, a complete response to treatment has been observed in 11.1% of patients, a partial response in 22.2% of patients, stable disease in 55.6% of patients, and progressive disease in 11.1% of patients.

20.4 Expert Commentary

MRgFUS is an alternative noninvasive method for reducing the pain in skeletal metastases.[33] The concentration of acoustic energy on the intact surface of cortical bone produces a rapid temperature increase that mediates critical thermal damage to the adjacent periosteum, the most innervated component of mature bone tissue. Such thermal ablation has been shown to be an extremely effective approach for pain management. This technique also has a potential role in achieving local tumour control, allowing de novo mineralisation of trabecular bone.[34] The effects of MRgFUS ablation on mechanical properties

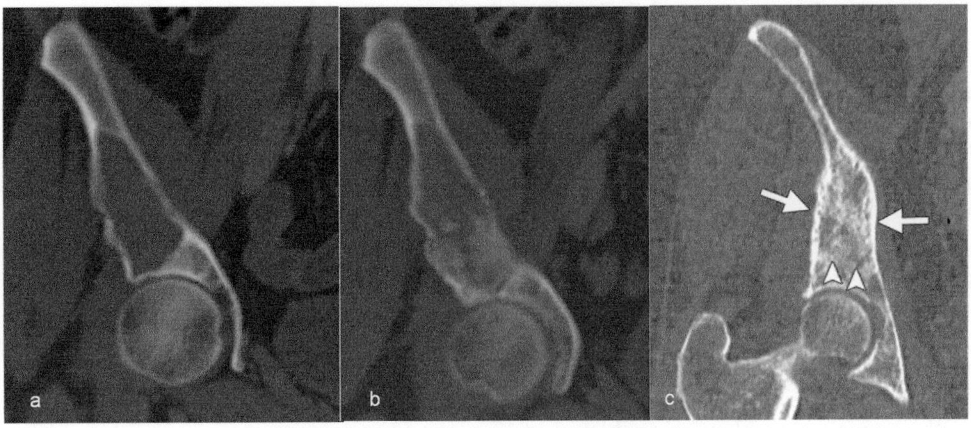

FIGURE 20.7 Coronal CT image of 42-year-old woman with breast cancer and diffuse metastatic skeletal involvement (stage IV). In **a,** lytic lesion located in the right iliac bone with evidence of cortical erosion without articular invasion. Coronal CT image obtained 2 months (**b**) and 4 months (**c**) after treatment demonstrates areas of de novo mineralisation (arrowheads) and increase of bone density within the treated area and restoration of cortical bone (arrows). This process achieves improvement in quality of life due to change of visual analogue pain score (VAS) from 9 to 0.

and modelling of bone or reduction in lesion size have been studied. Energy delivered during treatment and accumulated inside the pathological soft tissue of the metastases can create variable amounts of tissue necrosis, thus attempting local tumour control. The major advantages of MRgFUS include imaging guidance with three-dimensional visualisation MR for high accuracy treatment planning, real-time monitoring of thermal damage in the target zone using MR thermometry, continuous temperature mapping of treated tissue, and immediate post-treatment assessment of therapy. An additional advantage of MRgFUS over other ablative techniques is the totally non-invasive nature of the focused ultrasound intervention. During treatment, real-time multi-slice MR thermometry is used to evaluate the temperature rise in tissue, and, based on this feedback, portions of the periosteum and/or tumour that were not fully ablated may be retreated. Quantitative MR thermometry is a mapping technique that enables calculation of thermal dose and superimposes a representation of the regions in which the thermal dose has achieved cytotoxic levels on an anatomic MR image.[35–38] Usually, phase-difference fast spoiled gradient-echo sequences are acquired to provide temperature-dependent images and real-time mapping of the thermal dose in a preferred imaging plane during treatment. In the clinical application of bone metastasis pain treatment, MR thermometry does not measure temperature variations in the bone itself; in fact, the absence of mobile protons in cortical bone renders MR thermometry impossible in bone. However, the soft tissues immediately adjacent to the cortex respond linearly to bone temperature increase, thus allowing the bone temperature to be inferred. Exposure of tissue for 240 minutes at 43°C is considered to be the critical thermal dose, representing the threshold for 100% killing of the tissue cells. The real-time MR feedback also enables the physician to overcome misregistration, due to respiratory or bulk patient movement.[39]

MRgFUS can also be a feasible option for obtaining pain palliation in patients with benign bone tumours (such as osteoid osteoma) or non-tumoural conditions. A clinical trial performed in St. Mary's Hospital (London, UK) evaluated the safety and efficacy of MRgFUS for the treatment of low back pain due to facet joint arthropathy or degenerative arthritis, with 15 patients successfully treated with 62% pain decrease and disability decrease of 55%.[40]

In our experience, we have treated patients with limited joint function and reduced quality of life due to painful osteoid lesions confirmed at workup on MR and CT. In all subjects, symptoms were assessed before, and 1–3 months after, treatment on a 0–10 pain scale; in 83% of patients, complete clinical success after the MRgFUS procedure was reported, while a single patient with atypical medullary osteoid osteoma experienced symptom recurrence and underwent surgery with intralesional curettage 9 months after the MRgFUS procedure.

20.5 Summary

MR imaging–guided focused ultrasound ablation is an extremely promising alternative therapy for pain palliation and tumour control in patients suffering from bone metastases. In particular, MRgFUS ablation is indicated in patients who are considered to be radiation failures (those patients who received radiation without adequate symptom relief, those who can no longer undergo external beam radiation therapy for safety reasons, or those who refuse other therapy options). The absence of adverse events thus favours the use of the MRgFUS treatment option as a viable non-invasive alternative to standard primary palliative treatments, including EBRT, for painful bone metastases. In this regard, EBRT-related acute and long-term adverse effects (eg, skin and gastrointestinal reactions, loss of nerve function, pathological fractures, and bone marrow damage) can occur in up to 3% of cases as opposed to our study in which none of these adverse effects were observed. Furthermore, our personal experience shows that MRgFUS is also a safe and effective first line modality for pain palliation in skeletal metastases with complete clinical success achieved in 13 of the 18 patients treated (72.2%). MRgFUS treatment leads to complete ablation of the medullary boney component of skeletal metastases, necessary to reduce the risk for local recurrence, because occurrence of pain is preceded by metastatic involvement of the cortical bone.[3] The major advantages of the technique include its non-invasive nature, the ability to perform three-dimensional MR imaging visualisation for precise treatment planning, continuous temperature mapping of treated tissue with MR thermometry, which enables real-time monitoring of thermal damage in the target zone, and immediate post-treatment assessment of therapy. The concentration of acoustic energy on the intact surface of cortical bone produces a rapid temperature increase that mediates critical thermal damage to the adjacent periosteum, the most innervated component of mature bone tissue. Such thermal ablation has been shown to be an extremely effective approach for pain management. Energy delivered during MR–guided focused ultrasound ablation and accumulated inside the abnormal soft tissue of metastases can create a variable amount of tissue necrosis. This technique also has a potential role in achieving local tumour control, allowing remineralisation of medullary bone, or reduction in lesion size (complete or partial response in accordance with the MDA criteria for 33.3% of cases). Although MR thermal maps cannot be created directly inside the bone itself (as a result of the low MR signal from the cortical zone), heating due to conductive processes from the bone surface within adjacent soft tissue is measurable, and is considered adequate for treatment monitoring. At present, MRgFUS provides durable pain relief and improved function in patients who have failed to respond to radiation treatment for their pain, or those who are not candidates for, or have declined, radiation. Given the impact of these clinically significant results, MRgFUS should be considered a viable treatment option for painful bone metastases.

REFERENCES

1. Sze WM, Shelley MD, Held I, et al. Palliation of metastatic bone pain: Single fraction versus multifraction radiotherapy – a systematic review of randomized trials. Clin Oncol (R Coll Radiol) 2003;15:345Y352.
2. Ehara S, Khurana JS, Systematic approach to tumours and focal lesions of bone. Springer; 2010.
3. Napoli A, Anzidei M, Cavallo Marincola B, et al. Primary pain palliation and local tumour control in bone metastases treated with magnetic resonance-guided focused ultrasound. Invest Radiol 2013 Jun;48:6.
4. Kurup AN, Callstrom MR. Ablation of skeletal metastases: Current status. J Vasc Interv Radiol 2010;21(8 suppl):S242–50.
5. Mundy GR. Metastasis to bone: Causes, consequences and therapeutic opportunities. Nat Rev Cancer 2002;2(8):584–93.
6. Napoli A, Anzidei M, Cavallo Marincola B, et al. MR imaging–guided focused ultrasound for treatment of bone metastasis. Radiographics 2013;33:1555–68.
7. Rades D, Schild SE, Abrahm JL. Treatment of painful bone metastases. Nat Rev Clin Oncol 2010;7:220–9.
8. Konski A. Radiotherapy is a cost-effective palliative treatment for patients with bone metastasis from prostate cancer. Int J Radiat Oncol Biol Phys 2004;60:1373–8.

9. Frassica DA. General principles of external beam radiation therapy for skeletal metastases. Clin Orthop Relat Res 2003;415S:158–64.
10. Ahrar K. The role and limitations of radiofrequency ablation in treatment of bone and soft tissue tumours. Curr Oncol Rep 2004 Jul;6(4):315–20.
11. Callstrom MR, Charboneau JW, Goetz MP, et al. Image-guided ablation of painful metastatic bone tumours: A new and effective approach to a difficult problem. Skeletal Radiol 2006 Jan;35(1):1–15.
12. Saarto T, Janes R, Tenhunen M, et al. Palliative radiotherapy in the treatment of skeletal metastases. Eur J Pain 2002;6(5):323–30
13. Selvaggi G, Scagliotti GV. Management of bone metastases in cancer: A review. Crit Rev Oncol Hematol 2005 Dec;56(3):365–78.
14. Wu F, Wang ZB, Chen WZ, et al. Advanced hepatocellular carcinoma: Treatment with high-intensity focused ultrasound ablation combined with transcatheter arterial embolization. Radiology 2005 May;235(2):659–67
15. Gianfelice D, Khiat A, Amara M, et al. MR imaging-guided focused US ablation of breast cancer: Histopathologic assessment of effectiveness-initial experience. Radiology 2003 Jun;227(3):849–55.
16. Jenne JW. Non-invasive transcranial brain ablation with high-intensity focused ultrasound. Front Neurol Neurosci 2015;36:94–105.
17. Chen W, Zhu H, Zhang L. Primary bone malignancy: Effective treatment with high-intensity focused ultrasound ablation. Radiology 2010 Jun;255(3):967–78.
18. Kobus T, McDannold N. Update on clinical magnetic resonance–guided focused ultrasound applications. Magn Reson Imaging Clin N Am 2015 Nov;23(4):657–67
19. Tempany CM, McDannold NJ, Hynynen K, et al. Focused ultrasound surgery in oncology: Overview and principles. Radiology 2011 Apr;259(1):39–56.
20. Kang TW, Rhim H. Recent advances in tumour ablation for hepatocellular carcinoma. Liver Cancer 2015 Sep;4(3):176–87
21. Kovatcheva R, Guglielmina JN, Abehsera M, et al. Ultrasound-guided high intensity focused ultrasound treatment of breast fibroadenoma-a multicenter experience. J Ther Ultrasound 2015 Jan 22;3(1):1
22. Fornage BD, Hwang RF. Current status of imaging-guided percutaneous ablation of breast cancer. AJR 2014 Aug;203(2):442–8
23. Shehata IA. High intensity focused ultrasound: Imaging is the key! Diagn Interv Imaging 2014 Jun;95(6):569–72
24. Martin E, Jeanmonod D, Morel A, et al. High-intensity focused ultrasound for noninvasive functional neurosurgery. Ann Neurol 2009 Dec;66(6):858–61
25. Hurwitz MD, Ghanouni P, Kanaev SV, et al. Magnetic resonance–guided focused ultrasound for patients with painful bone metastases: Phase III trial results. JNCI 2014 Apr 23;106(5)
26. Huisman M, Lam MK, Bartels LW, et al. Feasibility of volumetric MRI-guided high intensity focused ultrasound (MR-HIFU) for painful bone metastases. J Ther Ultrasound 2014 Oct 10;2:16
27. Jolesz FA. MRI-guided focused ultrasound surgery. Annu Rev Med 2009;60:417–30
28. Catane R, Beck A, Inbar Y, et al. MR-guided focused ultrasound surgery (MRgFUS) for the palliation of pain in patients with bone metastases – preliminary clinical experience. Ann Oncol 2007;18:163–7
29. Napoli A, Anzidei M, Ciolina F, et al. MR-guided high-intensity focused ultrasound: Current status of an emerging technology. Cardiovasc Intervent Radiol 2013 Oct;36(5):1190–203
30. Gianfelice D, Gupta C, Kucharczyk W, et al. Palliative treatment of painful bone metastases with MR imaging-guided focused ultrasound. Radiology 2008;249:355–63.
31. Liberman B, Gianfelice D, Inbar Y, et al. Pain palliation in patients with bone metastases using MR-guided focused ultrasound surgery: A multicenter study. Ann Surg Oncol 2009;16:140–6
32. Costelloe CM, Chuang HH, Madewell JE, et al. Cancer response criteria and bone metastases: RECIST 1.1, MDA and PERCIST. J Cancer 2010;1:80–92
33. Joo B, Park MS, Lee SH, et al. Pain palliation in patients with bone metastases using magnetic resonance-guided focused ultrasound with conformal bone system: A preliminary report. Yonsei Med J 2015;56(2):503–9
34. Yeo SY, Arias Moreno AJ, van Rietbergen B, et al. Effects of magnetic resonance-guided high intensity focused ultrasound ablation on bone mechanical properties and modeling. J Ther Ultrasound 2015 Aug11;3:13

35. Sapareto SA, Dewey WC. Thermal dose determination in cancer therapy. Int J Radiat Oncol Biol Phys 1984;10(6):787–800.
36. Ishihara Y, Calderon A, Watanabe H, et al. A precise and fast temperature mapping using water proton chemical shift. Magn Reson Med 1995;34(6):814–23.
37. Mougenot C, Salomir R, Palussière J, et al. Automatic spatial and temporal temperature control for MR-guided focused ultrasound using fast 3D MR thermometry and multispiral trajectory of the focal point. Magn Reson Med 2004;52(5):1005–15.
38. Ramsay E, Mougenot C, Kazem M, et al. Temperature-dependent MR signals in cortical bone: Potential for monitoring temperature changes during high-intensity focused ultrasound treatment in bone. Magn Reson Med 2015;74:1095–102
39. Celicanin Z, Auboiroux V, Bieri O, et al. Real-Time Method for motion-compensated MR thermometry and MRgHIFU treatment in abdominal organs. Magn Reson Med 2014;72:1087–95
40. Weeks EM, Platt MW, Gedroyc W. MRI-guided focused ultrasound (MRgFUS) to treat facet joint osteoarthritis low back pain-case series of an innovative new technique. Eur Radiol 2012;22:2822–35

21

Clinical Application of MR-Guided Focused Ultrasound Therapy in the Brain

David Aum, Maya Harary, Nathan J. McDannold, and Travis S. Tierney

21.1 Introduction

Ultrasound has its modern origins in the discovery of the piezoelectric effect by Jacques and Pierre Curie, with their experiments on compressing crystals in 1880. Their development of piezoelectric transducers as both generators and sensors of ultrasonic waves were the foundation for ultrasound being developed as a therapy. The first therapeutic application for ultrasound presciently suggested its use for heating tissue in 1932.[1] In 1942, John Lynn et al. first demonstrated the use of focused ultrasound for producing lesions in animal brain tissue.[2] High-intensity focused ultrasound (HIFU) first emerged as a non-invasive ablative technique distinct from its use in diagnostic imaging with the early work of William Fry and colleagues at the University of Illinois on pioneering focused ultrasound systems capable of producing lesions in the brain. Their partial ablation of basal ganglia in 1955 showed that discrete ultrasonic lesions produced thermo-coagulative necrosis without evidence of haemorrhage in both grey and deep white matter structures.[3] In 1959, Fry's focused ultrasound instrumentation demonstrated well-circumscribed lesions in the brains of patients with Parkinson's disease.[4] Early clinical attempts to use HIFU for treating tumours were restricted by the lack of temperature feedback and limitations of imaging during the procedure. Further clinical progress using ultrasonic thermo-coagulation in the brain only came later with the advent of tomographic imaging techniques such as magnetic resonance imaging (MRI) to provide the real-time visualisation and thermal measurement required for the precise application of HIFU. The first North American patent for the use of focused ultrasound as a brain lesioning system was awarded to Francis Fry, the brother of William Fry, in 1990.[5] Although the first clinically approved applications of HIFU have been for conditions outside the central nervous system (CNS) – glaucoma in 1986, benign prostatic hyperplasia in 1994 and uterine fibroids in 2002 in Europe, followed by Food and Drug Administration (FDA) approvals in the United States in 2004 for uterine fibroids and the palliative treatment of bone metastases in 2007 – focused ultrasound continues to be intensively studied for its potential applications as a neurosurgical tool. Indeed, HIFU finally received FDA pre-market approval in 2015 for the treatment of essential tremor after completion of a large randomised multicentre trial.

21.2 Basic Mechanisms of Tissue Destruction Using Focused Ultrasound

The primary thermal effect of HIFU in tissue is coagulation necrosis due to heating. The "thermal dose" delivered to tissue depends on the magnitude and duration of temperature elevation. Focused ultrasound is capable of inducing local hyperthermia, which is characterised by a gradual increase in temperature over minutes, or of inducing thermal ablation during which temperature increases rapidly in seconds.[6] A temperature of 55°C–60°C held for more than 1 second is sufficient to cause protein denaturation and instant necrosis.[7] Temperatures at the focal point can reach 80°C–100°C.[8] The exposure time required to achieve thermal necrosis decreases with increasing temperature. Focused ultrasound

DOI: 10.1201/9780429162671-21

can also initiate apoptosis as a secondary mechanism for cell death. This has been found to occur at the lower temperatures lying outside of the focal coagulative zone and is thus an important consideration for the application of HIFU in sensitive areas such as the brain.[9] Other potential off-target secondary effects of HIFU-induced hyperthermia include thrombosis and arterial occlusion that may produce ischemic injury at unintended sites remote to the targeted tissue.[10]

The primary non-thermal effect of focused ultrasound is cavitation. At high pressure amplitudes, ultrasonic waves can nucleate small gas bodies to form microbubbles. These bubbles can expand in size by the process of rectified diffusion, and ultimately collapse violently, a phenomenon known as inertial cavitation. The bursting of these gas bubbles can cause forces strong enough to damage cell membranes. Stable microbubble oscillations can also result in bioeffects. For example, stable cavitation is thought to be the mechanism behind the disruption of the blood-brain barrier for enhancement of systemic drug delivery to the brain. The oscillation of bubbles can also cause rapid movement of fluids that can exert disruptive shear forces on cell membranes. The presence of microbubbles has been found to increase heating efficiency and thus reduce the power required to produce an ablative lesion.[11] The cavitation activity of these microbubbles can be therapeutically applied to disrupting the blood-brain barrier for the purposes of drug delivery.

Focused ultrasound for therapy is distinguished from diagnostic ultrasound by its much higher intensity and smaller area of effect. Diagnostic ultrasound transducers deliver time-average intensities of 0.1–100 mW/cm^2 compared to the much greater 100–10,000 W/cm^2 delivered by HIFU to the focal region.[12, 13] HIFU concentrates ultrasonic waves into a small volume to induce thermal and cavitation effects in tissue. Critically, tissue outside the focal region receives much lower intensity. Thus, the tissue between the ultrasound transducer array and the focus usually receives no biologically significant sonication. Bone represents a challenge in neurosurgical applications of HIFU due to its 30–60 times greater absorption of ultrasound energy and consequent rapid heating. Methods of compensating for overheating of the skull include the use of a lower frequency combined with active cooling of the scalp.[14] The high absorption characteristics of bone also significantly affect the propagation of ultrasonic waves, and result in less precise targeting of the focal volume because of reverberation and refraction.[12] An array of independently driven piezoelectric ultrasound transducers with separate phase offsets can correct for the different propagation delays induced to yield a more precise focal region.[15] In the brain, focused ultrasound is typically delivered in short pulses to minimise heat damage to tissues in the path of the beam, and to avoid cooldown effects in the target.[16]

21.3 Focused Ultrasound for Movement Disorders

Movement disorders such as essential tremor and Parkinson's disease have been treated historically either with neurostimulation, or by the creation of lesions using stereotactic surgical ablation in specific anti-tremor targets in the pallidum or thalamus.[17, 18] While deep brain stimulation has the advantage over ablation of reversibility, both techniques are invasive to some degree, and require the intracranial introduction of instruments. By comparison, transcranial HIFU offers a uniquely non-invasive surgical route to those same neural targets. MRI guidance provides real-time monitoring of temperature as well as precise localisation of the target tissue.

A number of recent studies have demonstrated the safety and efficacy of focused ultrasound in treating movement disorders. Like conventional stereotactic procedures, focused ultrasound therapy for movement disorders has been conducted under local anaesthesia and with the application of a stereotactic frame. A seminal pilot study conducted at the University of Virginia in 2011 targeted the ventral intermediate nucleus (Vim) of the thalamus with focused ultrasound in 15 patients with essential tremor.[19] Thermal ablation of this target with focused ultrasound produced long-term tremor control and significant improvements in quality-of-life scores in all patients. A similar study at the University of Toronto in 2013 yielded an 81% reduction in tremor score after 3 months, and a 51% reduction in perceived functional disability.[20] Two of the four patients in this study experienced paraesthesia, probably due to the lesion spreading slightly posteriorly into the sensory thalamus. One patient's paraesthesia disappeared immediately after each sonication, while the other's persisted for 3 months after the operation. In a third study, reported in 2015 from South Korea, 8 of 11 patients with essential tremor saw effective tremor control lasting more than 6 months, with minimal adverse effects.[21] Three patients in this study could not be effectively sonicated at the thalamic target due to high skull densities and poor acoustic transmission. In a retrospective study of 25 patients treated in clinical trials, the maximum temperature induced by HIFU was found to be negatively correlated with the area of the outer skull bone within the sonication field, while the "skull density ratio", a metric comparing the density of trabecular and cortical bone, was positively correlated.[22]

These three open label trials have motivated a large multicentre double-blinded trial of 72 patents with essential tremor ("A Pivotal Study to Evaluate the Effectiveness and Safety of ExAblate Transcranial MRgFUS Thalamotomy Treatment of Medication Refractory Essential Tremor Subjects, NCT01827904") designed to provide class I level evidence that MR-guided focused ultrasound (MRgFUS) thalamotomy is a safe and effective treatment for this condition. Based on a preliminary unpublished analysis of this data, the FDA issued Premarket Approval to the device maker for this indication, the first such approval for any intracranial application of this technology. Here, we briefly describe the procedure and clinical results of our two cases to provide an illustrative example of the concept of non-invasive transcranial ultrasound neurosurgery.

21.4 Methods for Performing a Thalamotomy with Focused Ultrasound and Two Case Reports

The procedure begins with clipping and shaving of the patient's entire head. Shaving reduces the possibility of hair-trapped air bubbles at the scalp surface that could impact on the ultrasound transmission. A modified Cosman-Roberts-Wells (CRW) MRI-compatible frame is fixed to the patient's head (Radionics Inc., Burlington, MA) after infiltrating the pin sites with 1% lidocaine. No pre-operative steroids, sedation, anti-epileptic medication or antibiotics are administered. The frame is then positioned on the table in a 3T MRI system (GE medical system, Milwaukee, Wisconsin, USA). The stereotactic frame is connected to a 30-cm-diameter hemispherical 1024-element phased-array transducer operating at 650 kHz. The ExAblate 4000 device uses a three-axis mechanical positioner attached to a flexible membrane that seals the space between the patient's head and the transducer. This space is then filled with degassed and chilled water (15–20°C) circulated between the head and the transducer. The water serves as an efficient acoustic coupler between the transducer array and scalp and mitigates skull heating.

In both patients, the sonication target was the left Vim nucleus of the thalamus in order to treat dominant right hand tremor. Traditional stereotactic coordinates for the Vim measured relative to a line at midsagittal plane of the brain connecting the anterior and posterior commissures (the AC-PC line): 14–15 mm left from midline, 6–7 mm anterior to the posterior commissure and at the intercommissural plane were used. In both cases, this point was approximately 11.5 mm from the wall of the third ventricle on the left side. For the first, but not the second case, we moved the sonication centre and performed a second lesion as described later. For both cases, lesion making began with several low-power (100 W delivered over 10 s) sonications to induce peak temperature rises of 40–42°C as seen on MR thermometry. These sonications revealed an initial position of thermal deposition within the motor thalamus and reduced tremor amplitude. Once the team was satisfied that the thermal energy had been deposited in an optimal location, a number of 10–20 second high-power sonications were applied with power raised in a stepwise fashion from 10,000–20,000 J while monitoring the patient clinically for tremor reduction. Each high-power sonication event achieved desired peak target temperatures between 55° and 60°C and was monitored acoustically for any cavitation events. Periodically, between high-energy sonications, T_2-weighted MR sequences were acquired to confirm the actual location of the evolving thalamotomy. Throughout the entire series of sonications, the patient was continuously examined to exclude the development of a focal neurological deficit and to assess tremor attenuation. An MRI scan was performed immediately following the procedure to confirm final lesion size and placement in the postero-ventral thalamus. After removing the head-frame, the patient was taken to the postoperative anaesthesia care unit for further recovery. The entire procedure required 4–5 hours to complete. Both patients were subject to sham surgery randomisation, but active treatment was drawn for both cases.

21.5 Illustrative Cases

21.5.1 Case 1

The first patient was a 58-year-old right-handed male with a personal and family history of essential tremor (ET) that limited his activities of daily living. He had been trialled on multiple medications, including primidone and propranolol, with unsatisfactory tremor control. The Movement Disorders Committee at the Brigham and Women's Hospital discussed many surgical options, including gamma knife thalamotomy, right frontal lesion (RFL) thalamotomy, and deep brain stimulation. The patient was determined to be a good candidate for MRgFUS Vim nucleus ablation. The risks and benefits of surgical intervention for the tremor were discussed with the patient and his wife. The patient was accepted for inclusion in the focused ultrasound trial and went on to receive a left Vim thalamotomy. Between sonications, T_2 sequences were acquired to confirm that the lesion was forming. In this patient, we decided to make two discrete overlapping sonication foci, the first at the previously mentioned target, and the second 2 mm posterior and 1 mm below the first, in an attempt to cover the entire theoretical volume of the Vim. On final post-operative imaging, a well-delineated lesion could be seen in the postero-ventral thalamus, and the patient had nearly complete tremor suppression (90%) by the end of the case, with a small degree of immediate right peri-oral numbness. However, over the first post-operative night, the area of paraesthesia progressed to include the right arm and leg. This was accompanied by the delayed development of a significant proprioceptive deficit and gait imbalance that lasted for several weeks. We placed him on a week of high-dose steroids and monitored his progress in the outpatient setting. Review of his imaging shows that the T_1 signal extended below the thalamus into the left cerebral peduncle (Figure 21.1B) with perilesional oedema out laterally to the internal capsule (Figure 21.1A, C). Eventually, he recovered full gait control but had residual finger paraesthesia at 3 months. His right hand tremor capture was complete at this last follow-up point, and he was highly satisfied with the outcome of the procedure.

21.5.2 Case 2

The second patient was a 73-year-old right-handed female, with a long history of action tremor, beginning on the right side and progressing to the left. She also had significant voice tremor and slight head

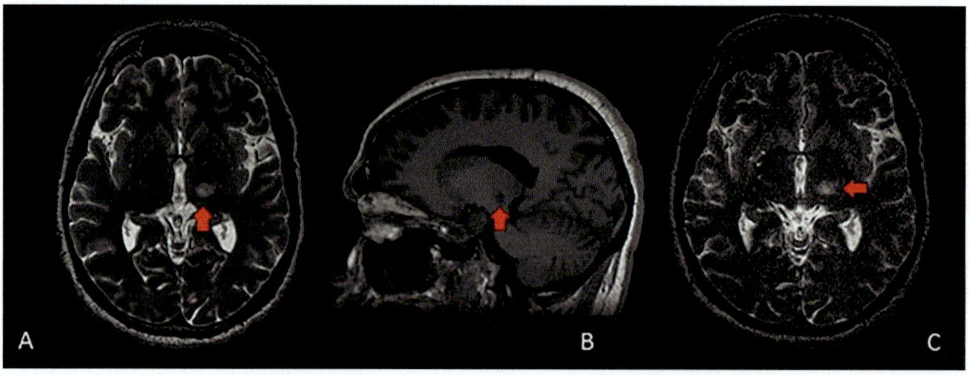

FIGURE 21.1 Post-treatment magnetic resonance images. (A, C) Axial T_2-weighted image, (B) T1-weighted image of patient 1, obtained immediately following treatment. Two overlapping sonication lesions of 3–5mm diameter were placed into the left Vim nucleus of the thalamus. The sagittal image shows that T1 hypointensity extends below the intercommissural plane into the left lateral cerebral peduncle.

tremor. She was diagnosed with ET. The patient received a number of medications, including propranolol and primidone, that did not give optimal tremor control. We discussed the risks and benefits of various surgical modalities to help control her tremor, including gamma knife thalamotomy, RFL thalamotomy and deep brain stimulation (DBS). The patient met the selection criteria for MRgFUS and was offered admission to the trial.

She received a left Vim thalamotomy centred on the coordinates mentioned. During this second case, we did not move the system to a separate, more inferoposterior sonication site, but focused all acoustic energy on the initial site. Serial testing over the course of several sonication events with spiral drawings showed that there was a decrease in tremor amplitude, but not quite complete tremor arrest (Figure 21.2). There were no significant adverse events, although at higher intensity sonication levels (20,000 J), she experienced a sense of dizziness and at one point, became nauseous but did not vomit. During the procedure she developed transient lip paraesthesia that resolved after 2 weeks. A postoperative MRI scan revealed an adequate-sized lesion in the postero-ventral thalamus (Figure 21.3). She was then taken to the postoperative anaesthesia care unit for further recovery. By the following postoperative day, she developed near-complete tremor arrest on the right, but also some gait instability. We did not prescribe a course of steroids, but chose to observe her recovery in the outpatient clinic. The gait disturbance resolved within several weeks, and her tremor control remained excellent at the 3-month follow up interval.

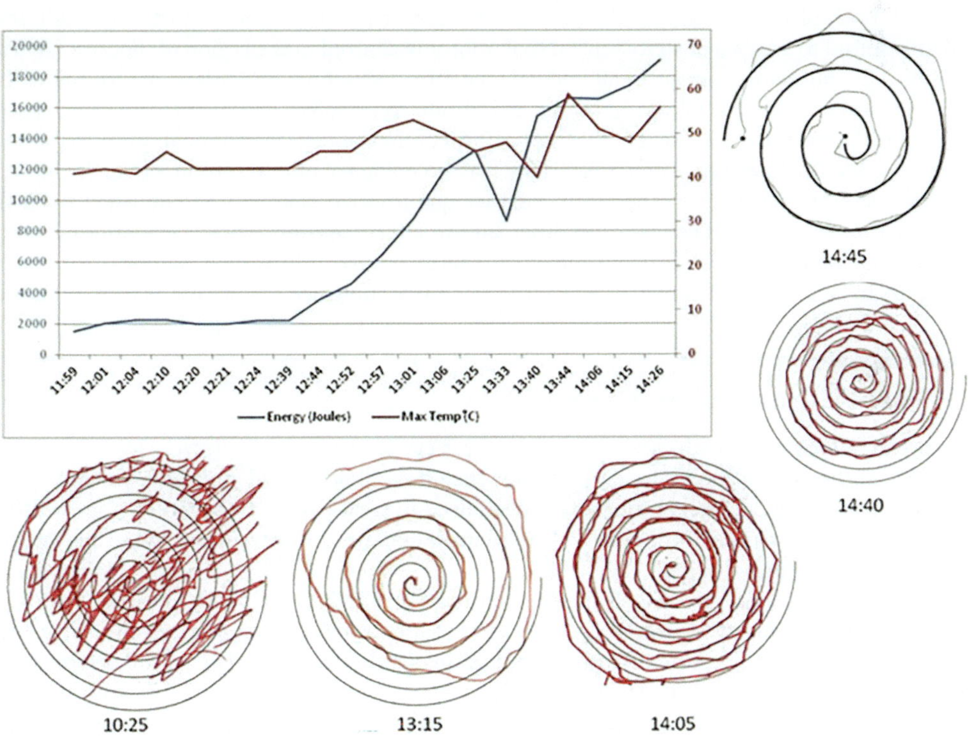

FIGURE 21.2 Intraoperative testing for Patient 2. Between sonication treatments, the subject drew Archimedes spirals to show progress of tremor reduction. The graph shows two distinct phases of treatment, with the first phase involving low energy sonications to define the target area followed by a steady increase in energy delivered to form the lesion. Maximum temperature achieved during each sonication increased overall and correlated to total energy delivered during each sonication; at no point did the temperature exceed cavitation threshold. Clinicians decreased energy at approximately 13:30 because the patient developed symptoms of nausea and dizziness. Sonication treatments continued after administration of anti-nausea medication. Archimedes spirals showed improvement over time and indicate correlation between relative degree of tremor capture and increase in energy delivered to produce the lesion.

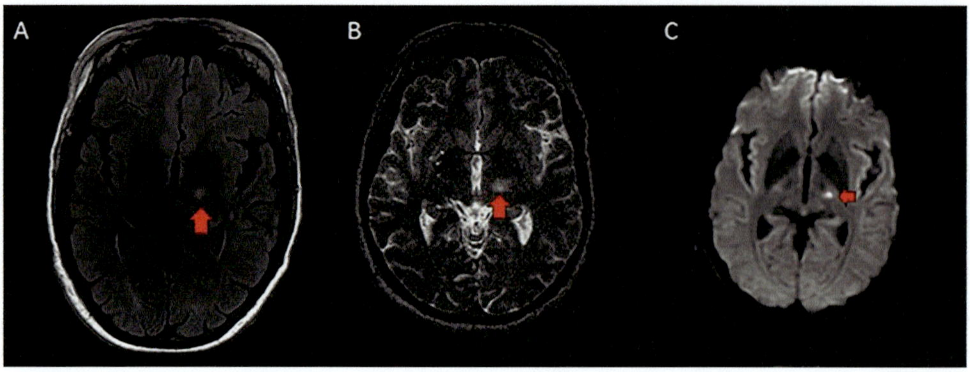

FIGURE 21.3 Patient 2 post-treatment axial magnetic resonance images. (A) Axial-T_1weighted image showing the lesion in the left thalamus, (B) Axial T_2-weighted image, and (C) diffusion weight image (DWI). A single 3- to 5-mm-diameter lesion is centred on the left Vim nucleus of the thalamus. The lesion is T_1 hypointense and T_2 hyperintense. There is no evidence of T_1 hyperintensity or abnormal signal within the lesion on the susceptibility-weighted images to suggest microhaemorrhage. The centre of the lesion is bright on DWI, suggesting immediate coagulation of tissue at the sonication epicentre, and is surrounded by a significantly larger area of perilesional oedema on the T_2 sequences.

In general, both of our patients achieved excellent tremor control when treated with high energy focused ultrasound to create a postero-ventral thalamotomy centred in the region of the Vim nucleus of the thalamus. Despite some transient gait and balance difficulties, both patients were satisfied with the procedure at the three-month follow up point. In addition to transient gait disturbance, both patients reported contralateral post-treatment paraesthesia. Both of these effects were probably due to the spread of oedema outside the intended lesion area. There was no evidence of microhaemorrhage either at the thalamotomy site or elsewhere in the brain. Further quantitative data will be published from these patients, together with the full cohort from other sites in a forthcoming article. Generally, our experience in treating tremor in these patients with high energy focused ultrasound suggests that the technique appears to be safe and effective, in line with previously published studies in the recent literature.

21.6 Focused Ultrasound for Chronic Pain

Chronic neuropathic pain, which can be caused by a variety of insults to the nervous system, affects an estimated 8% of the population.[23] Standard therapy includes opioids, antidepressants and antiepileptic medications. Neurosurgical interventions have been used to treat patients who suffer from treatment-refractory neuropathic pain.[24] Both ablative and neuromodulatory interventions target peripheral or central components of the condition.[25,26]

Jeanmonod and colleagues described the first application of MRgFUS for the central treatment of chronic, treatment-refractory neuropathic pain in 11 patients.[27,28] In this phase I clinical trial, the patients, aged 45–75 years old, suffered from chronic pain of either peripheral or central origin affecting a variety of physical locations, and all were non-responsive to standard therapy. The patients underwent a central lateral thalamotomy (CTL) using ultrasound. MRgFUS was used to ablate the posterior part of the central lateral thalamic nucleus (CLp), which is a recognised neurosurgical target for chronic pain relief using current stereotactic interventions.[28] The procedure was carried out bilaterally in six patients and unilaterally in five patients. The pain level was assessed pre- and post-operatively using a variety of measures, including the McGill pain questionnaire, a Visual Analog Scale (VAS) score of 1–100 for level of pain and a reporting of percentage pain relief compared to pre-procedure levels.

As a group, the patients reported an average 49% pain relief at 3 months, rising to 57% at a year following treatment. Similarly, the VAS score went from an average of 59.5/100 before the procedure to 35.3/100 at the 1-year follow-up mark. With the exception of one patient who suffered a small haemorrhage and ischemia to the nearby motor thalamus, causing partial paralysis that had almost completely subsided by the end of the follow-up year, all patients tolerated the procedure well. Five of the 11 patients were able to stop oral pain medication after treatment completely. These results suggest promise for the application of MRgFUS for the treatment of drug-refractory neuropathic pain, and further clinical trials are warranted.

21.7 Focused Ultrasound for Psychiatric Indications

Psychiatric conditions account for approximately 37% of healthy life years lost to disability.[29] Despite significant advances in the treatment of psychiatric disorders, medical therapy alone is insufficient in more than half of patients, and these cases require additional psychosocial intervention.[29] Unfortunately, between 10% and 30% of patients remain refractory to treatment altogether.[29–31] This subgroup of patients stands to benefit from targeted neurosurgical intervention. Indeed, some success has been reported with the application of DBS targeting the anterior limb of the internal capsule (ALIC) and the ventral capsule/ventral striatum (VC/VS) in patients with treatment refractory obsessive-compulsive disorder (OCD).[32–34] Although high-frequency stimulation of the anterior limb of the internal capsule for OCD received FDA approval under a humanitarian device exemption in 2009, one of the major problems with DBS in this target is the high energy required and the need for frequent battery exchanges, in addition to the psychological burden of implanted hardware. These drawbacks recently rekindled interest in thermal capsulotomies in this target using focused ultrasound.

Jung et al. (2014) reported the first attempt at bilateral thermal capsulotomy using MRgFUS in four patients with treatment refractory OCD.[35] The inclusion criteria were (1) a confirmed OCD diagnosis, (2) at least a 3-year history of OCD symptoms, (3) a minimum Yale-Brown Obsessive-compulsive scale (Y-BOCS) score of 28 and (4) a recorded resistance to pharmacological and cognitive-behavioural therapy. The four patients that fulfilled the inclusion criteria were three males and one female ages 22 to 44 years. Post-operative behavioural evaluation consisted of the Y-BOCS and the Hamilton Rating Scales for Anxiety and Depression (HAM-A and HAM-D, respectively). All four patients showed significant improvement that was detectable 1 week post-operatively, and was sustained until the end of the follow-up period 6 months later on each of these measures. The average percentage improvement in the Y-BOSC score was 33 ± 10.8% (Mean ± SD), constituting a change from extreme to moderate/severe clinical presentation.[36] The improvement for the HAM-A and HAM-D were 68.2 ± 19.8% and 61.1 ± 19.3%, respectively, constituting a change from severe to mild clinical presentation.[37, 38] With the exception of mild vestibular symptoms that occurred during the procedure, the patients did not report, or demonstrate, any transient or long-term physical, neurological or psychological complications following the procedure.

Since the patients remained on their antipsychotic medication regimen throughout the follow-up period, it will be important to acquire further long term outcome data to determine whether thermal capsulotomy with MRgFUS is sufficient on its own, or is effective exclusively in combination with ongoing medical treatment. Nevertheless, this report demonstrates the potential of MRgFUS to offer relief to treatment-refractory OCD patients and provides a basis for further clinical trials. To date, this is the only report of the application of MRgFUS for a psychiatric indication.

21.8 Focused Ultrasound for Brain Tumours

Early in vitro pilot data suggested that focused ultrasound may be used to target glioblastoma cells selectively. Hyperthermia was found to kill cultured glioblastoma cells held at 44°C for 24 minutes, with even shorter heating times being necessary for cells at lower pH.[39] As cancer cells are often in a low pH environment due to high metabolic activity, this difference in required heating time was of interest as a potential means of discriminating cancer cells. An early proof-of-concept study on focused ultrasound for patients with high-grade glioma at the University of Arizona in 1991 demonstrated that scanned focused ultrasound was capable of inducing hyperthermia of the tumour, with controllable heating over the tumour volume.[40] A decade later, the first pilot study with the intent to treat three patients with glioblastoma was launched at Brigham and Women's Hospital using transcranial MRgFUS. Unfortunately, tumour ablation was not achieved due to temperatures being below the critical threshold required for necrosis.[14] At the time, only 512 elements of the device were active and the power output was limited to 650–800 W. Based on the measured heating levels, the authors of the study hypothesised that sonication at a higher acoustic power level might have been able to reach the threshold temperature. Patient discomfort due to the thermoplastic mask used to fixate the head within the device also limited the treatment time. Nevertheless, the study demonstrated that non-invasive heating of neural tissue without craniectomy was feasible and could be monitored using MR temperature imaging, without overheating of the skull. This promise was supported by a case report demonstrating that high temperatures can be achieved in a human brain tumour.[41] These initial studies indicate that focused ultrasound could become an effective neurosurgical tool for brain tumours. Recently, recruitment has opened for several clinical trials using transcranial MRgFUS to treat centrally located metastatic and primary brain tumours (NCT00147056; NCT01473485) and to open the blood-brain barrier to deliver the chemotherapeutic agent doxorubicin (NCT02343991).

21.9 Preliminary Evidence for Further Applications

In addition to the main clinical applications of MRgFUS that have been discussed earlier, pre-clinical studies are currently under way to investigate other potential applications of this technology in the brain. MRgFUS shows potential in the treatment of epilepsy with the same advantages of non-invasive ablation as seen for other neurosurgical applications. Most focused ultrasound studies of epilepsy have been conducted in animal models thus far. One of the earliest such studies of induced epilepsy in cats found that focused ultrasound effectively eradicated the epileptogenic focal area, without destroying adjacent brain tissue.[42] A 2011 study on epilepsy in rats induced by pentylenetetrazol, a GABA receptor antagonist, found that low energy focused ultrasound could significantly suppress epileptic activity.[43] Similar low-energy focused ultrasound has demonstrated a modulating effect on neural activity, including modulation of the primary somatosensory cortex resulting in altered sensory discrimination.[44] A better understanding of these non-lesioning, neuromodulatory effects induced by low energy focused ultrasound may lead to a new paradigm for nonablative treatment of the epileptogenic network. More traditional ablative surgical destruction of the irritative zone, for example within the medial structures of the temporal lobe, near developmental malformations, or in brain tissue adjacent to epileptogenic tumours, would be obvious applications of MRgFUS.

The blood-brain barrier (BBB) regulates entry of haematogenous substances into the CNS and displays selective permeability to these substances based on a variety of factors including lipid solubility, molecular size and charge.[45] While conferring neuroprotection from infection and immune-reactivity, the BBB also hampers the entry of many pharmacological agents into the CNS and prevents active drug levels from being achieved.[46] This has been a substantial obstacle for the treatment of a variety of neurological conditions including brain neoplasms, where the BBB prevents the entry of chemotherapy agents. Even though the vasculature that forms via tumour-driven angiogenesis can display altered barrier properties and be inherently leakier than healthy BBB, primary and secondary brain tumours remain difficult targets for pharmacological agents.[47–50] This obstacle has perhaps frustrated clinicians the most in the case of brain tumours, for which there are evidence-based targeted therapies. An example of this is human epidermal growth factor receptor 2 positive (HER2+) breast cancer metastases which can be treated effectively with the monoclonal antibody-based drug Herceptin (trastuzumab; Genentech). Antibody-based drugs, such as Herceptin and Rituxan (rituximab) which target CD20+ B-cell lymphomas, are ~150kDa in size and are therefore almost wholly excluded from the CNS by the BBB.[51, 52] Thus, despite significant progress in the field of targeted therapy using antibody-based drugs, many brain tumours remain out of reach.

Pre-clinical trials show that MR-guided focused ultrasound (MRgFUS) can be used with circulating microbubbles to produce localised mechanical effects that can disrupt the BBB at the ultrasound focus and increase its permeability.[53] The microbubbles allow use of 100-fold lower energy sonications to achieve effective BBB opening, and consequently avoid the risks associated with higher energies such as haemorrhage, skull heating, thermal tissue-lesioning and cavitation-mediated damage.[53] Preclinical studies in rodents show that MRgFUS with microbubbles allow successful CNS-entry and subsequent tumour reducing effects for doxorubicin,[45, 54, 55] methotrexate,[46] 1,3-bis(chloroethyl)-1-nitrosourea (BCNU),[46] epirubicin,[46] and Herceptin.[46, 51] This technique also shows promise in the field of neurodegenerative disease where MRgFUS with microbubbles allowed the delivery of therapies ranging from neurotrophic factors and siRNA against mutant Huntington protein in a Huntington's disease animal model, to anti-amyloid antibodies in an Alzheimer's disease model and even stem cells for replacement of neuronal loss.[46] In a non-human primate model, McDannold and colleagues demonstrated the long-term safety of the procedure in a trial involving repeated opening of the BBB with microbubbles in the visual cortex and lateral geniculate by MRgFUS.[56] These findings suggest that repetitive BBB-opening by MRgFUS with microbubbles does not affect the neurological functionality of neural tissue surrounding the targeted vascular region. These preclinical safety data have justified the previously mentioned trial on BBB opening to deliver doxorubicin in humans with metastatic disease.

The yearly worldwide incidence of stroke, including both ischemic and haemorrhagic strokes, is estimated at 15 million, with stroke remaining a significant contributor to neurological burden of disease.[57] Intravascular and extravascular clots are associated with ischemic and haemorrhagic strokes, respectively. Thrombolysis is thus a therapeutic goal in both types of stroke, and early preclinical trials have tested the use of MRgFUS energy to induce inertial cavitation and mechanical disruption of the clot matrix. In cases of intracerebral haemorrhage, even after the initial bleeding is under control, the resulting clot may continue to contribute to neurological dysfunction through a mass effect or by seizure generation. This is attributable to the mechanical pressure exerted by the clot on surrounding neural tissue, which contributes to increasing intracerebral pressure, to decreased cerebral blood flow due to surrounding oedema, and to the neurotoxic effects of the clot breakdown products.[54] Reduced clot size tracks with improved clinical outcomes, and various neurosurgical interventions have been tested to improve the thrombolysis achieved by medical therapy alone.[57] Preclinical studies conducted on cadavers used MRgFUS to liquefy >95% of the clot which could then be cleared with MR-guided aspiration successfully.[58] More studies are needed to determine the efficacy of MRgFUS in thrombolysis, but this

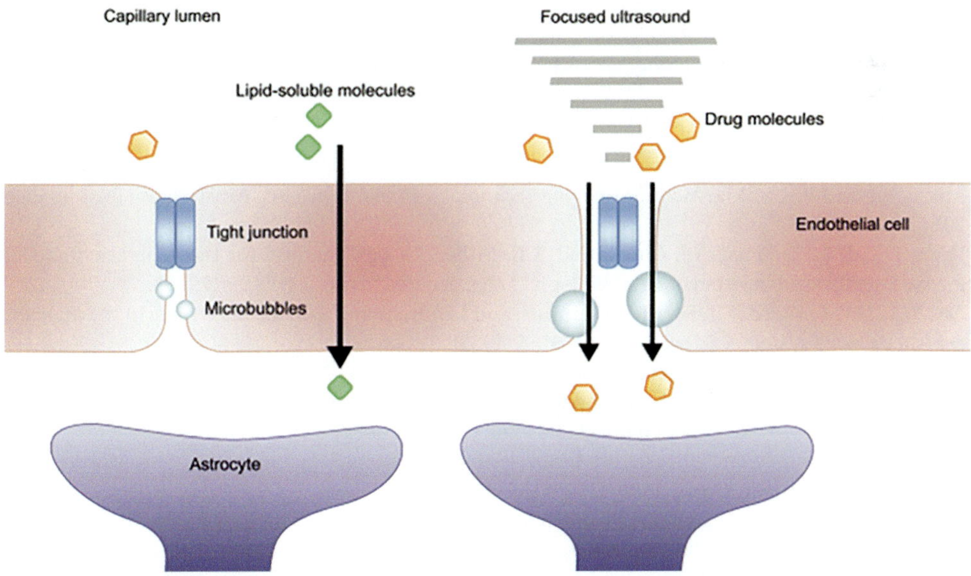

FIGURE 21.4 Disruption of blood-brain barrier using focused ultrasound. Sonication of microbubbles disrupts the tight junctions between endothelial cells and induces active transport, thereby creating transient openings in the blood-brain barrier. Ultrasound-induced disruption is reversible and does not appear to cause any long-term effects.

technique could prove particularly useful for patients with clots deep in the brain parenchyma or within the ventricles, where surgical removal of the clot may be more difficult. If, as the preclinical studies suggest, MRgFUS can accomplish >95% clot lysis on its own, then it could be used as a monotherapy in some patients, to selectively lyse the intracerebral clot while avoiding the risks associated with the administration of systemic thrombolytic medication. Another vascular application of MRgFUS under early stage preclinical investigation is the use of ultrasound for intravascular thrombolysis and recanalisation in ischemic stroke, with the goal of re-establishing blood flow to affected neural tissue and minimising ischemic damage.[57]

21.10 Expert Commentary

Medical applications of HIFU have deep historical roots in neurological applications. The major impediment to non-invasive intracranial clinical applications until recently was sound attenuation, and the defocusing properties of the human skull. This problem has largely been overcome with the use of large independently controlled phased array transducers coupled with MR thermography to track, in near real time, the evolution of the thermal lesion. The safety and efficacy of transcranial MR-guided focused ultrasound was first definitively demonstrated in patients with essential tremor where discrete lesions were created within the motor thalamus for long term tremor capture. Other clinical applications thus far have included central thalamotomy for the treatment of chronic pain, and thermal capsulotomy for the treatment of refractory obsessive compulsive disorder. Promising preliminary evidence for both conditions has been reported in open label trials. Ongoing investigations at the preclinical level are motivating further clinical trials for the treatment of intracranial tumours, epilepsy, and stroke.

21.11 Summary

Transcranial MRI-guided focused ultrasound (TcMRgFUS) is a highly accurate, non-invasive, non-ionising tool that is revolutionising brain surgery. It has deep historical roots, but has only recently emerged clinically as a treatment modality with the first application at the Brigham and Women's Hospital in Boston nearly a decade ago for glioma. Recent multicentre trials have established its safety and efficacy for ET and trials for Parkinson's disease have been initiated. TcMRgFUS is now being investigated for psychiatric, neuro-oncological and chronic pain conditions.

REFERENCES

1. Mikla, V.I. and V.V. Mikla. *Medical Imaging Technology, Elsevier Insights*. Amsterdam; Boston: Elsevier, 2014.
2. Lynn, J.G., R.L. Zwemer, A.J. Chick, and A.E. Miller, "A new method for the generation and use of focused ultrasound in experimental biology." *J Gen Physiol* 26, no. 2 (1942): 179–93.
3. Fry, W.J., J.W. Barnard, E.J. Fry, R.F. Krumins, and J.F. Brennan, "Ultrasonic lesions in the mammalian central nervous system." *Science* 122, no. 3168 (1955): 517–8.
4. Meyers, R., W.J. Fry, F.J. Fry, L.L. Dreyer, D.F. Schultz, and R.F. Noyes, "Early experiences with ultrasonic irradiation of the pallidofugal and nigral complexes in hyperkinetic and hypertonic disorders." *J Neurosurg* 16, no. 1 (1959): 32–54, doi:10.3171/jns.1959.16.1.0032.
5. Fry, F.J., Sanghvi, N.T. "Ultrasound brain lesioning system." Indianapolis, IN; Mooresville, IN: Laboratory Equipment, Corp., 1990. US4951653A.
6. Marmottant, P. and S. Hilgenfeldt, "Controlled vesicle deformation and lysis by single oscillating bubbles." *Nature* 423, no. 6936 (2003): 153–6, doi:10.1038/nature01613.
7. Nikfarjam, M., V. Muralidharan, and C. Christophi, "Mechanisms of focal heat destruction of liver tumours." *J Surg Res* 127, no. 2 (2005): 208–23, doi:10.1016/j.jss.2005.02.009.
8. Hill, C.R., I. Rivens, M.G. Vaughan, and G.R. ter Haar, "Lesion development in focused ultrasound surgery: A general model." *Ultrasound Med Biol* 20, no. 3 (1994): 259–69.

9. Qian, Z.W., L. Xiong, J. Yu, D. Shao, H. Zhu, and X. Wu, "Noninvasive thermometer for HIFU and its scaling." *Ultrasonics* 44, Suppl 1 (2006): e31–5, doi:10.1016/j.ultras.2006.06.036.
10. Wang, Y.N., T. Khokhlova, M. Bailey, J.H. Hwang, and V. Khokhlova, "Histological and biochemical analysis of mechanical and thermal bioeffects in boiling histotripsy lesions induced by high intensity focused ultrasound." *Ultrasound Med Biol* 39, no. 3 (2013): 424–38, doi:10.1016/j.ultrasmedbio.2012.10.012.
11. Yu, T., G. Wang, K. Hu, P. Ma, J. Bai, and Z. Wang, "A microbubble agent improves the therapeutic efficiency of high intensity focused ultrasound: A rabbit kidney study." *Urol Res* 32, no. 1 (2004): 14–9, doi:10.1007/s00240-003-0362-x.
12. Dubinsky, T.J., C. Cuevas, M.K. Dighe, O. Kolokythas, and J.H. Hwang, "High-intensity focused ultrasound: Current potential and oncologic applications." *AJR Am J Roentgenol* 190, no. 1 (2008): 191–9, doi:10.2214/AJR.07.2671.
13. Zhou, Y., L. Zhai, R. Simmons, and P. Zhong, "Measurement of high intensity focused ultrasound fields by a fiber optic probe hydrophone." *J Acoust Soc Am* 120, no. 2 (2006): 676–85.
14. McDannold, N., G.T. Clement, P. Black, F. Jolesz, and K. Hynynen, "Transcranial magnetic resonance imaging-guided focused ultrasound surgery of brain tumours: Initial findings in 3 patients." *Neurosurgery* 66, no. 2 (2010): 323–32; discussion 32, doi:10.1227/01.NEU.0000360379.95800.2F.
15. Hynynen, K. and F.A. Jolesz, "Demonstration of potential noninvasive ultrasound brain therapy through an intact skull." *Ultrasound Med Biol* 24, no. 2 (1998): 275–83.
16. Jolesz, F.A., "MRI-guided focused ultrasound surgery." *Annu Rev Med* 60 (2009): 417–30, doi:10.1146/annurev.med.60.041707.170303.
17. Aum, D.A. and T.S. Tierney, "Deep brain stimulation: Foundations and future trends." *Front Biosci (Landmark Ed)* 23, no. 1 (2018): 162–82.
18. Tierney, T.S., V.S. Vasudeva, S. Weir, and M.T. Hayes, "Neuromodulation for neurodegenerative conditions." *Front Biosci (Elite Ed)* 5 (2013): 490–9.
19. Elias, W.J., D. Huss, T. Voss, J. Loomba, M. Khaled, E. Zadicario, R.C. Frysinger, et al., "A pilot study of focused ultrasound thalamotomy for essential tremor." *N Engl J Med* 369, no. 7 (2013): 640–8, doi:10.1056/NEJMoa1300962.
20. Lipsman, N., M.L. Schwartz, Y. Huang, L. Lee, T. Sankar, M. Chapman, K. Hynynen, and A.M. Lozano, "MR-guided focused ultrasound thalamotomy for essential tremor: A proof-of-concept study." *Lancet Neurol* 12, no. 5 (2013): 462–8, doi:10.1016/S1474-4422(13)70048-6.
21. Chang, W.S., H.H. Jung, E.J. Kweon, E. Zadicario, I. Rachmilevitch, and J.W. Chang, "Unilateral magnetic resonance guided focused ultrasound thalamotomy for essential tremor: Practices and clinicoradiological outcomes." *J Neurol Neurosurg Psychiatry* 86, no. 3 (2015): 257–64, doi:10.1136/jnnp-2014-307642.
22. Chang, W.S., H.H. Jung, E. Zadicario, I. Rachmilevitch, T. Tlusty, S. Vitek, and J.W. Chang, "Factors associated with successful magnetic resonance-guided focused ultrasound treatment: Efficiency of acoustic energy delivery through the skull." *J Neurosurg* 124, no. 2 (2016): 411–6, doi:10.3171/2015.3.JNS142592.
23. Gilron, I., R. Baron, and T. Jensen, "Neuropathic pain: Principles of diagnosis and treatment." *Mayo Clin Proc* 90, no. 4 (2015): 532–45, doi:10.1016/j.mayocp.2015.01.018.
24. White, J.C. and W.H. Sweet. *Pain and the Neurosurgeon; a Forty-year Experience.* Springfield, IL: C. C. Thomas, 1969.
25. Jeraq, M., A. Bayoumi, E.M. Kasper, and T.S. Tierney, "Deep brain stimulation for refractory chronic pain," Chap., in *Surgical Pain Management: A Complete Guide to Implantable and Interventional Pain Therapies*, edited by Narang, S., E.L. Ross and A. Weisheipl. Oxford: Oxford University, 2015.
26. Moses, Z., B. McGinn, P. Dinakar, and T.S. Tierney, "Dorsal column stimulation," Chap., in *Surgical Pain Management: A Complete Guide to Implantable and Interventional Pain Therapies*, edited by Narang, S., E.L. Ross and A. Weisheipl. Oxford: Oxford University Press, 2015.
27. Martin, E., D. Jeanmonod, A. Morel, E. Zadicario, and B. Werner, "High-intensity focused ultrasound for noninvasive functional neurosurgery." *Ann Neurol* 66, no. 6 (2009): 858–61, doi:10.1002/ana.21801.
28. Jeanmonod, D., B. Werner, A. Morel, L. Michels, E. Zadicario, G. Schiff, and E. Martin, "Transcranial magnetic resonance imaging-guided focused ultrasound: Noninvasive central lateral thalamotomy for chronic neuropathic pain." *Neurosurg Focus* 32, no. 1 (2012): E1, doi:10.3171/2011.10.FOCUS11248.

29. Cleary, D.R., A. Ozpinar, A.M. Raslan, and A.L. Ko, "Deep brain stimulation for psychiatric disorders: Where we are now." *Neurosurg Focus* 38, no. 6 (2015): E2, doi:10.3171/2015.3.FOCUS1546.
30. Thase, M.E. and T.L. Schwartz, "Choosing medications for treatment-resistant depression based on mechanism of action." *J Clin Psychiatry* 76, no. 6 (2015): 720–7; quiz 27, doi:10.4088/JCP.14052ah2c.
31. Drubach, D.A., "Obsessive-compulsive disorder." *Continuum (Minneap Minn)* 21, no. 3 Behavioural Neurology and Neuropsychiatry (2015): 783–8, doi:10.1212/01.CON.0000466666.12779.07.
32. Greenberg, B.D., L.A. Gabriels, D.A. Malone, Jr., A.R. Rezai, G.M. Friehs, M.S. Okun, N.A. Shapira, et al., "Deep brain stimulation of the ventral internal capsule/ventral striatum for obsessive-compulsive disorder: Worldwide experience." *Mol Psychiatry* 15, no. 1 (2010): 64–79, doi:10.1038/mp.2008.55.
33. Tierney, T.S., M.M. Abd-El-Barr, A.D. Stanford, K.D. Foote, and M.S. Okun, "Deep brain stimulation and ablation for obsessive compulsive disorder: Evolution of contemporary indications, targets and techniques." *Int J Neurosci* 124, no. 6 (2014): 394–402, doi:10.3109/00207454.2013.852086.
34. Liu, K., H. Zhang, C. Liu, Y. Guan, L. Lang, Y. Cheng, B. Sun, et al., "Stereotactic treatment of refractory obsessive compulsive disorder by bilateral capsulotomy with 3 years follow-up." *J Clin Neurosci* 15, no. 6 (2008): 622–9, doi:10.1016/j.jocn.2007.07.086.
35. Jung, H.H., S.J. Kim, D. Roh, J.G. Chang, W.S. Chang, E.J. Kweon, C.H. Kim, and J.W. Chang, "Bilateral thermal capsulotomy with MR-guided focused ultrasound for patients with treatment-refractory obsessive-compulsive disorder: A proof-of-concept study." *Mol Psychiatry* 20, no. 10 (2015): 1205–11, doi:10.1038/mp.2014.154.
36. Goodman, W.K., L.H. Price, S.A. Rasmussen, C. Mazure, R.L. Fleischmann, C.L. Hill, G.R. Heninger, and D.S. Charney, "The Yale-Brown Obsessive Compulsive Scale. I. Development, use, and reliability." *Arch Gen Psychiatry* 46, no. 11 (1989): 1006–11.
37. Hamilton, M., "The assessment of anxiety states by rating." *Br J Med Psychol* 32, no. 1 (1959): 50–5.
38. Hamilton, M., "A rating scale for depression." *J Neurol Neurosurg Psychiatry* 23 (1960): 56–62.
39. Gerweck, L.E. and B. Richards, "Influence of pH on the thermal sensitivity of cultured human glioblastoma cells." *Cancer Res* 41, no. 3 (1981): 845–9.
40. Guthkelch, A.N., L.P. Carter, J.R. Cassady, K.H. Hynynen, R.P. Iacono, P.C. Johnson, E.A. Obbens, et al., "Treatment of malignant brain tumours with focused ultrasound hyperthermia and radiation: Results of a phase I trial." *J Neurooncol* 10, no. 3 (1991): 271–84.
41. Coluccia, D., J. Fandino, L. Schwyzer, R. O'Gorman, L. Remonda, J. Anon, E. Martin, and B. Werner, "First noninvasive thermal ablation of a brain tumour with MR-guided focused ultrasound." *J Ther Ultrasound* 2 (2014): 17, doi:10.1186/2050-5736-2-17.
42. Manlapaz, J.S., K.E. Astroem, H.T. Ballantine, Jr., and P.P. Lele, "Effects of Ultrasonic Radiation in Experimental Focal Epilepsy in the Cat." *Exp Neurol* 10 (1964): 345–56.
43. Min, B.K., A. Bystritsky, K.I. Jung, K. Fischer, Y. Zhang, L.S. Maeng, S.I. Park, Y.A. Chung, F.A. Jolesz, and S.S. Yoo, "Focused ultrasound-mediated suppression of chemically-induced acute epileptic EEG activity." *BMC Neurosci* 12 (2011): 23, doi:10.1186/1471-2202-12-23.
44. Legon, W., T.F. Sato, A. Opitz, J. Mueller, A. Barbour, A. Williams, and W.J. Tyler, "Transcranial focused ultrasound modulates the activity of primary somatosensory cortex in humans." *Nat Neurosci* 17, no. 2 (2014): 322–9, doi:10.1038/nn.3620.
45. Treat, L.H., N. McDannold, N. Vykhodtseva, Y. Zhang, K. Tam, and K. Hynynen, "Targeted delivery of doxorubicin to the rat brain at therapeutic levels using MRI-guided focused ultrasound." *Int J Cancer* 121, no. 4 (2007): 901–7, doi:10.1002/ijc.22732.
46. Burgess, A. and K. Hynynen, "Drug delivery across the blood-brain barrier using focused ultrasound." *Expert Opin Drug Deliv* 11, no. 5 (2014): 711–21, doi:10.1517/17425247.2014.897693.
47. Agarwal, S., R. Sane, R. Oberoi, J.R. Ohlfest, and W.F. Elmquist, "Delivery of molecularly targeted therapy to malignant glioma, a disease of the whole brain." *Expert Rev Mol Med* 13 (2011): e17, doi:10.1017/S1462399411001888.
48. Rapisarda, A. and G. Melillo, "Role of the VEGF/VEGFR axis in cancer biology and therapy." *Adv Cancer Res* 114 (2012): 237–67, doi:10.1016/B978-0-12-386503-8.00006-5.
49. Fukumura, D., "Balancing angiogenic pathways in solid tumours." *Microvasc Rev Commun* 7, no. 1 (2014): 23–23, doi:10.14532/mvrc.7.23.
50. van Tellingen, O., B. Yetkin-Arik, M.C. de Gooijer, P. Wesseling, T. Wurdinger, and H.E. de Vries, "Overcoming the blood-brain tumour barrier for effective glioblastoma treatment." *Drug Resist Updat* 19 (2015): 1–12, doi:10.1016/j.drup.2015.02.002.

51. Kinoshita, M., N. McDannold, F.A. Jolesz, and K. Hynynen, "Noninvasive localized delivery of Herceptin to the mouse brain by MRI-guided focused ultrasound-induced blood-brain barrier disruption." *Proc Natl Acad Sci U S A* 103, no. 31 (2006): 11719–23, doi:10.1073/pnas.0604318103.
52. Ponzoni, M., S. Issa, T.T. Batchelor, and J.L. Rubenstein, "Beyond high-dose methotrexate and brain radiotherapy: Novel targets and agents for primary CNS lymphoma." *Ann Oncol* 25, no. 2 (2014): 316–22, doi:10.1093/annonc/mdt385.
53. Hynynen, K., N. McDannold, N. Vykhodtseva, and F.A. Jolesz, "Noninvasive MR imaging-guided focal opening of the blood-brain barrier in rabbits." *Radiology* 220, no. 3 (2001): 640–6, doi:10.1148/radiol.2202001804.
54. Aryal, M., N. Vykhodtseva, Y.Z. Zhang, and N. McDannold, "Multiple sessions of liposomal doxorubicin delivery via focused ultrasound mediated blood-brain barrier disruption: A safety study." *J Control Release* 204 (2015): 60–9, doi:10.1016/j.jconrel.2015.02.033.
55. Aryal, M., J. Park, N. Vykhodtseva, Y.Z. Zhang, and N. McDannold, "Enhancement in blood-tumour barrier permeability and delivery of liposomal doxorubicin using focused ultrasound and microbubbles: Evaluation during tumour progression in a rat glioma model." *Phys Med Biol* 60, no. 6 (2015): 2511–27, doi:10.1088/0031-9155/60/6/2511.
56. McDannold, N., C.D. Arvanitis, N. Vykhodtseva, and M.S. Livingstone, "Temporary disruption of the blood-brain barrier by use of ultrasound and microbubbles: Safety and efficacy evaluation in rhesus macaques." *Cancer Res* 72, no. 14 (2012): 3652–63, doi:10.1158/0008-5472.CAN-12-0128.
57. Monteith, S.J., N.F. Kassell, O. Goren, and S. Harnof, "Transcranial MR-guided focused ultrasound sonothrombolysis in the treatment of intracerebral haemorrhage." *Neurosurg Focus* 34, no. 5 (2013): E14, doi:10.3171/2013.2.FOCUS1313.
58. Lipsman, N., T.G. Mainprize, M.L. Schwartz, K. Hynynen, and A.M. Lozano, "Intracranial applications of magnetic resonance-guided focused ultrasound." *Neurotherapeutics* 11, no. 3 (2014): 593–605, doi:10.1007/s13311-014-0281-2.

22

Sonoporation: Concept, Mechanisms and Application to Cancer Treatment

Junru Wu

22.1 Introduction

It was found in the late 1990s that encapsulated gas microbubbles (EMBs) could oscillate vigorously under ultrasound (US) excitation and could temporarily 'open' the membranes of nearby cells, allowing micro- and macro-molecules, such as DNA, peptides, proteins or genetic drugs (pDNA, siRNA, mRNA) contained within the microbubbles or existing in the extracellular fluid, to be delivered into cells.[1–5] Albunex (Molecular Biosystems, approved in 1994), Optison (GE Medical Diagnostics, Princeton, NJ, approved in 1997) and Definity spheres (Lantheus Medical Imaging, Billerica, NJ, approved in 2001) are ultrasound imaging contrast agents approved by the Food and Drug Administration (FDA) in the United States. These are micron-sized (mean diameter ~1–10 μm) denatured hollow albumin or polymer microbubbles of shell thickness greater than 10 nm, filled with air (Albunex) or with the inert gas octafluoropropane (Optison and Definity). The small size of these EMBs allows them to be infused intravenously and to circulate freely throughout the vasculature, including the capillaries of the human body; their resonant frequencies match the frequency spectrum (1–15 MHz) used in biomedical ultrasound.[6] The term 'sonoporation' (assisted by EMB) was first adopted by Miller et al.[3] and Ward et al.[5] in 1999. Later, Pepe et al.[7] found experimentally that electroporation and sonoporation have similar effects in the application of targeted drug delivery in vitro. The sonoporation process is usually transient. Cells may later 'reseal' themselves and remain viable after exposure if the US intensity is low or moderate. Where this is the case, the technique is called reparable sonoporation.[8] Since reparable sonoporation has unique capabilities of site specificity (US can easily be focused into a desired volume) and non-invasiveness in vivo, it has the potential to become a non-viral technology for the safe and efficient delivery of DNA or drugs to a targeted cancer cell or tissue.[2, 9–15]

Targeted drug delivery (TDD) assisted by US offers enormous advantages compared to conventional delivery methods. Since conventional methods lack target specificity, the highly toxic dose of anticancer drugs delivered may cause undesirable and severe damage to healthy tissues and organs. Targeted drug delivery not only increases drug efficacy but also minimises these possible side effects. Although it has great potential, TDD currently presents serious technical challenges. The main difficulties arise from the barriers presented by cell and nuclear membranes to DNA, antibody and drug transport, if their targets are inside the cell nuclei.

The gene transfection used in some cancer treatments is the process of introducing recombinant DNA into eukaryotic cells and subsequently integrating it into the recipient cell's chromosomal DNA. Current gene transfection techniques may be divided into two categories: viral and non-viral. The former achieves transfection using a virus,[16] while the latter does not. Several viral systems (adenovirus and retrovirus) have been used to deliver genes into primary cells from specific tissues in vitro, but their use for in vivo gene delivery has faced several obstacles, including an immune response against the virus.[17, 18] and serious side effects, due to the poor specificity of cell targets. Existing non-viral transfection approaches include calcium phosphate infusion, electroporation, particle bombardment and lipofection. Lack of target specificity is a major problem for most existing delivery techniques. Recently,

DOI: 10.1201/9780429162671-22

nanoparticles have been investigated as targeted drug delivery carriers.[19] Nanoparticles include nano-sized (<1000 nm) polymeric particles, liposomes and micelles. The application of liposomes has shown great potential in gene transfection[20] because of their small size, biocompatibility with cell membranes and the possible addition of special ligands to their surfaces and to internalised agents. A new non-viral and controllable transfection tool to deliver drug carrying liposomes and other nanoparticles, safely and efficiently, into targets in vivo and in vitro is urgently needed.

22.2 Physical Principles and Mechanisms

The possible mechanisms for sonoporation may include stable and inertial acoustic cavitation. Stable cavitation refers to the repeated periodic oscillations of bubbles in response to the acoustic pressure field. These oscillating bubbles may interact with cells during ultrasound exposure. These interactions can generate shear stresses which can produce small transient multi-pores in plasma membranes through which molecules may enter a cell.[21–23] They may also promote endocytosis,[24, 25] a process by which a cell takes up some extracellular fluid, including material dissolved or suspended in it, through its endogenous cellular machinery, e.g., surface receptor sites, such as caveoli. Unstable and violent bubble oscillations (also called inertial cavitation) may result in bubble rupture and can generate micro-jets and shock waves, which may produce relatively larger pores in the cell membrane in a short time. Most injured cells cannot repair themselves. In general, the time-averaged radius of EMBs during the sonoporation process associated with the stable cavitation is relatively stable, the associated TDD process is slow but controllable, with the US exposure-time needed being long (a few minutes or longer). The time-averaged radius of the EMBs during sonoporation associated with the unstable cavitation decreases with time because of bubble rupture, the accompanying TDD process is relatively fast, but the cell mortality rate is high.[26] The efficacy of sonoporation not only depends on acoustic field parameters such as acoustic pressure amplitude, frequency and exposure time but also on the molecular size of agents to be delivered: the smaller the size, the higher the efficacy.

22.2.1 Bubble-Cell Interaction Is a Short-Range Interaction

Since the microspheres are small, the bubble-cell interaction is essentially short-range, i.e., a cell must be somewhere in the proximity of the cavitation source (a bubble) in order to be affected by it. Ward et al.[12] performed an experiment to examine the consequences of varying the distance of cells (Jurkat lymphocytes) to Optison microspheres, which acted as the sources of acoustic cavitation, in suspension. This was done by varying cell concentration and the ratio of bubbles to cells in a given sample; the higher cell concentrations and higher bubble-to-cell ratios resulted in an increased number of observed sonoporation events under the same ultrasound conditions. Figure 22.1 shows the percentage of sonoporated cells, as indicated by fluorescent light emission, vs the effective cell-bubble spacing. The percentage of affected cells declined approximately as the inverse third power of the static spacing ($1/r^3$). Both sets of data (lethally damaged cells represented by 'diamonds' and reparable cells by 'squares') showed a steady increase in sonoporation as the bubble-cell spacing decreased. However, there was very little indication of sonoporation under the same US excitation in the absence of Optison (not shown). For lethal damage to occur, the nearest bubble-cell spacing was less than 45 μm (the cutoff spacing) under these experimental conditions. For reparable cells, there was no clear cutoff spacing. The higher cell concentration corresponded to smaller spacing between the nearest cavitation bubbles and cells and resulted in consistently higher percentages of sonoporation than the lower concentration. It should be noted that this is an example of relatively slow and controllable sonoporation (US frequency = 2 MHz; spatial negative peak acoustic pressure, p_- = 0.2 MPa; duty cycle = 10%; pulse repetition frequency = 10 kHz, exposure time = 5 min). In summary, to achieve controlled TD, tone-burst US of low duty cycle (<20%) and low acoustic negative peak pressure ($\approx$ 0.2 MPa) and longer exposure time (>1 min) should be used. The bubble to cell ratio should be approximately 200 (that is, each cell should 'see' 200 bubbles within a 45 μm range). In clinical application, the bubble concentration would be much lower. To achieve the same results, p_- needs to be higher than 0.2 MPa.

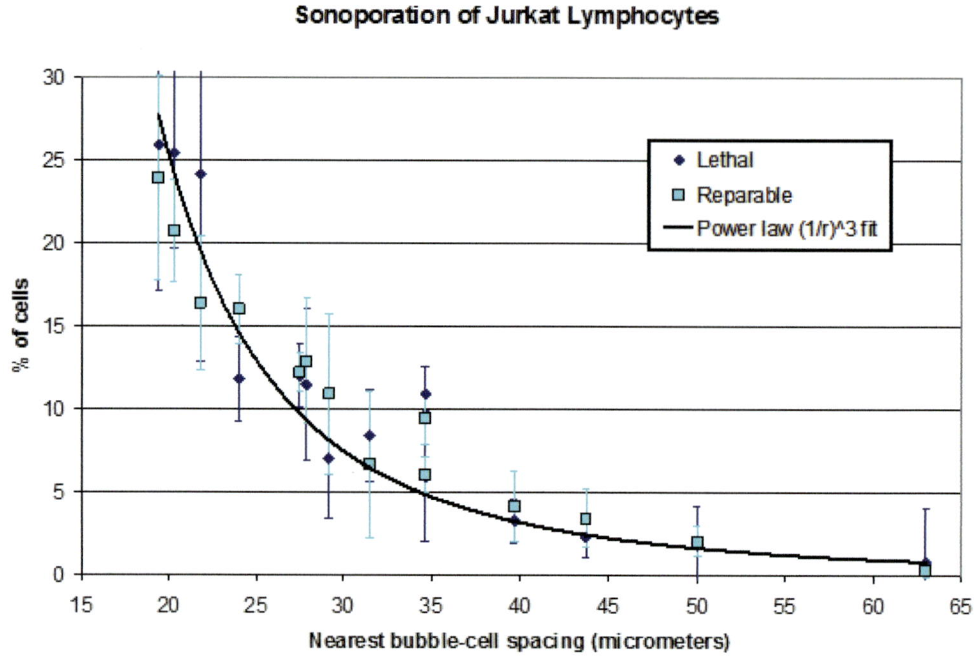

FIGURE 22.1 Percentage of sonoporated cells, as indicated by fluorescence, versus effective bubble spacing. Each data point represents the average and standard deviation of six measurements. Frequency = 2 MHz; the spatial peak acoustic pressure = 0.2 MPa; the duty cycle = 10%; the pulse repetition frequency = 10 kHz, exposure time = 5 min. (Adapted from Ward, M., Wu, J., Chiu, J. F., 2000, with permission.)

It is worth pointing out that acoustic radiation force may also play an important role in the TDD and sonoporation process.[6] In a traveling acoustic field, there is a 'push' force which moves microbubbles (bubble size << the wavelength) along the direction of the wave propagation, towards target cells. In a standing wave field, due to acoustic pressure gradient, the microbubbles will usually accumulate at the acoustic antinodes where the acoustic pressure reaches the local maximum.[6] If the cell diameter is also smaller than a wavelength, it is very likely that they are also be trapped at the antinodes, and that significant interaction between the oscillating bubble and cells would occur there.

22.2.2 Sonoporated Cells Repair Themselves

It is known that when cell-membranes suffer instant disruption, a 'resealing' process may be triggered. 'Resealing' is a complex and dynamic cell adaptation process which is needed for cell survival.[27–29] It has been reported that cell membrane disruption may trigger Ca^{2+} to enter the disrupted area and cause vesicles present in cytoplasm underlying the disruption site to fuse with one another rapidly and also with the adjacent plasma membrane.[27, 30] Lysosomes, membrane-bound organelles, have been recognised as playing an important role in repairing plasma membrane 'wounds'.[27] It has also been found that LAMP-1, a lysosomal-associated membrane protein which is not normally present at the plasma membrane surface, can become ubiquitously exposed on the cell surface[27, 28] when lysosomes were triggered to fuse with the plasma membrane under stressful conditions.

Yang et al.[31] (2008) performed an experiment to study the sonoporation self-sealing process. Reparable sonoporation of human breast cancer cells (MCF7 cell line) was achieved during exposure to moderate ultrasound (spatial peak acoustic pressure amplitude p_+= 0.25 MPa, 1 MHz tone-bursts, duty cycle = 20%, pulse repetition frequency = 10 kHz) for up to 40 s, assisted by the presence of EMBs. It was demonstrated that the shear stress generated by microstreaming around oscillating

EMBs near cell membranes may be as high as1000 Pa when US of frequency of 1 MHz, and acoustic pressure of p_+= 0.12 Pa is used.[14] This introduces small transient pores in membranes, through which cells are able to take up some extracellular agents in the fluid, and which also meanwhile triggered the repair process, through self-sealing, during sonoporation. It was also indicated, during post-sonoporation analysis using fluorescent microscopy, scanning electron microscopy and the Bradford assay, which determines the protein content in the cell supernatant, that the self-sealing might be established by lysosomal-associated membrane proteins, LAMP-1, fusing with the plasma membrane during the stressful conditions of sonoporation. Yang et al.[31] found that a similar process occurred during a reparable sonoporation experiment. That is, the shear-stress generated by oscillating EMBs at cell-membrane surfaces would trigger a similar resealing process to allow cells to repair themselves.[14, 23] Scanning electron microscope images (magnification 5,000) of MCF7 cells (a human breast cancer cell line) are shown in Figure 22.2. The pore sizes were estimated to be in the range of 0–94.3 nm, 10–533 nm, 786 nm–1.11µm and 2.03–4.31 µm, respectively, for Figures 22.2C, D, E and F. Rough regions and small pits started to be seen as the acoustic pressure amplitude increased, as shown in Figures 22.2C – F (spatial peak acoustic pressure amplitude, P_+ = 0.19, 0.25, 0.38 and 0.48 MPa, exposure for 40s with EMBs present, respectively for C–F). It is interesting to note that although the same P_+ (0.25 MPa) was used, Figure 22.2B looks different from Figure 22.2D. The presence of oscillating EMBs (Figure 22.2D) near cells introduced a few pits at the cell membrane. This difference in cell surface morphology indicates that US effects on cells were amplified by the presence of the nearby EMBs. It is noted that the 'holes' in Figure 22.2F are conspicuously 'large'. This suggests that the "hole" size might have reached a level beyond that which can be repaired by self-sealing, i.e., cell membranes may be ruptured.

The use of electron microscopy to gauge pore size is intrinsically limited to post-US measurements. The formation of transient pores has also been shown by measuring changes in ionic conductivity[32, 33] using the voltage-clamp technique to measure changes in the transmembrane current (TMC) of a single cell in order to monitor sonoporation in real time (Figure 22.3). Because the TMC is related to the diffusion of ions through pores on the membrane, it can provide information about the pore size generated during sonoporation. Using the relatively larger Xenopus laevis oocytes as the model system, the TMC of a single cell under a voltage clamp was measured in real time to assess the formation of pores on the membrane during sonoporation. The cells were exposed to US (0.2 s, p_- = 0.3 MPa, 1.075 MHz) in the presence of Definity microbubbles. Experiments were designed to determine the TMC corresponding to a single pore on the membrane (Figure 22.3). The size of the pores was estimated from an electro-diffusion model that relates the TMC to pore size from ion transport through the membrane pores. The mean radius of single pores was determined to be 110 nm, with a standard deviation of 40 nm. It should be noted that the pore size is a function of acoustic pressure amplitude, frequency, and exposure time. When the pore size reaches micrometer dimensions and larger, the cell would have difficulty in repairing itself.

22.3 Pre-clinical Results

Recent preclinical applications of sonoporation with microbubbles, often called sonochemotherapy, have increased significantly.[34] Most research focuses on treatments of tumours in tissues that are readily accessible to EMBs. The increasing knowledge of cellular and molecular mechanisms for human disease allows sonoporation to become a promising therapeutic alternative. Sonoporation for site-specific gene or drug delivery using EMBs has been extensively studied in cells in vitro. For example Duvshani-Eshet et al.[35, 36] pre-mixed plasmid DNA with Optison as the carrier and applied therapeutic ultrasound (TUS) of 1MHz, 30% duty cycle (DC), spatial and temporal averaged intensity of 2W/cm^2 for 0–30 min to mediate gene delivery. Their results revealed that

Optison microbubbles enhanced TUS-gene transfection by increasing the number of plasmids in the cells and also by distributing the plasmids to more cells, without significant decrease in cell viability. Their results also demonstrated that Optison mainly affects the cytoplasmatic membrane without

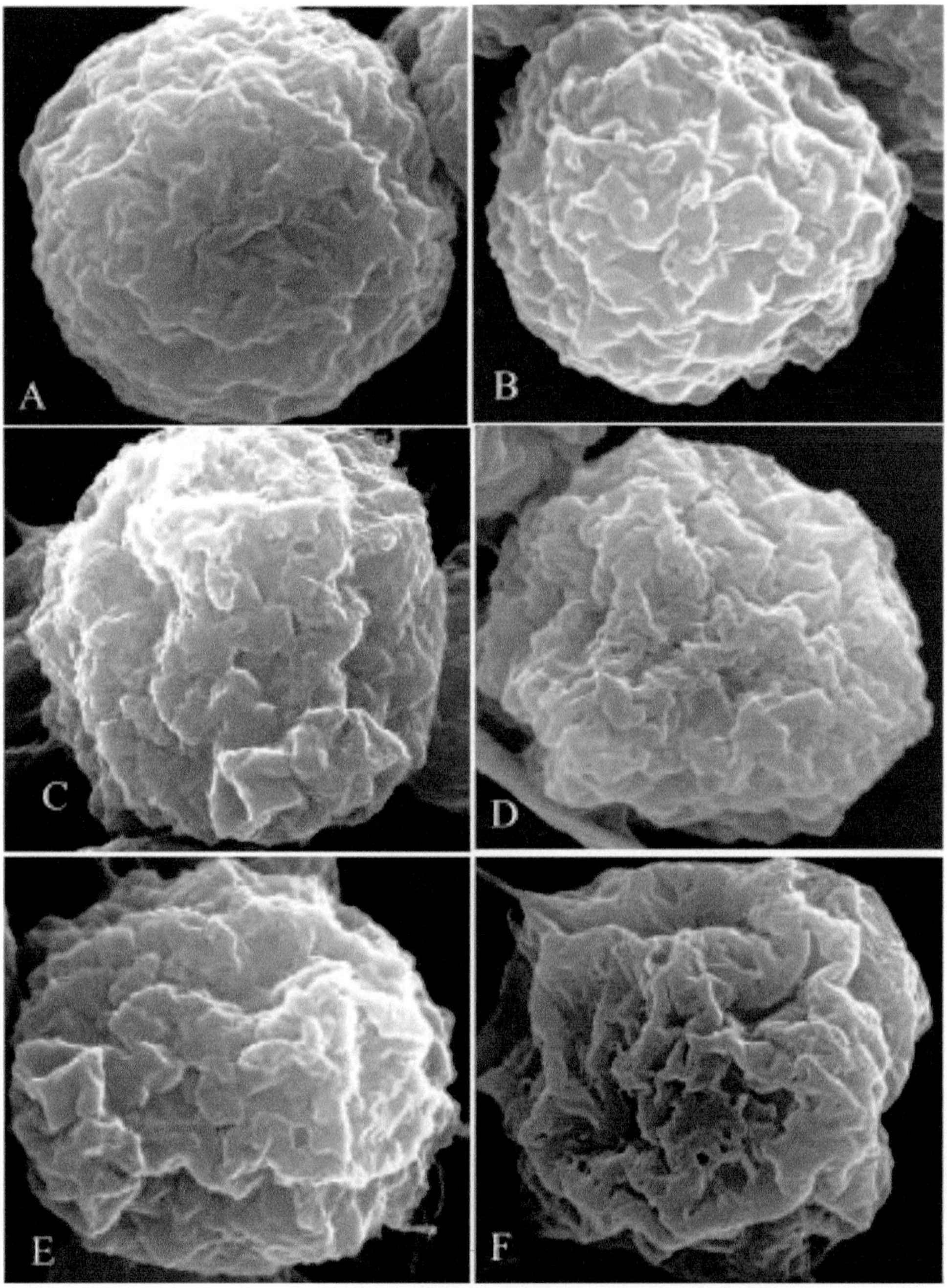

FIGURE 22.2 Scanning electron microscopic images (magnification × 5,000) of MCF7 cells (a human breast cancer cell line) irradiated with ultrasound in the presence of EMBs. A: No US; B: US but no EMBs presence; After spatial peak acoustic pressure Psp = 0.19, 0.25, 0.38 and 0.48 MPa exposure for 40 s with EGBs presence, respectively (C–F). The size of the pores were estimated to be in the range of 0–94.3 nm, 10–533 nm, 786–1.11 μm and 2.03–4.31μm, respectively, for C, D, E and F. (Adapted from Yang, F., Gu, N., Chen, D., Xi, X., Zhang, D., Li, Y., Wu, J., 2008, with permission.)

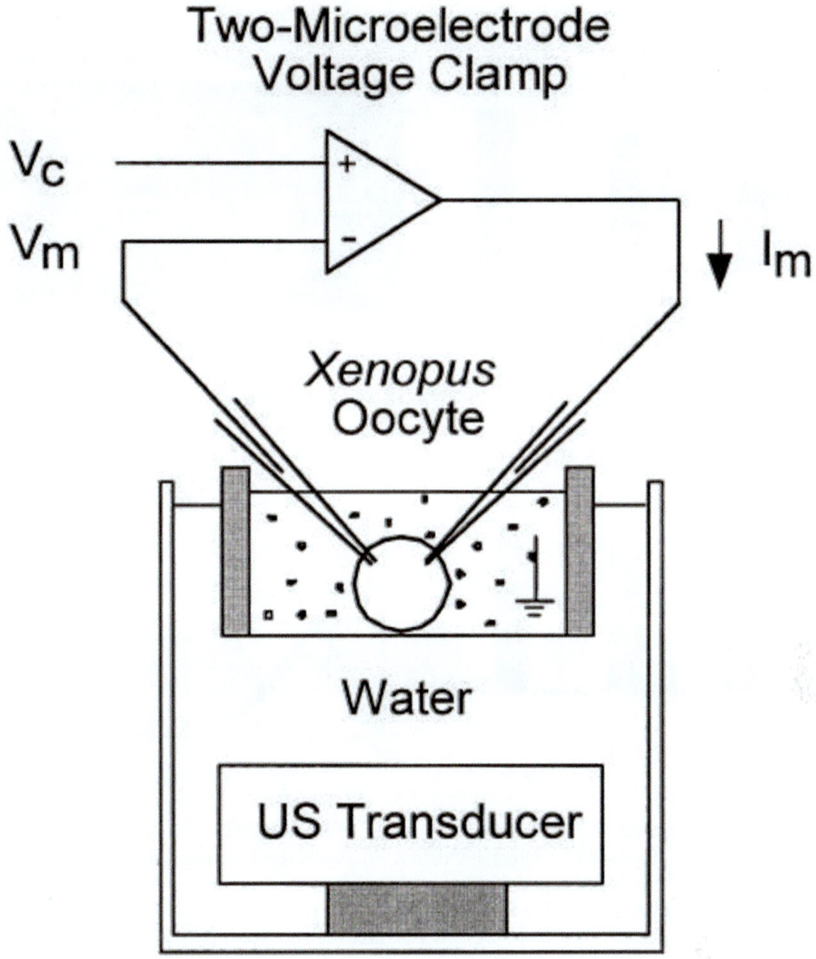

FIGURE 22.3 An experimental setup for monitoring the sonoporation of the plasma membrane of Xenopus oocytes.

Source: (Adapted from Deng, C.X., Sieling, F., Pan, H., Cui, J., 2004, with permission.)

interfering with intracellular DNA trafficking. As seen in Figure 22.4A, when DNA was first incubated with Optison, transfection efficiency was significantly higher than that achieved when TUS was applied alone for 10, 20 and 30 min ($p < 0.05$). This high transfection efficiency was also confirmed by fluorescent microscopy (Figure 22.4B), which demonstrated an increase in the number of cells expressing GFP when Optison was added. The total fluorescence level was also significantly enhanced ($p < 0.05$) when Optison was pre-incubated with the DNA compared with cells treated with TUS alone (Figure 22.4C). The results demonstrated that when TUS was applied for 30 min to cells in the presence of Optison pre-incubated with DNA, the percentage of cells expressing GFP increased from 28±6% to 44 ±8% (Figure 22.4D). From these studies it was also clear that the relative fluorescence enhancement indicates that more copies of plasmids entered cells.

Alter et al.,[37] mixed phosphorodiamidate morpholino oligomers and plasmids with three different kinds of EMB spheres for their studies. Other approaches included therapeutic agents which were durably bound into the microbubble structure: plasmids were incorporated into microbubbles during the synthesis of albumin-shelled agents[38] in an animal study. While the exact binding mechanism between the agent and the bubble was still elusive, the covalent bond is one possible stable linkage put forward. For example, it has been reported that plasmid DNA[39] and interfering RNA were covalently bound

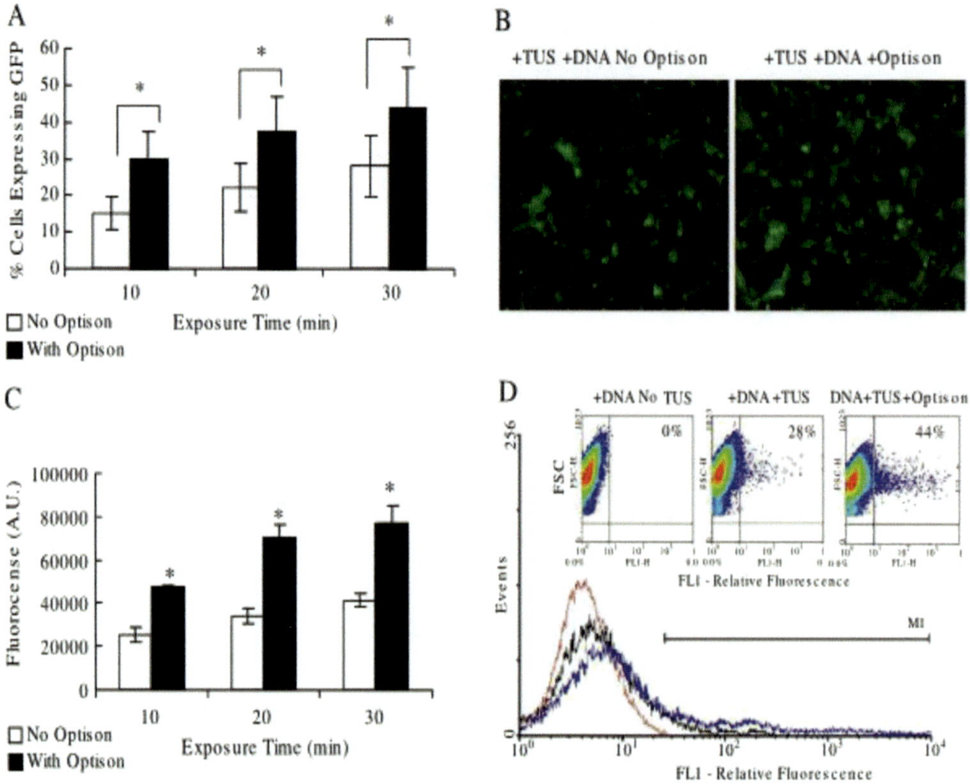

FIGURE 22.4 The effects of Optison on TUS transfection using pIRES-EGFP-BHK cells treated with 1 MHz TUS at 30% DC and 2 W/cm² with or without Optison (A). Effect of Optison (B). Fluorescent micrographs of cells expressing GFP 24 h post TUS transfection for 30 min with or without Optison. (C). Effects of Optison on total GFP expression post TUS. (D). FACS analysis of cells 24 h post TUS transfection for 30 min. FACS Dot-plot showing cell size (FSC) vs green fluorescence (FL1) and percentage of the number of cells with fluorescence greater than the control * $p < 0.05$. (Adapted from Duvshani-Eshet, M., Adam, D., Machluf, M., 2006, with permission.)

to phospholipid-shelled bubbles via biotin-avidin-biotin linkages.[40] Czarnota et al.[41] have shown that ultrasound-mediated microbubble vascular disruption can enhance tumour responses to ionising radiation in vivo. They demonstrated this effect using a human PC3 prostate cancer xenograft model. Results indicate that there is a synergistic effect in vivo, with combined single treatments of ultrasound-stimulated microbubble vascular perturbation with ionising radiation inducing a greater than 10-fold cell killing than with ionising radiation alone. Thus, in vivo experiments with ultrasound combined with bubbles allow radiation doses to be decreased significantly to give a comparable effect. In order to ensure that microbubbles replenished the microvasculature between the US pulses designed to cause microbubble disruption, the US pulse sequence for mouse treatments was a 10% duty cycle within a 50-ms window every 2 s for a total active insonification time of 750 ms over 5 min, with an overall duty cycle of 0.25%. Microbubble disruption was carried out using a diagnostic ultrasound exposure of $p_- = 570$ kPa and a low mechanical index (0.76). These parameters were chosen to minimise the thermal effects. The use of diagnostic instead of therapeutic ultrasound pulses is significant for safety reasons.

22.3.1 Thrombolysis and Stroke Treatment

Ischemic stroke is caused by the interruption of the blood flow to the brain. Stroke is a relatively common disease, particularly in senior citizens. Catheter-type ultrasound transducers have been used to aid release of therapeutic drugs such as urokinase carried by EMBs to increase the effectiveness of thrombolytic agents such as tissue plasminogen activator (t-PA).[42] In contrast, controls treated with either ultrasound (490 KHz, spatial and temporal averaged intensity of 0.13 W/cm^2) or microbubbles alone showed no reduction in thrombolysis. It is known that the efficacy of t-PA decreases dramatically 2 hours after a stroke has taken place. Intracranial clot lysis was also achieved by Culp et al.[43] in swine arteries using thrombolytic agents with intravenous microbubbles assisted by therapeutic ultrasound. Alexandrov et al.[44] performed a randomised clinical pilot safety study for acute ischemic stroke involving sonothrombolysis using perfutren-lipid microbubbles administered intravenously (IV) and assisted by ultrasound excitation (2 MHz pulsed ultrasound with output power less than 720mW measured by hydrophone; the detailed information of US parameter was not reported in literature). They reached the following conclusion: perflutren microbubbles reached and permeated beyond intracranial occlusions with no increase in symptomatic intracranial hemorrhage after systemic thrombolysis. This suggested the feasibility of further microbubble dose-escalation studies and the development of drug delivery to tissues with compromised perfusion. Molina et al.[45] demonstrated that when driven by ultrasound, microbubbles can reach intracranial occlusions, and that the radiation force and acoustic streaming generated by ultrasound and bubble oscillation increase the residual flow and promote recanalisation. The ultrasound used was 2MHz transcranial Doppler (TCD) from a diagnostic ultrasound system. The detailed parameters were not reported, but the ultrasound combined with microbubbles increased the ability of tPA to break up middle cerebral artery (MCA) thrombi.

22.3.2 Cancer Treatment

Numerous studies have been emerging for the treatment of cancer using sonoporation and TDD.[34] Compared with the serious adverse systemic side effects and low efficacy associated with the use of chemotherapeutic drugs alone, TDD and sonoporation can reduce the required dose of chemotherapeutic drugs and improve their efficacy significantly. Heath et al.[46] delivered cisplatin and cetuximab with microbubbles into cancer-bearing mice. A significant reduction in tumour size was observed; an increased number of apoptotic cells was seen following the treatment compared to that with chemotherapeutic agents used alone. Using tumour-bearing mice as a model, Sorace et al.[47] studied the effects of TDD on the efficiency of systemic drug uptake due to changing cell permeability by sonoporation. They reported that membrane permeability appeared to be dependent on ultrasound exposure parameters (acoustic amplitude, frequency, sonication time, etc.); the resultant cancer cell death rate increased by over 50% compared with that from the chemotherapy treatment alone.

22.3.3 Blood-Brain Barrier Disruption

Brain disorders such as Parkinson's disease and Alzheimer's disease (AD) are difficult to treat clinically. One hurdle is that neurons are tightly 'sealed' by endothelial cells which form the so-called blood-brain barrier (BBB). The BBB is a layer of tightly joined cells that line the blood vessels of the brain. It is used to prevent disease and preserve health by keeping harmful substances (such as toxins and infectious agents) from entering the brain. Unfortunately, this barrier also prevents some drugs from reaching adequate concentrations in their targets within the brain, and there are limited options for circumventing the BBB for their delivery. The BBB restricts the passage of substances from the bloodstream much more than do the endothelial cells in capillaries elsewhere in the body. Noninvasive, transient and local blood-brain barrier disruption (BBBD) has been demonstrated following focused ultrasound exposure in animal models.[48] Most studies have combined low pressure amplitude and low time-averaged acoustic power burst sonications with intravascular injection of pre-formed micro-bubbles to produce BBBD without damage to the neurons. For example, Samiotaki et al.[49] used pulsed US (centre frequency 1.5 MHz, pulse length between 67 μs and 6.7 ms, and acoustic pressure amplitude ranging from 0.30 to 0.60 MPa) and T1-weighted magnetic resonance imaging (MRI) to quantify permeability changes. The BBB has been shown to reseal within a few hours of the US exposure. MR image guided focused ultrasound beams allow precise anatomical targeting as demonstrated by the delivery of several marker molecules in different animal models. This method may in the future have a significant impact on the diagnosis and treatment of central nervous system (CNS) disorders. Most notably, the delivery of the chemotherapy agents (liposomal doxorubicin and Herceptin) has been demonstrated in a rat model. Noninvasive, transient and local image-guided BBBD has been accomplished using focused ultrasound exposure with intravascular injection of microbubbles. The delivery of several marker molecules has been demonstrated in different animal models with minimal or no damage to the brain tissue.

Amyloid-β (Aβ) peptide has been connected with the pathogenesis of AD. Ultrasound-assisted cavitation bubbles have been shown to be able to breach the BBB. By overcoming BBB, Leinenga et al.[50] applied repeated scanning ultrasound with bubbles to treat the mouse brain to remove Aβ without the need for any additional therapeutic agent such as anti-Aβ antibody. An integrated focused ultrasound system was used (TIPS, Philips Research), which consists of an annular array transducer with a natural focus of 80 mm, a radius of curvature of 80 mm, a spherical shell of 80 mm with a central opening 31 mm in diameter, a 3D positioning system, and a programmable motorised system to move the ultrasound focus in the x and y planes to cover the entire brain area. A coupler mounted to the transducer was filled with degassed water and placed on the head of the mouse with ultrasound gel for coupling, to ensure propagation of the ultrasound to the brain. The focal zone of the array was an ellipse of about 1.5 mm × 1.5 mm × 12 mm. They optimised the ultrasound settings and used $p_- = 0.7$ MPa, 10-Hz pulse repetition frequency, 10% duty cycle, and 6-s sonication time per spot. This method may potentially open a new era in CNS targeted drug delivery.

22.4 Clinical Treatments

To the author's knowledge, very few clinical treatments using sonoporation have been reported. One rare example is that of Kotopoulis et al.[51] who investigated the ability and efficacy to increase the patient's quality of life by inducing sonoporation in patients with pancreatic adenocarcinoma using a commercial clinical ultrasound scanner in a clinical setting over 31.5 min following standard chemotherapy treatment treated with gemcitabine chemotherapy in a pilot trial (five patients were involved). In two out of the five patients treated, the maximum tumour diameter was temporarily decreased to 80 ± 5%, and permanently to 70 ± 5% of their original size, while control patients treated with chemotherapy alone showed no tumour size reduction, although there was a decrease in tumour growth rate. Intravascular SonoVue (sulphur hexafluoride microbubbles, Bracco UK Ltd.) ultrasound contrast agent micro-bubbles were injected during the treatment. The ultrasound central frequency was 1.9 MHz, de-rated in situ negative acoustic peak pressure was 0.27 MPa, spatially and temporally averaged acoustic intensity was 0.20 mW/cm^2, ultrasound duty cycle was 1% and mechanical index MI = 0.20 measured in free field.

22.5 Expert Commentary

Systemic chemotherapy is still the mainstream standard regimen in the treatment of cancer. In routine clinical practice there are two major limitations to the use of chemotherapy. One is the poisonous effects on fast-growing normal cells, such as those in the bone morrow, digestive tract and hair follicles, resulting in serious side effects in patients. The other is the lack of tumour response to chemotherapeutic agents, which, in part, arises from the poorly organised tumour vasculature, irregular blood flow and high interstitial pressure within the tumour tissue.

Sonoporation is a new and minimally invasive modality which utilises the mechanical effects of ultrasound, mainly acoustic cavitation.[8] There are two types of sonoporation: one uses inertial (transient) cavitation and the other uses non-inertial (stable) cavitation. As far as targeted drug delivery is concerned, the former can generate higher yield than the latter, but also generates more irreparable sonoporated cells. Depending on the application, inertial cavitation may be preferable because it minimises sonication time, but its results are difficult to control. Non-inertial cavitation allows more control of sonoporation, but takes longer to achieve desirable results for drug delivery to targets.

Ultrasound-mediated drug delivery via sonoporation is a novel technique that has the clinical potential to improve the efficacy and specificity of systemic chemotherapy. As a non-invasive modality, it allows the targeted release, improved delivery and enhanced extravasation of chemotherapeutic agents into solid tumours. To date, the preclinical data have demonstrated its promising for enhancing localised drug delivery into tumours, while minimising systemic side effects. However, improvements in clinical translation are still needed, including (1) the development of a new generation of microbubbles that have longer circulation times and higher load capacities, without significant change in acoustic behaviour; (2) an investigation of ultrasound exposure parameters that optimise the efficiency of localised drug delivery, including exposure time, pressure, frequency and duty cycle; (3) the development of cavitation detection techniques such as passive cavitation mapping to improve the remote monitoring of ultrasound-mediated drug delivery; and (4) the assessment of therapeutic benefits in large animal models that are similar to human tumours.[52–55] Not until these issues have been resolved, and the results from prospective, worldwide randomised clinical trials become available, can ultrasound-mediated drug delivery be considered to be a candidate for conventional therapy, for widespread clinical application.

22.6 Summary

The goal of this chapter is to serve as a brief review of sonoporation and its applications in in vitro, in vivo, preclinical and clinical applications. However, since the sonoporation technique is a new modality and is rapidly developing, many excellent scientific papers are being published daily; it is not possible to include them all in this review. Up to now, the pre-clinical trials reported have mainly been performed on small animals. To expand pre-clinical research to human clinical treatment, there are still many obstacles and hurdles to overcome; very few human studies have been performed. The design of new microbubbles and liposomes that can carry an optimal therapeutic dose of drug and genes is an important step for the translation of this research on sonoporation to clinical applications. The intravascular route usually used in clinics is desirable for the administration of microbubble contrast agents in both superficial and deeper organs. Finally, the mechanisms discussed in this article are mostly biased towards those that are physical in origin; readers should also refer to other reviews[56–58] for further information.

REFERENCES

1. Bao, S., Thrall, B. D., Miller, D. L., 1997. Transfection of a reporter plasmid into cultured cells by sonoporation in vitro. Ultrasound Med Biol 23: 953–959.
2. Miller, D. L., Bao, S., Morris, J. E., 1999. Sonoporation of cultured cells in the rotating tube exposure system. Ultrasound Med Biol 25: 143–149.
3. Greenleaf, W. J., Bolander, M. E., Sarkar, G., Goldring, M. B., Greemleaf, J. F., 1998. Artificial cavitation nuclei significantly enhance acoustically induced cell transfection. Ultrasound Med Biol 24: 587–595.
4. Brayman, A., Coppage, M., Vaidya, S., Miller, M., 1999. Transient poration and cell surface receptor removal from human lymphocytes in vitro by 1 MHz ultrasound. Ultrasound Med Biol 25: 999–1008.
5. Ward, M., Wu, J., Chiu, J. F., 1999. Ultrasound-induced cell lysis and sonoporation by enhanced by contrast agents. J Acoust Soc Am 105: 2951–2957.
6. Wu, J., Nyborg, W. L., 2008. Ultrasound, cavitation bubbles and their interaction with cells, Invited Review Paper. Adv Drug Deliv Rev 60: 1103–1116.
7. Pepe, J., Mercede Ricon, M., Wu, J., 2004. Experimental comparison of sonoporation and electroporation in cell transfection applications. ARLO 5: 62–67.
8. Wu, J., 2007. Sonoporation, gene transfection, anticancer drug and antibody drug delivery using ultrasound, in Emerging Therapeutic Ultrasound, Wu, J., Nyborg, W. L., eds., Hackensack, NJ, World Scientific Co., 219–244.
9. Miller, D. L., Bao, S., Morris, J. E., 1999. Sonoporation of cultured cells in the rotating tube exposure system. Ultrasound Med Biol 25: 143–149.

10. Lu, Q. L., Liang, H. D., Partridge, T., Blomley, M. J., 2003. Microbubble ultrasound improves the efficiency of gene transduction in skeletal muscle in vivo with reduced tissue damage. Gene Ther 10: 396–405.
11. Lawrie, A., Brisken, A. F., Francis, S. E., 2000. Microbubble-enhanced ultrasound for vascular gene delivery. Gene Ther 7: 2023–7.
12. Ward, M., Wu, J., Chiu, J. F., 2000. Experimental study on effects of Optison concentration on sonoporation in vitro. Ultrasound Med Biol 26: 1169–1175.
13. Wu, J., Ross, J. R., Chiu, J. F., 2002. Reparable sonoporation generated by microstreaming. J Acoust Soc Am 111: 1460–1464.
14. Wu, J., 2002. Theoretical study on shear stress generated by microstreaming surrounding contrast agents attached to living cells. Ultrasound Med Biol 28: 125–129.
15. Miller, D. L., Dou, C., Song, J., 2003. DNA transfer and cell killing in epidermoid cells by diagnostic ultrasound activation of contrast agent gas bodies in vitro. Ultrasound Med Biol 29: 601–607.
16. Waehler, R., Russell, S. J., Curiel, D. T., 2007. Engineering targeted viral vectors for gene therapy. Nat Rev Genet 8: 573–587. Lehrman S., 1999. Virus treatment questioned after gene therapy death. Nature 401: 517–8.
17. Hartman, Z. C., Appledorn, D. M., Amalfitano, A., 2008. Adenovirus vector induced innate immune responses: Impact upon efficacy and toxicity in gene therapy and vaccine applications. Virus Res 132: 1–14.
18. Nayak, S., Herzog, R. W., 2010. Progress and prospects: Immune responses to viral vectors. Gene Ther 17: 295–304.
19. Vasir J. K., Reddy, M. K., Labhasetwar, V. D., 2005. Nanosystems in drug targeting: Opportunities and challenges. Curr Nanosci 1: 47–64.
20. Lassic, D. D., 1993. Liposomes: From Physics to Applications, Amsterdam, Elsevier Scientific Publishing Co.
21. Van Wamel, A. Bouakaz, A., Versluis, M., de Jong, N., 2004. Micromanipulation of endothelial cells: Ultrasound-microbubble-cell interaction. Ultrasound Med Biol 30: 1255–1258.
22. Tran, T. A., Roger, S., Le Guennec, J. Y., Tranquart, F., Bouakaz, A., 2005. Mechanisms of cell membrane permeabilization with ultrasound and contrast microbubbles. IEEE Ultrasonics Symposium: 5–8.
23. Wu, J. Shear stress in cells generated by ultrasound. Prog Biophy Mol Bio 2007; 93: 363–373.
24. Guzmán, H. Nguyen, D., Khan, S., Prausnitz, M., 2001. Ultrasound-mediated disruption of cell membranes. II. Heterogeneous effects on cells. J Acous Soc Am 110: 597–606.
25. Meijering, B., Juffermans, L., van Wamel, A., Henning, R., Zuhorn, I., Emmer, M., Versteilen, A., Paulus, W., van Gilst, W., Kooiman, K., de Jong, N., Musters, R., Deelman, L., Kamp, O., 2009. Ultrasound and microbubble-targeted delivery of macromolecules is regulated by induction of endocytosis and pore formation. Circ Res 104: 679–687.
26. Qiu, Y. Y., Luo, Y., Zhang, Y. L., Cui, W. C., Zhang, D., Wu, J., Zhang, J. F., Tu, J. A., 2010. The correlation between acoustic cavitation and sonoporation involved in ultrasound-mediated DNA transfection with polyethylenimine (PEI) in vitro. J Control Release 145: 40–48.
27. Reddy, A., Caler, E. V., Andrews, N. W., 2001. Plasma membrane repair is mediated by Ca2+-regulated exocytosis of lysosomes. Cell 106: 157–169.
28. McNeil, P. L., 2002. Repairing a torn cell surface: Make way, lysosomes to the rescue. J Cell Sci 115: 873–879.
29. McNeil, P. L., Kirchhausen, T., 2005. An emergency response team for membrane repair. Nat Rev Mol Cell Biol 6(6): 499–505.
30. Kumon, R. E., Parikh, P., Sabens, D., Aehle, M., Kourennyi, D., Deng, C. X., 2007. Ultrasound-induced calcium oscillations and waves in Chinese hamster ovary cells in the presence of microbubbles. Biophys J 93(6): L29–31.
31. Yang, F., Gu, N., Chen, D., Xi, X., Zhang, D., Li, Y., Wu, J., 2008. Experimental study on cell self-sealing during sonoporation. J Control Release 131: 205–210.
32. Deng, C. X., Sieling, F., Pan, H., Cui, J., 2004. Ultrasound-induced cell membrane porosity. Ultrasound Med Biol 30: 519–26.
33. Zhou, Y., Kumon, R., Cui, J., Deng, C. X., 2009, The size of sonoporation pores on the cell membrane. Ultrasound Med Biol 35: 1756–1760.

34. Lammertink, B. H. A., Bos, C., Deckers, R., Storm, G., Moonen, C. T. W., Escoffre, J-M., 2015. Sonochemotherapy: From bench to bedside (Review). Front Pharmacol 6(138): 1–17.
35. Duvshani-Eshet, M., Adam, D., Machluf, M., 2006. The effects of albumin-coated microbubbles in DNA delivery mediated by therapeutic ultrasound. J Control Release 112: 156–166.
36. Duvshani-Eshet, M., Machluf, M., 2007. Efficient transfection of tumours facilitated by long-term therapeutic ultrasound in combination with contrast agent: From in vitro to in vivo setting. Cancer Gene Ther 14: 306–315.
37. Alter, J., Sennoga, C. A., Lopes, D. M., Eckersley, R. J., Wells, D., 2009. Microbubble stability is a major determinant of the efficiency of ultrasound and microbubble mediated in vivo gene transfer. Ultrasound Med Biol 35: 976–984.
38. Fujii, H., Sun, Z., Li, S. H., Wu, J., Fazel, S., Weisel, R. D., Rakowski, H., Lindner, J., Li, R. K., 2009. Ultrasound-targeted gene delivery induces angiogenesis after a myocardial infarction in mice. J Am Coll Cardiol 2: 869–879.
39. Rahim, A. A., Taylor, S. L., Bush, N. L., ter Haar, G. R., Bamber, J. C., Porter, C. D., 2006. Spatial and acoustic pressure dependence of microbubble-mediated gene delivery targeted using focused ultrasound. J Gene Med 8: 1347–1357.
40. Xie, F., Matsunaga, T., Zutshi, R., Porter, T. R., 2009. Diagnostic ultrasound combined with glycoprotein IIb/IIIa-targeted microbubbles improves microvascular recovery after acute coronary thrombotic occlusions. Circulation 119: 1378–1385.
41. Czarnota, G. J., Karshafian, R., Burns, P. N., Wong, S., Mahrouki, A. A., Lee, J. W., Caissie, A., Tran, W., Kim, C., Furukawa, M., Wong, E., Giles, A., 2012. Tumour radiation response enhancement by acoustical stimulation of the vasculature. PNAS, online July 9, E2033–E2041.
42. Tachibana, K., Tachibana, S., 2007a. Emerging technologies using ultrasound for drug delivery, in Emerging Therapeutic Ultrasound, Wu, J., Nyborg, W. L., eds., Hackensack, NJ, World Scientific Co.
43. Culp, W. C., Porter, T. R., Lowery, J., Xie, F., Roberson, P. K., Marky, L., 2004. Intracranial clot lysis with intravenous microbubbles and transcranial ultrasound in swine. Stroke 35: 2407–2411.
44. Alexandrov, A. V., Mikulik, R., Ribo, M., Sharma, V. K., Lao, A. Y., Tsivgoulis, G., Sugg, R. M., Barreto, A., Sierzenski, P., Malkoff, M. D., Grotta, J. C., 2008. A Pilot randomized clinical safety study of sonothrombolysis augmentation with ultrasound-activated perflutren-lipid microspheres for acute ischemic stroke. Stroke 39: 1464–1469.
45. Molina, C. A., Barreto, A. D., Tsivgoulis, G., Sierzenski, P., Malkoff, M. D., Rubiera, M., Gonzales, N., Mikulik, R., Pate, G., Ostrem, J., Singleton, W., Manvelian, G., Unger, E. C., Grotta, J. C., Schellinger, P. D., Alexandrov, A. V., 2009. Transcranial ultrasound in clinical sonothrombolysis (TUCSON) trial. Ann Neurol 66: 28–38.
46. Heath, C. H., Sorace, A., Knowles, J., Rosenthal, E., Hoyt, K., 2012. Microbubble therapy enhances antitumour properties of cisplatin and cetuximab in vitro and in vivo. Otolaryngol Head Neck Surg 146: 938–945.
47. Sorace, A. G., Warram, J. M., Umphrey, H., Hoyt, K., 2012. Microbubble-mediated ultrasonic techniques for improved chemotherapeutic delivery in cancer. J Drug Target 20: 43–54.
48. Hynynen, K., 2008. Ultrasound for drug and gene delivery to the brain. Adv Drug Deliv Rev 60(10): 1209–17.
49. Samiotaki, G., Konofagou, E. E., 2013. Dependence of the reversibility of focused-ultrasound-induced blood–brain barrier opening on pressure and pulse length in vivo. IEEE Trans Ultrason Ferroelectr Freq Control 60(11): 2257–2265.
50. Leinenga, G., Götz, J., 2015. Scanning ultrasound removes amyloid-β and restores memory in an Alzheimer's disease mouse model. Sci Transl 7: 278ra33, DOI: 10.1126/scitranslmed.aaa2512.
51. Kotopoulis, S., Dimcevsk, G., Hoem, D., Postema, M., 2013. Treatment of human pancreatic cancer using combined ultrasound, microbubbles, and gemcitabine: A clinical case study. Med Phys 40(7): 072902-1-072902-9.
52. Chen, H., Hwang J. H., 2013. Ultrasound-targeted microbubble destruction for chemotherapeutic drug delivery to solid tumours. J Ther Ultrasound 2013 1: 10.
53. Mo, S., Coussios, C. C., Seymour, L., Carlisle, R. 2012. Ultrasound-enhanced drug delivery for cancer. Expert Opin Drug Deliv 9(12): 1525–38.
54. Udroiu, I., 2015. Ultrasonic drug delivery in oncology. J BUON 20(2): 381–90.

55. Waehler, R., Russell, S. J., Curiel, D. T., 2007. Engineering targeted viral vectors for gene therapy. Nat Rev Genet 8: 573–587.
56. Escoffre, J. M., Zeghimi, A., Novell, A., Bouakaz, A., 2013. In-vivo gene delivery by sonoporation: Recent progress and prospects. Curr Gene The 13(1): 2–14.
57. Delalande, A., Kotopoulis, S., Postema, M., Midoux, P., Pichon, C., 2013. Sonoporation: Mechanistic insights and ongoing challenges for gene transfer. Gene 525(2): 191–199.
58. Lentacker, I., De Cock, I., Deckers, R., De Smedt, S. C., Moonen, C. T. W., 2014. Understanding ultrasound induced sonoporation: Definitions and underlying mechanisms. J Control Release 72: 49–64.

23

Nano/Microbubble-Assisted Ultrasound for Drug Delivery in Cancer

Natalya Rapoport

23.1 Introduction

For many types of cancer, chemotherapy remains the main treatment of choice. However, conventional chemotherapy is associated with severe side effects, due to the deleterious effects of the chemotherapeutic drug on the normal tissues. During the last decade, progress in nanomedicine has enabled *tumour-targeted* delivery of anticancer drugs, which has decreased side effects, and increased their concentration in tumour tissue. Advances in nanotechnology have allowed the combination of various functionalities in molecular or supramolecular constructs, i.e. nanoparticles. The family of nanoparticles includes polymeric micelles, liposomes, nano- or microemulsion droplets, polymerosomes, hollow particles, etc. Various chemotherapeutic drugs, imaging agents and targeting moieties may be encapsulated in the same nanoparticle. Drug encapsulation in nanocarriers has a number of advantages. It may dramatically increase the effective aqueous solubility of highly potent compounds which had previously been abandoned due to their low solubility. Encapsulation also prevents or decreases drug degradation under the action of body fluids.

However, while being very beneficial for tumour targeting, drug encapsulation in nanoparticles also creates some problems. Penetration through biological barriers on the way to the target is more problematic for nanoparticle encapsulated drugs than for small naked drug molecules. Moreover, after reaching the site of action, the drug must be released from the carrier. These problems can be solved by developing stimuli responsive drug carriers. Triggering factors may be internal (i.e. pH, hypoxia, enzymatic degradation) or external physical stimuli, e.g. ultrasound or light.[1] The application of ultrasound for targeted drug delivery is discussed later, with special emphasis on the role of a triggered phase-shift transition inside injected nanoparticles.

Ultrasound has a number of advantages when compared to other physical methods used in tumour therapy. It has been widely used for decades as an imaging modality. During the last two decades therapeutic applications of ultrasound have evolved, with the development of tumour ablation techniques.[2–4] Ultrasound is the most cost effective and accessible energy source and does not use ionising radiation. It can be directed towards deeply located body sites, and tumour sonication with millimetric precision is feasible. Sonication may be performed non-invasively or minimally invasively using intraluminal, laparoscopic or percutaneous means. For extracorporeal sonication, the transducer is placed in contact with a water-based gel or a water layer on the skin, with no insertion or surgery being required. Ultrasound has both thermal (i.e. local heating of tissue to hyperthermic or ablative temperatures) and non-thermal mechanisms (i.e. cavitation and radiation force). These mechanisms are expected to work synergistically to trigger drug release from carriers, increase extravasation and internalisation of carrier and drug and increase drug diffusion in tumour tissue, which ultimately results in enhanced treatment outcome. Moreover, development of real-time imaging methods, such as magnetic resonance (MR) or ultrasound imaging, allows precise spatiotemporal control of focused ultrasound (FUS)-mediated drug delivery. Indeed, imaging assists in identification of the target, guidance of ultrasound action and evaluation of therapeutic efficacy. In addition, real-time temperature measurements during treatment using

DOI: 10.1201/9780429162671-23

MRI thermometry provide data that can be used in a feedback controller to enable greater control of the energy delivery.

An ideal drug carrier for ultrasound-mediated drug delivery should satisfy a number of requirements: stability in circulation; drug retention until activated; a size that allows extravasation through defective tumour vasculature; ultrasound responsiveness. Among various suggested drug carriers, three types, namely liposomes, polymeric micelles and emulsions, have been the most extensively studied and developed. These are spherical nanoparticles with a core-shell structure. All three carrier types can be made ultrasound-responsive. Liposomes have an aqueous internal compartment sequestered by a phospholipid shell, which allows encapsulation of water-soluble drugs in the inner core. Use of temperature-sensitive liposomes is discussed in detail in Chapter 25. Polymeric micelles are characterised by hydrophobic cores and hydrophilic shells; hydrophobic micelle cores serve as reservoirs of lipophilic drugs. These micelles are formed by amphiphilic block copolymers composed of hydrophobic and hydrophilic blocks; each block copolymer molecule spans both a core and a shell of a micelle. Use of micelles in ultrasound-mediated drug delivery (UMDD) has recently been reviewed in detail in ref. [5] Emulsions are the oldest drug carriers and have been used in clinical practice for decades; in emulsions, oil droplets are stabilised by ionic or non-ionic surfactants or surfactant mixtures; in contrast to polymeric micelles, oil droplets in emulsion form a separate phase and are usually substantially larger than micelle cores. The size of emulsion droplets may be reduced to a nanoscale by the application of external energy and selection of appropriate surfactants and co-surfactants. Nanoemulsions formed by perfluorocarbon compounds differ from other emulsions because of the high solubility of ambient gases. Perfluorocarbon nanoemulsions for use as ultrasound-responsive drug carriers are the main topic of the current chapter.

23.2 Physical Principles and Mechanisms

23.2.1 Achilles' Heels of Tumours: A Brief Overview

Tumours are usually highly heterogeneous structures, with necrotic cores and perfused shells. While the heat-induced ablation of a core is relatively effective, that of a shell is problematic since circulating blood carries the heat away. However, enhanced perfusion that hampers ablation favours drug delivery to the tumour periphery, which is an area of active tumour growth. As shown later, at non-ablative energies, ultrasound can enhance tumour-directed drug delivery and overall therapeutic response.

Tumour tissue is characterised by poorly organised vascular architecture, irregular blood flow and reduced lymphatic drainage. Leaky blood vessels and the lack of a lymphatic system result in an increased interstitial fluid pressure, which hinders convectional transport of drug carriers across blood vessel walls. Still, nanoparticles of appropriate size accumulate in tumour tissue via the enhanced permeability and retention (EPR) effect[6] because of the defective tumour microvasculature. A characteristic pore cutoff size range of 380–780 nm has been shown in a variety of tumours, although in some tumours this may be up to 2 μm. This allows extravasation of drug-loaded nanoparticles through large inter-endothelial gaps,[6–8] while the poor lymphatic drainage of tumours results in longer retention of extravasated particles in tumour tissue. In contrast to tumours, blood vessels in normal tissues have tight inter-endothelial junctions, which do not allow extravasation of nanoparticles (Figure 23.1). Effective tumour accumulation of nanoparticles via the EPR effect requires sufficient particle residence time in circulation. To provide for this, nanoparticles are commonly coated with poly(ethylene oxide) chains that decrease blood protein adsorption and particle recognition by the cells of the reticuloendothelial system.

23.2.2 Ultrasound as a Component of a Drug Delivery System: Mechanisms of Action

Several mechanisms of ultrasound action in drug delivery have been discussed[9–17]; both ultrasound-triggered localised drug release from carriers and effects of ultrasound on biological tissue should be considered.

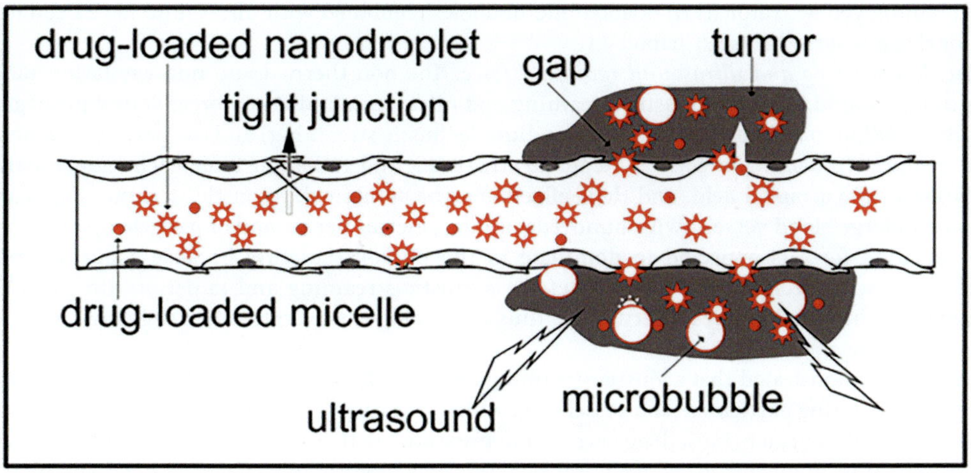

FIGURE 23.1 Schematic representation of the EPR effect. Nanoparticles cannot cross tight junctions in normal tissues, but extravasate into tumour tissue through large inter-endothelial gaps in the defective tumour microvasculature. Under the action of tumour-directed ultrasound, nanodroplets are converted into microbubbles.

Thermal effects. Ultrasound produces localised tissue heating. Tissue heating depends on its absorption of energy, and rates of thermal diffusion and convection. Absorption of ultrasound energy is frequency dependent and increases approximately monotonically with frequency.

Even a moderate temperature increase may have serious biological consequences, e.g. significantly increased permeability of blood capillaries[18–20] and/or lead to cell membrane fluidisation,[21, 22] which facilitates drug extravasation and internalisation. In addition, thermal effects of ultrasound may be used to release encapsulated drugs from temperature-sensitive carriers. Temperature-sensitive liposomes that rapidly release their contents at physiologically tolerated tissue temperatures have been developed.[10, 19, 23–34] Heating produces a gel-to-fluid phase transition in the phospholipid membrane that enhances release and diffusion of drug in the target region. Doxorubicin-loaded liposomes have been commercialised (ThermoDox, Celsion Corp.) and are undergoing clinical trials in combination with radiofrequency thermal ablation.[25, 35]

Mechanical effects (cavitation). Cavitation phenomena may exert substantial effects on biological tissues and drug carriers. Cavitation can be enhanced by the introduction of gas-filled microbubbles. In current clinical practice, microbubbles have been used as ultrasound contrast agents for cardiovascular imaging[36, 37] and for molecular imaging.[38] During the last decade, these bubbles have attracted attention as drug carriers and enhancers of drug and gene delivery. In the ultrasound pressure field, microbubbles grow and collapse in a process of inertial cavitation. This motion of microbubbles creates microjets and shock waves that can create holes in blood vessels and cell membranes (sonoporation), thus increasing the permeability of biological barriers for drugs, genes and their carriers. At ultrasound energies that do not induce inertial cavitation, microbubbles oscillate stably in the ultrasound field. Stable cavitation of systemically injected microbubbles can induce alternating invagination and distention of blood vessel walls, which, in turn, can cause damage to the endothelial lining, and temporarily increase blood vessel permeability.[39–42] For blood vessels that are large in comparison to microbubble sizes, invagination appears to be a major vessel damaging factor; for small blood capillaries, both invagination and distention result in endothelial damage and increased permeability.[40]

Several research groups have concentrated their efforts on developing microbubble-based drug delivery systems.[12, 43–45] The biological effects of microbubbles are based on the enhanced penetration of various nanoscaled particles or drugs through biological barriers.[46, 47] Microbubble cavitation has been used successfully for opening the blood-brain barrier to allow effective delivery of drugs to the brain[48–52] (see Chapter 26). Drug-loaded microbubbles have also been developed for targeting intravascular targets;

tissue plasminogen activator (tPA)–loaded microbubbles combined with ultrasound have been developed for thrombolysis [53–59] (see Chapter 24).

Acoustic streaming and ultrasound radiation force. The non-thermal and non-cavitation mechanisms of ultrasound relate to acoustic streaming and ultrasound radiation force. Sound propagating through a medium produces a force on the medium (acoustic streaming) and the particles suspended in the medium (radiation force).[60, 61] Acoustic streaming and radiation force each induce particle translation in the acoustic field, and their effects may be combined. Acoustic streaming appears to dominate in large blood vessels (with hundreds of micrometres per second of particle displacement), while radiation force is expected to dominate in the microvasculature because acoustic streaming decreases with decreasing vessel diameter.[61] Acoustic streaming and radiation force can push nanoparticles through blood capillary walls, thus enhancing extravasation of drug carriers or macromolecular drugs.[11, 60–64]

It has been demonstrated that acoustic streaming and/or radiation force provide a means of localising and concentrating particles near a vessel wall, which may assist the delivery of targeted agents. The radiation force pulses can bring a drug carrier into proximity with a cell, which can facilitate adhesion of the carrier or its fragments to cell membranes.[65] This may be especially effective for enhancing active targeting that is based on ligand/receptor interaction. Actively targeted acoustically active lipospheres were used to deliver paclitaxel (PTX) to HUVEC cells overexpressing $\alpha_v\beta_3$-integrins.[66] Circulating drug-loaded particles were first deflected by radiation force to a vessel wall and were subsequently fragmented by stronger pulses.[60] A similar strategy was used for enhancing the cellular interaction of targeted lipid-coated perfluorooctylbromide (PFOB) nanoparticles with melanoma cells.[67] The authors hypothesised that the ultrasound facilitated drug transport from the perfluorocarbon nanoparticles into cells due to direct cell/nanoparticle interactions that stimulated lipid exchange and drug delivery. In an interesting novel application, ultrasound radiation force has been used to modulate ligand exposure on the surface of actively targeted contrast agents.[68]

For perfluorocarbon microbubbles, the mismatch between acoustic impedances of water or tissue (1.4 MRayl) and perfluorocarbon (approx. 0.3 MRayl) may promote generation of shear stresses. This in turn would increase inter-endothelial gaps and extra-cellular spaces, resulting in increased extravasation and diffusion of drug carriers and drugs in sonicated tissues as will be exemplified later.[69–75]

For ultrasound-triggered localised drug delivery, carriers that are sensitive to either mechanical factors, thermal factors or both may be used.[5, 11, 61, 76–89] Ultimately, ultrasound affects both drug carriers and biological tissues. Effects on drug carriers are associated with triggered drug release. Effects on biological tissues are related to enhanced perfusion, increased extravasation of drug carriers and drugs, facilitated drug penetration through biological barriers, enhanced drug diffusion throughout tumour tissue and enhanced internalisation. Combined, these factors result in significantly enhanced conventional therapeutic outcomes (see later).[16, 46, 90–97]

23.2.3 Microbubbles as Drug Carriers for UMBB

The most straightforward and cost-effective way to develop ultrasound-responsive drug delivery systems would be to load drugs into Food and Drug Administration (FDA)–approved ultrasound contrast agents, such as Optison (Amersham, Inc.) or Definity (Lanteus Medical Imaging, Inc.). In principle, drug may be encapsulated within the carrier core, incorporated within the shell or a conventional (not ultrasound-responsive) nanoparticle may be attached to the microbubble surface.

Though drug delivery from micelles, liposomes or emulsions may be ultrasonically enhanced even without microbubbles,[1, 61, 83, 84, 98, 99] the presence of microbubbles dramatically increases intracellular uptake of drugs or genes.[43, 100–102] The use of microbubbles as drug carriers is very attractive because it can allow the combination of cost-effective ultrasound imaging with ultrasound-mediated therapy. Due to mismatch in acoustic impedance, both droplets and bubbles exhibit echogenic properties in biological tissue[103]; however bubbles have much higher echogenicity than droplets, thus creating better contrast in ultrasound images. Even more importantly, only bubbles undergo inertial cavitation (growth and collapse of bubbles in an ultrasound field), which concentrates ultrasound energy and substantially enhances ultrasound-mediated drug delivery.

Using drug-loaded microbubbles may be very beneficial for targeting intravascular targets. However, currently used ultrasound contrast agents present a number of inherent problems as *tumour-targeted* drug carriers. The very short circulation time (minutes) of commercially available microbubbles, and their large size (two to ten microns), do not allow effective extravasation into tumour tissue, thus preventing effective drug targeting. To solve this problem, drug-loaded nanoscaled microbubble precursors that accumulate in tumours via passive or active targeting have been developed. The microbubble precursors are perfluorocarbon (PFC) nanoemulsions. After tumour accumulation, they convert into microbubbles in situ under the action of ultrasound as discussed next.

23.2.4 Perfluorocarbon Nano-emulsions as Microbubble Precursors: Manufacture and Structure

Nano-emulsion droplets are spherical particles with hydrophobic cores made of oil; cores are stabilised with surfactants, forming droplet shells. Due to very low water solubility, PFC nano-emulsions are stable in circulation and biologically inert; for low boiling temperature PFCs, the in vivo excretion route is via the capillaries of lungs.[104, 105] Perfluorocarbon micro- and nanodroplets are manufactured by emulsification of a water/surfactant/perfluorocarbon mixture. In order to decrease droplet sizes, crude emulsions are usually additionally processed through a microfluidizer.[106]

23.2.4.1 Nano-emulsion Compositions

The composition of the shell is based on the type of a surfactant used; shell composition affects the droplet half-life in circulation and its acoustic properties. Various surfactants, perfluorocarbons and emulsification means have been explored.

Among surfactants, lipids, proteins and polymers have been the most investigated. In the studies by Fowlkes' group, dodecafluoropentane (also called perfluoropentane, PFP) was used as a droplet core, with albumin used as a droplet shell; emulsification was performed in a high-speed shaker.[103] In the work of Ferrara's group, PFC mixtures were used, with a lipid mixture used for droplet stabilisation.[61] Polymer-coated "nanocapsules" were prepared using perfluoro-octyl bromide (PFOB), with a poly(lactic-glycolic acid) (PLGA)copolymer used as a shell. PLGA was co-dissolved with PFOB in an organic solvent; the mixture was then pre-emulsified in a high-speed shaker and additionally emulsified by ultrasound; organic solvent was removed by evaporation.[107] For delivering water soluble compounds (e.g. fluorescein or thrombin), a double emulsion technique has been developed.[108]

A new approach for the generation of highly acoustically active perfluorocarbon droplets has recently been suggested.[109, 110] The authors formulated droplets from highly volatile decafluorobutane (DFB) (boiling point about −2 °C). Micrometre size droplets were generated from the condensed DFB gas by extrusion with a lipid formulation in HEPES buffer, thus generating nanoscaled droplets (200 nm to 300 nm diameter). Nanodroplets were stable at physiological temperatures, but were activated by ultrasound *in vivo* using pressures within the FDA guidelines for diagnostic imaging.[110] Acoustic characterisation of the PLGA-stabilised PFOB nanodroplets also suggested that vaporisation may be induced by diagnostic 7.5 MHz ultrasound at a mechanical index in the diagnostic range (MI <1).[107] Nanodroplet activation by the FDA-approved ultrasound energies is very important for the clinical translation of this technology.

A new approach to generation of drug-loaded PFC nanodroplets has been suggested by Rapoport's group. Drug-loaded polymeric micelles formed by amphiphilic block copolymers were used as a starting point for generating nanoemulsions.[15, 16, 95, 96, 101, 111, 112] Block copolymer micelles are formed by self-assembly of amphiphilic block copolymer molecules in aqueous milieu. The self-assembly occurs when copolymer concentration reaches some critical value called the critical micelle concentration (CMC). Below the CMC, block copolymer molecules exist in solution in the form of individual molecules (unimers). Manufacture simplicity, absence of toxic solvents and increased drug loading capacity are attractive features of this technology. In addition, amphiphilic block copolymer unimers (if they are preserved in a formulation) may exert extremely important biological effects by preventing development of drug resistance.[113–117]

To produce nanodroplets, a PFC compound was introduced into a micellar solution formed by an amphiphilic block copolymer. The mixture was emulsified on ice under low-frequency ultrasound. A chemotherapeutic drug (doxorubicin [DOX] or PTX) was pre-loaded into a micellar solution.[1, 14, 16, 101, 111]

These systems are extremely versatile. A large variation of perfluorocarbon compounds (and/or their mixtures) and amphiphilic block copolymers (and/or their mixtures) may be utilised. Any PFC compound or mixture may be emulsified into a nanoemulsion in this way.

In the work of the Rapoport's group, the PFC compounds tested were PFP and perfluoro-15-crown-5-ether (PFCE). PFCE has a high boiling temperature (146 °C) and generates more stable and easier to handle nanoemulsions than PFP (boiling temperature 29 °C, which is close to room temperature); in addition, PFCE offers a possibility of monitoring in vivo nanodroplet biodistribution using ^{19}F-MRI because the PFCE molecule has 20 equivalent fluorine nuclei that generate a sharp peak in MR spectra.

The amphiphilic block copolymers tested by the Rapoport's group were poly(ethylene oxide)-co-poly(L-lactide) (PEG-PLLA), poly(ethylene oxide)-co-poly(D,L-lactide) (PEG-PDLA), poly(ethylene oxide-co-polycaprolactone (PEG-PCL) or their mixtures.

23.2.4.2 Phase State of Block Copolymer Stabilised PFC Nanoemulsions

The phase diagram of the block copolymer stabilised PFC nanoemulsions is presented schematically in Figure 23.2. At low concentrations, PFC dissolves in micelle cores (Figure 23.2, zone 1). When the PFC concentration is increased to exceed a limit of solubility in micelle cores, nanodroplets evolve into a separate phase. In this process, a former micelle core turn into droplet shell. A nanodroplet shell contains two layers: the inner layer is formed by a hydrophobic block of a block copolymer (e.g. polylactide or polycaprolactone); the outer layer is formed by a hydrophilic block, usually PEG. The structure of a nanodroplet is shown schematically in Figure 23.3A. A lipophilic drug moves with the hydrophobic block of a block copolymer into the inner layer of a droplet shell. Figure 23.3B shows the laser confocal imaging of DOX encapsulating PFP droplets stabilised with PEG-PLLA block copolymer (Figure 23.3B).

In some ranges of PFC/copolymer concentration ratios, micelles coexist with nanodroplets (zone 2, Figure 23.2). As PFC concentration increases, all of the block copolymer is used for droplet stabilisation and micelles disappear; only droplets are observed in zone 3.

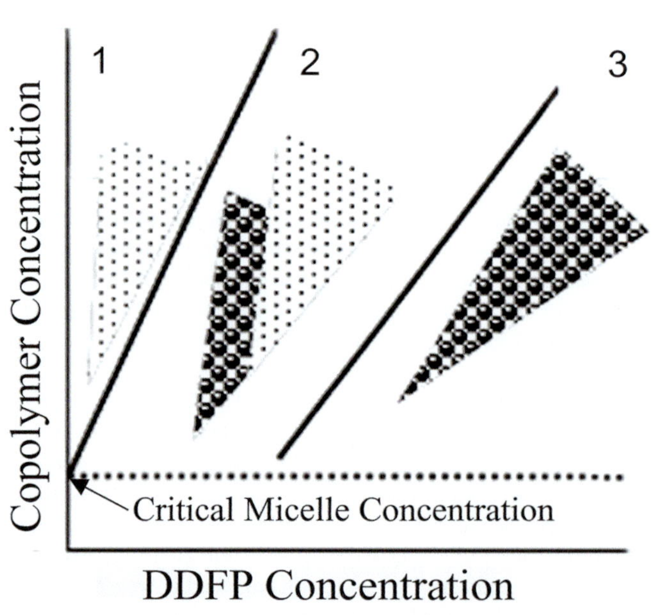

FIGURE 23.2 Schematic representation of the phase diagram of a PFC/block copolymer formulation in aqueous solution. Reprinted with permission from ref. [111]

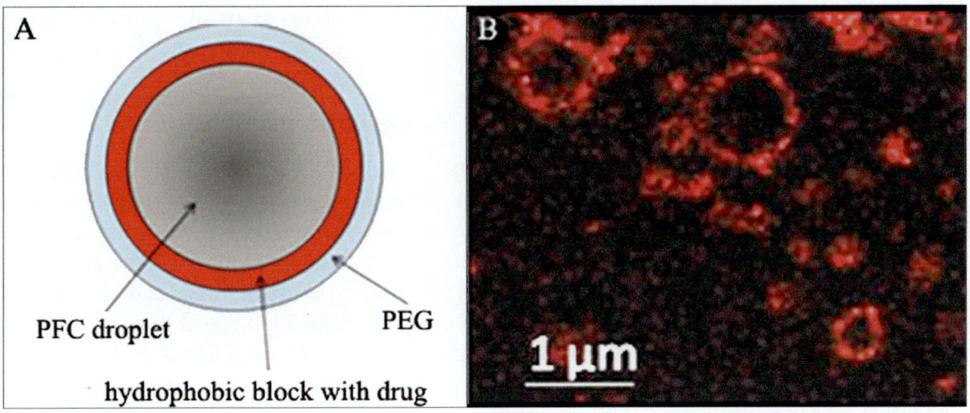

FIGURE 23.3 Schematic representation of a drug-loaded nanodroplet (A) and laser confocal image of DOX-loaded PFP/PEG-PLLA droplets; scale bar 1 μm (B); micron-sized droplets were produced to better visualise drug location on the droplet surface. Reprinted with permission from ref. [97]

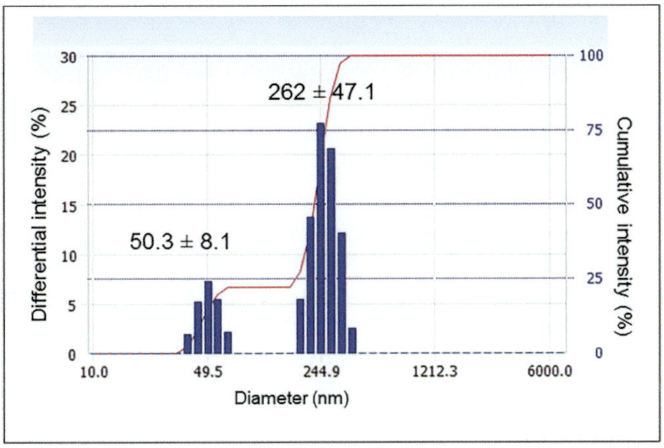

FIGURE 23.4 Particle size distribution in a 1% PECE/5% PEG-PDLA formulation (zone 2 of the phase diagram, see Figure 23.14); left peak – PEG-PDLA micelles with dissolved PFP; right peak – PFCE nanodroplets. Only one (micelle) peak would be observed in zone 3 (i.e. at higher PFP concentrations). Particle sizes in all zones depend on PFCE and PEG-PDLA concentrations and concentration ratios. Reprinted with permission from ref. [118]

The droplet size in PFC nanoemulsions ranges from 200 nm to 750 nm depending on the type of the stabilising copolymer, perfluorocarbon-to-copolymer concentration ratio and emulsification conditions.[111] An example of the size distribution for a 1%PFCE/5%PEG-PDLA formulation is presented in Figure 23.4, revealing coexisting micelles and nanodroplets (corresponding to zone 2 of the phase diagram).

23.2.5 Perfluorocarbon Nanoemulsions as Nano-scale Microbubble Precursors

Starting with the pioneering work of Apfel, it has been shown that perfluorocarbon droplets can be converted into microbubbles under ultrasound irradiation.[119] This effect, called acoustic droplet vaporisation (ADV), has been thoroughly investigated by the Fowlkes group,[103, 108, 120–129] the de Jong and Versluis' groups[106, 130–140] and Rapoport's group.[15, 16, 88, 89, 111, 112, 141] In medical applications, ADV has been tested for temporal and spatial control of tissue occlusion,[122, 123, 127] for cavitation nucleation in non-thermal ultrasound therapy,[128, 142] for enhancing gene transfer, for phase aberration correction[122] and for ultrasound-enhanced drug delivery.

23.2.5.1 Droplet-to-Bubble Transition in PFP Nanoemulsions: Mechanism

It has been found that micrometre-sized albumin-coated PFP droplets vaporised into gas bubbles with the application of short tone bursts in the diagnostic frequency range of 1.5 to 8 MHz.[103] The resulting bubbles were 20 to 80 μm in diameter. The threshold for vaporisation decreased with increasing ultrasound frequency and sonication time, and in the presence of microbubbles as nucleating agents.[103, 125] The vaporisation threshold was higher for smaller droplets.[121] These experiments were complemented with the optical imaging of the droplet-to-bubble transition using the ultra-high-speed imaging camera.[143]

Physico-chemical aspects of the PFP droplet vaporisation have been discussed by Rapoport et al.[15, 16, 112] PFP has a boiling temperature of 29 °C at atmospheric pressure and therefore has a high propensity for vaporisation under heating. However, for small droplets stabilised by elastic copolymer shells, the Laplace pressure (i.e. the pressure difference between the inside and outside of a droplet) may substantially increase boiling temperature. This effect is caused by the surface tension at the interface between a droplet and a bulk liquid. The Laplace pressure is given by

$$\Delta P = P_{inside} - P_{outside} = \frac{2\sigma}{r} \tag{23.1}$$

where P_{inside} is the pressure inside a droplet, P_{outside} is the pressure outside a droplet, σ is the surface tension and r is a droplet radius.

Excessive pressure inside a droplet results in an increase in PFP boiling temperature. This phenomenon has important consequences for drug delivery. Laplace pressure is inversely proportional to droplet size according to Eq. 23.1, meaning smaller droplets have higher boiling temperatures than larger droplets. The surface tension at the PFP/water interface for "naked" (i.e. not surfactant-coated) PFP droplets is 56 ± 1 mN/m. Using the known parameters of the Antoine equation for the pressure dependence of PFP vaporisation temperature,[144] the dependence of the PFP droplet vaporisation temperature on droplet size was calculated for two values of the interfacial tension (30 mN/m and 50 mN/m, which are typical values for PEG-coated colloid particles) [145] (Figure 23.5).[15] As indicated in Figure 23.5, the PFP boiling point in

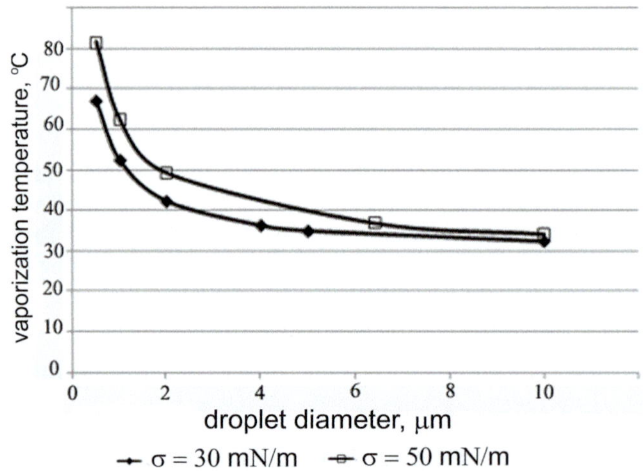

FIGURE 23.5 Dependence of the RFP boiling temperature in nanodroplets on droplet size calculated for two characteristic values of interfacial energy, 30 mN/m and 50 mN/m. Reprinted with permission from ref.[16]

droplets smaller than 4 μm is higher than normal physiological temperatures. These droplets remain in the liquid state at physiological temperatures, while droplets larger than 4 μm vaporise. Therefore, droplets larger than 4 μm should be excluded from pharmaceutical PFP emulsion formulations as they would prematurely vaporise upon systemic injection. The fact that micron-sized droplets would not extravasate is equally important. Hence, in Rapoport's studies, drug-loaded nanodroplets with an average size of 250 to 300 nm and relatively low polydispersity were prepared.[101, 111, 146, 147]

Upon complete PFP droplet vaporisation inside a copolymer wall, particle diameter increases 5-fold due to a 125-fold density difference between liquid and gaseous PFP phases.[101, 103, 111] Therefore, a 500-nm diameter droplet would generate a 2.5-μm bubble upon complete vaporisation. However, bubbles of much larger sizes were observed upon heating or ultrasound-induced PFP droplet vaporisation.[15, 16, 103, 125] These were secondary bubbles formed from primary 2.5-μm bubbles (Figure 23.6).

At least two different mechanisms of bubble growth beyond the size of primary bubbles may be considered: bubble coalescence with droplets or between themselves; i.e. diffusion of dissolved air and/or PFP from small bubbles into larger bubbles (i.e. Oswald ripening). Oswald ripening may also play a predominant role in gel or solid matrices, where droplet and bubble diffusion and collisions are restricted or stalled.

The increase of bubble size upon ultrasound-induced vaporisation was tested in embolotherapy. Experiments performed on the externalised rabbit kidney using albumin-coated PFP microdroplets with an initial diameter less than 6 μm showed more than a 70% perfusion reduction following ADV.[123] The authors hypothesised that this effect may be sufficient for cell death and possible for tumour treatment via ischemic necrosis. It was also suggested that radiofrequency ablation of tumours might also

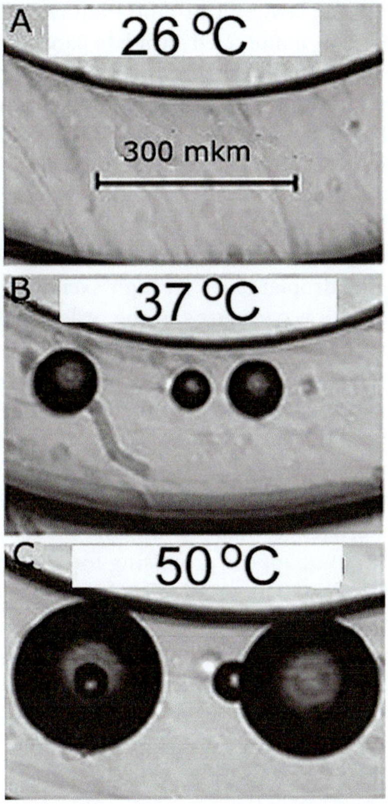

FIGURE 23.6 Bubble generation in the PFP nanodroplet suspension upon heating. At the microscope resolution used, nanodroplets are invisible in the initial suspension; bubbles appear and grow upon heating by coalescence with adjacent droplets/bubbles or due to Oswald ripening.

benefit from ADV due to reduced perfusion and heat loss. These experiments were later extended to externalised canine kidneys.[127] Substantial reduction of cortex perfusion was achieved in some cases.

To elucidate physical mechanisms behind acoustic vaporisation of PFP droplets, the relationship between ADV and inertial cavitation (IC) thresholds was studied.[120, 125, 148–150] Most of these experiments were performed with albumin- or lipid-coated microbubbles and showed that the ADV threshold was lower than the inertial cavitation threshold, indicating that the droplet-to-bubble transition preceded inertial cavitation. Measurements of the inertial cavitation threshold were performed for micrometre-sized albumin-shelled droplets containing various PFC cores, including those with higher boiling temperatures than that of PFP (i.e. perfluorohexane and perfluoromethylcyclohexane).[148] The authors found that inertial cavitation thresholds did not noticeably depend on perfluorocarbon molecular weights and boiling temperatures, and thus, the droplets did not need to be in a superheated state to be cavitated by ultrasound bursts. This was later confirmed in experiments with nanosized perfluoro-15-crown-5-ether (PFCE) droplets that effectively converted into bubbles at ultrasound pressures that were only slightly higher than those for PFP nanodroplets.[96] The mechanism of a droplet-to-bubble conversion with high boiling temperature perfluorocarbon compounds is most probably fundamentally different from true vaporisation (see later).

It was also found that nanometre-sized droplets containing a mixture of PFP and 2H,3H-perfluoropentane could be vaporised at diagnostic ultrasound frequencies (4 MHz to 7.8 MHz) and that the vaporisation threshold could be changed by altering relative concentrations of the two PFCs in the droplet.[151] The authors hypothesised that the vaporisation of a higher boiling temperature 2H,3H-perfluoropentane may have been caused not only by directly delivered ultrasound energy, but also by the energy deposited by ultrasonically induced PFP bubbles. Indeed, droplet-to-bubble transition in PFP nanodroplets was shown to be catalysed by pre-existing larger droplets or microbubbles. The catalytic effect was stronger and longer-ranging at lower ultrasound frequencies[15, 16] (Figure 23.7). This suggested that the droplet-to-bubble transition in nanoscaled droplets can be effectively catalysed not only by mixing PFCs of various boiling temperatures, but also by using a bimodal or broad droplet size distribution in initial formulations given that the conversion of larger droplets at lower power levels would catalyse droplet-to-bubble transition of smaller droplets.

Given that there is a large mismatch between the ultrasound wavelength and the droplet size, the detailed physical mechanisms for droplet vaporisation today remain elusive. A new mechanism has recently been proposed.[106, 138, 140] The authors concluded that droplet vaporisation is initiated by a combination of two phenomena: highly nonlinear distortion of the acoustic wave before it hits the droplet, and focusing of the distorted wave by the droplet itself. At high excitation pressures, nonlinear distortion causes significant superharmonics with wavelengths of the order of the droplet size. These superharmonics may strongly contribute to the focusing effect; therefore, this proposed mechanism also explains the observed pressure thresholding effect. This interpretation is validated with experimental data on the positions of the nucleation spots captured with an ultrahigh-speed camera; good agreement with the theoretical predictions was observed. The authors suggested a number of ways to decrease ultrasound pressure required for droplet vaporisation: to mix different liquids to vary the acoustic impedance; to use dual or multiple frequency transducers to optimise the amplitudes and phases of the transmitted waves for maximal constructive interference, thus maximising the focusing on the droplet.

The conclusions of the paper[140] did not appear promising for triggering the release of nanodroplet-loaded drugs into tumour interstitium using the ADV effect because nucleation of vaporisation strongly depended on droplet sizes and had a low probability for nanosized droplets. Small droplets would require higher ultrasound frequencies for vaporisation; the latter do not penetrate deep into the interior of the body due to enhanced attenuation. On the other hand, micron-sized droplets that require lower ultrasound frequencies for nucleation and have a higher probability of vaporisation would not extravasate. Despite these apparent issues, excellent therapeutic results were obtained with drug-loaded nanosized droplets and ultrasound (see Section 23.3). Note that droplet-to-bubble transition is not necessarily associated with true perfluorocarbon vaporisation as discussed in the next section.

Note of warning: Droplet-to-bubble transition in PFP nanoemulsions may be induced not only by ultrasound but also by shear stresses generated during injection through small-diameter (high-gauge)

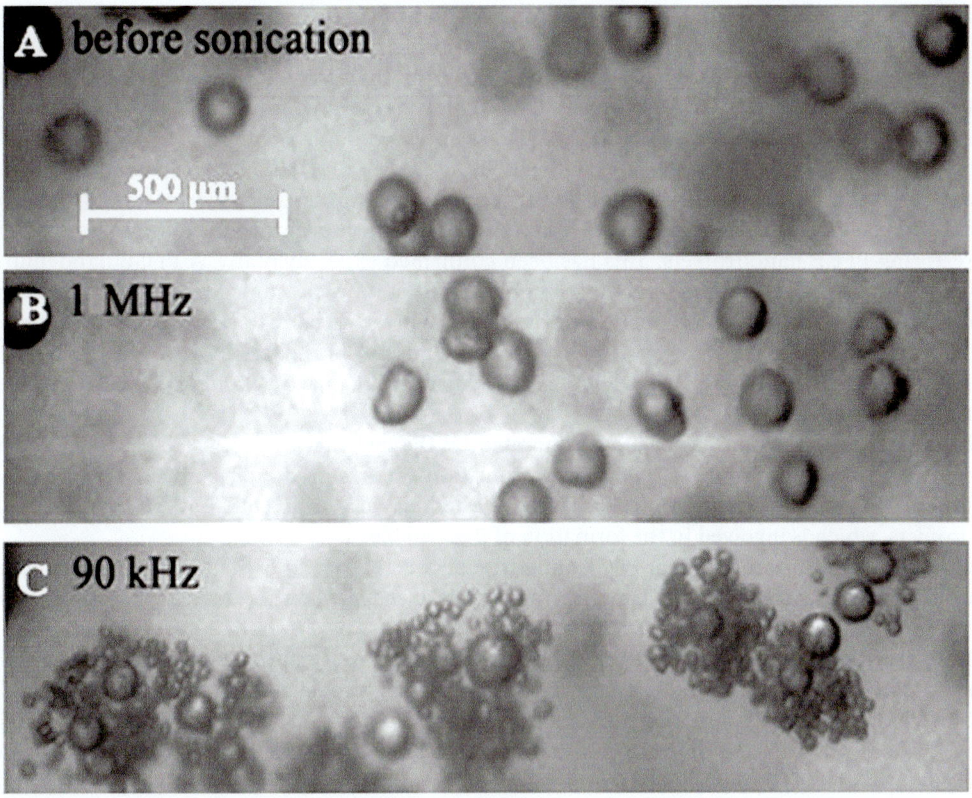

FIGURE 23.7 The catalytic effect of pre-existing microbubbles on the acoustic vaporisation of PFP nanodroplets inserted in the fibrin clot used as a tissue model. A – initial suspension of invisible tiny nanodroplets; B – after sonication with 1-MHz ultrasound; new bubbles are formed adjacent to pre-existing microbubbles; C – after sonication with 90-kHz ultrasound; new bubbles are formed and grow around pre-existing bubbles on much larger scale than at 1-MHz ultrasound. Reprinted with permission from ref.[16]

needles.[15, 16] Though some generation of microbubbles in the vascular bed may be beneficial for increasing ultrasound-induced vascular permeability,[39, 40, 42, 63, 152–155] massive transition of nanodroplets into microbubbles inside blood vessels should be avoided unless occlusion therapies have been considered. For safety reasons, PFP nanoemulsions should be injected either by infusion or through low-gauge needles.

23.2.6 Droplet-to-Bubble Transition in Perfluoro-15-Crown-5-Ether (PFCE) Nanoemulsions: Mechanism

PFCE has a much higher boiling temperature than PFP (146 °C at atmospheric pressure). However, initiating droplet-to-bubble transition in PFCE nanodroplets required only slightly higher ultrasound energies than those for PFP,[96] confirming the previously reported data.[148] The droplet-to-bubble transition in PFCE nanodroplets was induced by either continuous wave or pulsed ultrasound; the latter caused insignificant heating,[96] confirming that the mechanism of droplet-to-bubble transition in a PFCE nanoemulsion was non-thermal. A possible mechanism of ultrasound-induced droplet-to-bubble transition in PFCE has been suggested.[96] Perfluorocarbon emulsions differ from other emulsions by having very high gas solubility, particularly of oxygen. This feature has allowed the use of perfluorocarbon emulsions as blood substitutes.[156] According to Henry's law, the solubility of gases increases with pressure. It has been hypothesised that a pressure drop during a rarefactional phase of ultrasound led to the evolution of PFC-dissolved oxygen in a gas phase inside the nanodroplet shell, followed by rectified diffusion of dissolved gases from the surrounding liquid into the resulting nanobubble. According to this hypothesis, PFCE bubbles should predominantly contain a mixture of oxygen and other ambient gases, rather than PFCE vapour (though a bubble will also contain a low fraction of PFCE vapour in equilibrium with PFCE liquid phase). The bubbles formed this way are transient in nature; when the ultrasound is turned off, the equilibrium between nanodroplets and surrounding medium is restored; gases with super-equilibrium concentrations diffuse out of bubbles, thus restoring PFCE nanodroplets. This has been confirmed experimentally. A PFCE nanoemulsion was placed in a long test tube, but only the lower part of a test tube was sonicated. Bubbles that formed in the ultrasound field moved up due to buoyancy, but converted back to heavy droplets upon leaving the ultrasound field. On the way down towards the bottom of the test tube, droplets entered the ultrasound field and converted back to bubbles. Ultimately, nanoparticles "danced" at the border of the ultrasound field.

This proposed mechanism has been corroborated by the fact that degassing PFCE nanoemulsions inhibited the droplet-to-bubble transition; the transition was restored after contact with air was re-established. The bubble formation mechanism suggested above is different from true vaporisation of nanodroplets, which is involved in the formation of PFP bubbles.

Bubbles formed from either PFP or PFCE nanodroplets were shown to cavitate in the ultrasound field, as manifested by the generation of harmonic frequencies in the fast Fourier transform (FFT) spectra of the scattered ultrasound beam.[16, 96, 112] Stable cavitation was observed in both an aqueous environment and the agarose gel used as a tissue phantom (Figure 23.8A). However, broadband noise (thought to be characteristic of inertial cavitation) was not generated by PFCE droplets (Figure 23.8B).

Because biological effects are mediated by bubble cavitation, the exact mechanism of bubble generation is not as important as the very fact that bubbles are formed and cavitate. Cavitation of microbubbles formed via ADV of perfluorocarbon nanodroplets both in the liquid and gel phases supports expectations that drug-loaded PFC nanoemulsions combined with tumour-directed ultrasound would efficiently extravasate from the vasculature into tumour tissue and deliver drugs to tumour cells. In vivo studies described in the next section strongly sustained this assumption.

23.3 Preclinical Studies

23.3.1 In Vitro Studies of Ultrasound-Enhanced Drug Delivery to Cancerous Cells

On the way to its target, systemically injected drug has to overcome several biological barriers. The first barrier is the endothelial lining of blood vessels. Because drug targets are usually located in cell interiors, a second barrier is the plasma membrane (i.e. external membrane of the cell). Finally, if the target is located inside the cell nucleus, as it is for anthracycline chemotherapeutic drugs, nuclear membranes present the third barrier to successful therapy. In the ex vivo cellular experiments described later, the first barrier – the endothelial lining of vasculature – is absent. This is a clear shortcoming of these studies. However, plasma and nuclear membranes are present in cellular experiments. Therefore efficient killing of cancerous cells in cellular studies is the first step to successful therapy, upon which in vivo studies that involve drug extravasation, non-specific uptake by the liver or spleen etc. can be based.

Successful in vitro ultrasound-triggered delivery of PTX to monolayers of prostate cancer cells has been reported for a phospholipid-coated perfluorohexane nanoemulsion developed by ImaRx.[61] Promising in vitro results have also been obtained for delivery of a chemotherapeutic drug camptothecin to melanoma and ovarian cancer cells. Ultrasound-activated perfluorocarbon nanodroplets of diameters 220 to 420 nm were stabilised by phospholipids and/or Pluronic F68, and confocal laser scanning microscopy confirmed nanoemulsion uptake by the cells.[157] Albumin/soybean oil-coated PFP microdroplets were tested in vitro for the delivery of a lipophilic drug chlorambucil.[126] Application of ultrasound almost doubled cell killing by the drug.

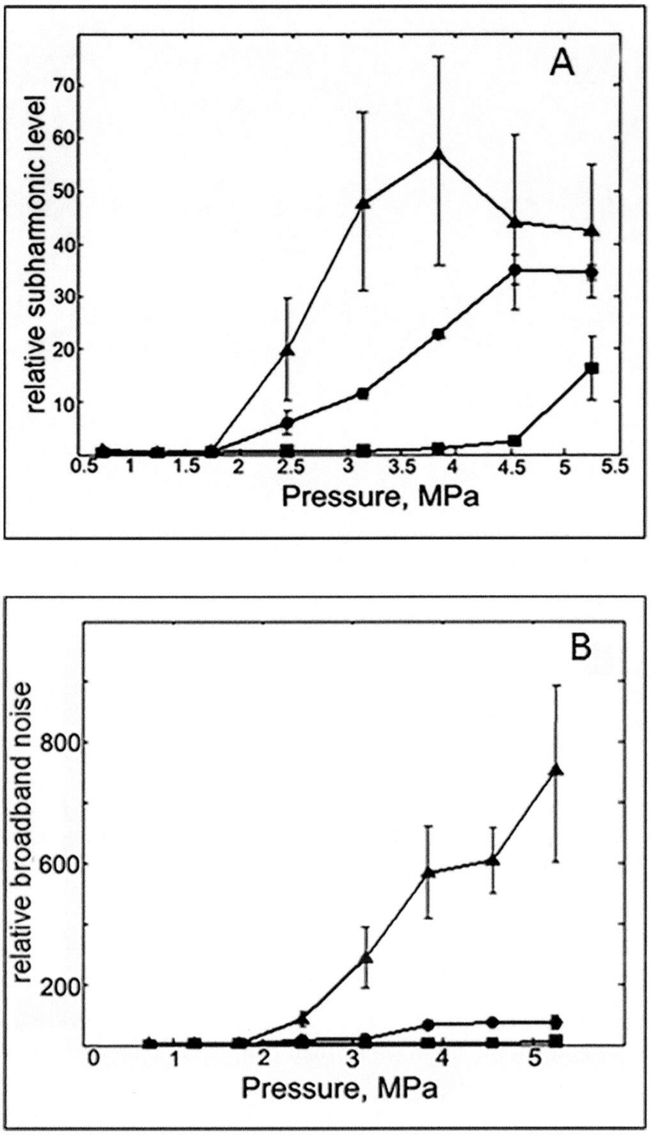

FIGURE 23.8 Relative subharmonic (A) and broadband noise (B) levels generated under the action of 1-MHz focused ultrasound (HIFU) at room temperature by PFP and PFCE nanodroplets inserted into 0.6% agarose gel. Nanodroplets were stabilised by a mixture of 0.25% PEG-PLAA/0.25% PEG-PCL copolymer. Triangles – PFP droplets; circles – PFCE droplets; squares – pure agarose gel. Reprinted with permission from ref.[96]

23.3.2 Ex Vivo Studies of Ultrasound-Enhanced Extravasation

The effect of ultrasound on the penetration of fluorescent PFCE nanodroplets through a vascular wall was studied ex vivo using mouse carotid arteries as model blood vessels[47, 64]; the near field of a1-MHz ultrasound beam dramatically enhanced nanodroplet penetration (Figure 23.9). At the same delivered ultrasound energy, the effect of continuous wave (CW) ultrasound (left panel) was much greater than that of pulsed ultrasound (right panel). Under the action of pulsed ultrasound, nanodroplets accumulated near the vessel wall but did not effectively penetrate through the wall. CW ultrasound efficiently

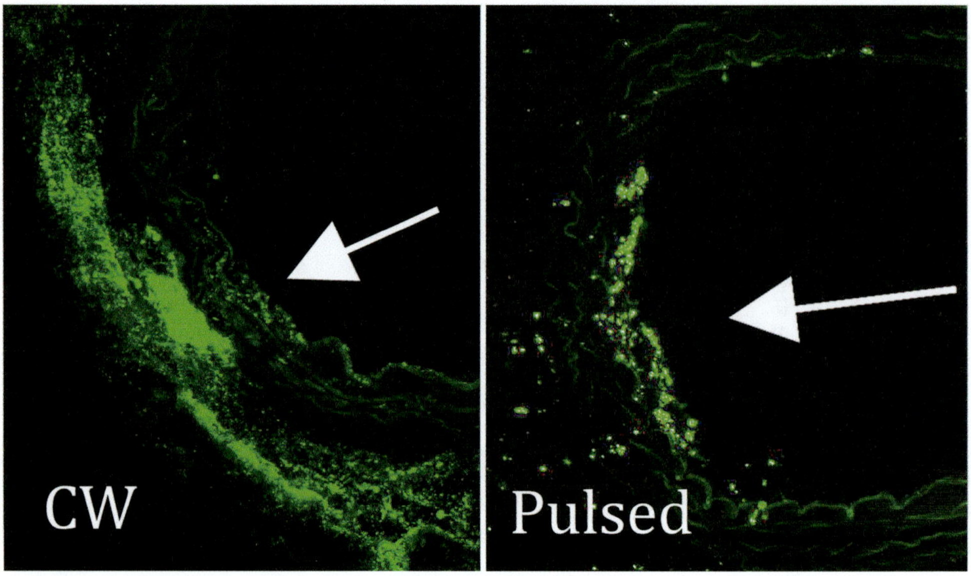

FIGURE 23.9 Fluorescence images of carotid arteries incubated with the fluorescent PFCE nanodroplets and irradiated with CW (left) or pulsed US (right). Arrows indicate anticipated direction of the ultrasound beam. Scale bar (0.1 mm) applies to both images. Reprinted with permission from ref.[64]

"pushed" droplets through the artery's wall. The effect of ultrasound was always directional, which implied that radiation force played an important role in enhancing nanodroplet extravasation, as was shown earlier for the extravasation of microbubbles.[11, 78]

23.3.3 Intravital Laser Fluorescence Microscopy of Nanodroplet Extravasation and Tissue Accumulation in Tumour-Bearing Live Mice

Intravital laser fluorescence microscopy of tumour-bearing mice confirmed that nanodroplets selectively extravasated into tumour tissue, upon which their conversion into microbubbles was triggered by tumour-directed ultrasound.[46]

Experiments were first performed with the microscope focused on the normal tissue of the subcutaneous muscle and adipose tissue in the mouse thigh (Figure 23.10A). The extravasation of the unimers (individual molecules with molecular weight about 2,000 Da) occurred extremely fast (Figure 23.10, B and C); 10 minutes after the arrival of fluorescently labelled particles to the thigh vasculature, blood vessels were empty, while the muscle tissue and adipose cells in the muscle were brightly fluorescent. The tissue fluorescence increased five-fold during the first 10 minutes after the injection. In contrast, the extravasation of PEG-PDLA stabilised PFCE nanodroplets into the normal tissue was extremely slow and vasculature fluorescence was maintained during an hour of observation (Figure 23.19 D and E); this is beneficial for tumour targeting.

Nanodroplet extravasation was much faster in the tumour than in muscle. In contrast to the muscle tissue where the vascular fluorescence was maintained during 60 minutes of observation, in the tumour, this dropped by 25% within 18 minutes of the formulation's arrival.

The fluorescence time curves for nanodroplets in vasculature and tumour tissue are presented in Figure 23.11. Vascular fluorescence decreased with time while tissue accumulation proceeded at a relatively constant rate. The total number of nanoparticles remained constant in the field of view during the period of observation.

Extravasation and tissue accumulation of nanodroplets was compared with those of the nanodroplet encapsulated drug (fluorescently labelled paclitaxel, F-PTX). A significantly faster vascular clearance

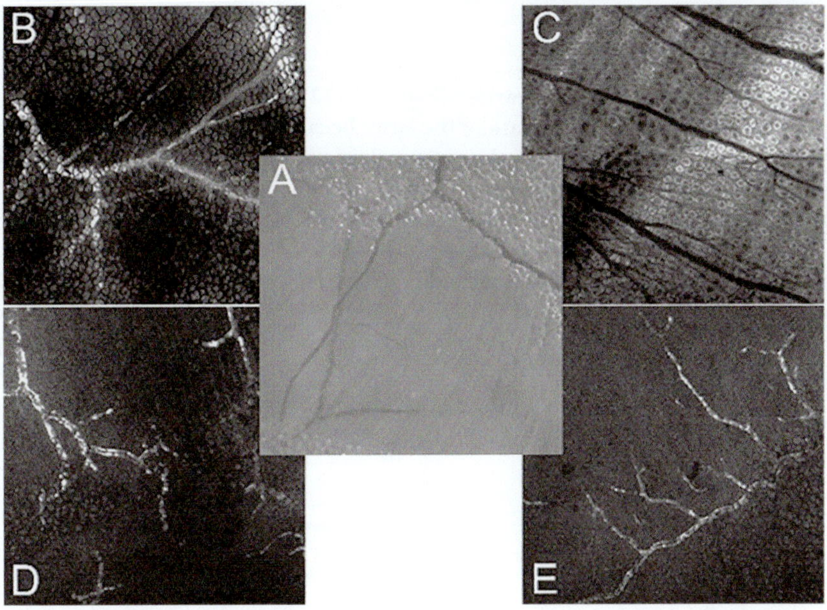

FIGURE 23.10 Bright field image of adipose and thigh muscle tissue (A). Extravasation of unimers (B – 0 min; C – 10 min after injection); vasculature lost fluorescence while tissue fluorescence increased during the first 10 minutes after injection. In contrast, for nanodroplets (D, E), blood vessel fluorescence was retained for an hour of observation (D – 30 min; E – 60 min). Reprinted with permission from ref.[46]

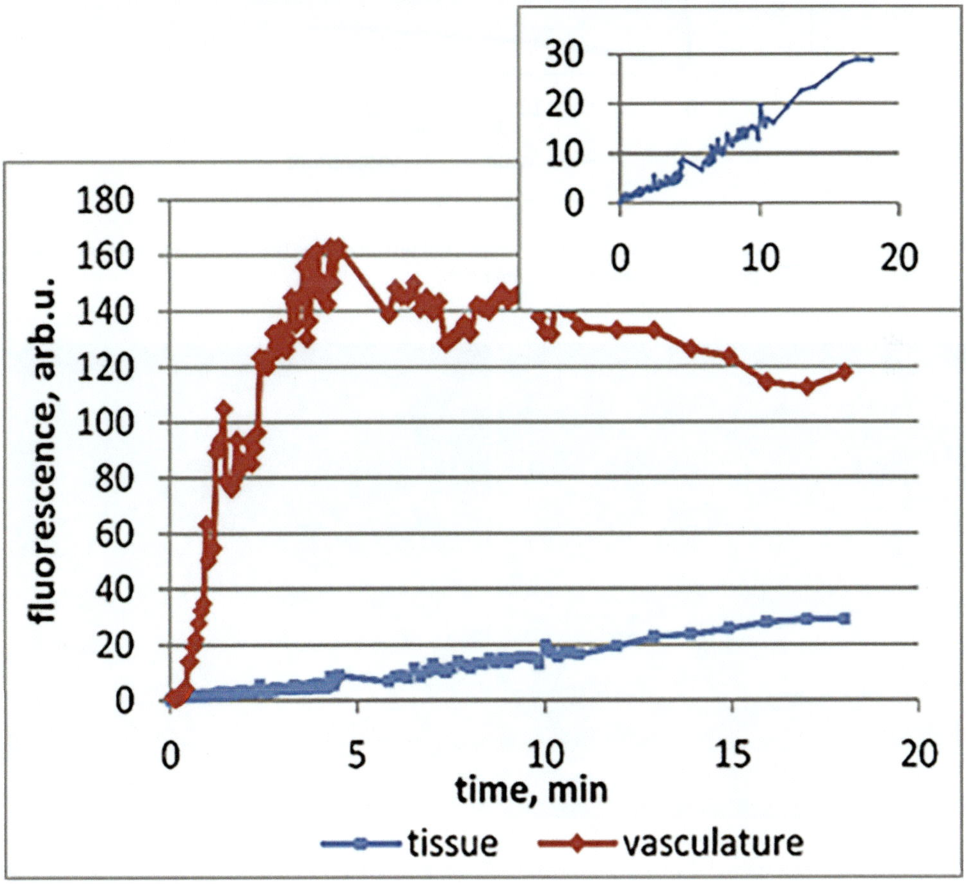

FIGURE 23.11 Nanodroplet time curves in the vasculature (rhombi) and tumour tissue (squares). Inset: magnification of the tissue accumulation curve. Reprinted with permission from ref. [46]

was observed for the drug than for the carrier (Figure 23.12); the initial vascular clearance was not associated with noticeable tissue accumulation; the latter became evident only later in the experiment. The fast vascular clearance of F-PTX pointed to a premature release of at least some fraction of the drug into the circulation.

The application of ultrasound accelerated the rate of nanodroplet extravasation 4.7-fold; following sonication, the fluorescence of blood vessels dropped, while that of adjacent tumour tissue increased and became more uniform (Figure 23.13); as an example, following ultrasound, the mean fluorescence of a selected blood vessel dropped from 165 to 126 arb.u. while that of the adjacent tissue increased from 47.7 to 69.1 arb. u. (as measured using ImageJ software). This is advantageous for the therapeutic applications of nanodroplets as drug carriers for UMDD.

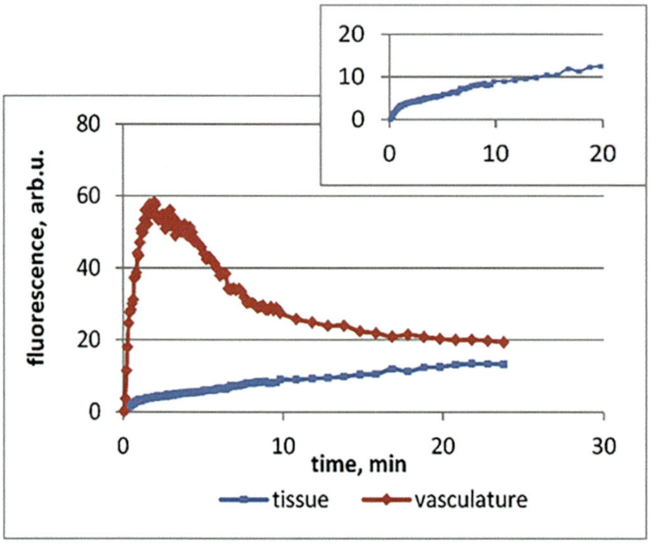

FIGURE 23.12 F-PTX time curves in the vasculature (rhombi) and tumour tissue (squares). Inset: a magnification of the tissue accumulation curve. Reprinted with permission from ref.[46]

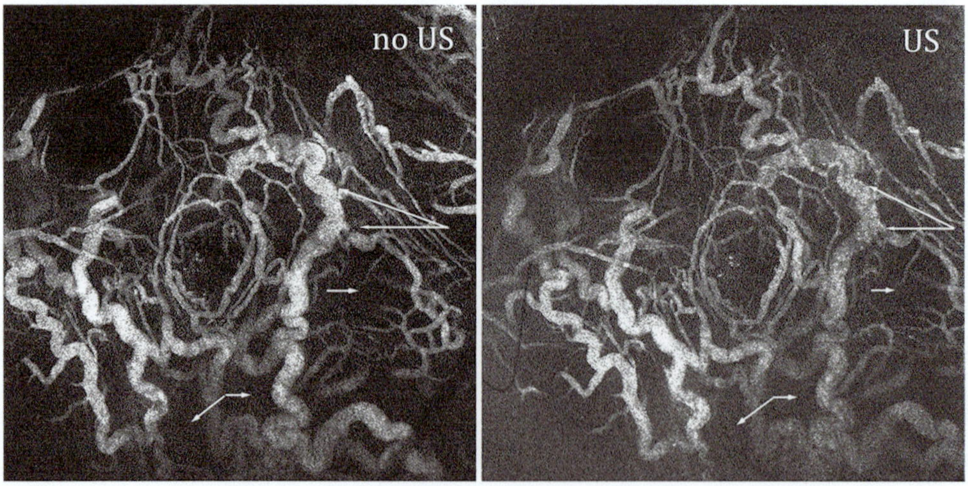

FIGURE 23.13 Effect of ultrasound on the extravasation of nanodroplets. Fluorescence micrographs were taken before (left panel) and 3 min after the application of ultrasound (right panel). Fluorescence of blood vessels dropped (long arrows) while that of the surrounding tissues increased (short arrows). Reprinted with permission from ref.[46]

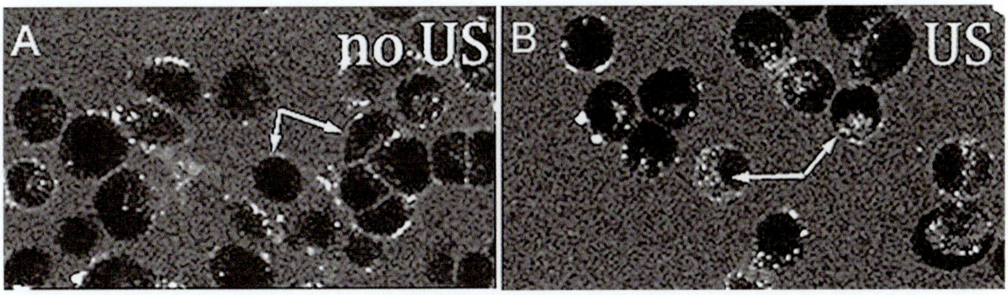

FIGURE 23.14 Scanning laser fluorescence micrographs of the nanodroplet internalisation by MiaPaCa2 pancreatic cancer cells. (A) – the internalisation was ineffective without ultrasound; even after a 24-h cell incubation, nanodroplets accumulated around the cells but were not internalised; arrows point to nanodroplets located on the cell surface; (B) – application of ultrasound dramatically enhanced nanodroplet internalisation; arrows point to internalised nanodroplets.

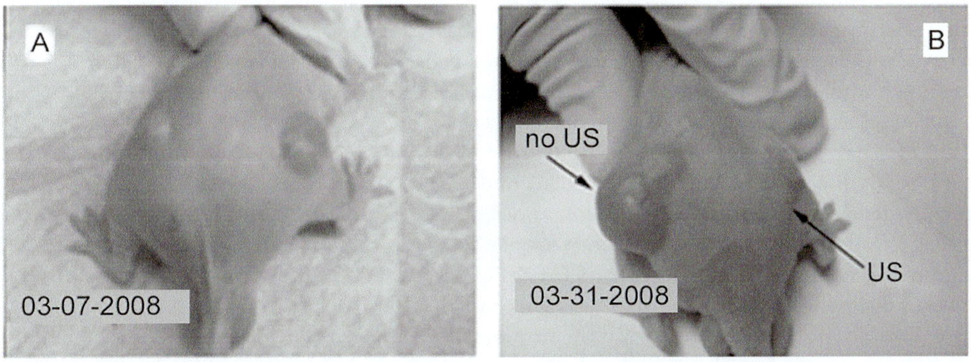

FIGURE 23.15 Photographs of a mouse bearing two ovarian carcinoma tumours (A) – immediately before and (B) – three weeks after the treatment; mouse treated by four systemic injections of nanodroplets encapsulating PTX (20 mg/kg as PTX) given twice weekly; the right tumour was sonicated by 1-MHz CW ultrasound (nominal output power density 3.4 W/cm^2, exposure duration 1 min) delivered 4h after the injection of the drug formulation. Ultrasound was delivered through a water bag coupled to a transducer and mouse skin by Aquasonic coupling gel. Reprinted with permission from ref.[16]

The ultrasound-induced droplet-to-bubble conversion occurred in vivo, which was confirmed by ultrasound imaging.[110, 158]

Moreover, ultrasound enhanced not only extravasation but also the intracellular uptake of nanodroplets by tumour cells (Figure 23.14).

In conclusion, the material presented here implies that drug-loaded nanodroplets accumulate in tumour tissue due to their nanoscale size, are effectively internalised by tumour cells under the action of tumour-directed ultrasound and undergo ultrasound-induced droplet-to-bubble transition in situ. These features make them attractive drug carriers for UMDD. Using this approach, successful therapy for a variety of cancerous tumours was achieved in pre-clinical studies as described next.

23.3.4 Therapeutic Outcomes of Ultrasound-Mediated Drug Delivery with Perfluorocarbon Nanoemulsions as Drug Carriers

23.3.4.1 Drug Retention in Nanodroplets in Vivo

To achieve efficient targeting, a nanocarrier should retain drug until externally triggered at a desired time and location in the body. In vivo, the drug PTX was shown to be tightly retained in PEG-PLLA stabilised PFP nanodroplets, as manifested by the experiments with bilateral ovarian carcinoma tumours (Figure 23.15).[16] A mouse was treated with four systemic injections of PTX-loaded nanodroplets

(20 mg/kg PTX) twice weekly for 2 weeks; only one tumour (right side) was sonicated by unfocused 1-MHz continuous wave (CW) ultrasound at a nominal output intensity of 3.4 W/cm^2 with an exposure duration of 1 min. The non-sonicated tumour (left side) grew at the same rate as control tumours, indicating that the drug did not reach this tumour in therapeutic concentrations. In contrast, the size of the sonicated tumour decreased dramatically, and the tumour appeared completely resolved after the treatment. This data suggested that without ultrasound, PTX was tightly retained by the PFP droplets but was effectively released under the action of tumour-directed therapeutic ultrasound. Tight drug retention by the nanodroplet carrier in vivo provides protection for healthy tissues, while effective ultrasound-induced localised drug release into the tumour, resulting in efficient tumour regression.

23.3.4.2 Therapeutic Effects of Combined Therapy with Nanodroplet-Encapsulated Drugs and Ultrasound

Very promising results on the therapeutic action of drug-loaded block copolymer stabilised PFP or PFCE nanoemulsions combined with 1- or 3-MHz ultrasound were obtained in experiments with breast and pancreatic tumours.[16, 96] Effective therapy of pancreatic ductal adenocarcinoma (PDA) is especially important because other treatment modalities tested for this devastating disease have so far proved ineffective. In these experiments, pancreatic tumour cells were transfected with red fluorescent protein to allow monitoring of tumour size and cell survival in orthotopically inoculated PDA tumours using intravital fluorescence imaging. In initial experiments, PTX was encapsulated in PEG-PLLA stabilised PFP nanodroplets. Tumours were treated with unfocused 1-MHz ultrasound.[16, 95] A significantly extended life span, decreased metastasis and ascites were observed. However, drug resistance was quickly developed during the treatment, and repeated treatments with the same regimens proved ineffective. In subsequent experiments, both droplet core and shells were replaced and focused 3-MHz ultrasound delivered under the MRI control (MRgFUS) was used.[96, 97] The temperature rise during treatment was monitored using MRI thermometry,[17] as shown schematically in Figure 23.16. The ultrasound beam was steered in a single plane within the tumour; hence the treated volume was much smaller than the whole tumour volume. The nanodroplet formulation included a core of PFCE (rather than PFP) and a less rigid block copolymer PEG-PDLA (rather than PEG-PLLA). As mentioned earlier, one of the advantages of using PFCE is that its molecule contains 20 equivalent fluorine nuclei that generate a sharp single resonance peak in ^{19}F magnetic resonance spectra,[159–161] which allows the use of ^{19}F MRI for monitoring nanodroplet biodistribution.[96] The PEG-PDLA stabilised PFCE formulation had a number of important improvements over the PFP/PEG-PLLA formulation used earlier. These were provided by both a different composition of the droplet core, and a different structure of the block copolymer that formed elastic rather than solid shells. Importantly, in these experiments, the development of drug resistance was prevented, presumably due to the action of PEG-PDLA unimers that were in equilibrium with the small fraction of PEG-PDLA micelles that was present in the formulation[97]; as shown in the

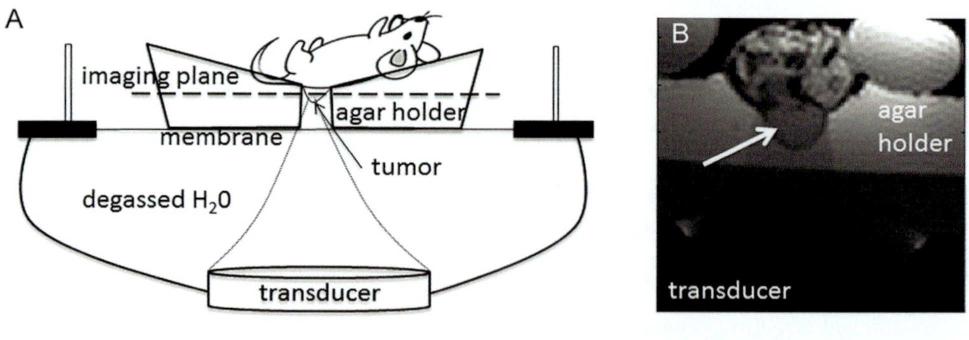

FIGURE 23.16 Schematic representation of mouse positioning on the small animal MRgFUS device. (A) An axial image of a mouse on the small animal MRgFUS device. (B) The white arrow indicates the tumour (initial size 455 mm^3). Reprinted with permission from ref.[118]

work of Kabanov's group, amphiphilic block copolymer unimers prevent the development of the drug resistance and sensitise drug-resistant cells.[114, 117, 162]

This study revealed a number of important factors involved in successful UMDD. (i) The time span between the drug injection and ultrasound application: Ultrasound irradiation before the drug injection or a short time (2 hours) after injection proved ineffective. It appears that efficient nanodroplet accumulation in the tumour before the application of ultrasound is a pre-requisite of successful therapy. It is possible that a large fraction of non-extravasated nanodroplets circulating in the vasculature scatter ultrasound, thus preventing effective tumour focusing. (ii) Ultrasound power level: For the experimental setting used in the study, optimal ultrasound pressure levels were between 3.4 and 4.2 MPa. Below and above the optimal ultrasound levels, the therapeutic effect was diminished; increasing ultrasound pressure above 4.6 MPa exerted a clear detrimental effect on tumour growth and animal survival. It is important to underline that the ultrasound power levels used in this study were always subablative.

Four mice treated with PTX-loaded PFCE/PEG-PDLA nanodroplets and MRgFUS with optimal ultrasound parameters, had their pancreatic tumours completely resolved after a single treatment and were long-term survivors. Another eight mice treated with optimal ultrasound parameters had their life span substantially extended compared with the treatment without ultrasound (Table 23.1).

Pulsed ultrasound had no positive effect on the tumour growth or mouse life span; the latter did not differ from that of mice treated with the same drug formulation without ultrasound (Table 23.1).

The treatment with empty droplets, with or without ultrasound, did not produce any positive effect; moreover, treatment with empty droplets combined with MRgFUS was detrimental when ultrasound pressure was increased above 4.6 MPa; tumour growth was accelerated and animal survival decreased.

These data indicate that the main therapeutic effect of the nanodroplet/ultrasound combination was caused by the drug, and not by ultrasound; even without ultrasound, treatment with PTX-loaded PFCE/PEG-PDLA nanodroplets considerably extended mouse life span (Table 23.1). Still, the application of ultrasound with optimal parameters significantly enhanced the action of the drug.

It is noteworthy that despite only a small fraction of the total tumour being treated by ultrasound, a significant delay in tumour growth was observed, which suggests that drug was effectively disseminated from the sonicated areas by enhanced convection or diffusion.

23.3.4.3 Possible Mechanisms of Combined Therapy with Nanodroplet-Encapsulated Drugs and Ultrasound

For lipid-coated nanodroplets, the mechanism of the ultrasound-enhanced therapy suggested by Lanza and Wicklin's group is based either on the enhanced molecular recognition of nanodroplets or the enhancement of droplet/cell contacts under the action of radiation force, which facilitates fusion between cell membranes and phospholipid-coated nanodroplets. This results in drug transfer from nanodroplets into the interior of the cells[67, 163–169]; the role of ultrasound radiation force in enhancing droplet or bubble contacts with cell surface was suggested earlier in works from Ferrara's group.[65, 68, 170, 171] This mechanism can be valid for lipid-coated particles but would be unlikely to pertain for block copolymer-stabilised

TABLE 23.1

Average mouse life span for various treatment parameters. MRgFUS was applied 8h after the drug injection. Reprinted with permission from ref.[118]

Treatment Group	Average Life Span, Weeks
Control	3.5 ± 0.5
No injection, MRgFUS (N = 6)	4.8 ± 2.3
Empty droplets, MRgFUS (N = 6)	3.5 ± 2.1
PTX droplets, no MRgFUS (N = 7)	7 ± 0.8
PTX droplets, MRgFUS CW (N = 8)	10.3 ± 1.6
PTX droplets, MRgFUS pulsed (N = 4)	6 ± 1.4

nanodroplets that expose protective PEG chains on their surfaces. An alternative mechanism has been proposed by Rapoport et al.[16] based on the ultrasound-induced droplet-to-bubble transition as presented schematically in Figure 23.17. Upon the droplet-to-bubble transition, the nanoparticle volume increases dramatically, while the thickness of the droplet shell, as well as block copolymer concentration on the particle surface, decreases correspondingly. This allows the drug to be "ripped off" the droplet surface under the ultrasound action. Drug transition from droplets to cells under the action of ultrasound has been observed in model experiments.[101]

23.4 Expert Commentary

The material presented here implies that ultrasound may exert both positive and negative effects on biological tissue. Positive effects may be related to ultrasound-enhanced drug carrier extravasation, ultrasound-triggered drug release from carrier, and enhanced nanocarrier and drug internalisation by tumour cells. On the other hand, vasodilation or vasoconstriction in response to ultrasound and especially to cavitating microbubbles may result in inflammation, oedema, haemorrhaging effects, etc. With empty microbubbles, these deleterious effects are not compensated for by the positive action of drug.

Tissue response to ultrasound-induced heating is also multifaceted. In the absence of drug, the response to sub-ablative heating may be negative due to enhanced perfusion that promotes tumour growth. In contrast, in the presence of drug, enhanced perfusion is a positive factor that promotes drug delivery to tumour tissue. In addition, hyperthermia increases vascular wall and plasma membrane permeability, thus increasing drug internalisation by a tumour cell. The ultimate biological response to ultrasound presumably depends on the prevalence of positive or negative factors, which is expected to depend on the treatment protocol.

Taken together, these results suggest that drug-loaded perfluorocarbon nanoemulsion in combination with optimal protocols of ultrasound treatment can provide an efficient therapy for a broad spectrum of diseases. An important additional advantage of these systems is the opportunity to monitor their location and distribution in the body using ultrasound and/or MR imaging.[95, 101, 163, 172–175]

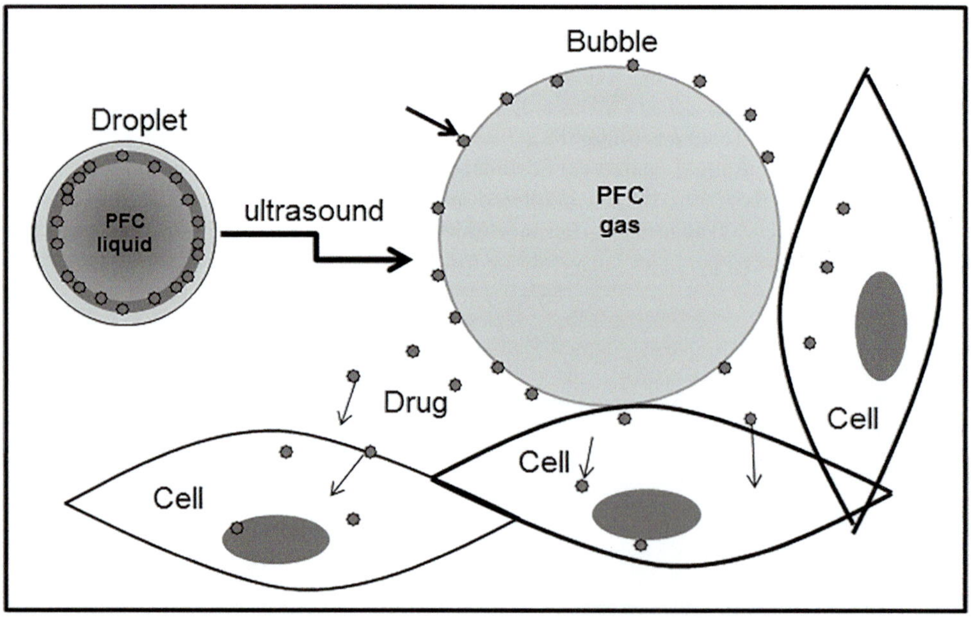

FIGURE 23.17 Schematic representation of the mechanism of drug release from a perfluorocarbon nanodroplet triggered by ultrasound-induced phase shift. Reprinted with permission from ref.[16]

23.5 Conclusions and Future Prospects

Targeted drug delivery has been a goal of the bioengineering community ever since the "magic bullet" concept was introduced by Paul Ehrlich over a century ago. During the last two decades, this formerly elusive goal has been turning into medical reality. The unprecedented opportunity to localise drug delivery is associated with developing stimuli responsive drug carriers, particularly ultrasound-responsive phase-shift perfluorocarbon nanoemulsions. Their important properties combine simple manufacturing, drug carrying, tumour-targeting, enhancing intracellular drug delivery and enhancing the ultrasound contrast of tumours. This novel technology has demonstrated excellent therapeutic potential in murine cancer models.

Much preclinical work remains to be done before the introduction of phase-shift nanoparticles into clinical practice. Transition to experiments in larger animal models is a critical task. Passive targeting of nanoparticles may prove more challenging in larger animals (and humans) than in small animal models due to much smaller tumour-to-body volume ratio in larger animals. Actively targeted phase-shift nanoemulsions may be required for efficient tumour accumulation. For this, identifying selective surface receptors on tumour cells is a crucial task.

The current nanoemulsions described here appear to lose some fraction of encapsulated drug into the circulation. Development of formulations with tighter drug retention is needed for increasing tumour-targeting efficiency. More research needs to be carried out on biodistribution and pharmacokinetics of components in nanoemulsion formulations, tracking delivery systems in the body, guidance of therapy, monitoring of immediate and delayed therapeutic responses, as well as optimisation of ultrasound parameters and time of ultrasound application. These problems remain to be addressed in future translational studies.

REFERENCES

1. Rapoport N. Physical stimuli-responsive polymeric micelles for anti-cancer drug delivery. *Prog Polym Sci.* 2007;32:962–990.
2. Manthe RL, Foy SP, Krishnamurthy N, Sharma B, Labhasetwar V. Tumour ablation and nanotechnology. *Mol Pharm.* Dec 6 2010;7(6):1880–1898.
3. McWilliams JP, Lee EW, Yamamoto S, Loh CT, Kee ST. Image-guided tumour ablation: Emerging technologies and future directions. *Semin Interv Radiol.* Sep 2010;27(3):302–313.
4. Lubner MG, Brace CL, Hinshaw JL, Lee FT, Jr. Microwave tumour ablation: Mechanism of action, clinical results, and devices. *J Vasc Interv Radiol.* Aug 2010;21(8 Suppl):S192–203.
5. Rapoport N. Ultrasound-mediated micellar drug delivery. *Int J Hyperthermia.* 2012;28(4):374–385.
6. Iyer AK, Khaled G, Fang J, Maeda H. Exploiting the enhanced permeability and retention effect for tumour targeting. *Drug Discov Today.* Sep 2006;11(17–18):812–818.
7. Campbell RB. Tumour physiology and delivery of nanopharmaceuticals. *Anticancer Agents Med Chem.* Nov 2006;6(6):503–512.
8. Hobbs SK, Monsky WL, Yuan F, et al. Regulation of transport pathways in tumour vessels: Role of tumour type and microenvironment. *Proc Natl Acad Sci USA.* Apr 14 1998;95(8):4607–4612.
9. Dalecki D. Mechanical bioeffects of ultrasound. *Annu Rev Biomed Eng.* 2004;6:229–248.
10. Deckers R, Moonen CT. Ultrasound triggered, image guided, local drug delivery. *J Control Release.* Aug 12 2010;148(1):25–33.
11. Ferrara KW. Driving delivery vehicles with ultrasound. *Advan Drug Deliv Rev.* Jun 30 2008;60(10):1097–1102.
12. Frulio N, Trillaud H, Deckers R, Lepreux S, Moonen C, Quesson B. Influence of ultrasound induced cavitation on magnetic resonance imaging contrast in the rat liver in the presence of macromolecular contrast agent. *Invest Radiol.* May 2010;45(5):282–287.
13. Miller MW, Miller DL, Brayman AA. A review of in vitro bioeffects of inertial ultrasonic cavitation from a mechanistic perspective. *Ultrasound Med Biol.* 1996;22(9):1131–1154.
14. Rapoport N, Nam KH, Gupta R, et al. Ultrasound-mediated tumour imaging and nanotherapy using drug loaded, block copolymer stabilized perfluorocarbon nanoemulsions. *J Control Release.* Jul 15 2011;153(1):4–15.

15. Rapoport NY, Efros AL, Christensen DA, Kennedy AM, Nam KH. Microbubble generation in phase-shift nanoemulsions used as anticancer drug carriers. *Bub Sci Eng Tech.* 2009;1(1–2):31–39.
16. Rapoport NY, Kennedy AM, Shea JE, Scaife CL, Nam K-H. Controlled and targeted tumour chemotherapy by ultrasound-activated nanoemulsions/microbubbles. *J Control Release.* Sep 2009;138(3):268–276.
17. Rapoport N, Payne A, Dillon C, Shea J, Scaife C, Gupta R. Focused ultrasound-mediated drug delivery to pancreatic cancer in a mouse model. *J Ther Ultrasound* 2013;1.
18. Dreher MR, Liu W, Michelich CR, Dewhirst MW, Yuan F, Chilkoti A. Tumour vascular permeability, accumulation, and penetration of macromolecular drug carriers. *J Natl Cancer Inst.* Mar 1 2006;98(5):335–344.
19. Kong G, Braun RD, Dewhirst MW. Hyperthermia enables tumour-specific nanoparticle delivery: Effect of particle size. *Cancer Res.* 2000;60(16):4440–4445.
20. Kong G, Braun RD, Dewhirst MW. Characterization of the effect of hyperthermia on nanoparticle extravasation from tumour vasculature. *Cancer Res.* 2001;61(7):3027–3032.
21. Hayat H, Friedberg I. Heat-induced alterations in cell membrane permeability and cell inactivation of transformed mouse fibroblasts. *Int J Hyperthermia.* 1986;2(4):369–378.
22. Krupka T, Dremann D, Exner A. Time and dose dependence of pluronic bioactivity in hyperthermia-induced tumour cell death. *Exp Biol Med (Maywood).* 2009;234(1):95–104.
23. Dewhirst MW, Vujaskovic Z, Jones E, Thrall D. Re-setting the biologic rationale for thermal therapy. *Int J Hyperthermia.* Dec 2005;21(8):779–790.
24. Gaber MH, Wu NZ, Hong K, Huang SK, Dewhirst MW, Papahadjopoulos D. Thermosensitive liposomes: Extravasation and release of contents in tumour microvascular networks. *Int J Radiat Oncol Biol Phys.* Dec 1 1996;36(5):1177–1187.
25. Hauck ML, LaRue SM, Petros WP, et al. Phase I trial of doxorubicin-containing low temperature sensitive liposomes in spontaneous canine tumours. *Clin Cancer Res.* Jul 2006;12(13):4004–4010.
26. Kong G, Anyarambhatla G, Petros WP, et al. Efficacy of liposomes and hyperthermia in a human tumour xenograft model: Importance of triggered drug release. *Cancer Res.* Dec 2000;60(24):6950–6957.
27. Kong G, Dewhirst MW. Hyperthermia and liposomes. *Int J Hyperthermia.* Sep–Oct 1999;15(5):345–370.
28. Needham D, Anyarambhatla G, Kong G, Dewhirst MW. A new temperature-sensitive liposome for use with mild hyperthermia: Characterization and testing in a human tumour xenograft model. *Cancer Res.* Mar 1 2000;60(5):1197–1201.
29. Negussie AH, Yarmolenko PS, Partanen A, et al. Formulation and characterisation of magnetic resonance imageable thermally sensitive liposomes for use with magnetic resonance-guided high intensity focused ultrasound. *Int J Hyperthermia.* 2011;27(2):140–155.
30. Vujaskovic Z, Kim DW, Jones E, et al. A phase I/II study of neoadjuvant liposomal doxorubicin, paclitaxel, and hyperthermia in locally advanced breast cancer. *Int J Hyperthermia.* 2010;26(5):514–521.
31. Yarmolenko PS, Zhao Y, Landon C, et al. Comparative effects of thermosensitive doxorubicin-containing liposomes and hyperthermia in human and murine tumours. *Int J Hyperthermia.* 2010;26(5):485–498.
32. Dromi S, Frenkel V, Luk A, et al. Pulsed-high intensity focused ultrasound and low temperature-sensitive liposomes for enhanced targeted drug delivery and antitumour effect. *Clin Cancer Res.* May 1 2007;13(9):2722–2727.
33. Stone MJ, Frenkel V, Dromi S, et al. Pulsed-high intensity focused ultrasound enhanced tPA mediated thrombolysis in a novel in vivo clot model, a pilot study. *Thromb Res.* 2007;121(2):193–202.
34. Staruch R, Chopra R, Hynynen K. Localised drug release using MRI-controlled focused ultrasound hyperthermia. *Int J Hyperthermia.* 2011;27(2):156–171.
35. Poon RTP, Borys N. Lyso-thermosensitive liposomal doxorubicin: A novel approach to enhance efficacy of thermal ablation of liver cancer. *Expert Opin Pharmacother.* February 2009;10(2):333–343.
36. Becher H, Burns PN. *Handbook for contrast echocardiograqphy.* Frankfurt and New York: Springer Verlag; 2000.
37. Becher H, Lofiego C, Mitchell A, Timperley J. Current indications for contrast echocardiography imaging. *Eur J Echocardiogr.* Dec 2005;6 Suppl 2:S1–5.
38. Klibanov AL. Ultrasound molecular imaging with targeted microbubble contrast agents. *J Nucl Cardiol.* Nov–Dec 2007;14(6):876–884.
39. Chen H, Brayman AA, Bailey MR, Matula TJ. Blood vessel rupture by cavitation. *Urol Res.* Aug 2010;38(4):321–326.

40. Chen H, Kreider W, Brayman AA, Bailey MR, Matula TJ. Blood vessel deformations on microsecond time scales by ultrasonic cavitation. *Phys Rev Lett.* Jan 21 2011;106(3):034301.
41. Gaitan DF, Tessien RA, Hiller RA, et al. Transient cavitation in high-quality-factor resonators at high static pressures. *J Acoust Soc Am.* Jun 2010;127(6):3456–3465.
42. Matula T, Guan J. Using optical scattering to measure properties of ultrasound contrast agent shells. *J Acoust Soc Am.* Mar 2011;129(3):1675.
43. Hernot S, Klibanov AL. Microbubbles in ultrasound-triggered drug and gene delivery. *Advanced drug delivery reviews.* Jun 30 2008;60(10):1153–1166.
44. Klibanov AL, Shevchenko TI, Raju BI, Seip R, Chin CT. Ultrasound-triggered release of materials entrapped in microbubble-liposome constructs: A tool for targeted drug delivery. *J Control Release.* Aug 4 2010;148(1):13–17.
45. Burke CW, Klibanov AL, Sheehan JP, Price RJ. Inhibition of glioma growth by microbubble activation in a subcutaneous model using low duty cycle ultrasound without significant heating. *J Neurosurg.* Jan 7 2011;114(6):1654–1661.
46. Rapoport N, Gupta R, Kim YS, O'Neill BE. Polymeric micelles and nanoemulsions as tumour-targeted drug carriers: Insight through intravital imaging. *J Control Release.* May 28 2015;206:153–160.
47. Thakkar D, Gupta R, Mohan P, Monson K, Rapoport N. Overcoming biological barriers with ultrasound. *AIP Conf Proc.* Jan 1 2012;1481:381–387.
48. Aryal M, Arvanitis CD, Alexander PM, McDannold N. Ultrasound-mediated blood-brain barrier disruption for targeted drug delivery in the central nervous system. *Advan Drug Deliv Rev.* Jun 15 2014;72C:94–109.
49. Hynynen K, McDannold N, Sheikov NA, Jolesz FA, Vykhodtseva N. Local and reversible blood-brain barrier disruption by noninvasive focused ultrasound at frequencies suitable for trans-skull sonications. *Neuroimage.* Jan 1 2005;24(1):12–20.
50. Hynynen K, McDannold N, Vykhodtseva N, et al. Focal disruption of the blood-brain barrier due to 260-kHz ultrasound bursts: A method for molecular imaging and targeted drug delivery. *J Neurosurg.* Sep 2006;105(3):445–454.
51. McDannold N, Arvanitis CD, Vykhodtseva N, Livingstone MS. Temporary disruption of the blood-brain barrier by use of ultrasound and microbubbles: Safety and efficacy evaluation in rhesus macaques. *Cancer Res.* Jul 15 2012;72(14):3652–3663.
52. Park J, Zhang Y, Vykhodtseva N, Jolesz FA, McDannold NJ. The kinetics of blood brain barrier permeability and targeted doxorubicin delivery into brain induced by focused ultrasound. *J Control Release.* Aug 20 2012;162(1):134–142.
53. Sutton JT, Ivancevich NM, Perrin SR, Jr., Vela DC, Holland CK. Clot retraction affects the extent of ultrasound-enhanced thrombolysis in an ex vivo porcine thrombosis model. *Ultrasound Med Biol.* May 2013;39(5):813–824.
54. Sutton JT, Haworth KJ, Pyne-Geithman G, Holland CK. Ultrasound-mediated drug delivery for cardiovascular disease. *Expert Opin Drug Deliv.* May 2013;10(5):573–592.
55. Hitchcock KE, Ivancevich NM, Haworth KJ, et al. Ultrasound-enhanced rt-PA thrombolysis in an ex vivo porcine carotid artery model. *Ultrasound Med Biol.* Aug 2011;37(8):1240–1251.
56. Laing ST, Moody M, Smulevitz B, et al. Ultrasound-enhanced thrombolytic effect of tissue plasminogen activator-loaded echogenic liposomes in an in vivo rabbit aorta thrombus model-brief report. *Arterioscler Thromb Vasc Biol.* Jun 2011;31(6):1357–1359.
57. Hitchcock KE, Holland CK. Ultrasound-assisted thrombolysis for stroke therapy: Better thrombus break-up with bubbles. *J Stroke.* Oct 2010;41(10 Suppl):S50–53.
58. Smith DA, Vaidya SS, Kopechek JA, et al. Ultrasound-triggered release of recombinant tissue-type plasminogen activator from echogenic liposomes. *Ultrasound Med Biol.* Jan 2010;36(1):145–157.
59. Shaw GJ, Meunier JM, Huang SL, Lindsell CJ, McPherson DD, Holland CK. Ultrasound-enhanced thrombolysis with tPA-loaded echogenic liposomes. *Thromb Res.* Jul 2009;124(3):306–310.
60. Dayton P, Klibanov A, Brandenburger G, Ferrara K. Acoustic radiation force in vivo: A mechanism to assist targeting of microbubbles. *Ultrasound Med Biol.* 1999;25(8):1195–1201.
61. Dayton PA, Zhao S, Bloch SH, et al. Application of ultrasound to selectively localize nanodroplets for targeted imaging and therapy. *Mol Imaging.* Jul 2006;5(3):160–174.
62. Holland CK, McPherson DD. Echogenic lipsomes for targeted drug delivery. *Proc IEEE Int Symp Biomed Imaging.* 2009;2009:755–758.

63. Stieger SM, Caskey CF, Adamson RH, et al. Enhancement of vascular permeability with low-frequency contrast-enhanced ultrasound in the chorioallantoic membrane model. *Radiology.* Apr 2007;243(1):112–121.
64. Thakkar D, Gupta R, Monson K, Rapoport N. Effect of ultrasound on the permeability of vascular wall to nano-emulsion droplets. *Ultrasound Med Biol.* Oct 2013;39(10):1804–1811.
65. Shortencarier MJ, Dayton PA, Bloch SH, Schumann PA, Matsunaga TO, Ferrara KW. A method for radiation-force localized drug delivery using gas-filled lipospheres. *IEEE Trans Ultrason Ferroelectr Freq Control.* Jul 2004;51(7):822–831.
66. Tartis MS, McCallan J, Lum AF, et al. Therapeutic effects of paclitaxel-containing ultrasound contrast agents. *Ultrasound Med Biol.* Nov 2006;32(11):1771–1780.
67. Soman NR, Marsh JN, Hughes MS, Lanza GM, Wickline SA. Acoustic activation of targeted liquid perfluorocarbon nanoparticles does not compromise endothelial integrity. *IEEE Trans Nanobioscience.* Jun 2006;5(2):69–75.
68. Lum AF, Borden MA, Dayton PA, Kruse DE, Simon SI, Ferrara KW. Ultrasound radiation force enables targeted deposition of model drug carriers loaded on microbubbles. *J Control Release.* 2006;111(1–2):128–134. Epub 2005 Dec 2027.
69. Frenkel V, Etherington A, Greene M, et al. Delivery of liposomal doxorubicin (Doxil) in a breast cancer tumour model: Investigation of potential enhancement by pulsed-high intensity focused ultrasound exposure. *Acad Radiol.* Apr 2006;13(4):469–479.
70. Frenkel V, Kimmel E, Iger Y. Ultrasound-facilitated transport of silver chloride (AgCl) particles in fish skin. *J Control Release.* Aug 10 2000;68(2):251–261.
71. Frenkel V, Kimmel E, Iger Y. Ultrasound-induced intercellular space widening in fish epidermis. *Ultrasound Med Biol.* Mar 2000;26(3):473–480.
72. Hancock H, Dreher MR, Crawford N, et al. Evaluation of pulsed high intensity focused ultrasound exposures on metastasis in a murine model. *Clin Exp Metastasis.* 2009;26(7):729–738.
73. Hancock HA, Smith LH, Cuesta J, et al. Investigations into pulsed high-intensity focused ultrasound-enhanced delivery: Preliminary evidence for a novel mechanism. *Ultrasound Med Biol.* Oct 2009;35(10):1722–1736.
74. O'Neill BE, Vo H, Angstadt M, Li KP, Quinn T, Frenkel V. Pulsed high intensity focused ultrasound mediated nanoparticle delivery: Mechanisms and efficacy in murine muscle. *Ultrasound Med Biol.* Mar 2009;35(3):416–424.
75. Yuh EL, Shulman SG, Mehta SA, et al. Delivery of systemic chemotherapeutic agent to tumours by using focused ultrasound: Study in a murine model. *Radiology.* Feb 2005;234(2):431–437.
76. Borden MA, Kruse DE, Caskey CF, Zhao S, Dayton PA, Ferrara KW. Influence of lipid shell physicochemical properties on ultrasound-induced microbubble destruction. *IEEE Trans Ultrason Ferroelectr Freq Control.* Nov 2005;52(11):1992–2002.
77. Borden MA, Zhang H, Gillies RJ, Dayton PA, Ferrara KW. A stimulus-responsive contrast agent for ultrasound molecular imaging. *Biomaterials.* Feb 2008;29(5):597–606.
78. Ferrara K, Pollard R, Borden M. Ultrasound microbubble contrast agents: Fundamentals and application to gene and drug delivery. *Annu Rev Biomed Eng.* 2007;9:415–447.
79. Gao Z, Fain HD, Rapoport N. Ultrasound-enhanced tumour targeting of polymeric micellar drug carriers. *Mol Pharm.* Jul–Aug 2004;1(4):317–330.
80. Kheirolomoom A, Dayton PA, Lum AF, et al. Acoustically-active microbubbles conjugated to liposomes: Characterization of a proposed drug delivery vehicle. *J Control Release.* Apr 23 2007;118(3):275–284.
81. Kheirolomoom A, Mahakian LM, Lai CY, et al. Copper-doxorubicin as a nanoparticle cargo retains efficacy with minimal toxicity. *Mol Pharm.* Dec 6 2010;7(6):1948–1958.
82. Qin S, Caskey CF, Ferrara KW. Ultrasound contrast microbubbles in imaging and therapy: Physical principles and engineering. *Phys Med Biol.* Mar 21 2009;54(6):R27–57.
83. Schroeder A, Avnir Y, Weisman S, et al. Controlling liposomal drug release with low frequency ultrasound: Mechanism and feasibility. *Langmuir.* Mar 27 2007;23(7):4019–4025.
84. Schroeder A, Honen R, Turjeman K, Gabizon A, Kost J, Barenholz Y. Ultrasound triggered release of cisplatin from liposomes in murine tumours. *J Control Release.* Mar 19 2009;137(1):63–68.
85. Unger EC, Porter T, Culp W, Labell R, Matsunaga T, Zutshi R. Therapeutic applications of lipid-coated microbubbles. *Advan Drug Deliv Rev.* May 7 2004;56(9):1291–1314.

86. Wheatley MA, Forsberg F, Oum K, Ro R, El-Sherif D. Comparison of in vitro and in vivo acoustic response of a novel 50:50 PLGA contrast agent. *Ultrasonics*. Nov 2006;44(4):360–367.
87. Zheng H, Kruse DE, Stephens DN, Ferrara KW, Sutcliffe P, Gardner E. A sensitive ultrasonic imaging method for targeted contrast microbubble detection. *Conf Proc IEEE Eng Med Biol Soc*. 2008;2008:5290–5293.
88. O'Neill BE, Rapoport N. Phase-shift, stimuli-responsive drug carriers for targeted delivery. *Ther Deliv*. Sep 2011;2(9):1165–1187.
89. Rapoport N. Phase-shift, stimuli-responsive perfluorocarbon nanodroplets for drug delivery to cancer. Wiley Interdisciplinary Reviews: Nanomedicine and Nanobiotechnology. 2012 Sep;4(5):492–510.
90. McDannold N, Vykhodtseva N, Hynynen K. Effects of acoustic parameters and ultrasound contrast agent dose on focused-ultrasound induced blood-brain barrier disruption. *Ultrasound Med Biol*. 2008;34(6):930–937. Epub 2008 Feb 2021.
91. McDannold NJ, Vykhodtseva NI, Hynynen K. Microbubble contrast agent with focused ultrasound to create brain lesions at low power levels: MR imaging and histologic study in rabbits. *Radiology*. 2006;241(1):95–106.
92. Treat LH, McDannold N, Vykhodtseva N, Zhang Y, Tam K, Hynynen K. Targeted delivery of doxorubicin to the rat brain at therapeutic levels using MRI-guided focused ultrasound. *Int J Cancer*. 2007;121(4):901–907.
93. Vykhodtseva N, McDannold N, Hynynen K. Induction of apoptosis in vivo in the rabbit brain with focused ultrasound and Optison. *Ultrasound Med Biol*. 2006;32(12):1923–1929.
94. Vykhodtseva N, McDannold N, Hynynen K. Progress and problems in the application of focused ultrasound for blood-brain barrier disruption. *Ultrasonics*. 2008;48(4):279–296. Epub 2008 Apr 2014.
95. Rapoport N, Kennedy AM, Shea JE, Scaife CL, Nam KH. Ultrasonic nanotherapy of pancreatic cancer: Lessons from ultrasound imaging. *Mol Pharm*. Feb 1 2010;7(1):22–31.
96. Rapoport N, Nam K-H, Gupta R, et al. Ultrasound-mediated tumour imaging and nanotherapy using drug loaded, block copolymer stabilized perfluorocarbon nanoemulsions. *J Control Release*. 2011;153:4–15.
97. Gupta R, Shea J, Scafe C, Shurlygina A, Rapoport N. Polymeric micelles and nanoemulsions as drug carriers: Therapeutic efficacy, toxicity, and drug resistance. *J Control Release*. Aug 28 2015;212:70–77.
98. Rapoport N, Marin A, Christensen DA. Ultrasound-activated micellar drug delivery. *Drug Delivery Syst Sci*. 2002;2(2):37–46.
99. Rapoport N, Marin A, Luo Y, Prestwich GD, Muniruzzaman MD. Intracellular uptake and trafficking of Pluronic micelles in drug-sensitive and MDR cells: Effect on the intracellular drug localization. *J Pharm Sci*. Jan 2002;91(1):157–170.
100. Mehier-Humbert S, Yan F, Frinking P, Schneider M, Guy RH, Bettinger T. Ultrasound-mediated gene delivery: Influence of contrast agent on transfection. *Bioconjug Chem*. May–Jun 2007;18(3):652–662.
101. Rapoport N, Gao Z, Kennedy A. Multifunctional nanoparticles for combining ultrasonic tumour imaging and targeted chemotherapy. *J Natl Cancer Inst*. Jul 18 2007;99(14):1095–1106.
102. Suzuki R, Takizawa T, Negishi Y, et al. Gene delivery by combination of novel liposomal bubbles with perfluoropropane and ultrasound. *J Control Release*. Jan 22 2007;117(1):130–136.
103. Kripfgans OD, Fowlkes JB, Miller DL, Eldevik OP, Carson PL. Acoustic droplet vaporization for therapeutic and diagnostic applications. *Ultrasound Med Biol*. Sep 2000;26(7):1177–1189.
104. Wu H, Rognin NG, Krupka TM, et al. Acoustic characterization and pharmacokinetic analyses of new nanobubble ultrasound contrast agents. *Ultrasound Med Biol*. Nov 2013;39(11):2137–2146.
105. Krafft MP. Fluorocarbons and fluorinated amphiphiles in drug delivery and biomedical research. *Advan Drug Deliv Rev*. Apr 25 2001;47(2–3):209–228.
106. Reznik N, Lajoinie G, Shpak O, et al. On the acoustic properties of vaporized submicron perfluorocarbon droplets. *Ultrasound Med Biol*. Jun 2014;40(6):1379–1384.
107. Reznik N, Williams R, Burns PN. Investigation of vaporized submicron perfluorocarbon droplets as an ultrasound contrast agent. *Ultrasound Med Biol*. Aug 2011;37(8):1271–1279.
108. Fabiilli ML, Lee JA, Kripfgans OD, Carson PL, Fowlkes JB. Delivery of water-soluble drugs using acoustically triggered perfluorocarbon double emulsions. *Pharm Res*. Dec 2010;27(12):2753–2765.
109. Sheeran PS, Luois S, Dayton PA, Matsunaga TO. Formulation and acoustic studies of a new phase-shift agent for diagnostic and therapeutic ultrasound. *Langmuir*. Sep 6 2011;27(17):10412–10420.

110. Matsunaga TO, Sheeran PS, Luois S, et al. Phase-change nanoparticles using highly volatile perfluorocarbons: Toward a platform for extravascular ultrasound imaging. *Theranostics*. 2012;2(12):1185–1198.
111. Gao Z, Kennedy AM, Christensen DA, Rapoport NY. Drug-loaded nano/microbubbles for combining ultrasonography and targeted chemotherapy. *Ultrasonics*. Aug 2008;48(4):260–270.
112. Rapoport N, Christensen DA, Kennedy AM, Nam KH. Cavitation properties of block copolymer stabilized phase-shift nanoemulsions used as drug carriers. *Ultrasound Med Biol*. Mar 2010;36(3):419–429.
113. Alakhov V, Moskaleva E, Batrakova EV, Kabanov AV. Hypersensitization of multidrug resistant human ovarian carcinoma cells by pluronic P85 block copolymer. *Bioconjug Chem*. Mar–Apr 1996;7(2):209–216.
114. Alakhova DY, Rapoport NY, Batrakova EV, et al. Differential metabolic responses to pluronic in MDR and non-MDR cells: A novel pathway for chemosensitization of drug resistant cancers. *J Control Release*. Feb 25 2010;142(1):89–100.
115. Batrakova E, Lee S, Li S, Venne A, Alakhov V, Kabanov A. Fundamental relationships between the composition of pluronic block copolymers and their hypersensitization effect in MDR cancer cells. *Pharm Res*. Sep 1999;16(9):1373–1379.
116. Batrakova EV, Li S, Alakhov VY, Elmquist WF, Miller DW, Kabanov AV. Sensitization of cells overexpressing multidrug-resistant proteins by pluronic P85. *Pharm Res*. Oct 2003;20(10):1581–1590.
117. Batrakova EV, Li S, Elmquist WF, Miller DW, Alakhov VY, Kabanov AV. Mechanism of sensitization of MDR cancer cells by Pluronic block copolymers: Selective energy depletion. *Br J Cancer*. Dec 14 2001;85(12):1987–1997.
118. Rapoport N, Payne A, Dillon C, Shea J, Scaife AR, Gupta R. Focused ultrasound-mediated drug delivery to pancreatic cancer in a mouse model. *J Ther Ultrasound*. 2013;1.
119. Apfel RE, Inventor. Activatable Infusable Dispersions Containing Drops of a Superheated Liquid for Methods of Therapy and Diagnosis, 1998. US5840276A
120. Fabiilli ML, Haworth KJ, Fakhri NH, Kripfgans OD, Carson PL, Fowlkes JB. The role of inertial cavitation in acoustic droplet vaporization. *IEEE Trans Ultrason Ferroelectr Freq Control*. May 2009;56(5):1006–1017.
121. Kripfgans OD, Fabiilli ML, Carson PL, Fowlkes JB. On the acoustic vaporization of micrometer-sized droplets. *J Acoust Soc Am*. Jul 2004;116(1):272–281.
122. Kripfgans OD, Fowlkes JB, Woydt M, Eldevik OP, Carson PL. In vivo droplet vaporization for occlusion therapy and phase aberration correction. *IEEE Trans Ultrason Ferroelectr Freq Control*. Jun 2002;49(6):726–738.
123. Kripfgans OD, Orifici CM, Carson PL, Ives KA, Eldevik OP, Fowlkes JB. Acoustic droplet vaporization for temporal and spatial control of tissue occlusion: A kidney study. *IEEE Trans Ultrason Ferroelectr Freq Control*. Jul 2005;52(7):1101–1110.
124. Lo AH, Kripfgans OD, Carson PL, Fowlkes JB. Spatial control of gas bubbles and their effects on acoustic fields. *Ultrasound Med Biol*. Jan 2006;32(1):95–106.
125. Lo AH, Kripfgans OD, Carson PL, Rothman ED, Fowlkes JB. Acoustic droplet vaporization threshold: Effects of pulse duration and contrast agent. *IEEE Trans Ultrason Ferroelectr Freq Control*. May 2007;54(5):933–946.
126. Fabiilli ML, Haworth KJ, Sebastian IE, Kripfgans OD, Carson PL, Fowlkes JB. Delivery of chlorambucil using an acoustically-triggered perfluoropentane emulsion. *Ultrasound Med Biol*. Aug 2010;36(8):1364–1375.
127. Zhang M, Fabiilli ML, Haworth KJ, et al. Initial investigation of acoustic droplet vaporization for occlusion in canine kidney. *Ultrasound Med Biol*. Oct 2010;36(10):1691–1703.
128. Miller DL, Kripfgans OD, Fowlkes JB, Carson PL. Cavitation nucleation agents for nonthermal ultrasound therapy. *J Acoust Soc Am*. Jun 2000;107(6):3480–3486.
129. Wong Z, Kripfgans OD, Qamar, Fowlkes JB, Bull J. Bubble evolution in acoustic droplet vaporization at physiological temperature via ultra-high speed imaging. *Soft Matter*. 2011;7:4009–4011.
130. Chen X, Wang J, Versluis M, de Jong N, Villanueva FS. Ultra-fast bright field and fluorescence imaging of the dynamics of micrometer-sized objects. *Rev Sci Instrum*. Jun 2013;84(6):063701.
131. Faez T, Emmer M, Kooiman K, Versluis M, van der Steen A, de Jong N. 20 years of ultrasound contrast agent modeling. *IEEE Trans Ultrason Ferroelectr Freq Control*. Jan 2013;60(1):7–20.
132. Kokhuis TJ, Garbin V, Kooiman K, et al. Secondary Bjerknes forces deform targeted microbubbles. *Ultrasound Med Biol*. Mar 2013;39(3):490–506.

133. Maresca D, Renaud G, van Soest G, et al. Contrast-enhanced intravascular ultrasound pulse sequences for bandwidth-limited transducers. *Ultrasound Med Biol.* Apr 2013;39(4):706–713.
134. Reznik N, Shpak O, Gelderblom EC, et al. The efficiency and stability of bubble formation by acoustic vaporization of submicron perfluorocarbon droplets. *Ultrasonics.* Sep 2013;53(7):1368–1376.
135. Shpak O, Kokhuis TJ, Luan Y, et al. Ultrafast dynamics of the acoustic vaporization of phase-change microdroplets. *J Acoust Soc Am.* Aug 2013;134(2):1610–1621.
136. Ten Kate GL, van den Oord SC, Sijbrands EJ, et al. Current status and future developments of contrast-enhanced ultrasound of carotid atherosclerosis. *J Vasc Surg.* Feb 2013;57(2):539–546.
137. Thomas DH, Sboros V, Emmer M, Vos H, de Jong N. Microbubble oscillations in capillary tubes. *IEEE Trans Ultrason Ferroelectr Freq Control.* Jan 2013;60(1):105–114.
138. Kooiman K, Vos HJ, Versluis M, de Jong N. Acoustic behavior of microbubbles and implications for drug delivery. *Advan Drug Deliv Rev.* Jun 15 2014;72C:28–48.
139. Segers T, Versluis M. Acoustic bubble sorting for ultrasound contrast agent enrichment. *Lab Chip.* May 21 2014;14(10):1705–1714.
140. Shpak O, Verweij M, Vos HJ, de Jong N, Lohse D, Versluis M. Acoustic droplet vaporization is initiated by superharmonic focusing. *Proc Natl Acad Sci USA.* Feb 4 2014;111(5):1697–1702.
141. Nam KH, Christensen DA, Kennedy AM, Rapoport N. Acoustic droplet vaporization, cavitation, and therapeutic properties of copolymer-stabilized perfluorocarbon nanoemulsions. *Am Inst Phys Conf Proc.* 2009;1113(1):124–128.
142. Miller DL, Song J. Lithotripter shock waves with cavitation nucleation agents produce tumour growth reduction and gene transfer in vivo. *Ultrasound Med Biol.* Oct 2002;28(10):1343–1348.
143. Wong Z, Krifgans O, Qamar, Fowlkes J, Bull J. Bubble evolution in acoustic droplet vaporization at physiological temperature via ultra-high speed imaging. *Soft Matter.* 2011;7:4009–4016.
144. Barber EJ, Cady GH. Vapor pressures of perfluoropentanes. *J Phys Chem.* 1956;60(4):504–505.
145. Alexandridis P, Holzwarth JF, Hatton TA. Micellization of Poly(ethylene oxide)-Poly(propylene oxide)-Poly(ethylene oxide) Triblock Copolymers in Aqueous Solutions: Thermodynamics of Copolymer Association. *Macromolecules.* 1994;27(9):2414–2425.
146. Rapoport NY, Efros AL, Christensen DA, Kennedy AM, Nam KH. Microbubble generation in phase-shift nanoemulsions used as anticancer drug carriers. *Bubble Sci Eng Technol.* 2009;1(1–2):31–39.
147. Rapoport NY, Kennedy AM, Shea JE, Scaife CL, Nam KH. Controlled and targeted tumour chemotherapy by ultrasound-activated nanoemulsions/microbubbles. *J Control Release.* Sep 15 2009;138(3):268–276.
148. Giesecke T, Hynynen K. Ultrasound-mediated cavitation thresholds of liquid perfluorocarbon droplets in vitro. *Ultrasound Med Biol.* Sep 2003;29(9):1359–1365.
149. Kawabata K, Yoshizawa A, Asami R. Site-specific contrast imaging with locally induced microbubble from liquid precursors. *IEEE Int. Ultrasonic Symp.* 2006:517–520.
150. Schad KC, Hynynen K. In vitro characterization of perfluorocarbon droplets for focused ultrasound therapy. *Phys Med Biol.* Sep 7 2010;55(17):4933–4947.
151. Kawabata K, Sugita N, Yoshikawa H, Azama T, Umemura S. Nanoparticles with multiple perfluorocarbons for controllable ultrasound-induced phase shift. *J Appl Physics.* 2005;44:4548–4552.
152. Caskey CF, Qin S, Dayton PA, Ferrara KW. Microbubble tunneling in gel phantoms. *J Acoust Soc Am.* May 2009;125(5):EL183–189.
153. Caskey CF, Qin S, Ferrara KW. Ultrasound mediated drug delivery: The effect of microbubbles on a gel boundary. *Conf Proc IEEE Eng Med Biol Soc.* 2009;2009:134–136.
154. Caskey CF, Stieger SM, Qin S, Dayton PA, Ferrara KW. Direct observations of ultrasound microbubble contrast agent interaction with the microvessel wall. *J Acoust Soc Am.* Aug 2007;122(2):1191–1200.
155. Kinoshita M, McDannold N, Jolesz FA, Hynynen K. Noninvasive localized delivery of Herceptin to the mouse brain by MRI-guided focused ultrasound-induced blood-brain barrier disruption. *Proc Natl Acad Sci USA.* Aug 1 2006;103(31):11719–11723.
156. Cohn CS, Cushing MM. Oxygen therapeutics: Perfluorocarbons and blood substitute safety. *Crit Care Clin.* Apr 2009;25(2):399–414, Table of Contents.
157. Zhou HF, Chan HW, Wickline SA, Lanza GM, Pham CT. Alphavbeta3-targeted nanotherapy suppresses inflammatory arthritis in mice. *FASEB J.* Sep 2009;23(9):2978–2985.
158. Wilson K, Homan K, Emelianov S. Biomedical photoacoustics beyond thermal expansion using triggered nanodroplet vaporization for contrast-enhanced imaging. *Nat Commun.* 2012;3:618.

159. Ahrens ET, Flores R, Xu H, Morel PA. In vivo imaging platform for tracking immunotherapeutic cells. *Nat Biotechnol.* Aug 2005;23(8):983–987.
160. Yu JX, Kodibagkar VD, Cui W, Mason RP. 19F: A versatile reporter for non-invasive physiology and pharmacology using magnetic resonance. *Curr Med Chem.* 2005;12(7):819–848.
161. Noth U, Morrissey SP, Deichmann R, et al. Perfluoro-15-crown-5-ether labelled macrophages in adoptive transfer experimental allergic encephalomyelitis. *Artif Cells Blood Substit Immobil Biotechnol.* May 1997;25(3):243–254.
162. Batrakova EV, Han HY, Miller DW, Kabanov AV. Effects of pluronic P85 unimers and micelles on drug permeability in polarized BBMEC and Caco-2 cells. *Pharm Res.* Oct 1998;15(10):1525–1532.
163. Kaneda MM, Caruthers S, Lanza GM, Wickline SA. Perfluorocarbon nanoemulsions for quantitative molecular imaging and targeted therapeutics. *Ann Biomed Eng.* Oct 2009;37(10):1922–1933.
164. Lanza GM. Theranostic agents: From micro to nano in seconds. *Nat Nanotechnol.* Apr 2015;10(4):301–302.
165. Soman NR, Baldwin SL, Hu G, et al. Molecularly targeted nanocarriers deliver the cytolytic peptide melittin specifically to tumour cells in mice, reducing tumour growth. *J Clin Invest.* Sep 2009;119(9):2830–2842.
166. Soman NR, Lanza GM, Heuser JM, Schlesinger PH, Wickline SA. Synthesis and characterization of stable fluorocarbon nanostructures as drug delivery vehicles for cytolytic peptides. *Nano Lett.* Apr 2008;8(4):1131–1136.
167. Tran TD, Caruthers SD, Hughes M, et al. Clinical applications of perfluorocarbon nanoparticles for molecular imaging and targeted therapeutics. *Int J Nanomed.* 2007;2(4):515–526.
168. Winter PM, Cai K, Caruthers SD, Wickline SA, Lanza GM. Emerging nanomedicine opportunities with perfluorocarbon nanoparticles. *Expert Rev Med Devices.* Mar 2007;4(2):137–145.
169. Winter PM, Schmieder AH, Caruthers SD, et al. Minute dosages of alpha(nu)beta3-targeted fumagillin nanoparticles impair Vx-2 tumour angiogenesis and development in rabbits. *FASEB J.* Aug 2008;22(8):2758–2767.
170. Borden MA, Sarantos MR, Stieger SM, Simon SI, Ferrara KW, Dayton PA. Ultrasound radiation force modulates ligand availability on targeted contrast agents. *Mol Imaging.* Jul 2006;5(3):139–147.
171. Gessner RC, Streeter JE, Kothadia R, Feingold S, Dayton PA. An in vivo validation of the application of acoustic radiation force to enhance the diagnostic utility of molecular imaging using 3-d ultrasound. *Ultrasound Med Biol.* Apr 2012;38(4):651–660.
172. Sheeran PS, Dayton PA. Phase-change contrast agents for imaging and therapy. *Curr Pharm Des.* 2012;18(15):2152–2165.
173. Zhao S, Kruse DE, Ferrara KW, Dayton PA. Selective imaging of adherent targeted ultrasound contrast agents. *Phys Med Biol.* Apr 21 2007;52(8):2055–2072.
174. Chen J, Lanza GM, Wickline SA. Quantitative magnetic resonance fluorine imaging: Today and tomorrow. *Wiley Interdiscip Rev Nanomed Nanobiotechnol.* Jul–Aug 2010;2(4):431–440.
175. Lanza GM, Moonen C, Baker JR, Jr., et al. Assessing the barriers to image-guided drug delivery. *Wiley Interdiscip Rev Nanomed Nanobiotechnol.* Jan–Feb 2014;6(1):1–14.

24

Anaesthesia, Ventilation and Immobilisation Strategies for Focused Ultrasound Therapy (with Special Reference to High-Frequency Ventilation)

Shaun H. Scott, Amy K. Swinson, and Daniel Y.F. Chung

24.1 Introduction

Focused ultrasound (FUS) Therapy includes ablative and non-ablative treatment modalities and presents a range of challenges for the anaesthetist. Foremost is the opportunity for anaesthetic ventilatory management to provide optimal immobilisation of targets in the upper abdomen in order to facilitate high fidelity imaging and precise, safe treatment.

High-frequency jet ventilation (HFJV) provides reliable and sustainable immobilisation of upper abdominal viscera during extracorporeal FUS treatment and permits incremental controlled displacement of hepatic targets into optimal planes of view relative to the ribcage. This anaesthetic technique facilitates clear imaging, accurate planning and precise, continuous treatment, while reducing risk of inadvertent collateral damage.

HFJV may be delivered under light general anaesthesia without muscle relaxation, obviating the need for apnoea or bronchial isolation. This greatly improves the simplicity and patient safety profile of lung-immobilisation anaesthesia, compared with conventional methods. Since 2007, this has been the standard lung immobilisation technique at our institution for extracorporeal FUS chemotherapeutic procedures as well as for percutaneous ablative therapy of hepatic, pulmonary and renal tumours.

24.2 Background

General considerations: FUS therapy includes diverse ablative and non-ablative treatment regimens, including direct tissue destruction (by high-intensity FUS, or HIFU) and local drug delivery (by hyperthermia or cavitation phenomenon, see Chapter 25), and presents a plethora of different requirements for the anaesthetist.[1] Patient demographics include a wide age range and varied co-morbidity, including advanced oncological disease, chronic pain and complex polypharmacy. Extracorporeal FUS procedures are often protracted and may necessitate awkward positioning to allow access to targets within the abdomen,[2–4] pelvis,[5] cranium[6–8] or elsewhere. FUS treatment of targets in the lung (necessitating unilateral or lobar flooding[9]) may be a possibility in the future.

Extracorporeal FUS therapy is typically conducted in remote suites or in MRI facilities, which may be confined, hazardous and/or isolated from anaesthetic support, post-operative care units and other services.[1] Proximity to resuscitation equipment, knowledge of emergency protocols and means of obtaining assistance is essential. Delivery of anaesthesia necessitates an anaesthetic machine with standard monitoring, suction, ventilator and vaporisers, as well as intravenous infusion pumps and, where treatment indicates it, a high-frequency jet ventilator. A mains gas supply is ideal, and uninterruptible mains power supply is mandatory where HFJV is employed. This large assortment of equipment, cabling and tubing, in addition to personnel and the patient, contribute significantly to overall hazard.

DOI: 10.1201/9780429162671-24

Induction of anaesthesia takes place on the HIFU/MRI table or on a tilting trolley. An appreciation of ergonomic, handling and positional risk factors and a precautionary practice is necessary. If the procedure is likely to be of lengthy duration, consideration must be given to patient warming, bladder catheterisation (particularly for patients undergoing trans-rectal prostatic HIFU[1]) and thrombo-prophylaxis, according to local operating procedures, hospital protocols and patient-specific indications.

Sedation or general anaesthesia: The patient's experience of pain during and after the procedure may range from minimal to severe.[1, 10–12] The type of procedure dictates the patient's position and this, the duration and intensity of the procedure, as well as other patient factors, determine whether sedation or general anaesthesia is appropriate.[1] Anaesthetic requirements range from sedation with analgesia (e.g. HIFU for uterine fibroids[11]) to general anaesthesia, and may include neuraxial blockade[1] (e.g. for trans-rectal prostatic HIFU).

In a subset of less painful FUS procedures of tolerable duration, it is beneficial to maintain patient awareness with voluntary immobilisation[10] under conscious sedation and analgesia (SA) to allow early indication of inadvertent non-target injury and to reduce this risk due to inadvertent movement (e.g. lumbo-sacral nerve irritation,[2, 3] skin burn,[13] and bowel and bladder injuries reported during FUS ablation of uterine fibroids[5, 12]) or to monitor cerebral function, treatment efficacy and detect pain or febrile seizures during FUS therapy of brain targets (e.g. to treat chronic pain[6, 7] or tremor[8]).

In cases where assurance of immobilisation is required or the treatment more protracted or painful, general anaesthesia is indicated. The choice of drugs for sedation, analgesia and anaesthesia is largely dictated by local availability and operator preference; steady-state intravenous infusions of short-acting drugs delivered by pharmacokinetic algorithm target-controlled infusion pumps provide ideal conditions which are beneficial in most circumstances, and essential when HFJV (which precludes volatile anaesthesia) is employed.

Monitoring and temperature control. Basic monitoring requirements for general anaesthesia are standard,[14] with consideration to MRI-specific requirements where applicable. Where HFJV is used, adequacy of ventilation is confirmed by either intermittent side-stream sampling of end-tidal alveolar carbon dioxide (etCO_2), or continuous transcutaneous CO_2 monitoring (TCM).

During HIFU treatment, the cumulative heat energy delivered to the target may reach 100–10 000 W/cc[1], while the patient's initial core thermal redistribution due to vasodilative anaesthesia,[15] compounded by conductive and convective heat loss (due to exposure of the patient's skin during positioning, as well as contact with the skin-cooling coupling device or water bath) may result in significant core hypothermia. In most cases, these factors may negate each other such that they are of little consequence. however, during FUS-mediated drug delivery by targeted hyperthermia, for example using thermo-sensitive liposomal chemotherapeutic drug release (e.g. Thermodox, see TARDOX study in Chapter 25), control of the patient's core temperature within the normal range is vital to allow controlled localised hyperthermia and drug release at the target site without unwanted systemic release. Accurate core thermometry (most reliably by distal oesophageal or urinary bladder thermometry probe placement) is therefore essential in these circumstances, as are vigilant anticipation of clinical changes and means of warming and cooling the patient.

MR-guided HIFU (MRgHIFU) provides non-invasive treatment-site proton resonance frequency-based MR-thermometry[16] to guide local treatment efficacy, but USgHIFU devices do not currently have this capability.

FUS planning: During the planning phase of abdominal FUS procedures, real-time imaging (US or MRI) is typically correlated with pre-acquired imaging, to plan the treatment of single or multiple targets. Feasibility of accessing each target with FUS is assessed and the target's volume and three-dimensional treatment perimeter are planned. For USgFUS, the treatment volume is divided into treatment units (depending on device-specific protocols) comprising arrays of individual target voxels (each approximately the size of a grain of rice). As non-ablative FUS treatment does not alter tissue echogenicity, the progress and completeness of the procedure is assured by reference to this initial treatment array.

It is important to note that ribs absorb and reflect ultrasound, resulting in acoustic interference which may both obstruct the US view and impair the FUS treatment[17] of a subcostal target, if there is no means of relocating the target into a more favourable position within an intercostal 'window' or beyond the costal margin. Lung parenchyma overlying a target near the dome of the liver may be displaced by creating a hydrothorax with 0.9% saline via an intercostal Touhy needle.[1]

Abdominal visceral motion: During spontaneous breathing or conventional tidal-volume ventilation, upper abdominal viscera are displaced by diaphragmatic movement by as much as 30–40 mm[4, 18–24] or up to 80 mm with deep inspiration.[25] Moreover, the liver is subject to curvilinear bulk movement and complex internal rotational[26] and plastic deformation[25, 27] during the respiratory cycle. The bulk position of an intra-hepatic target migrates cranio-caudally, laterally and antero-posteriorly, by up to 40, 20 and 13 mm, respectively,[20, 26] and its axial orientation rotates during each inspiratory phase.[26] Any variability of tidal volume, frequency or rhythm pattern adds further complexity and unpredictability to this displacement, compounded by the development of atelectasis and hysteretic re-inflation during intermittent apnoea manoeuvres.

24.3 Relative Target Immobilisation and Controlled Displacement

The technical success and procedural safety of abdominal FUS procedures depends upon the maintenance of the optimal spatial alignment of the target within the imaging and treatment axes. Inaccuracy or instability leads to the loss of thermal dose[25] and the risk of damage to adjacent structures, as discussed earlier. For upper abdominal targets, relative immobilisation may be achieved by 'gating' (where sonication occurs only when the target position rests within these axes during a pre-determined phase of the ventilatory cycle[4, 28]), 'tracking' (when ventilatory pattern is stable, the MR-gUS beam is steering to match real-time visceral movement[23, 29, 30]) or by direct minimisation of visceral movement, which is here the subject of further discussion.

Direct reduction of upper abdominal visceral respiratory movement, whilst facilitating planning, optimal target positioning and accuracy of treatment, presents a potential challenge for safe anaesthetic care in the FUS environment. Conventional methods of achieving relative immobilisation of the liver, pancreas or kidney include voluntary apnoea, bradypnoea under SA and general anaesthesia with either intermittent apnoea or lung isolation by bronchial blocker or double-lumen endotracheal tube.[31] Each of these standard methods, though familiar, present disadvantages for FUS and ablative therapies (vide infra)

High-frequency jet ventilation. The physiology of polypnoea has been the subject of investigation for more than a century, after Henderson noted[32] in 1915 that "there may easily be a gaseous exchange sufficient to support life even when the tidal volume is considerably less than the dead space". Lung immobilisation techniques have an even older heritage, as a sustained insufflation technique was demonstrated by Melzer[33] in 1909, based in part on Hooke's experiments[34] in 1667. Experimental high frequency delivery systems[35–37] rapidly evolved into clinical high-frequency ventilation (HFV) strategies,[38] which are now well-established in a wide range of clinical practice, including surgery[39, 40] and intensive care medicine.[41, 42]

As a subset of HFV, HFJV is conventionally utilised under general anaesthesia for laryngeal,[43–46] tracheal[47, 48] or thoracic surgery,[49–52] where the benefit of continuous surgical-site immobilisation has long been appreciated.[43, 46] During HFJV, liver excursion is observed to be less than 3–4 mm[53–55] and renal excursion 2–4 mm.[18, 56] With minor adaptations to the HFJV delivery system, this immobilisation method has proved to be safe outside of the operating theatre environment[57] and provides similar advantages for percutaneous microwave or radiofrequency tumour ablation under CT or US guidance (improving accuracy, broadening of inclusion criteria to include the treatment of smaller targets and reducing procedural duration, as well as CT fluoroscopy radiation dose[58–61]), intra-cardiac electrophysiological investigations and ablation (requiring fewer ablations by reduction in variability of atrial blood volume and velocity, thus reducing wall position variability[57, 62–65]) and similarly benefitting lithotripsy[18, 66, 67] and stereotactic radiation therapy.[54, 68]

24.4 Clinical Use

Establishment of steady-state immobilisation. The conduct of anaesthesia with HFJV for upper abdominal FUS procedures at our institution is as follows: after establishment of venous access and full monitoring, intravenous induction of anaesthesia and airway management with an endotracheal tube, HFJV is delivered by a Monsoon Jet Ventilator (Acutronic Medical Systems AG, Hirzel, Switzerland) via a jet swivel adapter[1] (Figure 24.1). This is interposed between the airway and a standard breathing circuit including heat and moisture exchange filter (HMEF). HFJV is started at a frequency of 120 cycles per minute (cpm; 2Hz) with initial driving pressure (DP) ranging between 0.6 and 1.0 bar. This DP is then adjusted to maintain CO_2 within an acceptable range (usually 4.5–6kPa) as determined by TCM (Radiometer, Copenhagen, Denmark) or intermittent sampling of $etCO_2$. Inspired oxygen fraction (FiO_2) is adjusted to match the patient's requirements. The breathing circuit and HMEF remain in situ, connected to the jet swivel, both to prevent heat and moisture loss from the patient's airway, and to allow swift resumption of manual ventilation and oxygenation, should it be necessary. The adjustable pressure-limiting (APL) valve of the anaesthetic breathing circuit remains fully open, but may be adjusted to generate a slight positive end-expiratory pressure (PEEP) if required (vide infra). Within a few minutes of commencement, a steady-state lung volume is established and, by sonographic view, abdominal organs will be observed to move through an almost imperceptible excursion, at a frequency of 2Hz. Maintenance of muscle relaxant, if administered to facilitate intubation, is usually not required.

As FUS planning and treatment proceeds, interruption of steady-state HFJV is necessary only infrequently, to measure $etCO_2$ (if TCM is not employed, and this is usually necessary only a few times during the first 15 minutes, thereafter only once per 15 minutes or less often) by delivering tidal volume ventilation. The FUS operators' view of this tidal manoeuvre will be of an excursion of 2–4 cm or more (so co-operative timing is essential), after which the HFJV steady state is re-established and targets revert to their initial positions, remaining virtually constant relative to the axis of the initially planned anatomical treatment volume for the duration of HFJV.

Improved access by incremental target displacement. If an abdominal target is situated unfavourably relative to overlying ribs, it may be possible to displace target (liver or kidney) into a more favourable position. In our experience, the addition of 5–10 cmH_2O PEEP increases lung volume by an increment that will result in a caudal displacement of 1–2 cm, which is then maintained as a new steady state (unpublished).

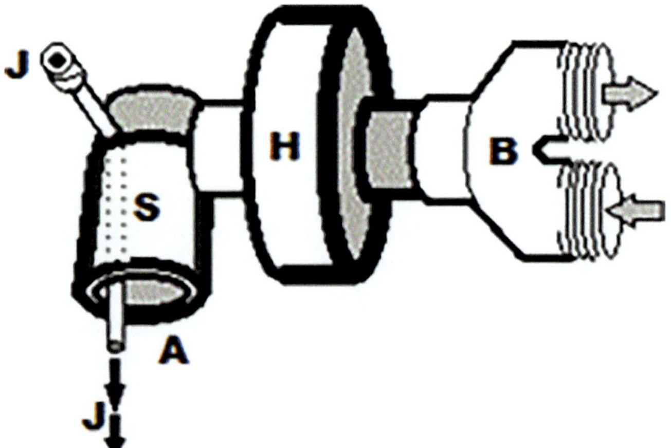

FIGURE 24.1 Schematic of jet swivel connector (S) and heat and moisture exchange filter (H) interposed between endotracheal tube airway (A, not shown) and the anaesthetic machine breathing circuit (B). Luer-lock connection of jet tubing (J) and direction of jet gas stream are shown.

24.5 Post-HIFU Management

Rapid recovery after GA with HFJV is usual, as the depth of anaesthesia is light, due to favourable drug offset characteristics and absence of maintenance muscle relaxant. After pre-dosing with suitable analgesia to minimise postoperative discomfort and emergence from anaesthesia, the patient is transferred to a suitable recovery area, ideally within close proximity to the FUS treatment location and with access to support services. Overnight stay is necessary for some procedures, but same-day discharge is not precluded by GA or HFJV.

24.6 Expert Commentary

Conventional methods of lung immobilisation include voluntary apnoea, bradypnoea under analgesia-sedation, and general anaesthesia with either intermittent apnoea or lung isolation by bronchial blocker or double-lumen endotracheal tube.[1] While these are familiar to most anaesthetists, they each present disadvantages for FUS (as well as to percutaneous and other similar ablative therapies).

FUS procedures for moderately large target volumes tend to be protracted, and the patient may experience pain related to the treatment procedure or awkward positioning. Pain intensity is variable during the procedure, influenced by patient factors such as location of target site (superficial, or close to sensitive capsule, intercostal nerves or skin) and treatment intensity, and is therefore difficult to predict.

The maintenance of episodic voluntary breath-hold is neither sustainable, for these reasons, nor reliable, as the breath-hold position is likely to vary between attempts. Spontaneous breathing under SA presents several disadvantages, even for fit healthy patients, for any extracorporeal or percutaneous procedure, especially if prolonged or painful. SA incurs a significant delay before initial 'steady-state' conditions are reached or after any alteration in depth of sedation.[4] Since the duration of each voluntary respiratory pause is brief, gated FUS imaging and sonication would be limited to these brief, discrete periods, thus prolonging total treatment duration. Longer pauses (up to 10 seconds or more) are possible but at the expense of greater depth of sedation and are associated with elevation of CO_2 with respiratory acidosis.[4] Furthermore, in this state, the patient is neither prevented from coughing nor making inadvertent movement. The likelihood of unwanted movement is directly related to the intensity of procedural stimulation perceived by the patient. This is often difficult to predict, prevent or control. The risks, related to deeper sedation, of airway obstruction, hypoxia and hypercarbia, or to poor immobilisation, have relegated this method to being unpopular for this type of procedure in our institution and the stable control that general anaesthesia affords is preferred. This is particularly true in patients in prone or inaccessible positions, or with significant cardio-respiratory co-morbidity.

Conventional lung immobilisation techniques to stabilise the operative field under GA (intermittent apnoea, or lung isolation by bronchial blocker or double-lumen endotracheal tube) are familiar and have well-established safety profiles in the context of surgery.[1, 31] However, they are relatively invasive and necessitate either a deep plane of anaesthesia or the use of muscle relaxant, or both, not only to facilitate initial airway management but also to guarantee the maintenance of this immobility. Whilst this is not necessarily difficult to achieve, it does contribute significantly to the complexity and risk of the anaesthetic in this environment, compared to the light anaesthetic that is possible with effective normoventilation that is achieved with HFJV.

The risk of movement during apnoea is most crucial at the onset of the FUS sonication phase. Any displacement of the target from view (due to cough or other movement) hampers the FUS process, risks injury to adjacent structures and reduces operator confidence. In this patient population, periods of apnoea are often not well tolerated, as desaturation may occur rapidly in those with poor gas exchange and hypercarbia may result in cardiovascular instability, while target position during apnoea may 'drift' (during and between sonications) as atelectasis develops in dependent and hypo-ventilated lung zones, is cumulative, and re-expansion is hysteretic and requires large-volume recruitment manoeuvres.

In addition, one-lung ventilation (OLV) causes a ventilation-perfusion mismatch and shunt,[31] which is exacerbated if the non-ventilated lung is dependent. This mismatch results in hypoxia in some patients (particularly the frail or those with poor lung function, though it is difficult to predict which patients will be most susceptible) and may necessitate re-inflation or ventilation of the non-ventilated lung, thus hampering the FUS planning or treatment.

By contrast, HFJV safely maintains effective gas exchange for prolonged periods,[69] allowing a steady state of target immobilisation to be maintained at light planes of anaesthesia without necessitating maintenance muscle relaxant. HFJV facilitates FUS treatment primarily by assuring optimal immobilisation of single or multiple targets in real time, as well as over the course of a treatment period. Further benefits to the patient are notable, particularly in the isolated setting of the FUS treatment suite: reduced anaesthetic dosing requirements; simplified airway management (without carinal or bronchial stimulation); and avoidance of the physiological challenges of apnoea and/or hypercarbia.

Clinical practice in this field has advanced experientially, with a relative lack of comparative evidence of benefit to support 'best practice' of anaesthetic care for FUS treatment, particularly of ventilatory control. We have presented here surrogate lines of evidence, mostly drawn from the analogous fields of percutaneous ablative therapy (radio-frequency and microwave ablation) and other extracorporeal treatment modalities, in the treatment of lung, liver and kidney tumours. Our experience of using HFJV for extracorporeal and percutaneous procedures spans a decade and now includes more than 600 patient encounters. We confidently achieve satisfactory target immobilisation under conditions of light general anaesthesia while maintaining adequate ventilatory gas exchange. In most cases, if necessary, we can displace 'hidden' targets into more favourable positions, e.g. to move liver tumour into an intercostal window, by the application of PEEP to the breathing circuit. As the confidence of our team has advanced over this decade, our scope of practice has expanded to include patients with more complex comorbidity, such as emphysema and obesity, and treatment targets that are smaller[60] or more awkwardly situated.

In the context of the growing field of extracorporeal FUS in abdominal organs for ablative and drug delivery indications, HFJV offers a practical and physiological solution for stable immobilisation and optimal repositioning of target volumes and can be safely sustained for treatments of prolonged duration.

NOTE

1 The Acutronic Jet Swivel is not MRI compatible, but suitable non-ferromagnetic catheters are available that may be passed through the aperture of an appropriate angle-piece. The jet DP tubing may be extended by several meters to allow the HFJ ventilator to be positioned at a safe distance from the MRI.

REFERENCES

1. Yao, C-L. et al. "Anaesthesia for high intensity focused ultrasound (HIFU) therapy." Anaesthesia 63, no. 8 (2008): 865–872.
2. Shi, Y. et al. "High-intensity focused ultrasound treatment for intra-abdominal desmoid tumors: A report of four cases." Journal of Medical Ultrasound 43, no. 2 (2016): 279–284.
3. Stewart, E. A. et al. "Clinical outcomes of focused ultrasound surgery for the treatment of uterine fibroids." Fertility and Sterility 85, no. 1 (2006): 22–29.
4. van Breugel, J. M. M. et al. "Procedural sedation and analgesia for respiratory-gated MR-HIFU in the liver: A feasibility study." Journal of Therapeutic Ultrasound 4, no.1 (2016): 19–31
5. Coakley, F. V. et al. "Pelvic applications of MR-guided high intensity focused ultrasound." Abdominal Imaging 38, no. 5 (2013): 1120–1129.
6. Martin, E. et al. "High-intensity focused ultrasound for noninvasive functional neurosurgery." Annals of Neurology 66, no. 6 (2009): 858–861.
7. McDannold, N. et al. "Transcranial MRI-guided focused ultrasound surgery of brain tumors: Initial findings in three patients." Neurosurgery 66, no. 2 (2010): 323–332.
8. Elias, W. J. et al. "A pilot study of focused ultrasound thalamotomy for essential tremor." New England Journal of Medicine 369, no. 7 (2013): 640–648.
9. Lesser, T. G. "One-lung flooding reduces the ipsilateral diaphragm motion during mechanical ventilation." European Journal of Medical Research 21, no. 1 (2016): 9.

10. Stewart, E. A. et al. "Focused ultrasound treatment of uterine fibroid tumors: Safety and feasibility of a noninvasive thermoablative technique." American Journal of Obstetrics and Gynecology 189, no. 1 (2003): 48–54.
11. Roberts, A. "Magnetic resonance-guided focused ultrasound for uterine fibroids." Seminars in Interventional Radiology 25, no. 4 (2008): 394–405.
12. Pron, G. "Magnetic resonance–guided high-intensity focused ultrasound (MRgHIFU) treatment of symptomatic uterine fibroids: An evidence-based analysis." Ontario Health Technology Assessment Series 15, no. 4 (2015): 1–86.
13. Leon-Villapalos, J. et al. "Full thickness abdominal burn following magnetic resonance guided focused ultrasound therapy." Burns 31, no. 8 (2005): 1054–1055.
14. Checketts, M. R. et al. "Recommendations for standards of monitoring during anaesthesia and recovery 2015: Association of Anaesthetists of Great Britain and Ireland." Anaesthesia 71, no. 1 (2016): 85–93.
15. Buggy, D. J. and A. W. Crossley. "Thermoregulation, mild perioperative hypothermia and post-anaesthetic shivering." British Journal of Anaesthesia 84, no. 5 (2000): 615–628.
16. de Senneville, B. D. et al. "MR thermometry for monitoring tumor ablation." European Radiology 17, no. 9 (2007): 2401–10.
17. Gélat, P., G. ter Haar and N. Saffari. "The optimization of acoustic fields for ablative therapies of tumours in the upper abdomen." Physics in Medicine and Biology 57, no. 24 (2012): 8471.
18. Warner, M. A. et al. "Clinical efficacy of high frequency jet ventilation during extracorporeal shock wave lithotripsy of renal and ureteral calculi: A comparison with conventional mechanical ventilation." J Urol. 139, no. 3 (1988): 486–487.
19. Davies, S. C. et al. "Ultrasound quantitation of respiratory organ motion in the upper abdomen." The British Journal of Radiology 67, no. 803 (1994): 1096–1102.
20. Bussels, B. et al. "Respiration-induced movement of the upper abdominal organs: A pitfall for the three-dimensional conformal radiation treatment of pancreatic cancer." Radiotherapy and Oncology 68, no. 1 (2003): 69–74.
21. Brandner, E. D. et al. "Abdominal organ motion measured using 4D CT." International Journal of Radiation Oncology, Biology, Physics 65, no. 2 (2006): 554–560.
22. von Siebenthal, M. et al. "4D MR imaging of respiratory organ motion and its variability." Physics in Medicine and Biology 52, no. 6 (2007): 1547–1564.
23. Ries, M. et al. "Real-time 3D target tracking in MRI guided focused ultrasound ablations in moving tissues." Magnetic Resonance in Medicine 64, no. 6 (2010): 1704–1712.
24. Hallman, J. L. et al. "A four-dimensional computed tomography analysis of multi-organ abdominal motion." International Journal of Radiation Oncology Biology Physics 83, no. 1 (2012): 435–441.
25. Muller, A. et al. "Management of respiratory motion in extracorporeal high-intensity focused ultrasound treatment in upper abdominal organs: Current status and perspectives." Cardiovascular and Interventional Radiology 36, no. 6 (2013): 1464–1476.
26. Shimizu, S. et al. "Three-dimensional movement of a liver tumor detected by high-speed magnetic resonance imaging." Radiotherapy and Oncology 50, no. 3 (1999): 367–70.
27. Roujol, S. et al. "Real-time MR-thermometry and dosimetry for interventional guidance on abdominal organs." Magnetic Resonance in Medicine 63, no. 4 (2010): 1080–1087.
28. Kubo, H. D. and B. C. Hill. "Respiration gated radiotherapy treatment: A technical study." Physics in Medicine and Biology 41, no. 1 (1996): 83.
29. De Luca, V., G. Székely and C. Tanner. "Gated-tracking: Estimation of respiratory motion with confidence." In: *International Conference on Medical Image Computing and Computer-Assisted Intervention*, pp. 451–458. Springer International Publishing, 2015.
30. Tanner, C. et al. "In vivo validation of spatio-temporal liver motion prediction from motion tracked on MR thermometry images." International Journal of Computer Assisted Radiology and Surgery 11, no. 6 (2016): 1143–1152.
31. Benumof, J. L. "One-lung ventilation and hypoxic pulmonary vasoconstriction: Implications for anesthetic management." Anesthesia & Analgesia 64, no. 8 (1985): 821–33
32. Henderson, Y., F. P. Chillingworth and J. L. Whitney. "The respiratory dead space." American Journal of Physiology 38, no. 1 (1915): 1–19.
33. Meltzer, S. J. and J. Auer. "Continuous respiration without respiratory movements." The Journal of Experimental Medicine 11, no. 4 (1909): 622.

34. Hooke, R. "An account of an experiment made by Mr. Hook [sic], of preserving animals alive by blowing through their lungs with bellows." Philosophical Transactions of the Royal Society of London 2 (1667): 539–540.
35. Briscoe, W. A., R. E. Forster and J. H. Comroe. "Alveolar ventilation at very low tidal volumes." Journal of Applied Physiology 7, no. 1 (1954): 27–30.
36. Jonzon, A. et al "High-frequency positive-pressure ventilation by endotracheal insufflation." Acta Anaesthesiologica Scandinavica 15, s43 (1971): 1–43.
37. Lunkenheimer, P. P. et al. "Application of transtracheal pressure oscillations as a modification of diffusion respiration." British Journal of Anaesthesia 44, no. 6 (1972): 627.
38. Bryan, A. C. "Historic and future development of high-frequency ventilation." Annals of Biomedical Engineering 12, no. 4 (1984): 353–356.
39. Heijman, K. et al. "High frequency positive pressure ventilation during anaesthesia and routine surgery in man." Acta Anaesthesiologica Scandinavica 16, no. 3 (1972): 176–187.
40. Klain, M. and H. Keszler. "High-frequency jet ventilation." The Surgical clinics of North America 65, no. 4 (1985): 917
41. Klain, M. and R. B. Smith. "High frequency percutaneous transtracheal jet ventilation." Critical Care Medicine 5, no. 6 (1977): 280–287.
42. Bohn, D. J. et al. "Ventilation by high-frequency oscillation." Journal of Applied Physiology 48, no. 4 (1980): 710–716.
43. Carden, E. and W. Crutchfield. "Anaesthesia for microsurgery of the larynx." Canadian Journal of Anesthesia 20, no. 3 (1973): 378–389.
44. Babinski, M., R. B. Smith and M. Klain. "High-frequency jet ventilation for laryngoscopy." The Journal of the American Society of Anesthesiologists 52, no. 2 (1980): 181–183.
45. Shikowitz, M. J., A. L. Abramson and L. Liberatore. "Endolaryngeal jet ventilation: A 10-year review." The Laryngoscope 101, no. 5 (1991): 455.
46. Bourgain, J. L. et al. "Transtracheal high frequency jet ventilation for endoscopic airway surgery: A multicentre study." British Journal of Anaesthesia 87, no. 6 (2001): 870–875.
47. Magee, M. J. et al. "Nasotracheal jet ventilation for rigid endoscopy." The Annals of Thoracic Surgery 57, no. 4 (1994): 1031.
48. Ratzenhofer-Komenda, B. et al. "Intraoperative application of high frequency ventilation in thoracic surgery." Acta Anaesthesiologica Scandinavica. Supplement 109 (1996): 149–53
49. Sanders, R. D. "Two ventilating attachments for bronchoscopes." Delaware Medical Journal 39 (1967): 170–5.
50. Hildebrand, P. J. et al. "High frequency jet ventilation – a method for thoracic surgery." Anaesthesia 39, no. 11 (1984): 1091–1095.
51. Perera, E. R., D. M. Vidic and J. Zivot. "Carinal resection with two high-frequency jet ventilation delivery systems." Canadian Journal of Anesthesia 40, no. 1 (1993): 59–63.
52. Misiolek, H. et al. "Comparison of double-lung jet ventilation and one-lung ventilation for thoracotomy." European Journal of Anaesthesiology 25, no. 1 (2008): 15.
53. Yin, F. F. et al. "Extracranial radiosurgery: Immobilizing liver motion in dogs using high-frequency jet ventilation and total intravenous anesthesia." International Journal of Radiation Oncology Biology Physics 49, no. 1 (2001): 211–216.
54. Fritz, P. et al "Technical note: Gold marker implants and high-frequency jet ventilation for stereotactic, single-dose irradiation of liver tumors." Technology in Cancer Research & Treatment 5, no. 1 (2006): 9–14.
55. Courbon, C. et al. "High-frequency jet ventilation for HIFU." Cardiovascular and Interventional Radiology 37, no. 5 (2014): 1397–8
56. Olive, D. J. and J. R. Cormack. "Kidney stone movement during lithotripsy under general anaesthesia: High frequency jet ventilation versus spontaneous ventilation." Anaesthesia and Intensive Care 34, no. 6 (2006): 832–834.
57. Raiten, J. et al. "Novel uses of high frequency ventilation outside the operating room." Anesthesia & Analgesia 112, no. 5 (2011): 1110–3.

58. Biro, P, D. R. Spahn and T. Pfammatter. "High-frequency jet ventilation for minimizing breathing-related liver motion during percutaneous radiofrequency ablation of multiple hepatic tumours." British Journal of Anaesthesia 102, no. 5 (2009): 650–4
59. Abderhalden, S. et al. "CT-guided navigation of percutaneous hepatic and renal radiofrequency ablation under high-frequency jet ventilation: Feasibility study." Journal of Vascular and Interventional Radiology 22, no. 9 (2011): 1275–1278.
60. Chung, D. Y. F. et al. "High-frequency jet ventilation under general anesthesia facilitates CT-guided lung tumor thermal ablation compared with normal respiration under conscious analgesic sedation." Journal of Vascular and Interventional Radiology 25, no. 9 (2014): 1463–1469.
61. Denys, A. et al. "Use of high-frequency jet ventilation for percutaneous tumor ablation." Cardiovascular and Interventional Radiology 37, no. 1 (2014): 140–6.
62. Goode J. S. et al. "High-frequency jet ventilation: Utility in posterior left atrial catheter ablation." Heart Rhythm 3, no. 1 (2006): 13–19.
63. Perkins, P. E. "High-frequency jet ventilation during radiofrequency ablation: A case report." AANA Journal 76, no. 3 (2008): 209.
64. Weiner M. M. "High frequency ventilation and atrial fibrillation ablation." Anesthesia & Analgesia 113, no. 4 (2011): 957.
65. Williams J. L. et al. "High frequency jet ventilation during ablation of supraventricular and ventricular arrhythmias: Efficacy, patient tolerance and safety." The Journal of Innovations in Cardiac Rhythm Management 2 (2011): 1–7.
66. Cormack J. R. et al. "Comparison of two ventilation techniques during general anesthesia for extracorporeal shock wave lithotripsy: High-frequency jet ventilation versus spontaneous ventilation with a laryngeal mask airway." Urology 70, no. 1 (2007): 7–10
67. Mucksavage, P. et al. "High-frequency jet ventilation is beneficial during shock wave lithotripsy utilizing a newer unit with a narrower focal zone." Canadian Urological Association Journal 4, no. 5 (2010): 333–335.
68. Fritz, P. et al. "High-frequency jet ventilation for complete target immobilization and reduction of planning target volume in stereotactic high single-dose irradiation of stage I non–small cell lung cancer and lung metastases." International Journal of Radiation Oncology Biology Physics 78, no. 1 (2010): 136–142.
69. Ihra, G. et al. "High-frequency jet ventilation in European and North American institutions: Developments and clinical practice." European Journal of Anaesthesiology 17, no. 7 (2000): 418–430.

25

Triggered Temperature-Sensitive Liposome Release by Focused Ultrasound for Localised Drug Delivery

Paul Lyon, Robert Carlisle, and Constantin C. Coussios

25.1 Introduction

In 2012 there were 14.1 million new cancer cases, 8.2 million cancer deaths and 32.6 million people living within 5 years of a cancer diagnosis worldwide. Lung, breast, colorectal, prostate and gastric cancer are the 5 most frequently occurring cancers.[1] The main cause of death is the development of metastases, with the liver being one of the most common sites of spread. Breast cancer affects 1 in 9 women and most commonly metastases to the lung, bone, liver and lymph nodes.[2] It is a leading cause of death in women and exemplifies the impact of such metastatic spread. Earlier detection and advanced treatments have dramatically improved outcomes in patients with primary localised breast cancer since the 1990s, reaching 5-year survival rates of 99%. However, those with regional disease have an 84% relative 5-year survival and once distant metastasis has occurred, this survival rate rapidly declines to just 24%.[3] Indeed, the presence of metastases is the single most important prognostic factor in these patients. Those having larger tumours at diagnosis, and thus increased risk of metastases including micro-metastases, are also associated with having a worse prognosis; in those patients with regional disease, 5-year relative survival rates are 95% for breast tumours under 2 cm at diagnosis, 83% for those 2.1–5 cm and 65% for those over 5 cm.

Whilst there have been great advances in minimally invasive surgery and ablative therapies for oligometastatic liver disease from a range of primary cancers, conventional chemotherapy remains the mainstay of treatment for patients with multi-focal liver disease. Despite advances in chemotherapy and its delivery, objective response in this patient group remains poor and represents a great economic cost across the globe. In the United States alone, the cost of all cancer care was $125 billion in 2010[4] and estimated to be $158 billion in 2020,[5] of which chemotherapy is a significant contributor with an estimated average price-tag of $161,000 for a typical chemotherapy regime for metastastic colorectal cancer in 2004.[6] In the United Kingdom, the current annual cost of chemotherapy to the NHS was estimated at ~£1.6 billion in 2021, a cost which could be greatly reduced if first-line treatments could be made more efficacious. The shortcomings of chemotherapy can be attributed both to the limitation of maximum dose, governed by systemic toxicity of intravenously injected agents, and to the challenge of achieving widespread intra-tumoural drug penetration to all tumour cells.[7]

25.1.1 Challenges in Drug Delivery to Tumours

For a cancer treatment to be curative, it must have access to all tumour cells or their micro-vasculature, as the survival of even minimal cell burden could form the focus of tumour recurrence. In 1955, using histological sections of bronchial carcinoma, Thomlinson and Gray first demonstrated that the quantity of necrotic tissue was related to the size of the tumour itself.[8] As central necrosis was observed in all tumours of radius greater than 200 μm, but never in tumours under 160 μm, it was concluded that this

 DOI: 10.1201/9780429162671-25

was due to an oxygen diffusion limit from the nearest blood vessel, with cells beyond that limit being anoxic and unable to proliferate. Furthermore, it was hypothesised that a rim of chronically hypoxic, but viable, cancer cells surrounds each necrotic core. Indeed hypoxic tumour cells in poorly perfused tumour regions have been shown to promote drug resistance, tumour progression and metastasis through several mechanisms[9] and thus are a dangerous target cell population which limit the effectiveness of systemic chemotherapy.

For any blood-borne therapeutic agent, there must be extravasation and penetration of the perivascular space to reach cancer cells.[10] Systemic chemotherapy relies on indiscriminate passive diffusion from vessels, and thus there is a trade-off between providing adequate dosage for tumour penetration and limiting the dose to avoid off-site, or adverse, effects. Several factors combine to make the tumour a challenging environment into which to deliver drugs. Tumour vasculature has a significantly different architecture from that found in normal tissue, having a highly heterogeneous, complex and dense branching pattern with enlarged vessels and absent lymphatic drainage.[11,12] Furthermore, tumour microvasculature has intercellular spaces of up to 500 nm, six times larger than fenestrated endothelia in the liver, and hundreds of fold larger than normal tissue beds, leading to a leaky microenvironment.[13–17] This, in turn, causes unregulated extravasation of fluid and solutes into the tumour interstitial space and increased interstitial fluid pressure (IFP).[18] Because the IFP is roughly equivalent to the pressure within the microvasculature (~20 mm Hg), convection from the vascularised regions to the rest of the tumour is very limited, and molecular movement through the tumour becomes entirely diffusion-driven.[19]

The maximum distance between a cell and the nearest blood vessel in healthy tissues rarely exceeds 100 μm, a remarkable feature of the human body. As tumour cells may proliferate more rapidly than the endothelial cells of blood capillaries, this has the effect of forcing vessels apart, increasing this distance to up to 180–200 μm in some tumour types.[7,8,20] This renders the passive, diffusion-driven delivery mechanism to these high pressure and hypoxic regions even more challenging and leads to perhaps the biggest barrier to successful delivery: poor drug penetration to tumour cells furthest from blood vessels. One in vivo study has shown that the concentration of systemically administered doxorubicin decreases exponentially with increasing distance from tumour vessels and falls to half its perivascular concentration at a distance of 40–50 μm.[21]

Finally, some particular tumour subtypes, including pancreatic cancer, have dense stroma which acts as a barrier, further limiting passive diffusion of chemotherapy.[22,23]

As a result of these features, systemically administered drugs will tend to concentrate around the periphery of solid tumours where perfusion is rich. However, in the more avascular central regions, rather than by convection, delivery becomes diffusion-limited due to low pressure gradients.[12] Indeed, the larger the agent, the more inefficient passive diffusion becomes.[24]

To date, therefore purely pharmacological approaches have failed to address what is essentially a three-fold challenge: (i) to deliver therapeutically significant concentrations of active agents to the tumour vasculature while minimising off-target effects; (ii) to release the therapeutic agent 'on-demand' at the target site; and (iii) to improve the distribution and spread of the therapeutic agent against the intratumoural pressure gradient in order to achieve a therapeutically relevant concentration throughout the entire tumour.

25.2 Physical Principles and Mechanisms

25.2.1 Introduction to Drug Delivery Systems

The use of macromolecular drug delivery systems (DDSs), such as those composed of liposomes,[25] polymers[26] or nanoparticles,[27] can enhance the pharmacological effect of chemotherapeutics by improving pharmacokinetics and pharmacodynamics.[28] The requirements of a targeted DDS are to (i) retain its content from manufacture to point of delivery, (ii) evade the innate defence mechanisms, (iii) target the specific tumour site and, only then, (iv) release its payload.[29]

25.2.2 Liposomal Drug Delivery Systems

In the early 1960s, Bangham et al. first identified the potential of a swollen phospholipid system, initially coined 'bangosome', which became known as the liposome.[30] Further pioneering research in the 1960–1970s by Gregoriadis and others[30–35] led to the realisation that liposomes could potentially be used as drug delivery vehicles due to their versatile biocompatible membranes and aqueous core, allowing incorporation of hydrophilic drugs. In early studies, liposomes were noted to suffer from rapid opsonisation and uptake by the mononuclear phagocyte system (MPS), resulting in rapid clearance from the circulation. The development of 'stealth liposomes' by incorporating PEG into the lipid membrane ('PEGylation'), has greatly extended circulation times, from minutes to hours or even days, due to evasion of uptake by the MPS.[36–38] A further optimisation has included the use of cholesterol in the membrane to reduce leakage of encapsulated content.[39, 40]

After decades of academic research efforts, liposomal formulations are under investigation for clinical use in intravascular delivery of anti-cancer, anti-fungal, gene therapy agents and vaccines by vascular, inhalational and topical delivery mechanisms. However, only a small minority of formulations have been approved for clinical use.[41] Liposomal DDS are currently approved for use in oncological clinical practice and there are many on-going clinical trials in this area (Table 25.1). The first human study to demonstrate the use of PEGylated liposomes for prolonged circulation was performed in 1994,[42] shortly after which the encouraging results of the first clinical study of PEGylated liposomal doxorubicin (Doxil) for Kaposi's sarcoma were published.[43] In 1995, Doxil became the first Food and Drug Administration (FDA)-approved liposomal pharmaceutical, or indeed nano-drug, and is indicated for

TABLE 25.1

Marketed Liposomal and Lipid-Based Products, plus a Section of Products in Clinical Development
Reprinted with permission from Elsevier, references available in original manuscript[43].

	Product	Drug	Indications	Year Approved/Study Phase
Approved Products	AmBisome (Gilead)	Amphotericin B	Fungal infections, Leishmaniasis	1990 (Europe), 1997 (USA), 2000
	Doxil/Caelyx (Johnson & Johnson)	Doxorubicin	Kaposi's sarcoma Ovarian cancer Breast cancer Multiple myeloma + Velcade	1995 1999 2003 (Europe, Canada) 2007
	DaunoXome (Galen)	Daunorubicin	Kaposi's sarcoma	1996 (Europe), 1996 (USA)
	Myocet (Cephalon)	Doxorubicin	Breast cancer + cyclophosphamide	2000 (Europe)
	Amphotec (Intermune)	Amphotericin B	Invasive aspergillosis	1996
	Abelcet (Enzon)	Amphotericin B	Aspergillosis	1995
	Visudyne (QLT)	Verteporphin	Wet macular degeneration	2000 (USA), 2003 (Japan)
	DepoDur (Pacira)	Morphine sulphate	Pain following surgery	2004
	DepoCyt (Pacira)	Cytosine Arabinoside	Lymphomatous meningitis Neoplastic meningitis	1999
	Diprivan (AstraZeneca)	Propofol	Anaesthesia	1986
	Estrasorb (King)	Oestrogen	Menopausal therapy	2003
	Lipo-Dox (Taiwan Liposome)	Doxorubicin	Kaposi's sarcoma, breast and ovarian cancer	2001 (Taiwan)
	Marciibo (Talon)	Vincristine	Acute lymphoblastic leukaemia	2012 (USA)

TABLE 25.1 (*Continued*)

Marketed Liposomal and Lipid-Based Products, plus a Section of Products in Clinical Development Reprinted with permission from Elsevier, references available in original manuscript[43].

	Product	Drug	Indications	Year Approved/Study Phase
Products in Clinical Trials	SPI-077 (Alza)	Cisplatin	Solid tumours	Phase II (development terminated)
	CPX-351 (Celator)	Cytarabine:daunorubicin	Acute myeloid leukaemia	Phase II
	CPX-1 (Celator)	kinotecan HCI:floxuridine	Colorectal cancer	Phase II
	MM-398 (Merrimack)	CPT-11	Gastric and pancreatic cancer Glioma and colon cancer	Phase II Phase I
	MM-302 (Merrimack)	ErbB2/ErbB3-targeted doxorubicin	ErbB2-positive breast cancer	Phase I
	MBP-436 (Mebiopharm)	Transferrin-targeted oxaliplatin	Gastric cancer and gastro-oesophageal junction	Phase II
	Brakiva (Talon)	Topotecan	Relapsed solid tumours	Phase I
	Alocrest (Talon)	Vinorelbine	Newly diagnosed or relapsed solid tumours	Phase I
	Lipoplatin (Regulon)	Cisplatin	Non-small cell lung cancer	Phase III
	L-annamycin (Callisto)	Annamycin	Adult relapsed ALL Paediatric relapsed ALL and acute myelogenous leukaemia Doxorubicin-resistant breast cancer	Phase I Phase I Phase II (development terminated)
	ThermoDox (Celsion)	Thermosensitive doxorubicin	Primary hepatocellular carcinoma Refractory chest wall breast cancer Colorectal liver metastases	Phase III Phase II Phase II
	Endo-Tag-1 (Medigene)	Cationic liposomal paclitaxel	Pancreatic cancer Triple negative breast cancer	Phase II Phase II
	ALN-TTR ALN-PCS	siRNA targeting transthyretin (TER)	TIR amyloidosis	Phase I
	ALN-VSP (Alnylam)	siRNA targeting PCSK9 RNAi targeting liver cancer	Hypercholesterolaemia Liver cancer and liver metastases	Phase I Phase I
	TKM-PLK1 TKM-ApoB (Tekmira)	RNAi targeting polo-like kinase 1 (POLO) RNAi targeting apoB	Liver tumours High levels of LDL cholesterol	Phase I Phase I
	Stimuvax (Oncothyreon/ Merck)	Anti-MUCI cancer vaccine	Non-small cell lung cancer	Phase III
	Exparel (Pacira)	Bupivacaine	Nerve block Epidural	Phase II Phase I

the treatment of metastatic breast and ovarian cancer.[44–47] Of note, FDA approval was based on equivalent therapeutic efficacy but reduced adverse effects. Other well-known chemotherapeutic liposomal formulations approved for use in Europe include Myocet (containing doxorubicin), also indicated for breast cancer,[48] and DaunoXome (containing daunorubicin) for Kaposi's sarcoma.[49]

Liposomal formulations of typical mean size 100 nm, such as Doxil, are of particular interest. By virtue of their size, such macromolecules will tend to preferentially accumulate across the leaky tumour vasculature due to a passive targeting phenomenon known as the enhanced permeability and retention (EPR) effect.[50] As a result of this process, macromolecules (defined as having a molecular size of more than 40 kDa), such as liposomes, are seen to accumulate in solid tumour and remain there for several days rather than minutes.[51] In particular, intravenously administered liposomes preferentially accumulate in the perivascular space of tumours, as they are unable to penetrate further.[52, 53] One study has shown Doxil distribution falling off rapidly further than 10 μm from the nearest vessel,[54] in contrast to bioavailable drugs, such as free doxorubicin, which may penetrate up to an order of magnitude further.[21] Consequently, these so-called non-temperature sensitive liposomes (NTSLs) are designed to degrade slowly following passive accumulation to reduce systemic toxicity, thus delivering sustained concentrations of bioavailable drug largely through the perivascular space.[55] Doxil is a stealthed NTSL, designed to accumulate by the EPR effect and slowly release its chemotherapeutic payload over days to weeks with peak bioavailability at 48 hours.[56] Despite FDA approval for Doxil, the mechanism for intratumoural release of doxorubicin still remains to be elicited.[57]

Key advantages of such liposomal preparations are longer circulation times and the ability to attenuate drug-related systemic toxicity, thus increasing the therapeutic index.[58, 59] However, despite great advances in the manufacture of clinically approved liposomes (Table 25.1), only modest improvements in clinical outcomes have been demonstrated in the treatment of cancer patients.[60]

Despite the EPR effect, a major limitation of systemically administered liposomal agents is their low therapeutic index: the dose required to produce a successful anti-tumour effect remains toxic to normal tissues, and, at lower doses, antitumour activity is hindered by a failure to penetrate significantly beyond the perivascular space.[61] Furthermore, as NTSL are primarily designed to be stable in circulation, they fail to release more than a third of their cargo upon reaching the perivascular space in the tumour.[62] Whilst the passive accumulation and slow release of PEGylated NTSLs may be efficacious in some circumstances such as schedule-dependent drugs,[63, 64] the activity of other drugs and in particular anti-cancer agents, such as doxorubicin, is dependent on peak concentrations.[65] In the absence of a triggered release mechanism, such passive release may create a situation whereby tumour cells are exposed to persistently low levels of mutagenic drugs rather than the rapid attainment of peak chemo-ablative levels. This passive approach may create conditions ideal for the development of resistance rather than treatment.

25.2.3 Heat-Triggered Liposomal Drug Delivery Systems

Since their introduction by Yatvin and Weinstein in the late 1970s,[66, 67] thermosensitive liposomes (TSLs), or traditional TSLs (TTSLs), have offered great promise as targeted delivery systems to improve on the passive release profiles of NTSLs. A large body of strategic work led by Needham and Dewhirst[41, 68] has since led to the development of novel low-temperature sensitive liposomes, also known as lysolipid thermally sensitive liposomes (LTSLs). Incorporation of a phospholipid, lysolecithin, facilitates opening of pores in the lipid bilayer at a transition threshold temperature which is above body temperature but below that which is intrinsically damaging to the cell.[69] Indeed, chemotherapy agents can now be packaged inside biocompatible LTSLs which are specifically formulated to be stable at 37 °C but release their content at temperatures as low as 40 °C. In addition, release is more rapid (near-instantaneous) and a higher percentage of drug release can be achieved over TTSLs.

When administered systemically, such LTSLs are also formulated to evade the MPS and remain in the blood stream for several hours. At peak circulating levels, if localised hyperthermia is sustained at a target tumour site, there is the potential for instantaneous and localised release of chemo-ablative levels of bioavailable drug, whilst avoiding rapid systemic off-target drug release. In using such a delivery system, the intratumoural concentration of delivered drug depends on several factors: (i) the plasma concentration of the LTSL, (ii) the liposomal drug-payload, (iii) the pharmacokinetic release profile of the liposome and (iv) the total exposure time to optimal levels of hyperthermia consequent with drug release.[70] LTSLs are now available for clinical use as investigational medicinal products. Such LTSLs rapidly release chemotherapeutic contents upon reaching levels of mild hyperthermia of around 40–42 °C.

25.2.4 Lyso-Thermosensitive Liposomal Doxorubicin

Doxorubicin is an anthracycline antibiotic with potent broad-spectrum cytotoxic properties which has been used clinically as an approved anti-cancer agent for almost four decades. When administered intravenously, doxorubicin is transported in the blood stream and enters cells to bind to DNA by intercalation, preventing further cell division. In addition free radical formation contributes to its anti-tumour effect, as well as adverse effects.[71] Doxorubicin's broad spectrum of anti-tumour activity and its inherent ability to fluoresce at low concentrations make it an excellent theranostic agent for both pre-clinical and clinical studies alike.

At the turn of the century Needham et al. developed a LTSL formulation containing doxorubicin, which, whilst stable at 37 °C, was optimised for rapid release of drug in conditions of only mild hyperthermia (39–40 °C).[72] Based on similar formulations, Celsion Corp., Columbia, MD, have developed lyso-thermosensitive liposomal doxorubicin (LTLD, LTSL-doxorubicin) for clinical use, under the commercial name of ThermoDox.[41] LTLD releases bioavailable doxorubicin when exposed to mild hyperthermia as the trigger. Release (80–100% of encapsulated drug) is rapid when heated to 41.3 °C for 20–40 seconds, whilst at 39 °C only minimal release (15%) is seen.[73] More recently Lindner et al. have developed a liposome with similar thermal release properties using a different formulation.[74, 75]

Many pre-clinical studies incorporating the use of LTLD for targeted delivery have already been completed, and a number of clinical studies are in the pipeline, in progress or near-completion. Early pre-clinical and clinical studies involving LTLD utilise fluorescence-based quantification assays to better understand its pharmacokinetics in the circulating plasma, and assess intratumoural delivery. Whilst doxorubicin remains encapsulated in liposomal form, its fluorescence emission is significantly quenched. Thus, in these studies, quantification assays will usually incorporate de-quenching steps, such as the use of heating, homogenisation, solvents or detergents, to achieve maximal liposomal release and determine total doxorubicin levels. This de-quenching effect is illustrated in vitro by heating in Figure 25.1(a).

LTLD is available for intravenous administration at the maximum tolerated dose of 50 mg/m^2 of the patient's body surface area over a 30-minute period. The pharmacokinetic profiles of encapsulated and

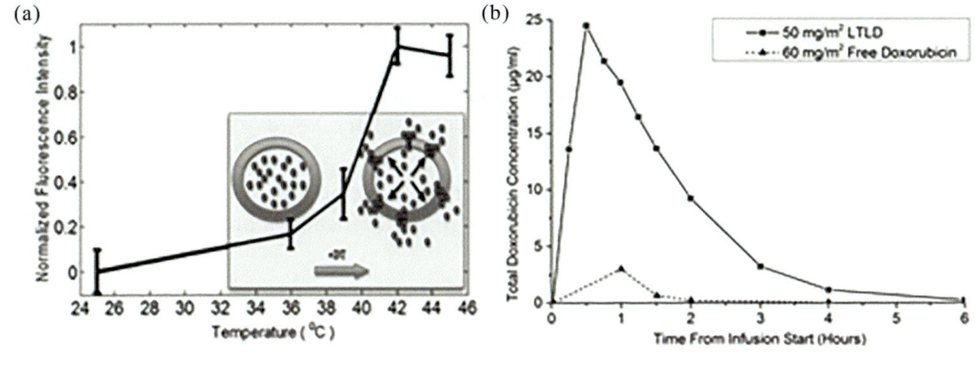

FIGURE 25.1 Pharmocokinetics of LTLD. (a): Plot of fluorescence intensity for LTLD for 6-minute exposures to varying degrees of hyperthermia in a water bath, figure provided courtesy of Dr. Eleonora Mylonopoulou, Institute of Biomedical Engineering, Oxford.[76] Doxorubicin fluorescence is quenched whilst in liposomal form and increases dramatically (dequenches) when released at the minimal threshold temperature of 39.5 °C, with no additional increase in release demonstrated at temperatures above 42 °C. (b): Plasma total doxorubicin in humans after intravenous injection of 50 mg/m^2 LTLD over 30 minutes (Poon et. al.[77]) or conventional doxorubicin at a slightly higher systemic dose of 60 mg/m^2 over 60 minutes (Swenson et. al.[78]), with the former demonstrating a much more favourable pharmacokinetic profile.

free doxorubicin in patients with liver tumours treated with LTLD and radio frequency ablation (RFA) have been evaluated in a previous study.[77] The LTLD pharmacokinetic data has been combined with data from another study, which performed pharmacokinetic analysis for conventionally administered doxorubicin.[78] LTLD circulation is extended for several hours over free doxorubicin due to its PEGylated liposomal carrier. The marked increase in the pharmacokinetic profile for LTLD over that of a slightly higher dose of systemically administered free doxorubicin is illustrated in Figure 25.1(b), due to free doxorubicin being rapidly cleared out of the circulation. Of note, the peak therapeutic levels in the first 2 hours post-infusion provide an optimal and clinically convenient window during which targeted heating modalities can be sustained.

25.2.5 Hyperthermia for Targeted Delivery of Lysolipid Thermally Sensitive Liposomes

When considering hyperthermia-mediated chemotherapeutic delivery to solid tumours using LTSLs, targeted hyperthermia of around 41–43 °C theoretically enhances efficacy by the following key mechanisms in synergy:

1) **Enhanced tumour blood flow**: Hyperthermia increases the potential flow for drug delivery using any systemically administered chemotherapeutic.[79, 80] However, at higher temperatures the converse becomes true and tumour perfusion may ultimately decrease below that of unheated tumour. The effect of decreased perfusion at temperatures of 43 °C and above has been demonstrated in several in vivo studies,[79, 81] emphasising the need for controlled levels of hyperthermia.
2) **Increased permeability of tumour vasculature**: Hyperthermia increases pore size in the microvasculature and thus increases permeability. In the presence of circulating liposomes, there is enhanced liposomal accumulation in the tumour interstitium and therefore delivery of a higher total payload than by EPR alone.[52, 60, 82] Up to a limit governed by the clearance of the LTSL from the circulation, the longer the duration of hyperthermia the more potential for liposomal accumulation.
3) **Instantaneous release of LTSLs**: Such release is thought to occur both intra-vascularly and in the tumour interstitium when the level of hyperthermia exceeds the release threshold. Such instantaneous release is thought to expose tumour cells to a rapid and lethal concentration gradient of chemotherapeutic, penetrating further than would be possible with systemic free drug or slower release from NTSLs. Key to current understanding is that the release time of LTSLs in a hyperthermic tumour matches the transit time through the microvasculature, where the majority of release is thought to happen.[60] Indeed, application of hyperthermia before or during the intravenous infusion which is then sustained whilst plasma levels are highest is optimal. This is in stark contrast to NSTLs which take 24–48 hours to accumulate and subsequently release.[55]
4) **Direct cytotoxic effect**: Sustained mild hyperthermia alone provides a direct cytotoxic effect even in the absence of chemotherapeutic, through mechanisms or protein denaturation or immune stimulation.[83]
5) **Enhanced chemotherapeutic effect**: The use of hyperthermia as a delivery mechanism is particularly attractive, as, when used simultaneously with specific chemotherapeutics, it is understood there is synergistic enhancement of chemotherapeutic effect, without increased systemic toxicity.[84–88] Specifically, in the case of doxorubicin, this enhanced cell kill effect[89] has been demonstrated in vivo[90] and is thought to be due to increased cellular uptake and due to mechanisms relating to inhibition of nucleic acid synthesis and DNA-repair.[91]
6) **Anti-angiogenic effect:** In addition to cytotoxic effects on the target cancer cells, it has been demonstrated that this rapid and localised delivery of high dose of chemotherapeutic agent via heated LTSLs has an anti-angiogenic effect with consequent tumour-regression, thought to be due to a direct cytotoxic effect on tumour vasculature endothelial cells.[92, 93]

25.2.6 Focused Ultrasound Devices for Hyperthermia

Different mechanisms for delivering thermal energy to the target site to release LTSLs are under investigation clinically; these include minimally invasive techniques including RFA to improve ablation margins and the non-invasive modality of focused ultrasound (FUS) to provide targeted hyperthermia alone. Given FUS has the potential to transmit energy and associated temperature rises into the body at precise locations non-invasively, safely and painlessly without the need for ionising radiation, it is an attractive modality for targeted drug delivery of solid tumours by localised volumetric hyperthermia.

Clinically approved extracorporeal high-intensity focused ultrasound (HIFU) therapeutic devices employ FUS, typically coupled through water or gel, to provide thermal and non-thermal tissue effects at a precise anatomical location, under MR (MRgFUS) or ultrasound guidance (USgFUS). When used at high intensity for typical ablative application, clinical HIFU devices produce a characteristic 'cigar-shaped' thermal lesion at the target, lying along the direction of ultrasound propagation. For example, a typical 0.94 MHz HIFU field used clinically for ablation, as produced by the Model JC-200 Focused Ultrasound Tumour Therapeutic System (Chongqing HAIFU Company, Chongqing, China), can generate focal peak acoustic intensities of up to 20 kW/cm^2, producing very small lesions of 10–20 mm along the beam axis and 1–2 mm transversely. Thus, in order to produce clinically relevant conformal and confluent volumes of ablation, such devices typically require placement of lesions side by side.[94]

Depending on the properties of the tissue medium,[95] at sufficiently high rarefactional pressure amplitudes, the ultrasound wave can lead to the formation of gas- and vapour-filled cavities, a process known as acoustically induced cavity nucleation.[96] These nucleated bubbles will then oscillate linearly or non-linearly in response to the ultrasound excitation, a process known as acoustic cavitation. Inertial cavitation is a process of rapid and unstable expansion during rarefaction, followed by a violent collapse during compression, which can occur over the course of a single acoustic cycle.[97] At the time of collapse, inertial cavities radiate part of the incident energy as broadband acoustic emissions into the surrounding tissue, which may result in dramatically enhanced heating at the focus.[96] Cavitation phenomena have been attributed to providing a wide range of desirable therapeutic effects in vivo, including at high intensities, histotripsy and cavitation-enhanced thermal ablation, and, at lower intensities, enhanced vascular permeability, improved drug extravasation and deeper penetration through challenging tissue targets such as tumours[98–102] or the blood-brain barrier.[103]

Subject to the appropriate regulatory approval, both USgFUS and MRgFUS therapeutic HIFU devices can potentially be utilised clinically at intensities below the ablative threshold in order to induce targeted localised hyperthermia for the purpose of safe and targeted drug delivery, without tissue destruction, through significant thermal or cavitation effects.[104] This said, depending on the FUS parameters, mechanical effects, namely cavitation and radiation force, may potentially play a role in release of the drug at the target site in addition to what is proposed to be a predominately thermal mechanism.[105]

In order to achieve a sub-ablative drug delivery regimen, strategies must be employed to significantly reduce the energy delivered to a given focal spot within the target volume, so as to avoid cytotoxic thermal levels of heat deposition within the target volume. This may be achieved by reducing acoustic power for a given transducer geometry, pulsing the ultrasound with a reduced duty cycle, or minimising dwell time in a particular tissue volume by continually moving the ultrasound beam during sonication either electronically (beam steering) or mechanically. In practice, a combination of these approaches may be required. Such strategies would ideally sustain hyperthermia, typically in the region of 40–43 °C, over clinically relevant tumour volumes for between tens to hundreds of minutes. The achievement of rapidly attained and sustained hyperthermia over a uniform as possible temperature range throughout a clinically relevant target volume (for example up to 100 cm^3) would be desirable for optimal efficacy. As significantly lower time-averaged ultrasound intensities are being delivered, the risks of off-target effects such as skin burns and damage to other vital structures is lower than for ablative HIFU.

Although the 'HIFU' acronym has historically received widespread use regardless of its intensity,[106] it is perhaps more accepted to use the term 'FUS' to describe sub-ablative regimens including targeted hyperthermia, although this more generic term can apply to devices used to generate both hyperthermia and ablation. For purposes of clarity, for the remainder of this chapter HIFU will be used to refer to ablative regimens and FUS for sub-ablative regimens, whereas USgFUS and MRgFUS will be used to refer to US- and MRI-guided devices respectively for either ablative or sub-ablative indications.

There have been several recent studies investigating the use of FUS to achieve prolonged targeted hyperthermia in vivo. A recent preclinical study demonstrated generation of 40 °C intratumoural hyperthermia using a 1.2 MHz 256-element phased array MRgFUS device (Sonalleve 1.5T, Philips Medical Systems, Vantaa, Finland) with a spatial peak, temporal average in situ focal intensity (I_{SPTA}) of 120 W/cm^2 at 7.5 W_{ac} and 55 W/cm^2 at 35 W_{ac}, at a focal depth of 15 mm in tissue (attenuation coefficient of 0.5 dB/cm/MHz).[107] Using concentric sonication subtrajectories with a binary feedback control algorithm over slices of 7 mm thickness, and powers of 20–35 W_{ac}, this device was used to tightly control volumetric intratumoural hyperthermia in ten tumour-bearing rabbits in vivo between 40.4 and 41.3 °C (SD 1.0–1.5 °C) at 10–18 mm focal depths from skin. The study did not evaluate for tissue damage using rigorous methods, but no macroscopically evident thermal damage was evident and thermal dose was well below the cumulative equivalent minutes at 43 °C threshold (CEM43). CEM43 is based on model by Sapareto and Dewey[108] and is a common standard used to define the transition from mild to ablative levels of hyperthermia.[109, 110]

Heating patterns may be affected by variability in the vascularity and perfusion of tumours between patients or even in the same patient.[111] Obtaining real-time spatiotemporal feedback from clinical FUS devices is of clinical relevance in ablative therapies and even more important in FUS-targeted drug delivery studies. For MRgFUS devices, such as the Sonalleve MR-HIFU (Philips Medical Systems, Vantaa, Finland),[112] non-invasive volumetric heating feedback is available in real time or cumulatively, providing a much sought after platform for non-invasive heating and monitoring by the same device. The Sonalleve is able to provide temperature measurements to an accuracy of 1 °C in stationary tissue and 2–3 °C in moving tissues such as liver; however, only temperature increases from baseline are interpretable, not absolute values.[113] Cumulative temperature measurements are derived from Sapareto and Dewey's thermal dose model.[108]

The Model JC200 Focused Ultrasound Tumour Therapeutic System (Chongqing Haifu, Chongqing, China) is a USgFUS device. A co-axially aligned diagnostic ultrasound B-mode probe of 3.5–5 MHz is used to monitor the appearance of hyperechoic greyscale changes in real time, which are consistent with tissue boiling.[96, 114] However, this monitoring capability alone has limited use in the context of drug delivery and cannot provide much-needed ultrasound thermography.[115] Despite many advances in the field of real-time ultrasound thermography,[116–122] although anticipated, such technology is not yet clinically available for USgFUS devices.[106]

The operating software for the FUS clinical devices can drive small movements of the transducer in an automated fashion, according to a pre-determined treatment plan. Parameters can be optimised to attain as uniform and as constant a bulk temperature rise as possible. For USgFUS devices, hyperthermia may typically be achieved by automated treatment plans to build up rows, slices and volumes through mechanical translation of the transducer. For MRgFUS systems which may incorporate electronic beam steering, typically spiral or circular raster paths are applied using closed-loop control algorithms.[106] For example, the Sonalleve system achieves volumetric sonication by an automated beam steering control algorithm that translates the focal point between specific locations following circular trajectories in an attempt to maximise heat diffusion for more uniform heat deposition. This method was developed following research efforts by Moonen et al.[123–126] and Köhler et al.[110]

More recently the JC200 USgFUS device has been utilised for sustaining large-volume (up to 70–80cm^3) intra-tumoural hyperthermia in liver tumours (TARDOX trial[127]), validated with a minimally invasive intratumoural thermometry device. The study was designed to demonstrate feasibility of attaining sustained intratumoural hyperthermia at sub-ablative levels consequent with liposomal release, and explored the use of USgFUS for targeted LTLD delivery in liver tumours.[128] Real-time thermometry data was acquired following insertion of a clinically approved thermometry device through a co-axial needle placed in the target tumour under ultrasound-guidance. It is anticipated that the thermometry and clinical data acquired in this early proof of concept study may lead to further similar USgFUS drug delivery studies performed non-invasively with FUS parameters based on patient-specific simulations, possibly in combination with ultrasound-based monitoring strategies.

25.3 Pre-clinical Results

Pre-clinical studies have played a crucial role in advancing the first LTSL and LTLD formulations into the clinical arena. The challenge of attaining peak levels of intratumoural free drug compatible with deep penetrance is key to successful treatment outcomes, and ease of tissue recovery in pre-clinical models has facilitated the assessment of doxorubicin delivery using a range of NTSLs, TSLs and various heating modalities for localised hyperthermia, including FUS. Doxorubicin's inherent fluorescence has proved extremely valuable in establishing both plasma and tumour pharmacokinetics using fluorescence-based assays, whilst fluorescence microscopy has been utilised for assessment of perivascular penetration depths.

As previously discussed, the peak distance of tumour cells from the closest blood vessel may be as much as 200 μm in tumour tissue, and consequently it follows that at adequate concentration, penetration depths greater than this would be therapeutic in the treatment of solid tumours. In respect of the therapeutic threshold of doxorubicin, there is variability, depending on the histological tumour type. A previous *in vitro* study has demonstrated *intracellular* doxorubicin concentrations of 60 ng/mg are required, in order to exceed a 99% cell kill in non-small cell lung cancer.[129] A total *intratumoural* doxorubicin concentration in excess of 20 μg/g of wet tumour mass would generally be considered to be therapeutic, although based on the fractional cell kill hypothesis,[130] multiple cycles are required for complete cell kill. Clinically, the use of FUS targeting to increase intra-tumoural concentration and penetration of delivered drug is aimed at improving therapeutic efficacy for the same systemic dose, and ultimately may render previously chemo-refractory tumours responsive, in addition to potentially reducing the required number of treatment cycles.

With regard to the third proposed mechanism regarding instantaneous release discussed previously, Gasselhuber et al. have developed a computational pharmacokinetic model to simulate tissue heating by FUS and consequent TSL-based doxorubicin delivery.[131] The model demonstrates increasing doxorubicin delivery with up to 2 hours of hyperthermia with maximal intracellular doxorubicin concentrations of ~15–23 μg/g in the target region. The simulated results were validated in an in vivo rabbit tumour model. The same group also performed pharmacokinetic simulations to compare delivery of doxorubicin in various forms: free, stealth liposomes and LTSL with intra- and extra-vascular triggered release, the former being released immediately after administration, and the latter being allowed to accumulate for 24 hours before release.[132] Simulated delivery to doxorubicin-sensitive cells in a mouse model revealed peak intracellular intratumoural drug concentrations of 3.4, 0.4, 100.6 and 15.9 μg/g and peak bioavailable intratumoural drug concentrations of 1.6, 0.2, 77.3 and 7.5 μg/g, respectively, correlating well with an in vivo study discussed later.[60] LTSL simulations assumed locally triggered release by a modality capable of providing 30 minutes of uniform hyperthermia. Simulations demonstrated that liposomal extravasation made a negligible contribution for LTSL when intra-vascular triggered release was applied. Mylonopoulou et al. developed and characterised a cell-embedding tissue-mimicking material with similar thermal and acoustic properties to liver for application to FUS-mediated drug delivery, validated using LTLD with an embedded hepatoma cell line (HuH-7).[133]

Due to significant effort from many research groups, there is now an established body of evidence from in vivo studies demonstrating that the combination of LTLD and FUS-mediated targeted hyperthermia selectively increases intratumoural concentration and penetration of doxorubicin over non-heated control tumours. Furthermore, several pre-clinical studies have demonstrated safe and efficacious targeted delivery using FUS with improved survival outcomes. These studies will be discussed in general chronological order.

As early as the mid-1970s, small animal models have been used to demonstrate enhanced outcomes attributable to liposomal DDS in the absence of hyperthermia.[134, 135] In 1978 Yatvin et al. developed the first traditional temperature sensitive liposomes (TTSL) and introduced the great clinical potential of hyperthermia-triggered release,[66] and further in vitro studies with improved formulations followed.[136, 137] In the 1990s, several pioneering small animal studies using TTSLs containing a range of chemotherapeutics including doxorubicin and cisplatin, delivered by targeted hyperthermia in the range of

42–45 °C for durations of up to an hour, evidenced both increased delivery and improved outcomes.[138–144] Whilst this pre-clinical research was groundbreaking, clinical translation of TTSLs for targeted tumour therapy was hindered by the difficulty in achieving uniform localised intratumoural hyperthermia of beyond 42 °C in the clinical setting. Notably, as these TTSL demonstrated relatively slow drug release, in order to achieve optimal drug release, exposure to these levels and durations of hyperthermia rapidly approach the thermal dose limit for complete cell death according to the thermal isoeffect dose (TID) model of Spareto and Dewey,[108, 145–147] and thus more physiologically relevant liposomal release profiles have been sought.

To address these limitations, the LTSL formulation developed by Needham et al. was validated in 2000 in a pre-clinical human tumour xenograft model.[60, 68] Free doxorubicin was compared with three long-circulating liposomal formulations given with and without tumour-bearing limb hyperthermia at 42 °C: i) NTSL, ii) TTSL releasing at 42–45 °C over a 30-minute exposure and iii) LTSL releasing at 39–40 °C in just seconds. In the presence of hyperthermia, the LTSL group showed the largest concentration of delivered drug (25.6 μg/g tumour, $P < 0.04$), was the only group to demonstrate significant DNA-bound doxorubicin ($P < 0.02$) and demonstrated both the most pervasive doxorubicin fluorescence on microscopy and the largest antitumour effect. The authors highlighted the importance of standardising factors influencing overall efficacy of the delivery mechanism, and distinguished hyperthermia-induced liposomal *delivery* from hyperthermia-triggered liposomal drug *release*. Of note, whilst in a liposomal DDS form, doxorubicin is non-bioavailable and cannot easily penetrate beyond the perivascular space, or bind to DNA, to achieve its cytotoxic effect. Key to this study, when comparing the LTSL group with TTSL and NTSL groups, the DNA-bound doxorubicin and the pervasive fluorescence both indicate higher levels of drug bioavailability and thus release.

In 2005, Laginha et al. explored doxorubicin pharmacokinetics in mice with orthotopically implanted mammary carcinoma injected with free doxorubicin or NTSLs with different release rates, including Doxil for its slow-release formulation.[62] Neither LTSLs nor hyperthermia were used in this study. For the group given Doxil, the time taken to reach the maximum intratumoural drug concentrations was 24–48 hours post-injection, compared to 30 minutes with free doxorubicin. This likely reflects both the rapid washout of free doxorubicin and the additional time taken for the larger liposomes to extravasate through the pores of the tumour vasculature to reach the interstitium by the EPR effect. The longer circulating time for Doxil was also highlighted, in stark contrast to free doxorubicin, with an area under the time-versus-concentration curve 87-fold higher at 7 days. Bioavailability was assessed using a nuclear extraction technique which showed 95% of free doxorubicin was nuclear-bound, and thus bioavailable, by no longer than 24 hours, whereas only 49% of Doxil was nuclear-bound at 7 days.

In 2006, Hauck et al. performed a phase I dose escalation study of LTSLs combined with local hyperthermia in dogs with spontaneous tumours (carcinomas or sarcomas) and included pharmacokinetic analysis.[148] Three treatments using a thirty-minute infusion of LTSL-doxorubicin were given at three weekly intervals. Hyperthermia was induced during, and for one hour after, infusion using a microwave device. Intratumoural thermometry probes were used to record temperature. The drug was tolerated well by most patients with dose-limiting toxicities of grade 4 neutropenia and acute death secondary to liver failure. Plasma total doxorubicin concentrations were shown to be maximal at the end of the infusion. Intratumoural doxorubicin concentration was significantly associated with intravenous drug dose administered ($P < 0.05$) but remained variable. The variability was attributed to the different vascular densities of tumours, and to potential sampling error from a single biopsy from a heterogenous tumour environment being used for drug quantification.

The first in vivo study to use of pulsed HIFU as a source of hyperthermia for triggered release of a LTSL was that of Dromi et al. in 2007.[98] Mice with subcutaneous tumours were injected with free doxorubicin, NTSLs or LTSLs. Each group was split into a subgroup that was either sacrificed immediately or 24 hours after injection for tumour recovery and further divided into those receiving HIFU or not immediately prior to sacrifice. Pulsed FUS (focus surgery, 120 pulses with pulse repetition frequency of 1 Hz, - mm raster spacing, each exposure giving a spatial average temporal average in situ focal intensity (I_{SATA}) of 1.3 kW/cm^2) at a 10% duty cycle was given for 2 minutes at each raster point, spanning the tumour. Although temperature rises were not monitored in this study, the same exposure variables had been previously shown to induce temperature elevations of 4–5 °C in a similar mouse model.[149]

The study demonstrated that the group of mice receiving LTSLs with HIFU simultaneously was the only group to benefit from a significant increase in the mean intratumoural doxorubicin concentration, which was over 3-fold greater than the mean concentration of the other groups. In addition, this treatment group demonstrated significantly enhanced antitumour effects compared with all other groups, suggested to be due to more rapid delivery of higher drug levels. Of the 2 groups receiving LTSL with or without HIFU at 24 hours, there was no significant difference in the mean intratumoural drug concentrations. This finding suggests that LTSLs were no longer circulating at sufficient concentrations to be released by HIFU and supports the hypothesis that the majority of LTSL release happens during peak circulating levels in the tumour microvasculature whilst the tumour is simultaneously under hyperthermic conditions.

In 2010, Staruch et al. made a breakthrough in the use of MR thermometry in a study of in vivo delivery of LTSLs to the thigh muscles of 10 rabbits.[150] A pre-clinical, custom-built and MR-compatible FUS rig was placed in the bore of a clinical 1.5T MRI device (Signa, GE Healthcare, Waukesha, WI, USA). Co-registration of the ultrasound focus with the MRI coordinate system was performed using MR thermometry in a gel-phantom. A closed-loop feedback system was used to heat in a circular trajectory. One thigh of each rabbit was used as an unheated control. Of the contralateral thighs, 6 rabbits received controlled hyperthermia whilst four received ablation. Of those rabbits receiving controlled hyperthermia, the drug concentrations in the heated tissues had a mean 15.8-fold increase over the controls, compared with a mean 9.7-fold increase seen in the ablated thigh tissue. This discrepancy may reflect decreased tumour perfusion resulting from ablation[151] and emphasises the importance of refined temperature monitoring and control.

In the same year, Yarmolenko et al. studied a range of human xenografts as well as a murine tumour line in a mouse model using the commercialised formulation of LTLD.[152] Of the mice treated with LTLD, tumours exposed to 1 hour of regional hyperthermia in a water bath (obtaining tumour temperatures of 43 °C) demonstrated a significant average total doxorubicin concentration increase in all 5 tumour types (FaDu, HCT116, PC-3, 4T07 and SKOV-3) and a significant increase in median growth time in three (FaDu, HCT116, PC-3), over LTLD alone. The study correlates variations in efficacy to *in vitro* cell doubling time and highlights the importance of the consideration of tumour types in studies assessing the efficacy of targeted delivery by tumour growth time or survival.

Theranostic LTSLs with co-encapsulated paramagnetic MRI contrast agents have already been developed, offering a surrogate marker of *release* using MRgFUS systems. Such a delivery and monitoring method offers the potential for more efficient optimisation of hyperthermia regimes in addition to avoiding the need for tissue sampling in early phase studies. Following in vivo studies using manganese-loaded LTSLs as a contrast agent for 'dose painting',[153, 154] de Smet et al. demonstrated delivery of LTSLs containing a gadolinium-based and clinically approved T_1-weighted MRI contrast agent in a rat model in 2011.[70] Using a 3T clinical MRgFUS device, the study demonstrated good correlation between T_1-weighted MRI mapping interleaved between FUS exposures and both doxorubicin and gadolinium concentrations present in the excised tumours. At around the same time, 2 further studies in this field were published, both testing novel formulations of LTSLs containing gadolinium-based contrast agents co-encapsulated with doxorubicin in vivo.[155, 156]

In 2011, Ranjan et al. came another step closer to clinical translation of targeted delivery of LTSLs.[157] Using a clinical MRgFUS system (Phillips Sonalleve, 1.5T) with MR thermometry, the study delivered clinical-grade LTSLs to rabbits with VX2 tumours. One group received free doxorubicin and the remaining 2 groups received LTSL with and without 30 minutes of MRgFUS, within 1 hour of drug infusion for non-invasive targeted hyperthermia. Rabbits were euthanised and tissues harvested to study the bio-distribution of drug. Tumours treated with LTSL and MRgFUS demonstrated a mean intratumoural doxorubicin concentration of 30 ± 9 μg/g tissue, a significant 7.6-fold increase over free doxorubicin and a significant 3.4-fold increase over LTSL alone ($p < 0.05$). Furthermore, the last treatment group demonstrated significantly more specific delivery to the target region, with a 43.5-fold increase in intratumoural concentration over adjoining muscle tissue, compared to a 12.5-fold increase for the LTSL group alone.

Following on from the earlier study, in 2012 Staruch et al. again used a pre-clinical MRgFUS system for FUS hyperthermia but this time to deliver LTLD to tumours in vivo in a VX2 rabbit model.[158]

Real-time MR thermometry was used to inform precise temperature control. Twelve rabbits with tumours transplanted to both thighs had a single tumour treated with FUS hyperthermia, using a feedback control loop based on MR thermometry. Doxorubicin delivery was assessed from fluorescence of tumour homogenates whilst microregional distribution was studied using fluorescence microscopy. The study revealed an impressive mean intra-tumoural doxorubicin concentration of 76.3 μg/g in the group treated with LTSD and targeted hyperthermia, which was over 26-fold higher than that in unheated tumours ($p < 0.017$). Furthermore, no significantly enhanced delivery was seen in heated tumours treated with free doxorubicin over those receiving doxorubicin alone. Fluorescence microscopy of snap-frozen sections from a heated tumour demonstrated co-localisation of a nuclear stain with doxorubicin fluorescence that penetrated beyond the perivascular space, indicating diffusion of bioavailable doxorubicin and thus validating release. In contrast, the unheated tumour sections demonstrated that penetration was confined to perivascular regions only, presumably largely in unreleased liposomal form. Tumour microscopy spatial distribution studies demonstrated a doxorubicin penetration depth of over 150 μm from the closest vessel in the LTSD/FUS group compared to around 50 μm in the group receiving LTSD alone.

Three years later the same group published a follow-up study focusing on therapeutic efficacy, using the same tumour model.[159] In this study a clinical MRgFUS system (Sonalleve[112]) was used for application of 20 minutes of localised hyperthermia at 42 °C using concentric circular trajectories for cylindrical volume coverage in a closed feedback control algorithm. Efficacy was evaluated using tumour progression, based on follow-up contrast-enhanced T1-weighted MRI scans and calculated tumour volumes. Of the 12 rabbits treated, at time of treatment the average tumour volume was 0.9 ± 0.35 cm^3 and the maximum dimension was 1.68 ± 0.75 cm. The 6 receiving LTLD alone had rapid tumour progression exceeding the allowed tumour size endpoint of maximal dimension greater than 6 cm at 24 days, whilst those receiving combined localised hyperthermia all saw at least a transient decrease in tumour volume, of which 4 survived to the study endpoint of 60 days. Of the remaining 2, one reached the tumour size endpoint whilst the final rabbit was sacrificed early due to hyperthermia-related toxicity.

Since 2010, groups have also been looking at novel LTLD formations in an attempt to improve on the thermo-responsiveness of the most clinically advanced formulation of LTSD (ThermoDox), used in several of the earlier studies. Tagami et al. presented a formulation with 90–100% release in 2.5 minutes at 40–42 °C in vitro, which demonstrated enhanced tumour regression in vivo when used in combination with regional hyperthermia via a water bath.[160] Park et al. described another formulation (STL) which showed over 95% release within 10 seconds at 42 °C in vitro and statistically significant tumour regression in the STL over LTSD when delivered with FUS in a murine tumour model.[161]

Finally, another group has observed benefit in use of a pulsed low intensity (under 10 W/cm^2) non-focused ultrasound regime (pLINFU) designed to sonoporate and extravasate intact liposomes from the tumour vascular prior to mechanical release by another non-thermal low intensity planar ultrasound-mediated regimen,[162] a method of release also explored by other studies.[163,164] These advanced studies are beyond the scope of this chapter and are not discussed further.

25.4 Clinical Application of Focused Ultrasound for Targeted Drug Delivery by Hyperthermia

In the 1980s, Lopez-Berestein et al. and then Gabizon et al. published the earliest clinical trials involving the use of liposomes in cancer patients,[165,166] ultimately leading to the clinical use of NTSLs for a range of different indications today.[44] Since the approval of LTLD (commercialised as ThermoDox) for investigational use, several studies involving microwave, radiofrequency (RFA-) and FUS-mediated targeted delivery of doxorubicin are in the development stage, are currently underway or have been completed.

To date, the most clinically advanced investigational programmes using targeted LTSL delivery have been based on attempts to improve survival outcomes in RFA of liver tumours. The individual studies seek to supplement localised tumour ablation by releasing doxorubicin in the surrounding hyperthermic tumour margins, thus extending the volume of cell kill, and, theoretically reducing recurrence.

In 2009, following phase I dose escalation studies for RFA/LTLD,[167, 168] Poon and Borys published the findings demonstrating a safety and a significant dose-response effect in the treatment of hepatocellular carcinoma (HCC).[77] In 2008, Celsion opened a randomised, double-blind, global multicentre phase III trial (Hepatocellular Carcinoma Study of RFA and ThermoDox, or HEAT[169]) comparing RFA + 50 mg/m^2 of ThermoDox versus RFA alone in over 700 patients with newly diagnosed and unresectable HCC. Although the primary endpoint of an improvement in progression free survival of at least 33% was not met in the HEAT trial, post hoc analysis demonstrated that LTLD treatment markedly improved progression-free survival and significantly improved overall survival in the subset of patients having optimal RFA for at least 45 minutes. A detailed analysis of the HEAT results were published in 2017 and the potential reasons for the shortcomings of the trial including choice of drug, the dosing regimen, the type of cancer and the study design itself have been discussed in detail.[170]

Consequently, the subsequent pivotal Phase III OPTIMA study, which enrolled 556 participants between 2014 and 2018, focused on the subset of HCC patients who are amenable to optimal RFA, with intermediate solitary lesions of 3–7 cm, and having standardised treatment times of over 45 minutes.[171] Again, the primary endpoint pertained to overall survival with progression free survival as a secondary endpoint. Unfortunately, the study follow-up was terminated by Celsion early in early 2021 following an earlier recommendation from the independent data monitoring committee for reasons of futility in June 2020, with no measurable survival benefit of RFA+LTLD over RFA alone.[172]

Investigators have raised the possibility that the combination of systemic LTLD and ablative therapies such as RFA is not an ideal approach physiologically due to high temperature gradients causing deleterious effects, such as vascular shunts leading to a reduction in drug delivery, and in fact it is homogenous hyperthermia which would best harness the true potential of LTLD,[172] and subsequent clinical studies are discussed next.

Extensive clinical data from the HEAT and OPTIMA studies has demonstrated that LTLD has a well-established and safe toxicity profile, not dissimilar to that of doxorubicin. The most frequent adverse events in patients treated with LTLD at a 50 mg/m^2 dose are myelosuppression (60%), haematological adverse event (related or unrelated) (45%) and alopecia (40%).[173] Other toxicities reported in greater than 5% of patients include pyrexia, fatigue, nausea and decreased appetite. To date, no significant hypersensitivity or anaphylactoid reactions have been reported in clinical studies using LTSD. Cumulative doxorubicin cardiotoxicity is a known serious risk, which limits lifetime exposure.[174, 175] Although formulations of pegylated liposomal doxorubicin reduce this risk, it remains significant, and consequently such pharmaceuticals typically have a maximum lifetime dose of ~600 mg/m^2.[176] Whilst not directly translatable to the FUS/LTLD delivery mechanism, the drug safety data captured from these large phase III studies has facilitated ethical approval for other early phase trials involving other heating modalities capable of inducing localised hyperthermia in the absence of ablation, such as FUS.

In 2014, Zagar et al. published the results of two phase I trials using LTLD in patients with chest wall recurrences of breast cancer, by definition an advanced and difficult-to-treat cohort of patients.[177] The study designs were similar, other than the permitted dose was higher (up to 50 mg/m^2 of LTLD) in the second study following dose escalation in the first. Hyperthermia was applied using superficial microwave or ultrasound hyperthermia devices with temperature monitoring by thermistor. The primary endpoint was identification of the maximum tolerated dose (MTD). Objective response was evaluated radiologically according to largest tumour diameter (RECIST criteria[178]). The study revealed a MTD of 50 mg/m^2 and an impressive overall local objective response in almost half of the 29 evaluable patients, with 5 demonstrating complete response.

The TARDOX phase I proof-of-concept study ran in Oxford, UK, from 2014 to 2016 and demonstrated safety, feasibility and efficacy of FUS-targeted drug delivery in 10 patients.[124, 179, 180] This first-in-man study evidenced enhanced delivery of LTLD to chemo-refractory metastatic and primary liver tumours at depth by use of extracorporeal USgFUS, delivered intercostally, to generate localised and sustained targeted hyperthermia, whilst avoiding FUS-induced ablation by remaining well below the thermal dose limit previously discussed (CEM43).[127, 181]

The primary endpoint of this study pertained to demonstration of enhanced delivery of intratumoural doxorubicin using the FUS/LTLD delivery strategy, for a single standard intravenous dose of 50 mg/m^2 LTLD. Core biopsies of the targeted tumour were taken pre-LTLD infusion, immediately post-LTLD and post-LTLD+FUS. Tumour samples were used to estimate total intratumoural doxorubicin concentration using a highly validated high-performance liquid chromatography (HPLC) quantification assay based on a previously published method.[182] The study exceeded its primary endpoint and demonstrated an average 3.7-fold increase in the concentration of total intra-tumoural doxorubicin from 2.34 μg/g post infusion, but prior to commensal of FUS hyperthermia, to 8.56 μg/g post-FUS+LTLD, with a maximum observed concentration of 21.8 μg/g.

In addition, biopsy samples were analysed for fluorescence using confocal microscopy to explore the bio-distribution of doxorubicin relative to nuclei and vessels. The study demonstrated drug intercalation with DNA at the cell nuclei (hypothesised to be a predominant site of the potent antiproliferative and cytotoxic effects of doxorubicin[183]), evidencing doxorubicin bioavailability and thus FUS-mediated liposomal release for the first time in man.

As per the mechanisms of cell kill previously outlined in section 1.2.5, it is hypothesised that in bulk-heating the tumour cells and tumour microenvironment, the tumour microvasculature is heated to beyond the minimal threshold release temperature (around 39.5 °C) and ideally to the optimal release temperatures (41–42 °C) in the presence of systemically circulating LTLD, and it is from these tiny blood vessels that the majority of liposomal release occurs. From these vessels free doxorubicin can then flood into the perivascular space and hence, by diffusion, penetrate deep into the tumour microenvironment down a steep concentration gradient, even in sparsely vascularised regions, before entering cancer cells at cytotoxic levels in combination with hyperthermia insult. An alternative hypothesis suggests that high dose doxorubicin disrupts the vasculature within the tumour, either by the coagulation cascade or inflammatory factors, and the heated tumour subsequently undergoes avascular necrosis due to impaired blood supply.[184] Whilst the former hypothesised mechanism relies on deep tumour penetrance of the free drug for enhanced cell kill, the latter mechanism conceivably induces cell death of cells downstream from the damaged vessels which are not necessarily exposed to cytotoxic levels of drug. In reality in the hyperthermia/LTLD paradigm, it is likely that a combination of both key mechanisms are working synergistically with added bioeffects of hyperthermia.

Tumour response was assessed by cross-sectional (contrast-enhanced CT and MRI) and functional imaging (^{18}F-FDG PET-CT) to assess efficacy radiologically. In the majority of patients, the study demonstrated a localised chemo-ablative cross-modality radiological response in the optimally heated tumour regions in the first 2 weeks, despite only a single standard cycle of LTLD, with absence of ablative change on the day 1 post-treatment MRI, further evidencing sub-ablative FUS heating regimens.

The ethos of the TARDOX protocol design was to gain, for the first time clinically, crucial total pharmacokinetic data of intratumoural doxorubicin concentrations at key timepoints, namely i) before LTLD administration (zero), ii) after LTDL infusion alone and iii) after LTLD and a prolonged duration (several minutes) of FUS hyperthermia (LTLD+FUS). It is unlikely that future clinical studies will quantify total intratumoural doxorubicin levels in such detail due to inherent technical challenges in heating and sampling the same tumour at such specific timepoints. Thus, by intentional design, the FUS-heating was commenced immediately following the 30-minute LTLD infusion when peak levels of LTLD are circulating and passive systemic uptake of doxorubicin by the tumour has already reached maximal levels, and after which doxorubicin begins to diffuse out of the tumour back into circulation. As in the clinical study there was a (volume-dependent) lag time of typically 5–10 minutes from the commensal of FUS hyperthermia treatment to the attainment of temperatures compatible with liposomal release, it is conceivable that if the FUS heating were commenced *before* the LTLD infusion, maintained during and sustained for some time after completion of infusion, even higher fold-increases of the delivered total intratumoural doxorubicin levels could be achieved,[185] and such heating protocols may be explored in future clinical studies.

As extracorporeal USgFUS does not provide temperature feedback, in the first 6 patient treatments of the TARDOX study, real-time thermometry with high temporal resolution of the bulk intratumoural temperature was obtained using an indwelling thermometry device (thermocouple or thermistor) implanted into the tumour via a co-axial needle shaft, placed percutaneously under ultrasound-guidance. The thermometry device may be regarded as a relatively crude single point temperature measurement and was intended for the early phase trial only. However, as well as providing crucial validated intratumoural temperature data (unavailable in HEAT and OPTIMA trials), the co-axial needle also permitted tumour sampling in the same region of tumour being heated and monitored.

The final 4 cases explored USgFUS delivery in the absence of real-time thermometry, in keeping with the clinical expectation for non-invasive FUS-targeted drug delivery. Optimal FUS parameters (including power, duty cycle) were predicted using a computational model incorporating anatomical measurements derived from CT data with attenuation coefficients and real-time thermometry data from the earlier cases and demonstrated similar drug delivery efficacy to the temperature-monitored cases.[179] The computational model incorporates patient factors (rib effects, tumour depth, volume and geometry) in addition to variable device factors (transducer translation speed, row and slice spacing).

Extracorporeal USgFUS/LTLD is cheaper, technically more straightforward and has practical advantages at the time of treatment over MRgFUS, which precludes the presence of metal in the room. However, real-time feedback of USgFUS is typically limited to that of the device's integrated B-mode, which can only identify grey-scale changes consequent with tissue boiling, and is not able to monitor levels of hyperthermia consistent with LTLD release.

In the TARDOX study, whilst sub-lethal levels of hyperthermia were sought as the primary delivery mechanism, it is conceivable that a small degree of cavitation, below the threshold for tissue boiling, may have occurred, in the absence of readily detectable B-mode changes. It is conceivable that cavitation may have acted synergistically with hyperthermia-triggered release to provide enhanced extravasation and penetration of released doxorubicin into the tumour by a further key hypothesis, namely cavitational microstreaming.[186, 187] This early clinical experience therefore highlights the clinical need for robust non-invasive methods of monitoring temperature and/or cavitation at depth within the body to fully explore these hypotheses. Future devices may potentially integrate both ultrasound-based methods for cavitation detection[100] and MRI methods for thermography (see Discussion).

Several other early phase FUS/LTLD clinical studies are currently in the pipeline, including phase 1 studies targeting primary breast cancer in late stage patients and relapsed solid tumours including sarcoma in paediatric patients, both using an MR-guided FUS device. Following a great body of preclinical work,[188, 189] most recently clinical studies have demonstrated safe transient opening of the blood-brain barrier non-invasively for the first time using phased array transcranial MRgFUS devices. This is typically achieved using intravenously administered ultrasound contrast agents (microbubbles) and may be used in combination with chemotherapeutic agents.[190–192] A more recent pre-clinical study has demonstrated how transcranial MRgFUS can be used to simultaneously open the blood-brain barrier with simultaneously localised hyperthermia,[193] paving the way for future clinical studies using trans-cranial targeting by FUS/LTSLs or other heat-sensitive liposomal agents.

25.5 Discussion

Despite a wealth of encouraging pre-clinical results for FUS-targeted delivery of LTSLs, clinical studies have only recently begun to gain momentum. In the author's opinion progress has been hindered due to several factors including:

1) The relatively slow uptake of widespread adoption of not inexpensive HIFU/FUS devices in general for clinical use, which is only now showing significant growth in most recent years. Further, the specialist training required to use such devices safely should not be neglected.
2) Despite an impressive worldwide collaborative research effort, the relatively immature and emerging technologies available for real-time monitoring of hyperthermia and cavitation using FUS devices in clinically relevant volumes, be it by MRI or ultrasound strategies, and the inevitable time-lag to achieve clinical approvals around such devices.
3) The great challenges in developing clinically approved LTSLs (and the tremendous efforts in getting ThermoDox to clinic deserve special recognition) and the paucity of clinically approved LTSLs with co-encapsulation of surrogate markers of release for radiological validation.
4) The challenges and huge expenses associated with later-phase randomised clinical trials in FUS therapies in cancer patients, which may be required to demonstrate efficacy and superiority before there is hope of any significant renumeration for the device and drug manufacturers.

25.5.1 Technological Advances

The use of FUS for drug delivery has been a highly anticipated area of clinical research for many years, and with the continued advances in technology and monitoring feedback academic and public interest continues to grow, perhaps exponentially in most recent years. It is anticipated that clinical FUS devices will advance further in their utility for drug delivery as well as ablative therapy, and this continues to represent an area of much active research highlighted by several reviews.[106, 194–200]

In order to achieve mainstream acceptance for such a novel targeted delivery technology, operator feedback from the device is of paramount importance in order to provide confidence in drug delivery and, more specifically, release from liposomes. Consequently, perhaps the most rapidly transforming technological advance of all would be the adoption of a clinically accepted method of non-invasive monitoring of LTSL delivery. MR thermometry[113, 201] has become established as the gold standard in monitoring temperature rises in tissue consequent with release, but comes at considerable expense, and has traditionally been hindered by lack of temporal and spatial resolution over a wide field of view as well its inability to detect cavitation directly. However, using a technique known as proton resonance frequency (PRF) shift,[201–203] one study has recently demonstrated rapid multi-plane MR thermometry in vivo at focal depths of up to 6 cm.[204] The technique achieved 2.5 mm resolution over a large field of view, over 5 coronal and 1 sagittal slice of 7 mm thickness with an acquisition time of less than 3 seconds, performed simultaneously with volumetric FUS exposure. Whilst spatially homogeneous temperature diffusion and regular temperature rises in the target region were used to evidence absence of cavitation, ultrasound-based methods presently remain superior. Research to further improve temporal resolution using the PRF shift method is on-going.[205]

Ultrasound-based monitoring methods, including passive acoustic mapping to monitor cavitation[100, 206–210] and ultrasound thermometry to monitor hyperthermia,[116–122] hold great promise due to their significantly reduced cost and improved resolution. However, there is a need for more formalised industry standards and integration of such technologies in clinical FUS devices before adoption. Other MR-based monitoring methods, such as co-loading of paramagnetic agents,[155, 156] or, alternatively, MR-spectroscopy techniques such as chemical exchange saturation transfer (CEST),[211] may hold the future for localisation of drug release in real time.

Obtaining the required regulatory approval for clinical studies involving both an investigational device and drug simultaneously, has understandably resulted in some inertia. However, the FUS/LTSL strategy addresses the drug delivery problem head-on and has potential to be highly impactful, thus justifying the huge amount of research effort and resources that have been, and continue to be, applied to this field. Success of such clinical studies could potentially revolutionise the future of chemotherapy delivery for ultrasound-accessible solid organ tumours; over the next decade, customised targeted chemotherapy regimens using LTSLs triggered non-invasively by FUS-targeted localised hyperthermia may become a reality in routine clinical practice, as may other FUS bioeffects in combination with systemic chemotherapies.

Future developments may see clinical approval of phased arrays for purposes of both faster and trans-cranial focusing,[212] development of defocused transducers which are more efficient for volumetric hyperthermia delivery and reduced treatment times[213, 214] and further advancement of ultrasound-based guidance and real-time monitoring techniques, including 3D ultrasound, dual-mode ultrasound and ultrasound thermography with higher spatial and temporal resolution than MRI thermometry can offer. There is even potential for the development of devices combining unique features of both MRgFUS and USgFUS.[106]

25.5.2 Pharmacological Advances

Advances in liposome formulations include antibody conjugation, leading to a new generation of 'immunoliposomes', which offer a unique opportunity for specific cellular targeting. Thermo-sensitive formulations are now beginning to emerge, such as the monoclonal antibody-targeted TSLs (TTSL-Ab),[215] which can provide targeting on both anatomical and molecular levels. Furthermore a wide range of hydrophilic chemotherapy agents could potentially be delivered by LTSLs and several thermo-sensitive formulations, including carriers for cisplastin[216] and melphalan,[217] have already been produced. Although this chapter has focused on cytotoxic FUS/LTSL targeted delivery in cancer patients, for which many studies have used doxorubicin as the benchmark agent, the potential scope for other classes of therapeutic agent to be delivered using LTSLs is large. Although not yet available in thermo-sensitive forms, a broad range of other liposomal therapeutic agents under investigation includes viral therapies (virosomes),[218-220] siRNA,[221, 222] rhematologics[223] and analgesics.[224]

Future developments in the FUS/LTSL delivery mechanism may include co-administration of liposomes with micron-sized cavitation-promoting agents in order to further increase penetration depth of the released drug.[225]

25.5.3 Clinical Translation

Overall, despite its early phase, the TARDOX study has provided powerful clinical findings, as the results strongly suggest efficacy of the combined FUS/LTLD technique for highly targeted chemo-ablation of liver tumours, even in metastatic colorectal subtypes previously thought chemo-refractory to doxorubicin therapy. In similar later phase efficacy trials, if optimised FUS devices can maintain a relatively uniform temperature distribution of around 41–42 °C across the target tumour volume, during and after LTLD infusion, it is likely that large volume chemo-ablation can be reliably achieved across a broad range of tumour subtypes and locations non-invasively with intratumoural doxorubicin increases in excess of the demonstrated 3.7-fold increase. Of note, temperatures in excess of 42 °C are unlikely to benefit from increased doxorubicin release from LTLD, and in fact temperatures beyond of 43 °C are likely to decrease drug delivery due to shutdown of the microvasculature.[79, 81]

In the clinical translation of this targeted drug delivery strategy to a clinically approved and accepted standard, there are several challenges yet to be overcome. Safety of both the drug and the device becomes of paramount importance and early phase studies will typically concentrate on these safety aspects, whilst the focus will shift to efficacy in later phase studies. Although it is fairly trivial to harvest the targeted tumour in pre-clinical studies, this is clearly not the case in clinical studies not least due to ethical considerations and the potential for patient harm with tissue sampling. In cases of neoadjuvant chemotherapy the study design affords tissue obtained following surgical resection, for example mastectomy after targeted delivery to a breast tumour. However for targeted delivery studies in unresectable tumours, endpoints involving intratumoural drug quantification and penetrance would necessitate biopsy, and tissue mass limits the extent of analysis (TARDOX study[128, 179]). Whilst non-invasive methods of quantifying surrogate markers of release are under investigation, they are not yet available for clinical use.[70, 155, 156] Some study designs have thus concentrated on anti-tumour efficacy quantified through survival outcomes and/or radiological response; for example, the primary endpoint of the HEAT and OPTIMA studies involve progression-free survival.[169, 171] Yarmolenko has discussed the difficulties associated with making comparisons of response across different tumour types and different patient groups.[152]

Despite these challenges, it is anticipated that the next decade will see results from a number of clinical studies using the FUS/LTSL model, demonstrating enhanced outcomes whilst minimising toxicity profiles, and ultimately leading to clinical approvals and more widespread usage worldwide.

25.6 Summary

We have summarised the continued advances in liposomal formulation since the conceptualisation of the liposome by Bangham et al. in 1965,[30] with focus on the FUS/LTSL model. Given the vast research effort, it is difficult to give credit to every individual contribution in this field in a single narrative. Several excellent reviews on this expanding field are available in areas of liposomal formulation,[226-228] ultrasound-mediated delivery mechanisms and technology[229-231] and paramagnetic liposomes for MR-guided drug delivery.[232]

With exclusion of chemotherapeutics that target on a molecular level, the use of targeted FUS offers the only truly non-invasive solution for the drug delivery problem to date. FUS-mediated delivery through thermal and/or cavitational mechanisms has the potential to deliver greater concentrations of therapeutic agents beyond the perivascular space to unsurpassed tumour penetration depths, without increasing systemic dose and in the absence of direct ablative effects. Coupled with radiological methods for non-invasive monitoring of delivery, release and subsequent clinical response, such optimised FUS device and drug combinations have the very real potential to transform the future of the management of solid cancers.

REFERENCES

1. Ferlay J, Soerjomataram I, Ervik M, Forman D, Bray F. GLOBOCAN 2012 v1.0, Cancer incidence and mortality worldwide. IARC CancerBase No. 11. Lyon, France: International Agency for Research on Cancer; 2013. Available from: http://globocan.iarc.fr.
2. Bathe OF, Kaklamanos IG, Moffat FL, Boggs J, Franceschi D, Livingstone AS. Metastasectomy as a cytoreductive strategy for treatment of isolated pulmonary and hepatic metastases from breast cancer. Surgical Oncology. 1999;8(1):35–42.
3. American Cancer Society. Breast Cancer Facts & Figures 2013–14. 2014. Available from: www.cancer.org/research/cancerfactsstatistics/breast-cancer-facts-figures.
4. Yabroff KR, Lund J, Kepka D, Mariotto A. Economic burden of cancer in the United States: Estimates, projections, and future research. Cancer Epidemiology, Biomarkers & Prevention: A publication of the American Association for Cancer Research, cosponsored by the American Society of Preventive Oncology. 2011;20(10):2006–14.
5. Mariotto AB, Yabroff KR, Shao Y, Feuer EJ, Brown ML. Projections of the cost of cancer care in the United States: 2010-2020. Journal of the National Cancer Institute. 2011 Jan 19;103(2):117–28.
6. Schrag D. The price tag on progress--chemotherapy for colorectal cancer. The New England Journal of Medicine. 2004;351(4):317–9.
7. Minchinton AI, Tannock IF. Drug penetration in solid tumours. Nature Reviews Cancer. 2006;6(8):583–92.
8. Thomlinson RH, Gray LH. The histological structure of some human lung cancers and the possible implications for radiotherapy. British Journal of Cancer. 1955;9(4):539–49.
9. Bennewith KL, Dedhar S. Targeting hypoxic tumour cells to overcome metastasis. BMC Cancer. 2011;11:504.
10. Jain RK. The next frontier of molecular medicine: Delivery of therapeutics. Nature Medicine. 1998;4(6):655–7.
11. Goel S, Duda DG, Xu L, Munn LL, Boucher Y, Fukumura D, et al. Normalization of the vasculature for treatment of cancer and other diseases. Physiological Reviews. 2011;91(3):1071–121.
12. Narang AS, Varia S. Role of tumor vascular architecture in drug delivery. Advanced Drug Delivery Reviews. 2011;63(8):640–58.
13. Jain RK. The Eugene M. Landis Award Lecture 1996. Delivery of molecular and cellular medicine to solid tumors. Microcirculation. 1997;4(1):1–23.
14. Jain RK. Delivery of molecular and cellular medicine to solid tumors. Advanced Drug Delivery Reviews. 2012;64(Suppl):353–65.
15. Dvorak HF, Nagy JA, Dvorak JT, Dvorak AM. Identification and characterization of the blood vessels of solid tumors that are leaky to circulating macromolecules. The American Journal of Pathology. 1988;133(1):95–109.
16. Jain RK. Transport of molecules across tumor vasculature. Cancer and Metastasis Reviews. 1987;6(4):559–93.
17. Gerlowski LE, Jain RK. Microvascular permeability of normal and neoplastic tissues. Microvascular Research. 1986;31(3):288–305.
18. Jain RK. Normalization of tumor vasculature: An emerging concept in antiangiogenic therapy. Science. 2005;307(5706):58–62.
19. Krol A, Maresca J, Dewhirst MW, Yuan F. Available volume fraction of macromolecules in the extravascular space of a fibrosarcoma: Implications for drug delivery. Cancer Research. 1999;59(16):4136–41.

20. Choi IK, Strauss R, Richter M, Yun CO, Lieber A. Strategies to increase drug penetration in solid tumors. Frontiers in Oncology. 2013;3:193.
21. Primeau AJ, Rendon A, Hedley D, Lilge L, Tannock IF. The distribution of the anticancer drug Doxorubicin in relation to blood vessels in solid tumors. Clinical Cancer Research: An Official Journal of the American Association for Cancer Research. 2005;11(24 Pt 1):8782–8.
22. Torphy RJ, Wang Z, True-Yasaki A, Volmar KE, Rashid N, Yeh B, et al. Stromal content is correlated with tissue site, contrast retention, and survival in pancreatic adenocarcinoma. JCO Precision Oncology. 2018;2:1–12.
23. Hosein AN, Brekken RA, Maitra A. Pancreatic cancer stroma: An update on therapeutic targeting strategies. Nature Reviews Gastroenterology & Hepatology. 2020;17:487–505. doi: 10.1038/s41575-020-0300-1
24. Pluen A, Boucher Y, Ramanujan S, McKee TD, Gohongi T, di Tomaso E, et al. Role of tumor-host interactions in interstitial diffusion of macromolecules: Cranial vs. subcutaneous tumors. Proceedings of the National Academy of Sciences of the United States of America. 2001;98(8):4628–33.
25. Schiffelers RM, Storm G. Liposomal nanomedicines as anticancer therapeutics: Beyond targeting tumor cells. International Journal of Pharmaceutics. 2008;364(2):258–64.
26. Lammers T, Hennink WE, Storm G. Tumour-targeted nanomedicines: Principles and practice. British Journal of Cancer. 2008;99(3):392–7.
27. Sajja HK, East MP, Mao H, Wang YA, Nie S, Yang L. Development of multifunctional nanoparticles for targeted drug delivery and noninvasive imaging of therapeutic effect. Current Drug Discovery Technologies. 2009;6(1):43–51.
28. Allen TM, Cullis PR. Drug delivery systems: Entering the mainstream. Science. 2004;303(5665):1818–22.
29. Needham D. Materials engineering of lipid bilayers for drug carrier performance. Mrs Bulletin. 1999;24(10):32–41.
30. Bangham AD, Standish MM, Watkins JC. Diffusion of univalent ions across the lamellae of swollen phospholipids. Journal of Molecular Biology. 1965;13(1):238–52.
31. Gregoriadis G. Drug entrapment in liposomes. FEBS Letters. 1973;36(3):292–6.
32. Gregoriadis G. The carrier potential of liposomes in biology and medicine (second of two parts). The New England Journal of Medicine. 1976;295(14):765–70.
33. Gregoriadis G. The carrier potential of liposomes in biology and medicine (first of two parts). The New England Journal of Medicine. 1976;295(13):704–10.
34. Gregoriadis G, Leathwood PD, Ryman BE. Enzyme entrapment in liposomes. FEBS Letters. 1971;14(2):95–9.
35. Gregoriadis G, Ryman BE. Liposomes as carriers of enzymes or drugs: A new approach to the treatment of storage diseases. The Biochemical Journal. 1971;124(5):58P.
36. Klibanov AL, Maruyama K, Torchilin VP, Huang L. Amphipathic polyethyleneglycols effectively prolong the circulation time of liposomes. FEBS Letters. 1990;268(1):235–7.
37. Papahadjopoulos D, Allen TM, Gabizon A, Mayhew E, Matthay K, Huang SK, et al. Sterically stabilized liposomes: Improvements in pharmacokinetics and antitumor therapeutic efficacy. Proceedings of the National Academy of Sciences of the United States of America. 1991;88(24):11460–4.
38. Senior J, Delgado C, Fisher D, Tilcock C, Gregoriadis G. Influence of surface hydrophilicity of liposomes on their interaction with plasma protein and clearance from the circulation: Studies with poly(ethylene glycol)-coated vesicles. Biochimica et biophysica acta. 1991;1062(1):77–82.
39. Cullis PR. Lateral diffusion rates of phosphatidylcholine in vesicle membranes: Effects of cholesterol and hydrocarbon phase transitions. FEBS Letters. 1976;70(1):223–8.
40. McIntosh TJ. The effect of cholesterol on the structure of phosphatidylcholine bilayers. Biochimica et biophysica acta. 1978;513(1):43–58.
41. Needham D, Dewhirst MW. The development and testing of a new temperature-sensitive drug delivery system for the treatment of solid tumors. Advanced Drug Delivery Reviews. 2001;53(3):285–305.
42. Gabizon A, Catane R, Uziely B, Kaufman B, Safra T, Cohen R, et al. Prolonged circulation time and enhanced accumulation in malignant exudates of doxorubicin encapsulated in polyethylene-glycol coated liposomes. Cancer Research. 1994;54(4):987–92.
43. James ND, Coker RJ, Tomlinson D, Harris JR, Gompels M, Pinching AJ, et al. Liposomal doxorubicin (Doxil): An effective new treatment for Kaposi's sarcoma in AIDS. Clinical Oncology. 1994;6(5):294–6.

44. Allen TM, Cullis PR. Liposomal drug delivery systems: From concept to clinical applications. Advanced Drug Delivery Reviews. 2013;65(1):36–48.
45. Markman M. Pegylated liposomal doxorubicin in the treatment of cancers of the breast and ovary. Expert Opinion on Pharmacotherapy. 2006;7(11):1469–74.
46. O'Brien ME, Wigler N, Inbar M, Rosso R, Grischke E, Santoro A, et al. Reduced cardiotoxicity and comparable efficacy in a phase III trial of pegylated liposomal doxorubicin HCl (CAELYX/Doxil) versus conventional doxorubicin for first-line treatment of metastatic breast cancer. Annals of Oncology: Official Journal of the European Society for Medical Oncology/ESMO. 2004;15(3):440–9.
47. Pisano C, Cecere SC, Di Napoli M, Cavaliere C, Tambaro R, Facchini G, et al. Clinical trials with pegylated liposomal Doxorubicin in the treatment of ovarian cancer. Journal of Drug Delivery. 2013;2013:898146.
48. Batist G, Barton J, Chaikin P, Swenson C, Welles L. Myocet (liposome-encapsulated doxorubicin citrate): A new approach in breast cancer therapy. Expert Opinion on Pharmacotherapy. 2002;3(12):1739–51.
49. Petre CE, Dittmer DP. Liposomal daunorubicin as treatment for Kaposi's sarcoma. International Journal of Nanomedicine. 2007;2(3):277–88.
50. Maeda H. The enhanced permeability and retention (EPR) effect in tumor vasculature: The key role of tumor-selective macromolecular drug targeting. Advances in Enzyme Regulation. 2001;41:189–207.
51. Maeda H. Tumor-selective delivery of macromolecular drugs via the EPR effect: Background and future prospects. Bioconjugate Chemistry. 2010;21(5):797–802.
52. Kong G, Braun RD, Dewhirst MW. Hyperthermia enables tumor-specific nanoparticle delivery: Effect of particle size. Cancer Research. 2000;60(16):4440–5.
53. Yuan F, Leunig M, Huang SK, Berk DA, Papahadjopoulos D, Jain RK. Microvascular permeability and interstitial penetration of sterically stabilized (stealth) liposomes in a human tumor xenograft. Cancer Research. 1994;54(13):3352–6.
54. Tailor TD, Hanna G, Yarmolenko PS, Dreher MR, Betof AS, Nixon AB, et al. Effect of pazopanib on tumor microenvironment and liposome delivery. Molecular Cancer Therapeutics. 2010;9(6):1798–808.
55. Drummond DC, Noble CO, Hayes ME, Park JW, Kirpotin DB. Pharmacokinetics and in vivo drug release rates in liposomal nanocarrier development. Journal of Pharmaceutical Sciences. 2008;97(11):4696–740.
56. Gabizon A, Shmeeda H, Barenholz Y. Pharmacokinetics of pegylated liposomal Doxorubicin: Review of animal and human studies. Clinical Pharmacokinetics. 2003;42(5):419–36.
57. Barenholz Y. Doxil(R)--the first FDA-approved nano-drug: Lessons learned. Journal of controlled release: Official journal of the Controlled Release Society. 2012;160(2):117–34.
58. Harris L, Batist G, Belt R, Rovira D, Navari R, Azarnia N, et al. Liposome-encapsulated doxorubicin compared with conventional doxorubicin in a randomized multicenter trial as first-line therapy of metastatic breast carcinoma. Cancer. 2002;94(1):25–36.
59. Ranson MR, Cheeseman S, White S, Margison J. Caelyx (stealth liposomal doxorubicin) in the treatment of advanced breast cancer. Critical Reviews in Oncology/Hematology. 2001;37(2):115–20.
60. Kong G, Anyarambhatla G, Petros WP, Braun RD, Colvin OM, Needham D, et al. Efficacy of liposomes and hyperthermia in a human tumor xenograft model: Importance of triggered drug release. Cancer Research. 2000;60(24):6950–7.
61. Sharma A, Sharma US, Straubinger RM. Paclitaxel-liposomes for intracavitary therapy of intraperitoneal P388 leukemia. Cancer Letters. 1996;107(2):265–72.
62. Laginha KM, Verwoert S, Charrois GJ, Allen TM. Determination of doxorubicin levels in whole tumor and tumor nuclei in murine breast cancer tumors. Clinical Cancer Research: An Official Journal of the American Association for Cancer Research. 2005;11(19 Pt 1):6944–9.
63. Hande KR. The importance of drug scheduling in cancer chemotherapy: Etoposide as an example. Stem Cells. 1996;14(1):18–24.
64. Janoff AS. Lipids, liposomes, and rational drug design. Laboratory Investigation; A Journal of Technical Methods and Pathology. 1992;66(6):655–8.
65. Gabizon A, Tzemach D, Mak L, Bronstein M, Horowitz AT. Dose dependency of pharmacokinetics and therapeutic efficacy of pegylated liposomal doxorubicin (DOXIL) in murine models. Journal of Drug Targeting. 2002;10(7):539–48.
66. Yatvin MB, Weinstein JN, Dennis WH, Blumenthal R. Design of liposomes for enhanced local release of drugs by hyperthermia. Science. 1978;202(4374):1290–3.

67. Weinstein JN, Magin RL, Yatvin MB, Zaharko DS. Liposomes and local hyperthermia: Selective delivery of methotrexate to heated tumors. Science. 1979;204(4389):188–91.
68. Needham D, Anyarambhatla G, Kong G, Dewhirst MW. A new temperature-sensitive liposome for use with mild hyperthermia: Characterization and testing in a human tumor xenograft model. Cancer Research. 2000;60(5):1197–201.
69. Anyarambhatla GR, Needham D. Enhancement of the phase transition permeability of DPPC liposomes by incorporation of MPPC: A new temperature-sensitive liposome for use with mild hyperthermia. Journal of Liposome Research. 1999;9(4):491–506.
70. de Smet M, Heijman E, Langereis S, Hijnen NM, Grull H. Magnetic resonance imaging of high intensity focused ultrasound mediated drug delivery from temperature-sensitive liposomes: An in vivo proof-of-concept study. Journal of Controlled Release: Official Journal of the Controlled Release Society. 2011;150(1):102–10.
71. Hortobagyi GN. Anthracyclines in the treatment of cancer. An overview. Drugs. 1997;54 Suppl 4:1–7.
72. Kong G, Dewhirst MW. Hyperthermia and liposomes. International Journal of Hyperthermia: The Official Journal of European Society for Hyperthermic Oncology, North American Hyperthermia Group. 1999;15(5):345–70.
73. Mills JK, Needham D. Lysolipid incorporation in dipalmitoylphosphatidylcholine bilayer membranes enhances the ion permeability and drug release rates at the membrane phase transition. Biochimica et biophysica acta. 2005;1716(2):77–96.
74. Lindner LH, Eichhorn ME, Eibl H, Teichert N, Schmitt-Sody M, Issels RD, et al. Novel temperature-sensitive liposomes with prolonged circulation time. Clinical Cancer Research: An Official Journal of the American Association for Cancer Research. 2004;10(6):2168–78.
75. Hossann M, Wiggenhorn M, Schwerdt A, Wachholz K, Teichert N, Eibl H, et al. In vitro stability and content release properties of phosphatidylglyceroglycerol containing thermosensitive liposomes. Biochimica et biophysica acta. 2007;1768(10):2491–9.
76. Mylonopoulou E. Enhancement and Mapping of Ultrasonic Drug Release for Thermosensitive Liposomes by Acoustic Cavitation. University of Oxford; 2011.
77. Poon RT, Borys N. Lyso-thermosensitive liposomal doxorubicin: A novel approach to enhance efficacy of thermal ablation of liver cancer. Expert Opinion on Pharmacotherapy. 2009;10(2):333–43.
78. Swenson CE, Bolcsak LE, Batist G, Guthrie TH, Jr., Tkaczuk KH, Boxenbaum H, et al. Pharmacokinetics of doxorubicin administered i.v. as Myocet (TLC D-99; liposome-encapsulated doxorubicin citrate) compared with conventional doxorubicin when given in combination with cyclophosphamide in patients with metastatic breast cancer. Anti-cancer Drugs. 2003;14(3):239–46.
79. Karino T, Koga S, Maeta M. Experimental studies of the effects of local hyperthermia on blood flow, oxygen pressure and pH in tumors. Journal of Japan Surgical Society. 1988;18(3):276–83.
80. Song CW, Park HJ, Lee CK, Griffin R. Implications of increased tumor blood flow and oxygenation caused by mild temperature hyperthermia in tumor treatment. International Journal of Hyperthermia: The Official Journal of European Society for Hyperthermic Oncology, North American Hyperthermia Group. 2005;21(8):761–7.
81. Brown SL, Hunt JW, Hill RP. Differential thermal sensitivity of tumour and normal tissue microvascular response during hyperthermia. International Journal of Hyperthermia: The Official Journal of European Society for Hyperthermic Oncology, North American Hyperthermia Group. 1992;8(4):501–14.
82. Kong G, Braun RD, Dewhirst MW. Characterization of the effect of hyperthermia on nanoparticle extravasation from tumor vasculature. Cancer Research. 2001;61(7):3027–32.
83. Hildebrandt B, Wust P, Ahlers O, Dieing A, Sreenivasa G, Kerner T, et al. The cellular and molecular basis of hyperthermia. Critical Reviews in Oncology/Hematology. 2002;43(1):33–56.
84. Storm FK. Clinical hyperthermia and chemotherapy. Radiologic Clinics of North America. 1989;27(3):621–7.
85. Cohen JD, Robins HI. Whole body hyperthermia and intraperitoneal carboplatin in residual ovarian cancer. Advances in Experimental Medicine and Biology. 1990;267:197–202.
86. Wiedemann GJ, Robins HI, Katschinski DM, Mentzel M, D'Oleire F, Kutz M, et al. Systemic hyperthermia and ICE chemotherapy for sarcoma patients: Rationale and clinical status. Anticancer Research. 1997;17(4B):2899–902.
87. Kowal CD, Bertino JR. Possible benefits of hyperthermia to chemotherapy. Cancer Research. 1979;39(6 Pt 2):2285–9.

88. Engelhardt R. Rational for clinical application of hyperthermia and drugs. Revista medico-chirurgicala a Societatii de Medici si Naturalisti din Iasi. 1987;91(2):347–52.
89. Herman TS. Temperature dependence of adriamycin, cis-diamminedichloroplatinum, bleomycin, and 1,3-bis(2-chloroethyl)-1-nitrosourea cytotoxicity in vitro. Cancer Research. 1983;43(2):517–20.
90. Overgaard J. Combined adriamycin and hyperthermia treatment of a murine mammary carcinoma in vivo. Cancer Research. 1976;36(9 pt.1):3077–81.
91. Hahn GM, Braun J, Har-Kedar I. Thermochemotherapy: Synergism between hyperthermia (42–43 degrees) and adriamycin (of bleomycin) in mammalian cell inactivation. Proceedings of the National Academy of Sciences of the United States of America. 1975;72(3):937–40.
92. Chen Q, Krol A, Wright A, Needham D, Dewhirst MW, Yuan F. Tumor microvascular permeability is a key determinant for antivascular effects of doxorubicin encapsulated in a temperature sensitive liposome. International Journal of Hyperthermia: The Official Journal of European Society for Hyperthermic Oncology, North American Hyperthermia Group. 2008;24(6):475–82.
93. Chen Q, Tong S, Dewhirst MW, Yuan F. Targeting tumor microvessels using doxorubicin encapsulated in a novel thermosensitive liposome. Molecular Cancer Therapeutics. 2004;3(10):1311–7.
94. Wu F. High intensity focused ultrasound: A noninvasive therapy for locally advanced pancreatic cancer. World Journal of Gastroenterology: WJG. 2014;20(44):16480–8.
95. Holland CK, Apfel RE. Thresholds for transient cavitation produced by pulsed ultrasound in a controlled nuclei environment. The Journal of the Acoustical Society of America. 1990;88(5):2059–69.
96. Coussios CC, Farny CH, Haar GT, Roy RA. Role of acoustic cavitation in the delivery and monitoring of cancer treatment by high-intensity focused ultrasound (HIFU). International Journal of Hyperthermia: The Official Journal of European Society for Hyperthermic Oncology, North American Hyperthermia Group. 2007;23(2):105–20.
97. Leighton T. The Acoustic Bubble. Academic Press; 2012.
98. Dromi S, Frenkel V, Luk A, Traughber B, Angstadt M, Bur M, et al. Pulsed-high intensity focused ultrasound and low temperature-sensitive liposomes for enhanced targeted drug delivery and antitumor effect. Clinical Cancer Research: An Official Journal of the American Association for Cancer Research. 2007;13(9):2722–7.
99. Evjen TJ, Hagtvet E, Moussatov A, Rognvaldsson S, Mestas JL, Fowler RA, et al. In vivo monitoring of liposomal release in tumours following ultrasound stimulation. European Journal of Pharmaceutics and Biopharmaceutics: Official Journal of Arbeitsgemeinschaft fur Pharmazeutische Verfahrenstechnik eV. 2013;84(3):526–31.
100. Choi JJ, Carlisle RC, Coviello C, Seymour L, Coussios CC. Non-invasive and real-time passive acoustic mapping of ultrasound-mediated drug delivery. Physics in Medicine and Biology. 2014;59(17):4861–77.
101. Graham SM, Carlisle R, Choi JJ, Stevenson M, Shah AR, Myers RS, et al. Inertial cavitation to non-invasively trigger and monitor intratumoral release of drug from intravenously delivered liposomes. Journal of Controlled Release: Official Journal of the Controlled Release Society. 2014;178:101–7.
102. Li T, Chen H, Khokhlova T, Wang YN, Kreider W, He X, et al. Passive cavitation detection during pulsed HIFU exposures of ex vivo tissues and in vivo mouse pancreatic tumors. Ultrasound in Medicine & Biology. 2014;40(7):1523–34.
103. Burgess A, Shah K, Hough O, Hynynen K. Focused ultrasound-mediated drug delivery through the blood-brain barrier. Expert Review of Neurotherapeutics. 2015;15(5):477–91.
104. Hynynen K. The threshold for thermally significant cavitation in dog's thigh muscle in vivo. Ultrasound in Medicine & Biology. 1991;17(2):157–69.
105. Novell A, Al Sabbagh C, Escoffre JM, Gaillard C, Tsapis N, Fattal E, et al. Focused ultrasound influence on calcein-loaded thermosensitive stealth liposomes. International Journal of Hyperthermia: The Official Journal of European Society for Hyperthermic Oncology, North American Hyperthermia Group. 2015;31(4):349–58.
106. Ebbini ES, ter Haar G. Ultrasound-guided therapeutic focused ultrasound: Current status and future directions. International Journal of Hyperthermia: The Official Journal of European Society for Hyperthermic Oncology, North American Hyperthermia Group. 2015;31(2):77–89.
107. Partanen A, Yarmolenko PS, Viitala A, Appanaboyina S, Haemmerich D, Ranjan A, et al. Mild hyperthermia with magnetic resonance-guided high-intensity focused ultrasound for applications in drug delivery. International Journal of Hyperthermia: The Official Journal of European Society for Hyperthermic Oncology, North American Hyperthermia Group. 2012;28(4):320–36.

108. Sapareto SA, Dewey WC. Thermal dose determination in cancer therapy. International Journal of Radiation Oncology, Biology, Physics. 1984;10(6):787–800.
109. Meshorer A, Prionas SD, Fajardo LF, Meyer JL, Hahn GM, Martinez AA. The effects of hyperthermia on normal mesenchymal tissues. Application of a histologic grading system. Archives of Pathology & Laboratory Medicine.1983;107(6):328–34.
110. Kohler MO, Mougenot C, Quesson B, Enholm J, Le Bail B, Laurent C, et al. Volumetric HIFU ablation under 3D guidance of rapid MRI thermometry. Medical Physics. 2009;36(8):3521–35.
111. Schramm W, Yang D, Wood BJ, Rattay F, Haemmerich D. Contribution of direct heating, thermal conduction and perfusion during radiofrequency and microwave ablation. The Open Biomedical Engineering Journal. 2007;1:47–52.
112. Köhler M, Enholm J, Mougenot C, Andreae T. Philips MR-guided High Intensity Focused Ultrasound (White Paper). Philips Healthcare; 2012.
113. de Senneville BD, Mougenot C, Quesson B, Dragonu I, Grenier N, Moonen CT. MR thermometry for monitoring tumor ablation. European Radiology. 2007;17(9):2401–10.
114. Coussios CC, Farny CH, Thomas CR, Cleveland RO, Holt RG, Roy RA. Cavitation detection during and following HIFU exposure in vitro. The Journal of the Acoustical Society of America. 2004;115(5):2448-%@ 0001–4966.
115. Rabkin BA, Zderic V, Vaezy S. Hyperecho in ultrasound images of HIFU therapy: Involvement of cavitation. Ultrasound in Medicine & Biology. 2005;31(7):947–56.
116. Seip R, Ebbini ES. Noninvasive estimation of tissue temperature response to heating fields using diagnostic ultrasound. IEEE Transactions on Bio-medical Engineering. 1995;42(8):828–39.
117. Simon C, Vanbaren P, Ebbini ES. Two-dimensional temperature estimation using diagnostic ultrasound. IEEE Transactions on Ultrasonics, Ferroelectrics, and Frequency Control. 1998;45(4):1088–99.
118. Arthur RM, Straube WL, Starman JD, Moros EG. Noninvasive temperature estimation based on the energy of backscattered ultrasound. Medical Physics. 2003;30(6):1021–9.
119. Arthur RM, Trobaugh JW, Straube WL, Moros EG. Temperature dependence of ultrasonic backscattered energy in motion-compensated images. IEEE Transactions on Ultrasonics, Ferroelectrics, and Frequency Control. 2005;52(10):1644–52.
120. Arthur RM, Straube WL, Trobaugh JW, Moros EG. In vivo change in ultrasonic backscattered energy with temperature in motion-compensated images. International Journal of Hyperthermia: The Official Journal of European Society for Hyperthermic Oncology, North American Hyperthermia Group. 2008;24(5):389–98.
121. Maass-Moreno R, Damianou CA, Sanghvi NT. Noninvasive temperature estimation in tissue via ultrasound echo-shifts. Part II. In vitro study. The Journal of the Acoustical Society of America. 1996;100(4 Pt 1):2522–30.
122. Maass-Moreno R, Damianou CA. Noninvasive temperature estimation in tissue via ultrasound echo-shifts. Part I. Analytical model. The Journal of the Acoustical Society of America. 1996;100(4 Pt 1):2514–21.
123. Mougenot C, Salomir R, Palussiere J, Grenier N, Moonen CT. Automatic spatial and temporal temperature control for MR-guided focused ultrasound using fast 3D MR thermometry and multispiral trajectory of the focal point. Magnetic Resonance in Medicine: Official Journal of the Society of Magnetic Resonance in Medicine/Society of Magnetic Resonance in Medicine. 2004;52(5):1005–15.
124. Quesson B, Vimeux F, Salomir R, de Zwart JA, Moonen CT. Automatic control of hyperthermic therapy based on real-time Fourier analysis of MR temperature maps. Magnetic Resonance in Medicine: Official Journal of the Society of Magnetic Resonance in Medicine/Society of Magnetic Resonance in Medicine. 2002;47(6):1065–72.
125. Salomir R, Palussiere J, Vimeux FC, de Zwart JA, Quesson B, Gauchet M, et al. Local hyperthermia with MR-guided focused ultrasound: Spiral trajectory of the focal point optimized for temperature uniformity in the target region. Journal of Magnetic Resonance Imaging: JMRI. 2000;12(4):571–83.
126. Mougenot C, Quesson B, de Senneville BD, de Oliveira PL, Sprinkhuizen S, Palussiere J, et al. Three-dimensional spatial and temporal temperature control with MR thermometry-guided focused ultrasound (MRgHIFU). Magnetic Resonance in Medicine: Official Journal of the Society of Magnetic Resonance in Medicine/Society of Magnetic Resonance in Medicine. 2009;61(3):603–14.
127. Gray MD, Lyon PC, Mannaris C, Folkes LK, Stratford M, Campo L, Chung DYF, et al. Focused ultrasound hyperthermia for targeted drug release from thermosensitive liposomes: Results from a phase I trial. Radiology. 2019 Apr;291(1):232–38. doi: 10.1148/radiol.2018181445. Epub 2019 Jan 15. PMID: 30644817.

128. Lyon PC, Gray M, Mannaris C, Carlisle R, Wu F, Middleton MR, et al. A Proof of Concept Study to Investigate the Feasibility of Targeted Release of Doxorubicin from Lyso-thermosensitive Liposomal (LTSL) Doxorubicin (ThermoDox®) Using Focused Ultrasound in Patients with Primary or Secondary Liver Tumours. ClinicalTrials.gov. University of Oxford; 2014 [updated 27 Feb 2015]. Available from: https://clinicaltrials.gov/ct2/show/NCT02181075.
129. Kerr DJ, Kerr AM, Freshney RI, Kaye SB. Comparative intracellular uptake of adriamycin and 4'-deoxydoxorubicin by non-small cell lung tumor cells in culture and its relationship to cell survival. Biochemical Pharmacology. 1986;35(16):2817–23.
130. Skipper HE. Perspectives in cancer chemotherapy: Therapeutic design. Cancer Research. 1964;24:1295–302.
131. Gasselhuber A, Dreher MR, Partanen A, Yarmolenko PS, Woods D, Wood BJ, et al. Targeted drug delivery by high intensity focused ultrasound mediated hyperthermia combined with temperature-sensitive liposomes: Computational modelling and preliminary in vivovalidation. International Journal of Hyperthermia: The Official Journal of European Society for Hyperthermic Oncology, North American Hyperthermia Group. 2012;28(4):337–48.
132. Gasselhuber A, Dreher MR, Rattay F, Wood BJ, Haemmerich D. Comparison of conventional chemotherapy, stealth liposomes and temperature-sensitive liposomes in a mathematical model. PloS One. 2012;7(10):e47453.
133. Mylonopoulou E, Bazan-Peregrino M, Arvanitis CD, Coussios CC. A non-exothermic cell-embedding tissue-mimicking material for studies of ultrasound-induced hyperthermia and drug release. International Journal of Hyperthermia: The Official Journal of European Society for Hyperthermic Oncology, North American Hyperthermia Group. 2013;29(2):133–44.
134. Kobayashi T, Tsukagoshi S, Sakurai Y. Enhancement of the cancer chemotherapeutic effect of cytosine arabinoside entrapped in liposomes on mouse leukemia L-1210. Gan. 1975;66(6):719–20.
135. Mayhew E, Papahadjopoulos D, Rustum YM, Dave C. Inhibition of tumor cell growth in vitro and in vivo by 1-beta-D-arabinofuranosylcytosine entrapped within phospholipid vesicles. Cancer Research. 1976;36(12):4406–11.
136. Magin RL, Niesman MR. Temperature-dependent drug release from large unilamellar liposomes. Cancer Drug Delivery. 1984;1(2):109–17.
137. Merlin JL. In vitro evaluation of the association of thermosensitive liposome-encapsulated doxorubicin with hyperthermia. European Journal of Cancer. 1991;27(8):1031–4.
138. Huang SK, Stauffer PR, Hong K, Guo JW, Phillips TL, Huang A, et al. Liposomes and hyperthermia in mice: Increased tumor uptake and therapeutic efficacy of doxorubicin in sterically stabilized liposomes. Cancer Research. 1994;54(8):2186–91.
139. Maruyama K, Unezaki S, Takahashi N, Iwatsuru M. Enhanced delivery of doxorubicin to tumor by long-circulating thermosensitive liposomes and local hyperthermia. Biochimica et biophysica acta. 1993;1149(2):209–16.
140. Unezaki S, Maruyama K, Takahashi N, Koyama M, Yuda T, Suginaka A, et al. Enhanced delivery and antitumor activity of doxorubicin using long-circulating thermosensitive liposomes containing amphipathic polyethylene glycol in combination with local hyperthermia. Pharmaceutical Research. 1994;11(8):1180–5.
141. Ning S, Macleod K, Abra RM, Huang AH, Hahn GM. Hyperthermia induces doxorubicin release from long-circulating liposomes and enhances their anti-tumor efficacy. International Journal of Radiation Oncology, Biology, Physics. 1994;29(4):827–34.
142. Nishimura Y, Ono K, Hiraoka M, Masunaga S, Jo S, Shibamoto Y, et al. Treatment of murine SCC VII tumors with localized hyperthermia and temperature-sensitive liposomes containing cisplatin. Radiation Research. 1990;122(2):161–7.
143. van Bree C, Krooshoop JJ, Rietbroek RC, Kipp JB, Bakker PJ. Hyperthermia enhances tumor uptake and antitumor efficacy of thermostable liposomal daunorubicin in a rat solid tumor. Cancer Research. 1996;56(3):563–8.
144. Gaber MH, Wu NZ, Hong K, Huang SK, Dewhirst MW, Papahadjopoulos D. Thermosensitive liposomes: Extravasation and release of contents in tumor microvascular networks. International Journal of Radiation Oncology, Biology, Physics. 1996;36(5):1177–87.

145. Dewey WC, Diederich CJ, Dewhirst MW. Hyperthermia classic commentary: 'Arrhenius relationships from the molecule and cell to the clinic' by William Dewey, Int. J. Hyperthermia, 10:457–483, 1994. International Journal of Hyperthermia: The Official Journal of European Society for Hyperthermic Oncology, North American Hyperthermia Group. 2009;25(1):21–4.
146. Sapareto SA. Thermal isoeffect dose: Addressing the problem of thermotolerance. International Journal of Hyperthermia: The Official Journal of European Society for Hyperthermic Oncology, North American Hyperthermia Group. 1987;3(4):297–305.
147. Sapareto SA, Hopwood LE, Dewey WC, Raju MR, Gray JW. Effects of hyperthermia on survival and progression of Chinese hamster ovary cells. Cancer Research. 1978;38(2):393–400.
148. Hauck ML, LaRue SM, Petros WP, Poulson JM, Yu D, Spasojevic I, et al. Phase I trial of doxorubicin-containing low temperature sensitive liposomes in spontaneous canine tumors. Clinical Cancer Research: An Official Journal of the American Association for Cancer Research. 2006;12(13):4004–10.
149. Frenkel V, Etherington A, Greene M, Quijano J, Xie J, Hunter F, et al. Delivery of liposomal doxorubicin (Doxil) in a breast cancer tumor model: Investigation of potential enhancement by pulsed-high intensity focused ultrasound exposure. Academic Radiology. 2006;13(4):469–79.
150. Staruch R, Chopra R, Hynynen K. Localised drug release using MRI-controlled focused ultrasound hyperthermia. International Journal of Hyperthermia: The Official Journal of European Society for Hyperthermic Oncology, North American Hyperthermia Group. 2011;27(2):156–71.
151. Ichihara M, Sasaki K, Umemura S, Kushima M, Okai T. Blood flow occlusion via ultrasound image-guided high-intensity focused ultrasound and its effect on tissue perfusion. Ultrasound in Medicine & Biology. 2007;33(3):452–9.
152. Yarmolenko PS, Zhao Y, Landon C, Spasojevic I, Yuan F, Needham D, et al. Comparative effects of thermosensitive doxorubicin-containing liposomes and hyperthermia in human and murine tumours. International Journal of Hyperthermia: The Official Journal of European Society for Hyperthermic Oncology, North American Hyperthermia Group. 2010;26(5):485–98.
153. Viglianti BL, Ponce AM, Michelich CR, Yu D, Abraham SA, Sanders L, et al. Chemodosimetry of in vivo tumor liposomal drug concentration using MRI. Magnetic Resonance in Medicine: Official Journal of the Society of Magnetic Resonance in Medicine/Society of Magnetic Resonance in Medicine. 2006;56(5):1011–8.
154. Ponce AM, Viglianti BL, Yu D, Yarmolenko PS, Michelich CR, Woo J, et al. Magnetic resonance imaging of temperature-sensitive liposome release: Drug dose painting and antitumor effects. Journal of the National Cancer Institute. 2007;99(1):53–63.
155. Negussie AH, Yarmolenko PS, Partanen A, Ranjan A, Jacobs G, Woods D, et al. Formulation and characterisation of magnetic resonance imageable thermally sensitive liposomes for use with magnetic resonance-guided high intensity focused ultrasound. International Journal of Hyperthermia: The Official Journal of European Society for Hyperthermic Oncology, North American Hyperthermia Group. 2011;27(2):140–55.
156. Tagami T, Foltz WD, Ernsting MJ, Lee CM, Tannock IF, May JP, et al. MRI monitoring of intratumoral drug delivery and prediction of the therapeutic effect with a multifunctional thermosensitive liposome. Biomaterials. 2011;32(27):6570–8.
157. Ranjan A, Jacobs GC, Woods DL, Negussie AH, Partanen A, Yarmolenko PS, et al. Image-guided drug delivery with magnetic resonance guided high intensity focused ultrasound and temperature sensitive liposomes in a rabbit Vx2 tumor model. Journal of Controlled Release: Official Journal of the Controlled Release Society. 2012;158(3):487–94.
158. Staruch RM, Ganguly M, Tannock IF, Hynynen K, Chopra R. Enhanced drug delivery in rabbit VX2 tumours using thermosensitive liposomes and MRI-controlled focused ultrasound hyperthermia. International Journal of Hyperthermia: The Official Journal of European Society for Hyperthermic Oncology, North American Hyperthermia Group. 2012;28(8):776–87.
159. Staruch RM, Hynynen K, Chopra R. Hyperthermia-mediated doxorubicin release from thermosensitive liposomes using MR-HIFU: Therapeutic effect in rabbit Vx2 tumours. International Journal of Hyperthermia: The Official Journal of European Society for Hyperthermic Oncology, North American Hyperthermia Group. 2015;31(2):118–33.

160. Tagami T, Ernsting MJ, Li SD. Efficient tumor regression by a single and low dose treatment with a novel and enhanced formulation of thermosensitive liposomal doxorubicin. Journal of Controlled Release: Official Journal of the Controlled Release Society. 2011;152(2):303–9.
161. Park SM, Kim MS, Park SJ, Park ES, Choi KS, Kim YS, et al. Novel temperature-triggered liposome with high stability: Formulation, in vitro evaluation, and in vivo study combined with high-intensity focused ultrasound (HIFU). Journal of Controlled Release: Official Journal of the Controlled Release Society. 2013;170(3):373–9.
162. Rizzitelli S, Giustetto P, Faletto D, Delli Castelli D, Aime S, Terreno E. The release of Doxorubicin from liposomes monitored by MRI and triggered by a combination of US stimuli led to a complete tumor regression in a breast cancer mouse model. Journal of Controlled Release: Official Journal of the Controlled Release Society. 2016;230:57–63.
163. Giustetto P, Castelli DD, Boffa C, Rizzitelli S, Durando D, Cutrin JC, et al. Release of a paramagnetic magnetic resonance imaging agent from liposomes triggered by low intensity non-focused ultrasound. Journal of Medical Imaging and Health Informatics. 2013;3(3):356–66.
164. Rizzitelli S, Giustetto P, Cutrin JC, Delli Castelli D, Boffa C, Ruzza M, et al. Sonosensitive theranostic liposomes for preclinical in vivo MRI-guided visualization of doxorubicin release stimulated by pulsed low intensity non-focused ultrasound. Journal of Controlled Release: Official Journal of the Controlled Release Society. 2015;202:21–30.
165. Lopez-Berestein G, Fainstein V, Hopfer R, Mehta K, Sullivan MP, Keating M, et al. Liposomal amphotericin B for the treatment of systemic fungal infections in patients with cancer: A preliminary study. The Journal of Infectious Diseases. 1985;151(4):704–10.
166. Gabizon A, Peretz T, Sulkes A, Amselem S, Ben-Yosef R, Ben-Baruch N, et al. Systemic administration of doxorubicin-containing liposomes in cancer patients: A phase I study. European Journal of Cancer & Clinical Oncology. 1989;25(12):1795–803.
167. Wood B. A Phase I Dose Escalation Study of Heat Activated Liposome Delivery of Doxorubicin and Radiofrequency Ablation of Primary and Metastatic Tumors of the Liver. ClinicalTrials.gov. National Institutes of Health Clinical Center; 2004 [updated 14 Mar 2012]. Available from: www.clinicaltrials.gov/ct2/show/NCT00093444.
168. Borys N. A Phase I Dose Escalation Tolerability Study of ThermoDox™ (Thermally Sensitive Liposomal Doxorubicin) in Combination with Radiofrequency Ablation (RFA) of Primary and Metastatic Tumors of the Liver. ClinicalTrials.gov. Celsion; 2007 [updated 16 Dec 2009]. Available from: www.clinicaltrials.gov/ct2/show/NCT00441376.
169. Celsion. A Phase III, Randomized, Double-Blinded, Dummy-Controlled Study of the Efficacy and Safety of ThermoDox® (Thermally Sensitive Liposomal Doxorubicin) in Combination with Radiofrequency Ablation (RFA) Compared to RFA-Alone in the Treatment of Non-Resectable Hepatocellular Carcinoma. ClinicalTrials.gov. Celsion; 2008 [updated 03 Feb 2014 (accessed 02 Jun 2015)]. Available from: www.clinicaltrials.gov/ct2/show/NCT00617981.
170. Dou Y, Hynynen K, Allen C. To heat or not to heat: Challenges with clinical translation of thermosensitive liposomes. Journal of Controlled Release. 2017;249:63–73.
171. Celsion. A Phase III, Randomized, Double Blind, Dummy-Controlled Study of ThermoDox® (Lyso-Thermosensitive Liposomal Doxorubicin-LTLD) in Hepatocellular Carcinoma (HCC) Using Standardized Radiofrequency Ablation (RFA) Treatment Time ≥ 45 Minutes for Solitary Lesions ≥ 3 cm to ≤ 7 cm. ClinicalTrials.gov. Celsion; 2014 [updated 05 May 2015]. Available from: www.clinicaltrials.gov/ct2/show/NCT02112656.
172. Regenold M, Bannigan P, Evans JC, Waspe A, Temple MJ, Allen C. Turning down the heat: The case for mild hyperthermia and thermosensitive liposomes. Nanomedicine: Nanotechnology, Biology and Medicine. 2021;102484.
173. Celsion. ThermoDox® Lyso-Thermosensitive Liposomal Doxorubicin (LTLD) Investigator's Brochure. Celsion, 07 Aug 2014. Report No.
174. Lefrak EA, Pitha J, Rosenheim S, Gottlieb JA. A clinicopathologic analysis of adriamycin cardiotoxicity. Cancer. 1973;32(2):302–14.
175. Floyd JD, Nguyen DT, Lobins RL, Bashir Q, Doll DC, Perry MC. Cardiotoxicity of cancer therapy. Journal of Clinical Oncology: Official Journal of the American Society of Clinical Oncology. 2005;23(30):7685–96.
176. Rahman AM, Yusuf SW, Ewer MS. Anthracycline-induced cardiotoxicity and the cardiac-sparing effect of liposomal formulation. International Journal of Nanomedicine. 2007;2(4):567–83.

177. Zagar TM, Vujaskovic Z, Formenti S, Rugo H, Muggia F, O'Connor B, et al. Two phase I dose-escalation/pharmacokinetics studies of low temperature liposomal doxorubicin (LTLD) and mild local hyperthermia in heavily pretreated patients with local regionally recurrent breast cancer. International Journal of Hyperthermia: The Official Journal of European Society for Hyperthermic Oncology, North American Hyperthermia Group. 2014;30(5):285–94.
178. Therasse P, Arbuck SG, Eisenhauer EA, Wanders J, Kaplan RS, Rubinstein L, et al. New guidelines to evaluate the response to treatment in solid tumors. European Organization for Research and Treatment of Cancer, National Cancer Institute of the United States, National Cancer Institute of Canada. Journal of the National Cancer Institute. 2000;92(3):205–16.
179. Lyon PC, Gray MD, Mannaris C, Folkes LK, Stratford M, Campo L, et al. Safety and feasibility of ultrasound-triggered targeted drug delivery of doxorubicin from thermosensitive liposomes in liver tumours (TARDOX): A single-centre, open-label, phase 1 trial. The Lancet Oncology. 2018 Aug;19(8):1027–39. doi: 10.1016/S1470-2045(18)30332-2. Epub 2018 Jul 11. PMID: 30001990; PMCID: PMC6073884.
180. Lyon PC, Griffiths LF, Lee J, Chung D, Carlisle R, Wu F, et al. Clinical trial protocol for TARDOX: A phase I study to investigate the feasibility of targeted release of lyso-thermosensitive liposomal doxorubicin (ThermoDox®) using focused ultrasound in patients with liver tumours. Journal of Therapeutic Ultrasound. 2017;5(1):1–8.
181. Lyon PC, Mannaris C, Gray M, Carlisle R, Gleeson FV, Cranston D, et al. Large-volume hyperthermia for safe and cost-effective targeted drug delivery using a clinical ultrasound-guided focused ultrasound device. Ultrasound in Medicine & Biology. 2021;47(4):982–97.
182. Urva SR, Shin BS, Yang VC, Balthasar JP. Sensitive high performance liquid chromatographic assay for assessment of doxorubicin pharmacokinetics in mouse plasma and tissues. Journal of Chromatography B: Biomedical Sciences and Applications. 2009;877(8–9):837–41.
183. Gewirtz DA. A critical evaluation of the mechanisms of action proposed for the antitumor effects of the anthracycline antibiotics adriamycin and daunorubicin. Biochemical Pharmacology. 1999;57(7):727–41.
184. Chen Q, Krol A, Wright A, Needham D, Dewhirst MW, Yuan F. Tumor microvascular permeability is a key determinant for antivascular effects of doxorubicin encapsulated in a temperature sensitive liposome. International Journal of Hyperthermia. 2008;24(6):475-82.
185. Needham D. Bringing research to clinical application lessons from thermodox (r): A thermal-sensitive liposome for treatment of cancer. In Drug Delivery. Fundamentals & Applications, 2nd ed.; Hillery, A., Park, K., Eds. 2016:523–85.
186. Bhatnagar S, Schiffter H, Coussios CC. Exploitation of acoustic cavitation-induced microstreaming to enhance molecular transport. Journal of Pharmaceutical Sciences. 2014;103(6):1903–12.
187. Arvanitis CD, Bazan-Peregrino M, Rifai B, Seymour LW, Coussios CC. Cavitation-enhanced extravasation for drug delivery. Ultrasound in Medicine & Biology. 2011;37(11):1838–52.
188. Liu HL, Huang CY, Chen JY, Wang HY, Chen PY, Wei KC. Pharmacodynamic and therapeutic investigation of focused ultrasound-induced blood-brain barrier opening for enhanced temozolomide delivery in glioma treatment. PLoS One. 2014 Dec 9;9(12).
189. Wei HJ, Upadhyayula PS, Pouliopoulos AN, Englander ZK, Zhang X, Jan CI, et al. Focused ultrasound-mediated blood-brain barrier opening increases delivery and efficacy of etoposide for glioblastoma treatment. International Journal of Radiation Oncology. 2021 Jun 1;110(2):539–50.
190. Carpentier A, Canney M, Vignot A, Reina V, Beccaria K, Horodyckid C, et al. Clinical trial of blood–brain barrier disruption by pulsed ultrasound. Science Translational Medicine. 2016;8:343re2.
191. Mainprize T, Lipsman N, Huang Y, Meng Y, Bethune A, Ironside S, et al. Blood–brain barrier opening in primary brain tumors with non-invasive MR-guided focused ultrasound: A clinical safety and feasibility study. Scientific Reports. 2019;9:321.
192. Idbaih A, Canney M, Belin L, Desseaux C, Vignot A, Bouchoux G, et al. Safety and feasibility of repeated and transient blood–brain barrier disruption by pulsed ultrasound in patients with recurrent glioblastoma. Clinical Cancer Research. 2019;25:3793–801.
193. Cheng B, Bing C, Chu TH, Alzahrani S, Pichardo S, Pike BG. Simultaneous localized brain mild hyperthermia and blood-brain barrier opening via feedback-controlled transcranial MR-guided focused ultrasound and microbubbles. IEEE Transactions on Biomedical Engineering. 2021 Nov 23;69(6):1880–8. doi: 10.1109/TBME.2021.3130164
194. Haar GT, Coussios C. High intensity focused ultrasound: Past, present and future. International Journal of Hyperthermia: The Official Journal of European Society for Hyperthermic Oncology, North American Hyperthermia Group. 2007;23(2):85–7.

195. Meng Y, Hynynen K, Lipsman N. Applications of focused ultrasound in the brain: From thermoablation to drug delivery. Nature Reviews Neurology. 2021;17:7–22. doi: 10.1038/s41582-020-00418-z
196. McClure A. Using high-intensity focused ultrasound as a means to provide targeted drug delivery: A literature review. Journal of Diagnostic Medical Sonography. 2016;32(6):343–50.
197. Hijnen N, Kneepkens E, de Smet M, Langereis S, Heijman E, Grüll H. Thermal combination therapies for local drug delivery by magnetic resonance-guided high-intensity focused ultrasound. Proceedings of the National Academy of Sciences. 2017;114(24):E4802–11.
198. Boissenot T, Bordat A, Fattal E, Tsapis N. Ultrasound-triggered drug delivery for cancer treatment using drug delivery systems: From theoretical considerations to practical applications. Journal of Controlled Release. 2016;241:144–63.
199. Tanbour R, Martins AM, Pitt WG, Husseini GA. Drug delivery systems based on polymeric micelles and ultrasound: A review. Current Pharmaceutical Design. 2016;22(19):2796–807.
200. Entzian K, Aigner A. Drug delivery by ultrasound-responsive nanocarriers for cancer treatment. Pharmaceutics. 2021;13(8):1135.
201. Rieke V, Butts Pauly K. MR thermometry. Journal of Magnetic Resonance Imaging: JMRI. 2008;27(2):376–90.
202. de Senneville BD, Mougenot C, Quesson B, Dragonu I, Grenier N, Moonen CT. MR thermometry for monitoring tumor ablation. European Radiology. 2007;17(9):2401–10.
203. Quesson B, Vimeux F, Salomir R, de Zwart JA, Moonen CT. Automatic control of hyperthermic therapy based on real-time fourier analysis of MR temperature maps. Magnetic Resonance in Medicine. 2002;47(6):1065–72.
204. Mougenot C, Andreae T, Köhler M, Enholm J. Philips MR-guided High Intensity Focused Ultrasound (white paper). Philips Healthcare, 2012.
205. Borman PTS, Bos C, de Boorder T, Raaymakers BW, Moonen CTW, Crijns SPM. Towards real-time thermometry using simultaneous multislice MRI. Physics in Medicine & Biology. 2016 Sep;61(17):N461–77.
206. Gyongy M, Coussios CC. Passive cavitation mapping for localization and tracking of bubble dynamics. The Journal of the Acoustical Society of America. 2010;128(4):EL175–80.
207. Gyongy M, Coussios CC. Passive spatial mapping of inertial cavitation during HIFU exposure. IEEE Transactions on Bio-medical Engineering. 2010;57(1):48–56.
208. Salgaonkar VA, Datta S, Holland CK, Mast TD. Passive cavitation imaging with ultrasound arrays. The Journal of the Acoustical Society of America. 2009;126(6):3071–83.
209. Coviello C, Kozick R, Choi J, Gyongy M, Jensen C, Smith PP, et al. Passive acoustic mapping utilizing optimal beamforming in ultrasound therapy monitoring. The Journal of the Acoustical Society of America. 2015;137(5):2573–85.
210. Jensen CR, Ritchie RW, Gyongy M, Collin JR, Leslie T, Coussios CC. Spatiotemporal monitoring of high-intensity focused ultrasound therapy with passive acoustic mapping. Radiology. 2012;262(1):252–61.
211. van Zijl PC, Yadav NN. Chemical exchange saturation transfer (CEST): What is in a name and what isn't? Magnetic Resonance in Medicine: Official Journal of the Society of Magnetic Resonance in Medicine/Society of Magnetic Resonance in Medicine. 2011;65(4):927–48.
212. McDannold N, Vykhodtseva N, Jolesz FA, Hynynen K. MRI investigation of the threshold for thermally induced blood-brain barrier disruption and brain tissue damage in the rabbit brain. Magnetic Resonance in Medicine: Official Journal of the Society of Magnetic Resonance in Medicine/Society of Magnetic Resonance in Medicine. 2004;51(5):913–23.
213. Sasaki K, Azuma T, Kawabata KI, Shimoda M, Kokue EI, Umemura SI. Effect of split-focus approach on producing larger coagulation in swine liver. Ultrasound in Medicine & Biology. 2003;29(4):591–9.
214. Patel PR, Luk A, Durrani A, Dromi S, Cuesta J, Angstadt M, et al. In vitro and in vivo evaluations of increased effective beam width for heat deposition using a split focus high intensity ultrasound (HIFU) transducer. International Journal of Hyperthermia: The Official Journal of European Society for Hyperthermic Oncology, North American Hyperthermia Group. 2008;24(7):537–49.
215. Al-Ahmady ZS, Chaloin O, Kostarelos K. Monoclonal antibody-targeted, temperature-sensitive liposomes: In vivo tumor chemotherapeutics in combination with mild hyperthermia. Journal of Controlled Release: Official Journal of the Controlled Release Society. 2014;196:332–43.
216. Iga K, Hamaguchi N, Igari Y, Ogawa Y, Gotoh K, Ootsu K, et al. Enhanced antitumor activity in mice after administration of thermosensitive liposome encapsulating cisplatin with hyperthermia. The Journal of Pharmacology and Experimental Therapeutics. 1991;257(3):1203–7.

217. Chelvi TP, Jain SK, Ralhan R. Hyperthermia-mediated targeted delivery of thermosensitive liposome-encapsulated melphalan in murine tumors. Oncology Research. 1995;7(7–8):393–8.
218. Kim HS, Park YS. Gene transfection by quantitatively reconstituted Sendai envelope proteins into liposomes. Cancer Gene Therapy. 2002;9(2):173–7.
219. Schneider J, Falk H, Hunsmann G. Virosomes constructed from lipid and purified Friend leukaemia virus glycoprotein. The Journal of General Virology. 1983;64 Pt 3:559–65.
220. Kaneda Y. Virosomes: Evolution of the liposome as a targeted drug delivery system. Advanced Drug Delivery Reviews. 2000;43(2–3):197–205.
221. Garbuzenko OB, Saad M, Betigeri S, Zhang M, Vetcher AA, Soldatenkov VA, et al. Intratracheal versus intravenous liposomal delivery of siRNA, antisense oligonucleotides and anticancer drug. Pharmaceutical Research. 2009;26(2):382–94.
222. Whitehead KA, Langer R, Anderson DG. Knocking down barriers: Advances in siRNA delivery. Nature reviews Drug Discovery. 2009;8(2):129–38.
223. Kapoor B, Singh SK, Gulati M, Gupta R, Vaidya Y. Application of liposomes in treatment of rheumatoid arthritis: Quo vadis. TheScientificWorldJournal. 2014;2014:978351.
224. Viscusi ER, Sinatra R, Onel E, Ramamoorthy SL. The safety of liposome bupivacaine, a novel local analgesic formulation. The Clinical Journal of Pain. 2014;30(2):102–10.
225. Kwan JJ, Myers R, Coviello CM, Graham SM, Shah AR, Stride E, et al. Ultrasound-propelled nanocups for drug delivery. Small. 2015;11(39):5305–14.
226. Kneidl B, Peller M, Winter G, Lindner LH, Hossann M. Thermosensitive liposomal drug delivery systems: State of the art review. International Journal of Nanomedicine. 2014;9:4387–98.
227. Grull H, Langereis S. Hyperthermia-triggered drug delivery from temperature-sensitive liposomes using MRI-guided high intensity focused ultrasound. Journal of Controlled Release: Official Journal of the Controlled Release Society. 2012;161(2):317–27.
228. Cho K, Wang X, Nie S, Chen ZG, Shin DM. Therapeutic nanoparticles for drug delivery in cancer. Clinical Cancer Research: An Official Journal of the American Association for Cancer Research. 2008;14(5):1310–6.
229. Schroeder A, Kost J, Barenholz Y. Ultrasound, liposomes, and drug delivery: Principles for using ultrasound to control the release of drugs from liposomes. Chemistry and Physics of Lipids. 2009;162(1–2):1–16.
230. Phenix CP, Togtema M, Pichardo S, Zehbe I, Curiel L. High intensity focused ultrasound technology, its scope and applications in therapy and drug delivery. Journal of Pharmacy & Pharmaceutical Sciences: A Publication of the Canadian Society for Pharmaceutical Sciences, Societe canadienne des sciences pharmaceutiques. 2014;17(1):136–53.
231. Mo S, Coussios CC, Seymour L, Carlisle R. Ultrasound-enhanced drug delivery for cancer. Expert Opinion on Drug Delivery. 2012;9(12):1525–38.
232. Langereis S, Geelen T, Grull H, Strijkers GJ, Nicolay K. Paramagnetic liposomes for molecular MRI and MRI-guided drug delivery. NMR in Biomedicine. 2013;26(7):728–44.

26

Transcranial Ultrasound–Mediated Blood-Brain Barrier Disruption for Targeted Drug Delivery

Stecia-Marie Fletcher, Thiele Kobus, Jonathan Sutton, and Nathan J. McDannold

26.1 Introduction

In the late 1800s, Paul Ehrlich observed that dyes injected into the blood stream did not reach the brain and spinal cord.[1] When his student, Edwin Goldmann, injected dye into the cerebrospinal fluid, this did not reach the blood circulation.[2] These experiments were the first proof of the existence of the blood-brain barrier. The blood-brain barrier consists of endothelial cells that are connected by tight junctions, and lined with pericytes, astrocytic endfeet, and a basement membrane (Figure 26.1). In contrast to the vascular endothelium of peripheral tissues,[3] the vasculature of the central nervous system excludes non-polar molecules and molecules greater than ~450 daltons from the brain parenchyma.[4] Molecules that can cross the blood-brain barrier either traverse the cytoplasm (transcellular) or the space between the epithelial cells, the tight junctions (paracellular).[5]

Since its discovery, the scientific community has aimed to develop methods of circumventing the blood-brain barrier and augmenting delivery of small molecules, biologicals, antibodies, immune therapies, and gene therapies to the brain. The methodologies that have been developed vary in their approach and invasiveness. One approach is to alter therapeutic agents, with, for example, Trojan horse and active transport strategies reliant upon receptor-mediated transcytosis.[7] Other methods use existing therapies and are based on modifying the permeability of the blood-brain barrier or on direct injection of the drug into the central nervous system parenchyma.[8] For the latter, a surgical approach is needed and may require a craniotomy to introduce drugs or drug-eluting implants intracerebrally or intraventricularly.[5] This strategy strongly relies on the passive and limited spread of molecules throughout the brain parenchyma by diffusion. Conversely, convection-enhanced diffusion techniques attempt to drive the spread of agent through the brain by bulk flow along fluid pressure gradients to achieve concentrations that are orders of magnitude higher.[9] However, convection-enhanced diffusion is inherently limited by the preferential flow of infused substances along white matter tracts.[10] Studies with viruses in the early- and mid-1900s revealed a direct entry route for viruses and other tracer materials to the brain trans-nasally, by moving via olfactory neurons.[11] The efficiency of this pathway is higher in rodents than in humans, possibly because of anatomical differences in the location and size of the olfactory epithelium in rats and mice.[11]

The most ubiquitous research method for increasing the permeability of the blood-brain barrier uses hyperosmotic shock.[12] Here, inert solutions are injected intra-arterially to render the cerebral blood volume hypertonic to endothelial cells, and to the brain parenchyma. Endothelial cells shrink, rendering the blood-brain barrier permeable to water soluble drugs for several minutes. Despite the appreciable increase in permeability of molecules, hyperosmotic shock is associated with vasculopathy and seizure.[13] Inorganic solvents, such as ethanol or dimethyl sulfoxide, can also modify blood-brain barrier permeability through direct solubility, but these, too, give rise to severe side effects.

Despite the progress of many of these strategies, no large molecule drugs that cross the blood-brain barrier are available to health care providers, nor have they been approved by the U.S. Food and Drug Administration.[14] Furthermore, methods such as hyperosmotic shock, convection-enhanced diffusion,

DOI: 10.1201/9780429162671-26

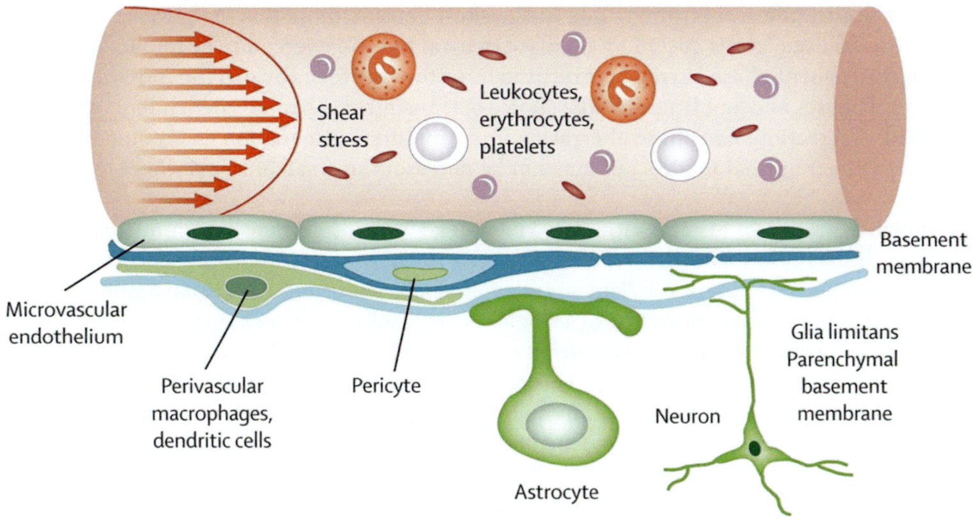

FIGURE 26.1 The blood-brain barrier consists of endothelial cells that are lined with a high concentration of pericytes embedded in the endothelial cell basement membrane, perivascular antigen-presenting cells, astrocytic endfeet, and associated parenchymal basement membrane and neurons. Reprinted from The Lancet Neurology, Vol. 7, Neuwelt et al., Strategies to Advance Translational Research into Brain Barriers, Pages 84–96, Copyright © 2008, with permission from Elsevier.[6]

and direct neurosurgical intervention are invasive and/or non-targeted. A method that can be combined with available approved drugs, and that can disrupt the blood-brain barrier non-invasively at targeted locations, would have a major impact on clinical neuroscience.

Ultrasound was introduced as an effective strategy for permeabilising the blood-brain barrier to large molecules in 2001.[15] To this end, microbubbles (small gas bubbles used as ultrasound contrast agent) were injected into the circulation, and acoustic energy was focused onto a region of the brain through the skull. In the ultrasound focus, the interaction between the acoustic waves and circulating microbubbles stimulated transient and reversible disruption of the blood-brain barrier, enabling targeted drug delivery.

26.2 Methods for Blood-Brain Barrier Disruption

This section covers important features that should be considered for focused ultrasound (FUS)-mediated blood-brain barrier disruption. This method has primarily been investigated in a preclinical setting. As such, this section will focus on preclinical data, but many aspects discussed herein are transferable to the clinical application of the technique (discussed in Section 26.5).

26.2.1 Ultrasound Delivery and Treatment Guidance

26.2.1.1 Focused Ultrasound Exposure

To deliver acoustic energy to the brain, an ultrasonic transmitter or *transducer* is needed. Chapter 4 discusses the influence of parameters such as the transducer F-number and frequency on the size and shape of the ultrasound focus. For applications in the brain, the intervening skull presents a significant challenge to precisely focusing the ultrasound beam. The skull is highly aberrative, causing amplitude attenuation and phase distortions, and in addition the thickness of the skull varies across the population and even across an individual's skull (Chapter 21).[16] At higher ultrasound frequencies, or for thicker skulls, phase aberrations due to the skull become more severe. Lower, sub-megahertz frequencies can be used, at the cost of an increase in focal size. To overcome the impact of focal aberrations, a multi-element phased array may be used to restore the focus by driving individual elements with optimised phases and amplitudes.[17] The choice of transducer is strongly dependent on the subject being studied. Corrections for phase aberration and amplitude attenuation are required in clinical settings and in larger animal models but may not be necessary in small animals where the skull bone is very thin.

The first demonstration of focused ultrasound combined with intravenously administered microbubbles to disrupt the blood-brain barrier was shown using a 16-element 1.63 MHz transducer in rabbits.[15] In this initial experiment, all transducer elements were driven in phase and with equal amplitude, thereby creating a single focus comparable to that of a single element, spherically focused transducer. The rabbits in the study underwent a craniotomy to create an acoustic window, to limit attenuation and to eliminate the need for phase correction. Measurements through excised bone at 1.08 MHz have shown that the rabbit skull attenuates the focal pressure amplitude by 84% compared to measurements made in water, without a skull.[18] Attenuation is frequency dependent. For example, in the rat skull, values of attenuation vary from 9% at 0.27 MHz to 43% at 2.53 MHz.[19] In the ex vivo mouse skull, the full width at half maximum of the focus is similar to that measured in water without the skull, indicating that a good focus can be obtained in mice using a single-element, spherically focused transducer at the relatively high frequency of 1.53 MHz, without phase corrections.[20] As such, a wide range of frequencies has been used to disrupt the blood-brain barrier in preclinical studies, ranging from 0.26 MHz in rabbits[21] to 8.0 MHz in mice.[22]

A craniotomy can be performed to create an acoustic window and eliminate the need for aberration corrections. However, transcranial disruption through the intact skull makes the technique minimally invasive and more attractive to patients and clinicians. Successful transcranial blood-brain barrier disruption has been achieved using a single-element, spherically focused transducer in mice and rats, but also in larger animals such as rabbits (0.26–1.08 MHz[18, 21]), pigs (1.0 MHz[23]), and monkeys (0.5 MHz[24–26]). At our lab, we have achieved successful blood-brain barrier opening in non-human primates using a hemispherical clinical focused ultrasound system designed for application in humans.[27] The device used in that study, the Exablate Neuro System (InSightec, Tirat Carmel, Israel) consists of a 1024-element phased array transducer operating at 220 KHz. It was observed that no aberration correction was needed for the primate skull. One of the advantages of this system is its large aperture, which helps in minimising standing waves.[28] Standing waves are most likely to occur at the skull interface, where reflected and incident waves interfere with each other and produce high amplitude, off-target effects.[29] There is a greater probability of standing wave formation at low frequencies and in preclinical models, when the focal length is comparable to the distance between the top and bottom of the skull.[29, 30]

26.2.1.2 Guidance Techniques

To achieve precise and targeted blood-brain barrier disruption, an accurate method is required to localise intra-cranial, anatomical structures. There are several options for guiding focused ultrasound therapies.

Currently, focused ultrasound ablations in the human brain are routinely performed using magnetic resonance imaging (MRI) guidance using a hemispherical multi-element transducer (Chapters 4 and 21). Computed tomography (CT) images of the skull are obtained prior to treatment and registered to MRIs acquired during the treatment. Density information from the CT images is used to calculate the optimal phase and amplitude corrections required to obtain a sharp focus for each transducer element. Typically, no aberration correction is applied in animal studies, eliminating the need for CT images. MRI has excellent soft tissue contrast, enabling visualisation of the different structures and regions in the brain. By relating the MRI coordinates to the ultrasound focus, the desired anatomical regions can be targeted with high accuracy and precision. Another advantage of using MRI for guiding blood-brain barrier disruption is the ability to confirm successful disruption after the sonication. To this end, an MRI-contrast agent is used, as will be discussed in detail in Section 26.2.2. The downside of MRI guidance is that the procedure becomes costly, since MR systems are expensive, and the procedure is generally time-consuming. Furthermore, all materials used in the procedure, including the ultrasound transducer, must be MRI-compatible.

It is also possible to perform focused ultrasound induced blood-brain barrier disruption without MRI guidance. Atlas-based, stereotactic-guided preclinical focused ultrasound devices have been used in preclinical studies for targeting.[31–33] This method has been utilised to achieve successful blood-brain barrier disruption in animals ranging from mice[34] to non-human primates,[32, 35] where, for example, a single-element spherical transducer (500 kHz) was attached to a stereotactic arm with 9 degrees of freedom.[32] In that study, the head of the monkey was fixed in a stereotactic frame and the stereotactic coordinates of the arm were related to sonication targets.

Ultrasound guidance may offer a low-cost and more accessible alternative than MRI-guidance but achieving transcranial ultrasound imaging remains a hindrance to the development of this technology. In animals that received a craniotomy, brain imaging is possible using a diagnostic ultrasound transducer. An imaging transducer placed in an opening in the centre of the therapeutic focused transducer[36] allows the focus to be located on the target. Others have used a similar transducer configuration in combination with a metal grid that was aligned with the sutures of the mouse skull.[20] However, the applicability of such an approach is limited, as the mice used require translucent skins. Raymond et al. used a Mylar window to set the location of the focus and guide animal alignment.[37] The localisation accuracy was poorer than for a MR-guided procedure, but much faster. Recently, Deng et al. developed a clinical-scale protype ultrasound-guided transcranial focused ultrasound system for microbubble-mediated brain therapy.[38] In that work, a high-frequency ultrasound skull localisation array was integrated into a transmit/receive phased array for therapy delivery and treatment monitoring.[39] The resultant targeting errors were found to be comparable to those achieved using gold-standard, landmark-based skull registration methods.

26.2.2 Detection of Blood-Brain Barrier Disruption

When disrupting the blood-brain barrier, robust methods of detection are needed to confirm successful disruption. In the case of animal experiments, where animals are immediately sacrificed, this can be achieved by the intravenous administration of a dye. However, in humans, or in animal survival studies, MRI and acoustics-based methods are better suited to providing this information.

26.2.2.1 Ex Vivo Detection Techniques

Ehrlich and Goldmann used dyes in their blood-brain barrier studies,[1, 2] and this method is still widespread in blood-brain barrier-related research. Trypan blue or Evans blue dyes are the most commonly used.[40] Both have a high affinity for plasma proteins in the serum, such as albumin, which does not leave the intact blood vessels. The permeability of the blood-brain barrier can therefore be studied by leaving the dye in circulation after its injection for a given amount of time (we use an hour at our institution) before perfusion with a fixative or saline to remove the blood from the brain vasculature. By sectioning the brain, an overview of the extent of blood-brain barrier disruption can be obtained from the extent of dye penetration in the brain (Figure 26.2).

Evans blue and Trypan blue are fluorescent, so they can also be used for quantitative evaluation of the disruption.[37, 41] Other fluorescent tracers available that do not leave the intact blood-brain barrier but do not bind to plasma proteins are also available. Several fluorescent tracers with sizes between 3 kDa and 70 kDa have been used to quantify the disruption.[41–43]

Horseradish peroxidase can be used to study the blood-brain barrier disruption in more detail. This is a 40-kDa enzyme that does not cross the intact blood-brain barrier. As it is electron dense, it can be observed using an electron microscope. After injection and circulation, the brain should be fixed by immersion to bind horseradish peroxidase to its location.[40] The use of electron microscopy makes it possible to study how the enzyme crosses the blood-brain barrier after disruption.[44, 45]

Besides injecting an exogenous tracer, it is also possible to perform immunohistochemistry on paraffin-embedded brain sections. This way, one can look at endogenous circulating proteins, such as

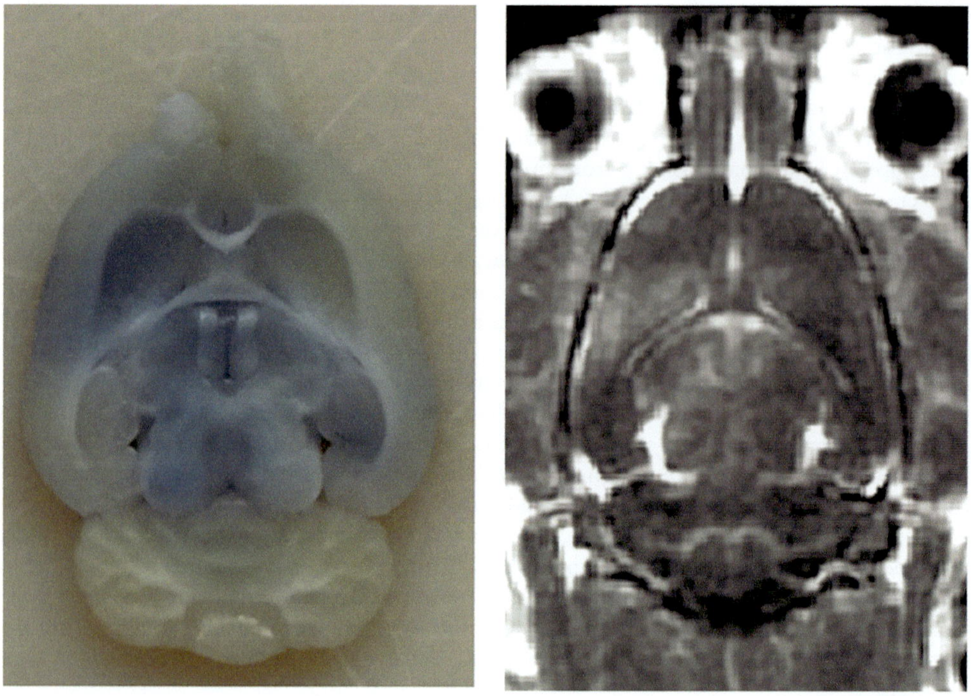

FIGURE 26.2 Example in a rat of good correlation between the extent of ultrasound-mediated blood-brain barrier disruption that was observed between Trypan blue extravasation (left) and the extent of hyper-intensity (right) on T1-weighted MR imaging, resulting from extravasation of gadolinium.

serum proteins. These processes can also be studied in greater detail under the electron microscope, by combining antibodies that target a specific antigen with gold-particles.

26.2.2.2 In Vivo Detection Techniques

MRI has been widely used to confirm successful blood-brain barrier disruption using T1-weighted imaging in combination with an intravenously administered MRI contrast agent. Gadolinium, the most commonly used MRI contrast agent, shortens the T1-relaxation time of the tissue. In the normal brain, gadolinium does not leave the capillaries and therefore only affects the contrast in vessels. However, after blood-brain barrier disruption, gadolinium can extravasate from the vessels and alter the T1-relaxation time of brain tissue, resulting in a hyperintense region on the T1-weighted image (Figure 26.2). There are several clinically used gadolinium chelates, with molecular weights in the range of 550–950 Da. Larger particles, such as gadolinium-labeled albumin with a molecular weight of ~74 kDa, are also available. Particles of different sizes make it possible to study the size dependence of the opening and closing of the blood-brain barrier.[46]

To confirm blood-brain barrier disruption at a desired location, a qualitative evaluation of the hyperintense region in post-contrast MRI is sufficient. To study blood-brain barrier disruption more quantitatively, pre- and post-contrast T1-weighted images can be subtracted to quantify the amount of signal enhancement.[47] For further quantification, the uptake of the MRI contrast agent can be studied dynamically. To this end, a fast T1-weighted imaging sequence is repeatedly and continuously acquired before, during and after injection of a contrast agent. A temporal map of the change in signal intensity due to the extravasation of the contrast agent can thus be obtained. From this curve, several semi-quantitative parameters can be determined, such as the area under the curve, or the time to maximum enhancement. These measures are difficult to interpret. Pharmacokinetic modelling has therefore been introduced to fit the change in signal intensity to physiological parameters. One of these models is the Tofts-Kermode model, which assumes exchange of the contrast agent between the blood plasma and the extracellular-extravascular compartment.[48] This model can be used to determine the transfer constant between blood plasma and the extracellular-extravascular space, K_{trans}, and the volume of extravascular extracellular space per unit volume of tissue, v_e. The blood plasma volume (v_p) is neglected, but has been added in the modified Tofts model.[49]

26.2.3 Treatment Monitoring Using Passive Cavitation Detection

The cavitation of microbubbles in an ultrasound field results in highly non-linear scattering of ultrasound with respect to the transmit frequency of the transducer, *f0*.[50] A real-time method for indirectly observing blood-brain barrier disruption detects the acoustic emissions of the microbubbles during the treatment using receive element(s) that are aligned with the focus of the therapeutic transducer. This is known as passive cavitation detection (see Chapter 3).

At very low pressures, bubbles will oscillate at the fundamental frequency (f_0) of the transducer. When the acoustic pressure is increased, stable volumetric oscillations produce ultrasound emissions at integer multiples of the fundamental frequency, known as harmonics ($2\,f_0$, $3\,f_0$, $4\,f_0$ . . .), while, beyond a threshold, nonlinear oscillations can result in scattering at half-integer multiples of the fundamental frequency, known as the sub- ($f_0/2$) and ultra-harmonics ($3\,f_0/2$, $5\,f_0/2$ . . .).[51] At high pressures, microbubbles can grow via rectified diffusion to a point where they collapse from the inertia of the surrounding medium. This is known as inertial cavitation. Inertial cavitation activity, including microbubble collapse and fragmentation, is associated with a shift from discrete frequency components at the harmonics to broadband acoustic emissions.[52] While under certain conditions it is possible for bubbles to repeatedly undergo inertial cavitation for extended periods, in the context of circulating contrast agents, authors often refer to "stable cavitation" as microbubble oscillations without inertial collapse.

The safe implementation of focused ultrasound and microbubble-mediated therapies, such as blood-brain barrier disruption, relies on the ability to passively monitor acoustic emissions from microbubbles to assess treatment effects, including successful barrier disruption and the potential for damage to the tissue. For the acoustic parameters typically used for blood-brain barrier disruption, the relationship between the spectral frequency content of recorded microbubble emissions and treatment bioeffects are well understood.[53, 54] This has been demonstrated in rabbits, where spectral signatures representing stable microbubble activity, such as harmonic signals, recorded during sonications have been associated with successful blood-brain barrier disruption as confirmed using MRI.[53] Furthermore, a relationship between the enhancement on contrast-enhanced MR images and the 2nd and 3rd harmonic has been demonstrated.[53] Spectral signatures indicating inertial cavitation, such as broadband emissions, that were recorded at higher acoustic pressures were related to extensive damage to the microvasculature.[53]

This understanding of the relationship between microbubble emissions and tissue bioeffects has been paramount for the development of emissions-based algorithms and controllers to promote blood-brain barrier disruption while minimising tissue damage in real time. The first such controller was described by O'Reilly and Hynynen in 2012.[55] It implements a fully automated, hybrid closed-loop/open-loop approach where pressures are incrementally ramped up until sub-/ultra-harmonic signals are detected, triggering a pressure drop by a pre-defined factor and maintained for the duration of the treatment. In that same year, Arvanitis et al. demonstrated that increasing the pressure level to a target value where strong 2nd or 3rd harmonic signals were observed was an effective way of effective blood-brain barrier disruption without adverse effects.[56, 57] Following these early control algorithms, Sun et al. developed a fully automated, closed-loop controller designed to sustain stable cavitation at a predetermined level, while suppressing inertial cavitation.[58] A major limitation of passive detection with single element acoustic receivers is the inability to localise microbubble activity. For example, microbubble cavitation at the focus cannot be differentiated from cavitation effects in the beam path. As such, researchers have used phased receive arrays to achieve source localisation and 3D transcranial passive acoustic mapping of microbubble activity during blood-brain barrier disruption.[59, 60]

26.2.4 Factors Affecting the Efficacy of Blood-Brain Barrier Disruption

The efficacy of blood-brain barrier disruption depends on several variables, such as the acoustic parameters, the type of microbubbles and the anesthesia protocol used. These factors are discussed here.

26.2.4.1 Acoustic Parameters

An important acoustic parameter that influences many aspects of the experiment is the frequency. This determines the size of the focus, the need for aberration correction, the probability of standing waves, and the threshold pressure for blood-brain barrier disruption. The acoustic pressure is also of major importance. For a wide range of frequencies (0.26–1.63 MHz), increasing the acoustic pressure has been found to lead to stronger hyperintensities on contrast-enhanced MRI, as more MRI contrast agent leaks from the vessels.[15, 21, 61] The pressure that yields a 50% probability of blood-brain barrier disruption increases with frequency.[62] However, the mechanical index, defined as the peak negative pressure amplitude divided by the square root of the frequency, has been found to be constant at 0.46 for blood-brain barrier disruption for a fixed set of parameters.[62] These results are in line with the underlying assumptions of the mechanical index that was developed for ultrasound imaging and showed a relationship between the frequency and expected degree of bio-effects.[63] More extensive bio-effects are expected for higher mechanical indices.

There are many possible combinations of acoustic settings that can result in good blood-brain barrier disruption. A burst length as short as 70 μs can result in good opening at both 1.5 and 5.7 MHz.[22, 64] By increasing the burst length, lower pressures are needed and longer-lasting disruptions are observed.[64, 65] This was found to be valid up to 10 ms at 1.63 MHz: increasing the burst length from 10 to 100 ms led to no significant increase in hyper-intensity observed on MR after contrast administration.[15] While longer continuous bursts have been found to disrupt the barrier successfully, pulses of 6 s and longer have led to extravasation of erythrocytes; vessel destruction and necrosis have been observed with 10 s bursts.[66] Along with the duration of the bursts, the pulse repetition frequency can also be adjusted. No effect of pulse repetition frequency was observed on contrast-enhanced MRI when frequencies between 0.5 and 5 Hz were used.[65]

26.2.4.2 Microbubbles

The original use of microbubbles was in diagnostic ultrasound imaging, as contrast agents. These microbubbles are filled with gas and have a lipid or protein shell. Several commercial microbubbles are available (e.g., SonoVue, Optison, and Definity), and their diameters are typically smaller than 5 μm. The resonant frequency (f_r) of a microbubble in a liquid is given by[67]:

$$f_r = \frac{1}{2\pi R}\sqrt{\frac{3\kappa P}{\rho}}$$

in which R is the diameter, κ is the ratio of the heat capacity at constant pressure to the heat capacity at constant volume (C_p/C_v), P the pressure, and ρ the density of the surrounding medium. The resonant frequency of a 4-μm bubble in water is around 1.6 MHz at normal atmospheric pressure. It has been observed that larger microbubbles (diameters of 4–5 or 6–8 μm) require a lower threshold pressure for disruption than smaller microbubbles (1–2 μm) at 1.5 MHz.[68, 69] The larger microbubbles also had a higher K_{trans}[68] and more fluorescence enhancement was seen.[69] Using large bubbles (4–5 or 6–8 μm), the blood-brain barrier could be disrupted at 1.5 MHz without inertial cavitation (as determined by the absence of broadband emissions); however, when 1–2 μm bubbles were used, the disruption went together with broadband emissions.[70] Furthermore, the duration of disruption lasted 24 hours for small bubbles and up to 5 days for the larger bubbles.[71] The resonant frequency is higher for small bubbles, and Fan et al. have shown that submicron microbubbles (~0.6 μm) can successfully disrupt the blood-brain barrier at 10 MHz.[72]

The dose of microbubbles used is often based on the recommended dose for contrast-enhanced ultrasound imaging: around 10 μl/kg for Definity and 50 μl/kg for Optison.[65,73,74] The effect of the dose has been studied, and although in one study no relationship between injected dose and enhancement on contrast-enhanced MR was found,[65] others have found increased enhancement,[75] increased Evans blue extravasation,[31,75,76] and increased concentrations of doxorubicin[77] with higher microbubble doses. However, more apoptotic cells[76] and extravasation of erythrocytes[77] were also observed at higher bubble doses.

26.2.4.3 Anaesthesia

In humans it has been observed that the circulation time for perfluorocarbon microbubbles decreased when oxygen was used as the carrier gas for isoflurane, compared to that for medical air.[78,79] This could potentially also affect the efficacy of blood-brain barrier disruption, as was demonstrated by McDannold et al. They showed, using contrast-enhanced MRI, that the hyperintensity on T1-weighted MRI was greater in animals that were anaesthetised with an intraperitoneal injection of ketamine/xylazine compared with those that inhaled oxygen and isoflurane.[47]

26.2.5 Safety of Blood-Brain Barrier Disruption

26.2.5.1 Histologic Evaluation

When an animal is sacrificed following ultrasound-induced blood-brain barrier disruption, the brain can be processed for histologic evaluation. The most common stain used is hematoxylin and eosin (H&E). This stain allows the study of short- and long-term effects of ultrasound induced blood-brain barrier disruption. If the animal is sacrificed shortly after the sonication, and the disruption has caused micro-haemorrhage, it can be seen on H&E-sections as extravasation of erythrocytes. An increase in the extravasation area has been observed with increasing pressure,[42,61,73] greater microbubble concentrations,[77,80] higher frequencies,[65] and longer exposures.[18] Ischemic neurons appear dark and shrunken on H&E-stained sections, but can also be studied with additional stains, such as TUNEL, which gives a measure for nuclear DNA fragmentation, an indicator of apoptosis. An increase in the number of apoptotic cells has been observed for increasing microbubble dose[31] and acoustic pressure.[61,81] Importantly, there is a safe window for barrier disruption without significant damage.[21,27,82,83] Several researchers have suggested that vascular damage is related to inertial cavitation, as characterised by broadband emissions. It has also been suggested that blood-brain barrier disruption using stable cavitation is possible, and can be performed without vessel damage.[53,55] This emphasises the importance of the use of cavitation detection in these experiments.

26.2.5.2 Functional Testing

Another important measure is the use of functional tests to compare results before and after ultrasound sonications. Behavioural tests have been performed in mice before, and after, the sonications, with no difference in outcome.[84] Performing these tests in non-human primates can provide important information for the translation of this technique to the clinic, since elaborate testing is possible. In these subjects, no difference was observed before or after one or more sonications in tests that assessed behaviour, visual deficits, and visual acuity[27] in reaction times or decision making[26] in non-human primates. Furthermore, 20 months after the procedure, there were still no negative physiological or neurological effects.[26]

26.3 Physical Principles of Ultrasound-Mediated Blood-Brain Barrier Disruption

26.3.1 Effects of Microbubbles on the Blood-Brain Barrier

A microbubble in an acoustic field experiences a time-varying force that causes successive compressions and rarefactions. Physical interactions of the oscillating microbubble with the blood-brain barrier include direct mechanical perturbation, shear stresses, radiation force, and fluid streaming (Figure 26.3).

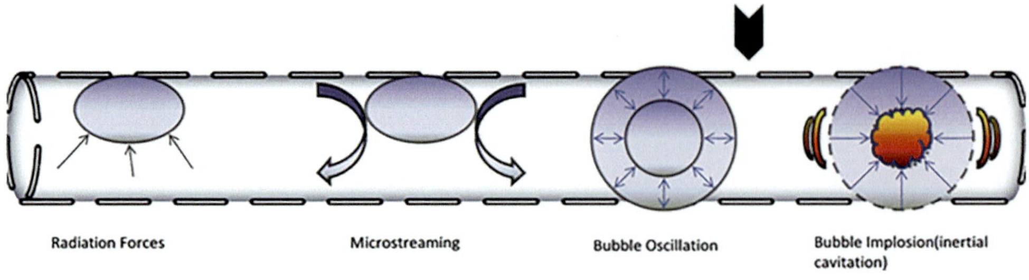

FIGURE 26.3 Possible mechanisms for ultrasound-mediated blood-brain barrier disruption using microbubbles. Radiation forces exert mechanical force on, and deform, the endothelium perpendicular to the direction of the blood flow and length of the vessel. Microstreaming results from eddying circular currents of fluid around the bubble. Focused ultrasound also causes the oscillation and the rapid growth of bubbles that, on implosion, unpredictably release stored energy in the form of shock waves. Reprinted from Neuroimaging Clinics of North America, Vol. 20, Colen and Jolesz, Future Potential of MRI-Guided Focused Ultrasound Brain Surgery, Pages 355–366, Copyright © 2010, with permission from Elsevier.[85]

A propagating wave interacting with a microbubble can influence nearby structures through acoustic radiation forces. The acoustic radiation force, which varies with the pulse repetition frequency, may directly drive drugs through porous membranes by induction of shear stresses up to 20 dynes/cm^2[2, 86] or position the microbubble for more efficient bubble activity near the walls of brain capilliaries.[87]

The shell of an oscillating microbubble near a vessel wall travels at speeds up to 250 m/s.[88] This nonlinear oscillation can either directly perturb endothelial cells or cause microstreaming[89] at the blood-brain barrier.

Bubble oscillations, microstreaming, radiation forces, and shock waves from bubble collapse and fragmentation result in shear stresses that cause stretching of cells and disruption of the tight junctions that characterise the blood-brain barrier. Using focused laser light and high-speed photography, Dijkink and Ohl found the shear stresses, on the order of kilopascals, to be highly focused at the vessel wall at the time of bubble collapse.[90] Following bubble collapse, a ring of much weaker stress can propagate radially. The magnitude of these effects depends strongly on the initial separation of the bubble and the nearby wall: bubbles more than a diameter away from the wall exert relatively little force compared to those pressed up against it.[90] This restriction could significantly reduce the contribution of shear stresses to blood-brain barrier disruption in large capillaries and arterioles, cerebral vessels much larger than the diameter of a microbubble.

The advent of computationally sophisticated software and hardware have enabled investigators to construct finite element models of bubble motion along the blood-brain barrier with the intention of simulating bubble interactions with sound, and the resulting forces on the blood-brain barrier.[91]

26.3.2 Mechanisms of Ultrasound-Mediated Blood-Brain Barrier Disruption

The exact mechanism by which the interaction of ultrasound and microbubbles induces blood-brain barrier disruption remains unknown. There is a general consensus within the research community that acoustic cavitation plays a role, due to the interaction of microbubbles with the nearby cerebrovascular wall. During, or as a result of this interaction, the transport of a substance across the blood-brain barrier—paracellularly or intracellularly[45]—is initiated. Three hypotheses have garnered the most attention: 1) tight junction breakdown from mechanical perturbation, 2) caveolin-dependent paracellular transport, and 3) p-glycoprotein-mediated efflux inhibition.

In capillaries, the breakdown of tight junction proteins from the direct mechanical perturbation during microbubble oscillation or from radiation forces may lead directly to an increase in paracellular permeability. Immunosignals from the proteins occludin, claudin-5, and ZO-1, which comprise tight junction complexes, decrease significantly in brains exhibiting blood-brain barrier disruption.[44]

Caveolin-1, a membrane protein, is particularly sensitive to shear stress along the endothelial surface, owing mainly to the presence of the small clefts in which they reside, called caveolae.[92] Capillaries and small arterioles have been shown to exhibit caveolin-dependent transcellular trafficking as a result of microbubble activity. Several investigators have documented evidence of this transcellular pathway during ultrasound exposure with microbubbles in rat brain and primary endothelial cells in vitro.[93–95] Further, caveolin-1 binds to endothelial-nitric oxide synthase (eNOS), which, upon cytoplasmic liberation, stimulates the production of nitric oxide, a potent vasodilator. Immunosignals from tight junction proteins occludin and claudin-5 have been shown to vanish only when intracellular caveolin-1 signals increase during blood-brain barrier disruption.[96] Likely to be a shear stress dependent mechanism, caveolin-dependent paracellular permeability may also play a role in blood-brain barrier disruption during acoustic exposure with microbubbles.

Transcellular trafficking evoked by ultrasound and microbubbles may also be increased by inhibition of p-glycoprotein mediated efflux. Known to play a role in multi-drug resistance of chemotherapeutic treatment by tumours, p-glycoprotein is a 170-kDa protein found in the plasma membrane that pumps hydrophobic compounds back out into the lumen,[97] preventing deposition and bioavailability within brain parenchyma. Zhang et al. have documented decreased p-glycoprotein at the protein and mRNA levels as a result of ultrasound exposure with microbubbles in rat glioma tumours.[98]

26.4 Therapeutic Effects in Preclinical Studies

The possibility of transferring agents that do not normally pass across the blood-brain barrier has been demonstrated using dyes, fluorescent markers, and MRI-contrast agents, using various acoustic settings within safe boundaries (see Section 26.2). As such, there have been many studies investigating the use of ultrasound-induced blood-brain barrier opening for therapeutic delivery to the brain. In animal studies, various therapeutic agents, including chemotherapeutic drugs,[77, 99–101] antibodies,[102–104] genes,[105–107] and stem cells.[108–111]

26.4.1 Enhanced Targeted Delivery of Therapeutic Agents to the Brain

An impression of the enhanced delivery of therapeutics can be obtained by comparing drug concentrations in the brain with and without focused ultrasound induced blood-brain barrier disruption. Using MRI-contrast agents of different sizes, it has been demonstrated that the permeability of the blood-brain barrier, and the duration of its opening, depend on the size of the agent for the same acoustic settings.[46] Therapeutic agents, such as chemotherapeutics, antibodies, and viral vectors, have different sizes and shapes which may affect efficacy of the treatment. When enhanced delivery is evaluated using dyes and MRI-contrast agents as surrogates for therapeutic agents, it is important to match the size of the drug and marker.[112]

In healthy animals, blood-brain barrier disruption has led to higher concentrations of chemotherapeutics with sizes between 214 and 580 Da.[66, 77, 99, 113] When doxorubicin was injected in its liposomal form (~100 nm), an increase in doxorubicin was also observed.[114] This also holds for tumour models where, despite their compromised vasculature, greater concentrations of chemotherapeutics were obtained with ultrasound treatment in rat glioma models.[99, 112] Higher doxorubicin concentrations can be obtained when the drug is injected shortly before the sonications, compared to injection 10 minutes afterwards.[114]

Antibodies, which have relatively large molecular weights, have successfully crossed the blood-brain barrier after focused ultrasound therapy, in normal and transgenic animal models.[37, 81, 102, 103] These large antibodies (~150 kDa) are not the limit for ultrasound-mediated drug delivery as 50–120 nm gold nanoparticles have also been successfully delivered to the brain of healthy animals and rats with gliomas.[115, 116] These gold particles have a wide applicability, including in enhancing local radiation effects, acting as thermotherapy agents, and delivering antibodies or chemotherapeutic agents. Magnetic nanoparticles (10–20 nm) have been conjugated with chemotherapeutics[117, 118] and increased accumulations of these have been seen. This enhancement was further increased by magnetic targeting of these nanoparticles.

Several other potential strategies for neurological diseases have been evaluated, including delivery across the blood-brain barrier of adeno-associated viruses,[105, 111] natural killer cells,[119, 120] and neural stem cells.[108]

26.4.2 Therapeutic Benefit

Improvement in outcome after successful delivery of a therapeutic agent across the blood-brain barrier has been demonstrated with varying levels of success, mainly in tumour and Alzheimer's disease models. An overview of selected studies and their therapeutic benefit is provided in Table 26.1. In none of the studies involving tumour models was an effect of the focused ultrasound treatment observed without administration of the therapeutics, suggesting that disruption of the blood-brain barrier alone has no

TABLE 26.1

Overview of Different Studies Investigating Treatment Benefit of Enhanced Drug Delivery by Focused Ultrasound-Mediated Blood-Brain Delivery in Several Diseases and the Primary Outcome

Disease	Model	Administered Therapy	Difference in Outcome of Therapy with and without Ultrasound	Reference
Primary brain tumour	C6 glioma	Chemotherapeutic BCNU (1×)	Tumour progression controlled and significant improvement in survival	Liu et al. 2010[99]
Primary brain tumour	C6 glioma	BCNU conjugated with magnetic nanoparticles	Lower dose necessary for tumour suppression	Chen et al. 2010[118]
Primary brain tumour	9L glioma	Chemotherapeutic temozolomide (2×)	Significantly better tumour progression control at lower dose	Wei et al. 2013[123]
Primary brain tumour	9L glioma	Chemotherapeutic liposomal doxorubicin (1×)	Modest increase in survival	Treat et al. 2012[121]
Primary brain tumour	9L glioma	Liposomal doxorubicin (3×)	100% increase in survival	Aryal et al. 2013[100]
Primary brain tumour	9L glioma	Chemotherapeutic liposomal doxorubicin (1×)	Significant increase in doxorubicin concentration in excised tumours 1 or 24 hours after treatment	Park et al. 2017[101]
Primary brain tumour	F98 glioma	Carboplatin	96% increase in tumour doubling time and 48% increase in median survival compared to the drug alone	McDannold et al. 2019[124]
Brain metastasis	BT-474	Antibody therapy trastuzumab (6×)	Improved survival and a complete response in part of the animals	Park et al. 2012[74]
Brain metastasis	MDA-361	Antibody therapy trastuzumab and pertuzumab (6×)	Improved survival and slowed tumour growth in 40% of animals treated with the combined treatment; 60% were non-responders	Kobus et al. 2016[104]
Alzheimer's disease	TgCRND8	Anti Aβ-antibodies (1×)	Plaque reduction	Jordão et al. 2010[103]
Alzheimer's disease	TgCRND8	Only ultrasound (1×)	Plaque reduction	Jordão et al. 2013[122]
Alzheimer's disease	TgCRND8	Nerve growth factor, tropomyosin receptor kinase A (TrkA)	Enhanced hippocampal neurogenesis	Xhima et al. 2022[110]
Parkinson's disease	MPTP-induced animal disease model	Glial cell line-derived neurotrophic factor (GDNF, gene therapy)	Increased GDNF expression in glial cells	Lin et al. 2016[107]

therapeutic effect.[74, 99, 100, 118, 121] However, in Alzheimer's disease models, a reduction in amyloid-beta plaques was observed without administration of an exogenous drug.[122] There, a temporary activation of microglia and astrocytes was observed, together with an increase of endogenous antibodies bound to the plaques.

26.5 Progress towards Ultrasound-Mediated Blood-Brain Barrier Disruption in a Clinical Setting

To date, as discussed in Section 26.4, there have been numerous studies of the safe and effective delivery of tracers and therapeutics to the brain in preclinical investigations. The progress made towards clinical translation, including device development, clinical trials, and relevant patient populations, will be discussed in this section.

26.5.1 Clinical Devices for Blood-Brain Barrier Disruption

Several clinical devices have reached the stage of clinical trials for ultrasound-mediated blood-brain barrier disruption. These include the implantable Carthera SonoCloud and SonoCloud-9, transcranial hemispherical arrays – the MRI-guided InSightec ExAblate Neuro (ExAblate Model 4000 Type-2) and the neuronavigation-guided NaviFUS, and an extracranial single-element transducer. A schematic diagram highlighting the ultrasonic devices developed for blood-brain barrier disruption is shown in Figure 26.4.

One of the first devices to enter clinical trials for disruption of the blood-brain barrier was the SonoCloud (CarThera, Paris, France). The original device is a single-element, 1.15-cm-diameter, unfocused 1.05-MHz transducer, designed to be implanted in a burr hole following a surgical procedure.[126]

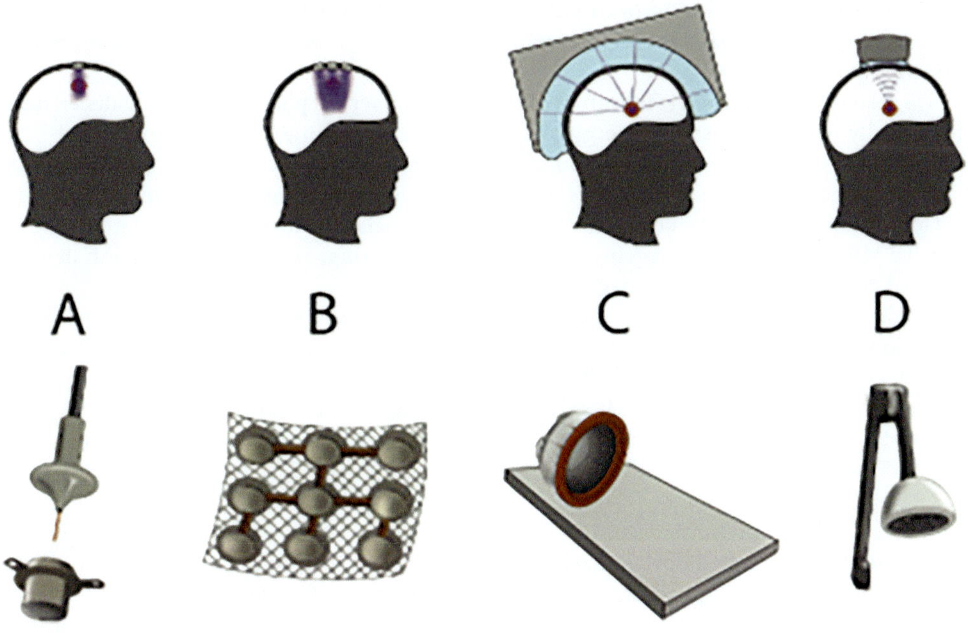

FIGURE 26.4 Schematic showing the clinical devices developed for ultrasound-induced blood-brain barrier disruption. ***A.*** Implantable, unfocused single-element emitter (SonoCloud). ***B.*** Implantable 9-element emitter (SonoCloud-9). ***C.*** Transcranial, focused, hemispherical arrays (ExAblate Neuro, NaviFUS). ***D.*** Transcranial single-element focused device. Reprinted from Cancer Letters, Vol. 479, Beccaria et al., Ultrasound-Induced Blood-Brain Barrier Disruption for the Treatment of Gliomas and other Primary CNS Tumours, Pages 13–22, Copyright © 2020, with permission from Elsevier.[125]

The second generation of this device, SonoCloud-9, is made up of 9 such 1-cm-diameter transducers on an implantable grid. Currently, the SonoCloud devices are the only implantable ultrasound transmitters that have been used for blood-brain barrier disruption in a clinical scenario. Implantable devices are highly suited to the treatment of large, infiltrative, and superficial lesions, such as extensive high-grade gliomas and diffuse intrinsic pontine gliomas.[125] Advantages of implantable devices include short procedures, large target volumes, and elimination of the need for head shaving that is associated with extracranial devices. However, there are drawbacks to these devices, which include the need for surgical implantation, the limitations of only treating within the device beam path and difficulty in treating deep targets.

Most clinical blood-brain barrier disruption devices are extracranial. These devices are non-invasive, appropriate for targeting multiple deep locations, and can be controlled in real time using MRI or neuronavigational control. Extracranial devices are well suited for treating multiple, deep-seated tumours and metastatic disease. The non-invasive nature makes them extremely attractive in patients where surgical intervention is not otherwise generally needed, such as Alzheimer's disease and epilepsy. However, these devices are limited to long procedure times when treating large volumes, the dependence on external and expensive additional hardware, like MRI, the possible need for general anesthesia in pediatric patients, difficulty treating superficial targets, and the need to remove hair to improve acoustic coupling and avoid trapping air bubbles.[125]

The most used device for transcranial focused ultrasound therapy is the InSightec ExAblate Neuro (InSightec, Tirat Carmel, Israel). This device was originally designed for thermal ablative ultrasound surgery[127, 128] and has been approved by the Food and Drug Administration (FDA) for thalamotomy in patients with essential tremor and pallidotomy in patients with Parkinson's disease. A low-frequency version of the device is currently undergoing clinical trials for blood-brain barrier disruption for several indications, including brain tumours,[129] Alzheimer's disease,[130] and amyotrophic lateral sclerosis (ALS).[131] The device consists of a 1024-element ultrasound helmet which operates at a centre frequency of 220 kHz. The helmet is attached to the patient using a stereotactic frame. MRI is used for targeting and treatment guidance, and CT images of the skull are registered with intraoperative MRI and used to calculate phase corrections for the transducer elements. The device includes embedded passive receivers which enable real-time acoustic feedback for determining sonication parameters.[129]

NaviFUS (NaviFUS, Inc., Taipei, Taiwan) is another hemispherical phased array transducer, designed to transcranially deliver ultrasound energy to the brain for blood-brain barrier disruption.[132–134] This device operates at a centre frequency of 500 kHz and is mounted on a semirigid mechanical arm to enable neuronavigation. A major advantage is that the procedure is completely frameless, eliminating the need for skull fixation and reduces patient discomfort associated with the use of a stereotactic frame. Preoperative MRI and CT images are used for treatment planning, and passive cavitation detection is implemented for real-time energy management.

The final device that has reached the stage of clinical trials for ultrasound-induced blood-brain barrier disruption is a 250-kHz neuronavigation-guided, single-element focused transducer that was first proposed by Pouliopoulos et al. at Columbia University.[135] This system incorporates passive cavitation detection for treatment monitoring. It is an attractive device for clinical adoption, as it offers a non-invasive, portable, and low-cost alternative to the other devices currently available for human use.

26.5.2 Clinical Trials

Since 2014, the aforementioned devices have been tested clinically for applications in a range of brain diseases and disorders. One of the first demonstrations of successful blood-brain barrier disruption in humans was performed in patients with primary brain tumours at Sunnybrook Research Institute (Toronto, ON, Canada) using the ExAblate Neuro.[129] A contrast-enhanced T1-weighted MRI from that clinical trial, confirming blood-brain barrier disruption is shown in Figure 26.5. In this safety trial, no evidence of petechiae, haemorrhage, oedema, or other adverse effects were observed using MRI and the disruption of the blood-brain barrier was reversible, completely resolving within one day of the treatment (Figure 26.6).

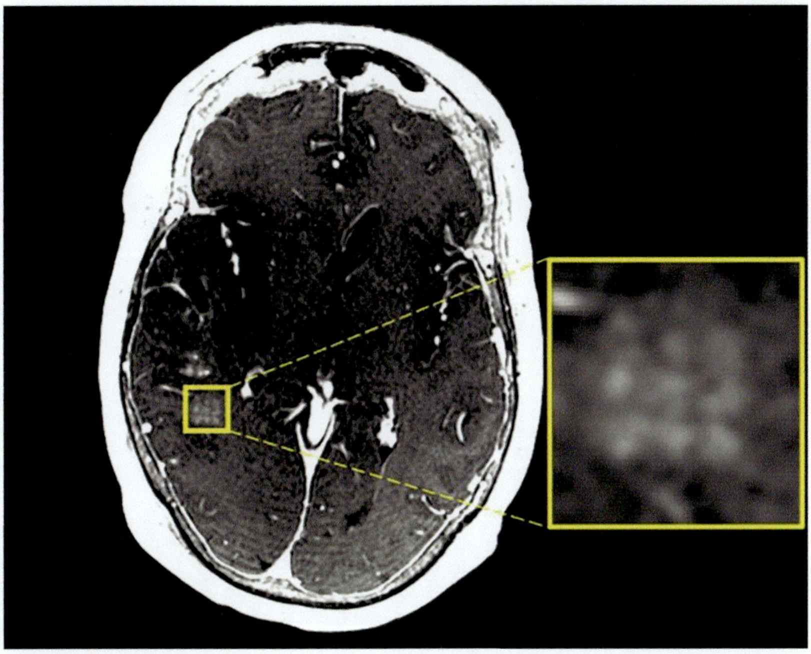

FIGURE 26.5 An example of contrast-enhanced T1-weighted MRI in one patient immediately following blood-brain barrier disruption. The image shows discrete and precise MRI contrast extravasation in the targeted grid pattern where the sonication was performed (inset). Reprinted from Scientific Reports, Vol. 9, Mainprize et al., Blood-Brain Barrier Opening in Primary Brain Tumours with Non-Invasive MR-Guided Focused Ultrasound: A Clinical Safety and Feasibility Study, Copyright © 2019 Mainprize et al.[129] [Publisher: Springer Nature, License: Creative Commons CC BY].

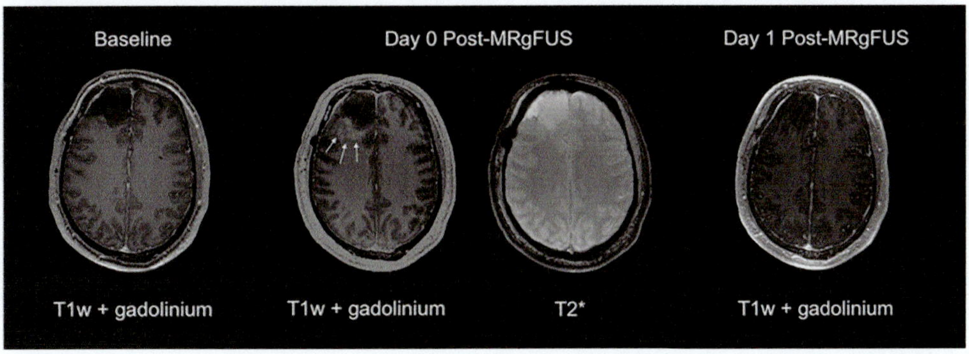

FIGURE 26.6 Example of a contrast-enhanced T1-weighted MRI from one patient obtained 30 days prior to ultrasound sonication (left), immediately following blood-brain barrier disruption (middle; white arrows) and 20 hours after blood-brain barrier disruption showing that the disruption has resolved (right). T2*-weighted MRI acquired immediately following blood-brain barrier disruption for this patient show no evidence of petechiae. Reprinted from Scientific Reports, Vol. 9, Mainprize et al., Blood-Brain Barrier Opening in Primary Brain Tumours with Non-Invasive MR-Guided Focused Ultrasound: A Clinical Safety and Feasibility Study, Copyright © 2019 Mainprize et al.[129] [Publisher: Springer Nature, License: Creative Commons CC BY].

Table 26.2 shows a comprehensive list of the clinical trials of ultrasound-induced blood-brain barrier disruption initiated from 2014 to date at centres across North America, Europe, and Asia. The purpose of most trials has been safety and feasibility, but some trials are also investigating efficacy. Large-scale demonstrations of enhanced therapeutic effects are still needed before clinical adoption of this technology. A range of brain diseases and disorders have been identified as potential indications

TABLE 26.2

A Comprehensive List of Clinical Trials Investigating Blood-Brain Barrier Disruption since 2014

Disease	Device	Administered Therapy [Purpose]	Trial Identifier (*clinicaltrials.gov*)	Institution(s)	Dates
Glioblastoma	SonoCloud	Blood-brain barrier disruption with carboplatin [Safety]	NCT02253212	Hôpital de la Pitié-Salpêtrière, Paris, France	2014–2018
Primary brain tumours	Transcranial ExAblate Neuro	Blood-brain barrier disruption with chemotherapeutic doxorubicin or temozolomide [Safety]	NCT02343991	Sunnybrook Health Sciences Centre, Toronto, ON, Canada	2014–2022
Alzheimer's disease (mild)	Transcranial ExAblate Neuro	Blood-brain barrier disruption alone [Safety]	NCT02986932	Sunnybrook Health Sciences Centre	2016–2018
Alzheimer's disease (mild)	SonoCloud	Blood-brain barrier disruption alone [Safety]	NCT03119961	Hôpital de la Pitié-Salpêtrière	2017–2020
Glioblastoma multiforme	NaviFUS	Blood-brain barrier disruption alone [Safety]	NCT03626896	Linkou Chang Gung Memorial Hospital Taoyuan City, Taiwan	2018–2019
Parkinson's disease with dementia	Transcranial ExAblate Neuro	Blood-brain barrier disruption alone [Safety]	NCT03608553	HM Hospitales Puerta del Sur – CINAC Móstoles, Madrid, Spain	2018–2021
Amyotrophic lateral sclerosis	Transcranial ExAblate Neuro	Blood-brain barrier disruption alone [Safety]	NCT03321487	Sunnybrook Health Sciences Centre	2018–2022
Alzheimer's disease	Transcranial ExAblate Neuro	Blood-brain barrier disruption alone [Safety, Efficacy]	NCT03739905	Sunnybrook Health Sciences Centre	2018–2022
Glioma glioblastoma multiforme	Transcranial ExAblate Neuro	Blood-brain barrier disruption (up to 6×) with adjuvant chemotherapeutic temozolomide [Safety]	NCT03551249, NCT03616860, NCT03712293	University of Maryland Brigham and Women's Hospital, Boston, MA, United States University of Virginia, Charlottesville, VA, United States West Virginia University, Morgantown, WV, United States Sunnybrook Health Sciences Centre Severance Hospital, Yonsei University Health System Seoul, S. Korea	2018–2024
Drug-resistant epilepsy	NaviFUS	Blood-brain barrier disruption with anti-epileptic drugs [Safety, Efficacy]	NCT03860298	Taipei Veterans General Hospital, Taipei, Taiwan	2019–2020
Melanoma with brain metastases	SonoCloud	Blood-brain barrier disruption with nivolumab (Anti PD-1) [Safety, Efficacy]	NCT04021420	Saint-Louis Hospital, Paris, France	2019–2020
Her2-positive breast cancer brain metastases	Transcranial ExAblate Neuro	Blood-brain barrier disruption (up to 6×) with trastuzumab [Safety]	NCT03714243	Sunnybrook Health Sciences Centre	2019–2022

Recurrent glioblastoma	SonoCloud-9	Blood-brain barrier disruption with carboplatin [Safety, Efficacy, Dose Escalation]	NCT03744026	Northwestern University, Chicago, IL, United States MD Anderson Cancer Center, Houston, TX, United States Centre Hospitalier Universitaire d'Angers, Angers, France Hôpital Neurologique Pierre Wertheimer, Bron, France Hôpital de La Timone, Marseille, France Hôpital de la Pitié-Salpêtrière	2019–2022
Alzheimer's disease	Transcranial ExAblate Neuro	Blood-brain barrier disruption alone (2x) [Safety]	NCT04526262	Yonsei University Medical Center, Seoul, S. Korea	2020
Alzheimer's disease	Neuronavigation-guided single-element focused ultrasound transducer	Blood-brain barrier disruption alone [Safety]	NCT04118764	Columbia University Irving Medical Center/New York-Presbyterian Hospital, New York, NY, United States	2020–2022
Parkinson's disease	Transcranial ExAblate Neuro	Biweekly blood-brain barrier disruption with Cerezyme [Safety, Dose Escalation]	NCT04370665	Sunnybrook Health Sciences Centre	2020–2022
Glioblastoma multiforme	NaviFUS	Biweekly blood-brain barrier disruption with Bevacizumab [Safety, Efficacy]	NCT04446416	Linkou Chang Gung Memorial Hospital	2020–2022
Recurrent glioblastoma multiforme	Transcranial ExAblate Neuro	Blood-brain barrier disruption (up to 6×) with carboplatin [Safety]	NCT04440358, NCT04417088	Sunnybrook Health Sciences Centre Sheba Medical Center, Tel Hashomer, Israel Fondazione IRCCS Neurologico Carlo Besta, Milano, Italy Yonsei University Medical Center Stanford University Palo Alto, CA, United States University of Maryland Brigham and Women's Hospital Cleveland Clinic Cleveland, OH, United States	2020–2023
Recurrent glioblastoma	SonoCloud	Repeated blood-brain barrier disruption with paclitaxel and carboplatin	NCT04528680	Northwestern Memorial Hospital, Chicago, IL, United States	2020–2025
Malignant glioma glioblastoma	Transcranial ExAblate Neuro	Blood-brain barrier disruption (up to 6×) with adjuvant chemotherapeutic temozolomide [Safety]	NCT04998864	Fondazione IRCCS Neurologico Carlo Besta HM Hospitales Puerta del Sur – CINAC Móstoles, Madrid, Spain	2021–2023

(Continued)

TABLE 26.2 (*Continued*)

A Comprehensive List of Clinical Trials Investigating Blood-Brain Barrier Disruption since 2014

Disease	Device	Administered Therapy [Purpose]	Trial Identifier (*clinicaltrials.gov*)	Institution(s)	Dates
Glioblastoma multiforme	SonoCloud	Blood-brain barrier disruption (up to 6×) with adjuvant chemotherapeutic temozolomide [Efficacy]	NCT04614493	Katholieke Universiteit Leuven, Leuven, Belgium Centre hospitalier Universitaire d'Angers Groupe Hospitalier Saint-André, Bordeaux, France Hôpital Neurologique Pierre Wertheimer Hôpital de La Timone Hôpital de la Pitié-Salpêtrière	2021–2024
Pediatric diffuse intrinsic pontine glioma Pediatric diffuse pontine and thalamic gliomas Pediatric diffuse midline glioma	Neuronavigation-guided single-element focused ultrasound transducer	Blood-brain barrier disruption and oral Panobinostat [Safety]	NCT04804709	Columbia University Irving Medical Center/New York-Presbyterian Hospital	2021–2025
Pediatric malignant brain tumours	SonoCloud-9	Blood-brain barrier disruption with carboplatin [Safety]	NCT05293197	Institut Curie, Paris, France Service de neurochirugie Pédiatrique – Hôpital Necker-Enfants Malades, Paris, France Institut Gustave Roussy, Villejuif, France	2022–2024
Non-small cell lung cancer brain metastases	Transcranial ExAblate Neuro	Blood-brain barrier disruption with pembrolizumab monotherapy [Safety, Efficacy]	NCT05317858	St. Joseph's Hospital and Medical Center, Phoenix, AZ, United States Miami Cancer Institute at Baptist Health, Miami, FL, United States University of Maryland, Baltimore, MD, United States Sunnybrook Health Sciences Centre	2022–2024
Pediatric diffuse intrinsic pontine gliomas	Transcranial ExAblate Neuro	Blood-brain barrier disruption with chemotherapeutic doxorubicin [Safety]	NCT05630209, NCT05615623	Children's National Medical Center, Washington, DC, United States Sunnybrook Health Sciences Centre	2022–2025
Alzheimer's disease with mild cognitive impairment	Transcranial ExAblate Neuro	Blood-brain barrier disruption with aducanumab [Safety]	NCT05469009	West Virginia University Rockefeller Neuroscience Institute, Morgantown, WV, United States	2022–2029

for ultrasound-enhanced blood-brain barrier disruption. These include brain tumours – primary and metastatic, Alzheimer's disease, Parkinson's disease, ALS, and epilepsy.

26.6 Other Applications in the Central and Peripheral Nervous Systems

This chapter, and much of the research in this field, has focused on microbubble-mediated ultrasound therapy as a means of therapeutic delivery across the blood-brain barrier, from the vasculature into the brain parenchyma. However, this mechanism of action can be translated for other applications. In this section, the adaption of microbubble-mediated ultrasound therapy for non-invasive liquid biopsy and for nervous system applications outside of the brain will be briefly discussed.

26.6.1 Focused Ultrasound-Enabled Non-Invasive Liquid Biopsy

Molecular biomarkers, such as, DNA mutations, changes in epigenetic makeup, and variations in gene expression, can provide valuable information for the diagnosis and monitoring of brain tumours.[136] These biomarkers are commonly examined by surgical resection and surgical tissue biopsy,[137] but there are many complications associated with these invasive procedures for transcranial tumours, especially when repeated biopsies are required.[138] Liquid biopsy, the detection of circulating cancer biomarkers in the blood plasma, has been established in patients with various types of cancer.[139] However, the progress of liquid biopsies for brain tumours has been challenging, as the blood-brain barrier limits the release of tumour biomarkers into the vasculature.[137, 140, 141]

Ultrasound has been used as a strategy for the amplification and localisation of blood biomarkers outside of the brain.[142–146] The Chen Ultrasound Laboratory at Washington University in St. Louis has shown that ultrasound-mediated blood-brain barrier disruption opens two-way trafficking between the brain and the vasculature. They developed "Sonobiopsy" – focused ultrasound–enabled brain tumour blood-based liquid biopsy – and demonstrated its safety and effectiveness in preclinical models.[147–149] In clinical trials (NCT03616860, NCT03739905), focused ultrasound-mediated blood-brain barrier disruption has been shown to enhance plasma cell-free DNA, neuron-derived extracellular vesicles, and brain-specific protein S100b in patients with glioblastoma multiforme.[150]

26.6.2 Other Blood–Nervous System Barriers: The Blood–Spinal Cord and Blood-Nerve Barriers

The blood-brain barrier, is one of a complex network of blood–central nervous system barriers, which include the blood–spinal cord and blood–cerebrospinal fluid barriers.[151, 152] Together, these barriers work to maintain the specialised environment within the central nervous system by limiting external molecules from passing from the bloodstream not just into the brain, but also the spinal cord. Axons, Schwann cells, and other cells of peripheral nerves function within the blood-nerve barrier. The blood-nerve barrier protects the endoneurial microenvironment by regulating the permeability of capillaries in the endoneurium and the investing perineurium.[153] Like the blood-brain barrier, these other blood–nervous system barriers pose a challenge to therapeutic delivery.

The feasibility and safety of using microbubble-mediated focused ultrasound for delivery tracers across the blood–spinal cord barrier has been demonstrated in small animals,[154–158] in rabbits following a laminectomy,[159] and through the intact spine in pigs.[160] Weber-Adrian et al. were the first to demonstrate therapeutic delivery, using focused ultrasound to deliver self-complementary adeno-associated virus serotype 9 (scAAV9) to the spinal cords of healthy rats.[161] Ultrasound-mediated blood–spinal cord barrier disruption has been shown to increase trastuzumab delivery in rats with HER2-positive leptomeningeal metastases around the spinal cord and suppress metastatic tumour growth.[162, 163] Given the complex structure of the human spine, new devices and methods of ultrasound exposure are necessary for clinical translation for spinal cord applications.[164, 165] Recently, one study has shown that ultrasound and microbubbles can facilitate blood-nerve barrier disruption, confirmed by the leakage of Evans blue dye, in the peripheral nervous system of rodents.[166] Further preclinical work and optimisation of acoustic parameters is required before this method can be clinically translated for drug delivery in diseases like peripheral nerve injury.

26.7 Outlook

In this chapter, different aspects if preclinical and clinical ultrasound-mediated blood-brain barrier disruption have been discussed. Over the last two decades, ultrasound and microbubble-mediated delivery of therapeutics to the brain has grown to become a fascinating field of research, with tremendous potential to revolutionise treatment options for patients with brain disease, including cancers, neurodegenerative diseases, and other neurological disorders. The major advantages of this approach compared with existing methods of bypassing the blood-brain barrier are that it is targeted, non-invasive, and reversible. Major technological advancements in acoustic signal analysis and device development have been able to ensure safe delivery of acoustic energy and robust systems of treatment monitoring.

Through preclinical trials, a range of potential clinical targets where this technology can be applied have been identified, and tracers and therapeutic agents, such as chemotherapeutics, gene therapies, antibodies, and stem cells, have been delivered across the blood-brain barrier with promising effects. Beginning in the mid-2010s, ultrasound-mediated blood-brain barrier disruption entered clinical trials for the treatment of a range of diseases, including primary brain tumours, brain metastases, Alzheimer's disease, Parkinson's disease, and epilepsy. Most of these trials have investigated device feasibility and safety in different clinical indications. If these procedures are deemed to be safe, the next step will be to assess the efficacy of the treatment in delivering therapeutic agents and to determine whether the enhanced delivery provides a benefit for patient outcomes.

The field of ultrasound-mediated blood-brain barrier disruption is still growing, and recent studies have shown promising technical advancements and clinical utilisation of this method. In light of the current state of the field, it is reasonable to imagine that this technology may soon be recognised as a life-changing for many patients, where the blood-brain barrier currently poses a hindrance to the delivery of otherwise effective therapeutic agents.

REFERENCES

1. Ehrlich, P. *Das Sauerstoff-Bedürfniss des organismus: Eine Farbenanalytische Studie* (A. Hirschwald, 1885).
2. Goldmann, E. E. *Vitalfärbung am Zentralnervensystem: Beitrag zur Physio-Pathologie des Plexus chorioideus und der Hirnhäute. No. 1* (Königl. Akademie der Wissenschaften, 1913).
3. Pardridge, W. M. Transport of insulin-related peptides and glucose across the blood-brain barrier. *Ann. N. Y. Acad. Sci.* **692**, 126–137 (1993).
4. Fischer, H., Gottschlich, R. & Seelig, A. Blood-brain barrier permeation: Molecular parameters governing passive diffusion. *J. Membr. Biol.* **165**, 201–211 (1998).
5. Pardridge, W. M. Drug transport across the blood–brain barrier. *J. Cereb. Blood Flow Metab.* **32**, 1959–1972 (2012).
6. Neuwelt, E. *et al.* Strategies to advance translational research into brain barriers. *Lancet Neurol.* **7**, 84–96 (2008).
7. Hendricks, B. K., Cohen-Gadol, A. A. & Miller, J. C. Novel delivery methods bypassing the blood-brain and blood-tumor barriers. *Neurosurg. Focus* **38**, E10 (2015).
8. Rizvi, S. & Kumar, K. History and present state of targeted intrathecal drug delivery. *Curr. Pain Headache Reports* **19**, 1–7 (2015).
9. Bobo, R. H. *et al.* Convection-enhanced delivery of macromolecules in the brain. *Proc. Natl. Acad. Sci.* **91**, 2076–2080 (1994).
10. Voges, J. *et al.* Imaging-guided convection-enhanced delivery and gene therapy of glioblastoma. *Ann. Neurol.* **54**, 479–487 (2003).
11. Illum, L. Transport of drugs from the nasal cavity to the central nervous system. *Eur. J. Pharm. Sci.* **11**, 1–18 (2000).

12. Abbott, N. J. & Romero, I. A. Transporting therapeutics across the blood-brain barrier. *Mol. Med. Today* **2**, 106–113 (1996).
13. Lossinsky, A. S., Vorbrodt, A. W. & Wisniewski, H. M. Scanning and transmission electron microscopic studies of microvascular pathology in the osmotically impaired blood-brain barrier. *J. Neurocytol.* **24**, 795–806 (1995).
14. Pardridge, W. M. Targeted delivery of protein and gene medicines through the blood–brain barrier. *Clin. Pharmacol. Ther.* **97**, 347–361 (2015).
15. Hynynen, K., McDannold, N., Vykhodtseva, N. & Jolesz, F. A. Noninvasive MR imaging-guided focal opening of the blood-brain barrier in rabbits. *Radiology* **220**, 640–646 (2001).
16. Ammi, A. Y. *et al.* Characterization of Ultrasound Propagation Through Ex-vivo Human Temporal Bone. *Ultrasound Med. Biol.* **34**, 1578–1589 (2008).
17. Hynynen, K. & Jolesz, F. A. Demonstration of potential noninvasive brain therapy through an intact skull. *Ultrasound Med. Biol.* **24**, 275–283 (1998).
18. Chopra, R., Vykhodtseva, N. & Hynynen, K. Influence of exposure time and pressure amplitude on blood-brain-barrier opening using transcranial ultrasound exposures. *ACS Chem. Neurosci.* **1**, 391–398 (2010).
19. O'Reilly, M. A., Muller, A. & Hynynen, K. Ultrasound insertion loss of rat parietal bone appears to be proportional to animal mass at submegahertz frequencies. *Ultraound Med. Biol.* **37**, 1930–1937 (2011).
20. Choi, J. J., Pernot, M., Small, S. A. & Konofagou, E. E. Noninvasive, transcranial and localized opening of the blood-brain barrier using focused ultrasound in mice. *Ultrasound Med. Biol.* **33**, 95–104 (2007).
21. Hynynen, K. *et al.* Focal disruption of the blood–brain barrier due to 260-kHz ultrasound bursts: A method for molecular imaging and targeted drug delivery. *J. Neurosurg.* **105**, 445–454 (2006).
22. Bing, K. F., Howles, G. P., Qi, Y., Palmeri, M. L. & Nightingale, K. R. Blood-brain barrier (BBB) disruption using a diagnostic ultrasound scanner and definity® in mice. *Ultrasound Med. Biol.* **35**, 1298–1308 (2009).
23. Xie, F. *et al.* Effects of transcranial ultrasound and intravenous microbubbles on blood brain barrier permeability in a large animal model. *Ultrasound Med. Biol.* **34**, 2028–2034 (2008).
24. Marquet, F., Tung, Y.-S., Teichert, T., Ferrera, V. P. & Konofagou, E. E. Noninvasive, transient and selective blood-brain barrier opening in non-human primates in vivo. *PLoS One* **6**, e22598 (2011).
25. Tung, Y. S., Marquet, F., Teichert, T., Ferrera, V. & Konofagou, E. E. Feasibility of noninvasive cavitation-guided blood-brain barrier opening using focused ultrasound and microbubbles in nonhuman primates. *Appl. Phys. Lett.* **98**, 163704 (2011).
26. Downs, M. E. *et al.* Long-term safety of repeated blood-brain barrier opening via focused ultrasound with microbubbles in non-human primates performing a cognitive task. *PLoS One* **10**, e0125911 (2015).
27. McDannold, N., Arvanitis, C. D., Vykhodtseva, N. & Livingstone, M. S. Temporary disruption of the blood-brain barrier by use of ultrasound and microbubbles: Safety and efficacy evaluation in rhesus macaques. *Cancer Res.* **72**, 3652–3666 (2012).
28. Song, J., Pulkkinen, A., Huang, Y. & Hynynen, K. Investigation of standing wave formation in a human skull for a clinical prototype of a large-aperture, transcranial MR-guided Focused Ultrasound (MRgFUS) phased array: An experimental and simulation study. *IEEE Trans. Biomed. Eng.* **59**, 435–444 (2012).
29. Deffieux, T. & Konofagou, E. Numerical study of a simple transcranial focused ultrasound system applied to blood-brain barrier opening. *IEEE Trans. Ultrason. Ferroelectr. Freq. Control* **57**, 2637–2653 (2010).
30. O'Reilly, M. A., Huang, Y. & Hynynen, K. The impact of standing wave effects on transcranial focused ultrasound disruption of the blood-brain barrier in a rat model. *Phys. Med. Biol.* **55**, 5251–5267 (2010).
31. Yang, F.-Y. *et al.* Quantitative evaluation of focused ultrasound with a contrast agent on blood-brain barrier disruption. *Ultrasound Med. Biol.* **33**, 1421–1427 (2007).
32. Marquet, F. *et al.* Real-time, transcranial monitoring of safe blood-brain barrier opening in non-human primates. *PLoS One* **9**, e84310 (2014).
33. Bing, C. *et al.* Trans-cranial opening of the blood-brain barrier in targeted regions using a stereotaxic brain atlas and focused ultrasound energy. *J. Ther. Ultrasound* **2** (2014).
34. Lapin, N. A., Gill, K., Shah, B. R. & Chopra, R. Consistent opening of the blood brain barrier using focused ultrasound with constant intravenous infusion of microbubble agent. *Sci. Rep.* **10** (2020).
35. Szczuzupak, D. *et al.* Non-invasive disruption of the blood-brain barrier in the marmoset monkey. *bioRxiv* (2022). doi:10.1101/2022.11.08.515696.

36. Goertz, D. E., Wright, C. & Hynynen, K. Contrast agent kinetics in the rabbit brain during exposure to therapeutic ultrasound. *Ultrasound Med. Biol.* **36**, 916 (2010).
37. Raymond, S. B. *et al.* Ultrasound enhanced delivery of molecular imaging and therapeutic agents in Alzheimer's disease mouse models. *PLoS One* **3**, e2175 (2008).
38. Deng, L., Yang, S. D., Oareilly, M. A., Jones, R. M. & Hynynen, K. An ultrasound-guided hemispherical phased array for microbubble-mediated ultrasound therapy. *IEEE Trans. Biomed. Eng.* **69**, 1776–1787 (2022).
39. Deng, L. *et al.* A multi-frequency sparse hemispherical ultrasound phased array for microbubble-mediated transcranial therapy and simultaneous cavitation mapping. *Phys. Med. Biol.* **61**, 8476–8501 (2016).
40. Nag, S. Blood-brain barrier permeability using tracers and immunohistochemistry. In *The Blood-Brain Barrier. Methods in Molecular Medicine™*. Vol. 89, 133–144 (Humana Press, 2003).
41. Raymond, S. B., Skoch, J., Hynynen, K. & Bacskai, B. J. Multiphoton imaging of ultrasound/Optison mediated cerebrovascular effects in vivo. *J. Cereb. Blood Flow Metab.* **27**, 393–403 (2007).
42. Baseri, B., Choi, J. J., Tung, Y. S. & Konofagou, E. E. Multi-modality safety assessment of blood-brain barrier opening using focused ultrasound and definity microbubbles: A short-term study. *Ultrasound Med. Biol.* **36**, 1445 (2010).
43. Nhan, T. *et al.* Drug delivery to the brain by focused ultrasound induced blood-brain barrier disruption: Quantitative evaluation of enhanced permeability of cerebral vasculature using two-photon microscopy. *J. Control. Release* **172**, 274–280 (2013).
44. Sheikov, N. *et al.* Brain arterioles show more active vesicular transport of blood-borne tracer molecules than capillaries and venules after focused ultrasound-evoked opening of the blood-brain barrier. *Ultrasound Med. Biol.* **32**, 1399–1409 (2006).
45. Sheikov, N., McDannold, N., Vykhodtseva, N., Jolesz, F. & Hynynen, K. Cellular mechanisms of the blood-brain barrier opening induced by ultrasound in presence of microbubbles. *Ultrasound Med. Biol.* **30**, 979–989 (2004).
46. Marty, B. *et al.* Dynamic study of blood-brain barrier closure after its disruption using ultrasound: A quantitative analysis. *J. Cereb. Blood Flow Metab.* **32**, 1948–1958 (2012).
47. McDannold, N., Zhang, Y. & Vykhodtseva, N. Blood-brain barrier disruption and vascular damage induced by ultrasound bursts combined with microbubbles can be influenced by choice of anesthesia protocol. *Ultrasound Med. Biol.* **37**, 1259–1270 (2011).
48. Tofts, P. S. & Kermode, A. G. Measurement of the blood-brain barrier permeability and leakage space using dynamic MR imaging. 1. Fundamental concepts. *Magn. Reson. Med.* **17**, 357–367 (1991).
49. Brix, G. *et al.* Microcirculation and microvasculature in breast tumors: Pharmacokinetic analysis of dynamic MR image series. *Magn. Reson. Med.* **52**, 420–429 (2004).
50. Simpson, D. H., Ting Chin, C. & Burns, P. N. Pulse inversion doppler: A new method for detecting nonlinear echoes from microbubble contrast agents. *IEEE Trans. Ultrason. Ferroelectr. Freq. Control* **46**, 372–382 (1999).
51. Neppiras, E. A. Acoustic cavitation. *Phys. Reports (Review Sect. Phys. Lett.)* **61**, 159–251 (1980).
52. Stride, E. Physical principles of microbubbles for ultrasound imaging and therapy. *Cerebrovasc. Dis.* **27**, 1–13 (2009).
53. McDannold, N., Vykhodtseva, N. & Hynynen, K. Targeted disruption of the blood–brain barrier with focused ultrasound: Association with cavitation activity. *Phys. Med. Biol.* **51**, 793–807 (2006).
54. Tung, Y.-S. *et al.* In vivo transcranial cavitation threshold detection during ultrasound-induced blood–brain barrier opening in mice. *Phys. Med. Biol.* **55**, 6141–6155 (2010).
55. O'Reilly, M. A. & Hynynen, K. Blood-brain barrier: Real-time feedback-controlled focused ultrasound disruption by using an acoustic emissions-based controller. *Radiology* **263**, 96–106 (2012).
56. Arvanitis, C. D., Livingstone, M. S., Vykhodtseva, N. & McDannold, N. Controlled ultrasound-induced blood-brain barrier disruption using passive acoustic emissions monitoring. *PLoS One* **7**, e45783 (2012).
57. Arvanitis, C. D., Livingstone, M. S. & McDannold, N. Combined ultrasound and MR imaging to guide focused ultrasound therapies in the brain. *Phys. Med. Biol.* **58**, 4749–4761 (2013).
58. Sun, T. *et al.* Closed-loop control of targeted ultrasound drug delivery across the blood-brain/tumor barriers in a rat glioma model. *Proc. Natl. Acad. Sci.* **114**, E10281–E10290 (2017).
59. Jones, R. M. *et al.* Three-dimensional transcranial microbubble imaging for guiding volumetric ultrasound-mediated blood-brain barrier opening. *Theranostics* **8**, 2909–2926 (2018).

60. Crake, C., Brinker, S. T., Coviello, C. M., Livingstone, M. S. & McDannold, N. J. A dual-mode hemispherical sparse array for 3D passive acoustic mapping and skull localization within a clinical MRI guided focused ultrasound device. *Phys. Med. Biol.* **63**, 065008 (2018).
61. Hynynen, K., McDannold, N., Sheikov, N. A., Jolesz, F. A. & Vykhodtseva, N. Local and reversible blood-brain barrier disruption by noninvasive focused ultrasound at frequencies suitable for trans-skull sonications. *Neuroimage* **24**, 12–20 (2005).
62. McDannold, N., Vykhodtseva, N. & Hynynen, K. Blood-brain barrier disruption induced by focused ultrasound and circulating preformed microbubbles appears to be characterized by the mechanical index. *Ultrasound Med. Biol.* **34**, 834 (2008).
63. Apfel, R. E. & Holland, C. K. Gauging the likelihood of cavitation from short-pulse, low-duty cycle diagnostic ultrasound. *Ultrasound Med. Biol.* **17**, 179–185 (1991).
64. Samiotaki, G. & Konofagou, E. E. Dependence of the reversibility of focused-ultrasound-induced blood-brain barrier opening on pressure and pulse length in vivo. *IEEE Trans. Ultrason. Ferroelectr. Freq. Control* **60**, 2257–2265 (2013).
65. McDannold, N., Vykhodtseva, N. & Hynynen, K. Effects of acoustic parameters and ultrasound contrast agent dose on focused-ultrasound induced blood-brain barrier disruption. *Ultrasound Med. Biol.* **34**, 930–937 (2008).
66. Mei, J. *et al.* Experimental study on targeted methotrexate delivery to the rabbit brain via magnetic resonance imaging–guided focused ultrasound. *J. Ultrasound Med.* **28**, 871–880 (2009).
67. de Jong, N., Emmer, M., van Wamel, A. & Versluis, M. Ultrasonic characterization of ultrasound contrast agents. *Med. Biol. Eng. Comput.* **47**, 861–873 (2009).
68. Choi, J. J. *et al.* Microbubble-size dependence of focused ultrasound-induced blood–brain barrier opening in mice in vivo. *IEEE Trans. Biomed. Eng.* **57**, 145 (2010).
69. Vlachos, F., Tung, Y. S. & Konofagou, E. Permeability dependence study of the focused ultrasound-induced blood–brain barrier opening at distinct pressures and microbubble diameters using DCE-MRI. *Magn. Reson. Med.* **66**, 821–830 (2011).
70. Tung, Y.-S., Vlachos, F., Feshitan, J. A., Borden, M. A. & Konofagou, E. E. The mechanism of interaction between focused ultrasound and microbubbles in blood-brain barrier opening in mice. *J. Acoust. Soc. Am.* **130**, 3059 (2011).
71. Samiotaki, G., Vlachos, F., Tung, Y. S. & Konofagou, E. E. A quantitative pressure and microbubble-size dependence study of focused ultrasound-induced blood-brain barrier opening reversibility in vivo using MRI. *Magn. Reson. Med.* **67**, 769–777 (2012).
72. Fan, C. H. *et al.* Submicron-bubble-enhanced focused ultrasound for blood–brain barrier disruption and improved CNS drug delivery. *PLoS One* **9**, e96327 (2014).
73. McDannold, N., Vykhodtseva, N. & Hynynen, K. Use of ultrasound pulses combined with Definity® for targeted blood-brain barrier disruption: A feasibility study. *Ultrasound Med. Biol.* **33**, 584 (2007).
74. Park, E. J., Zhang, Y. Z., Vykhodtseva, N. & McDannold, N. Ultrasound-mediated blood-brain/blood-tumor barrier disruption improves outcomes with trastuzumab in a breast cancer brain metastasis model. *J. Control. Release* **163**, 284 (2012).
75. Weng, J. C., Wu, S. K., Yang, F. Y., Lin, W. L. & Tseng, W. Y. I. Pulse sequence and timing of contrast-enhanced MRI for assessing blood–brain barrier disruption after transcranial focused ultrasound in the presence of hemorrhage. *J. Magn. Reson. Imaging* **31**, 1323–1330 (2010).
76. Yang, F. Y., Fu, W. M., Chen, W. S., Yeh, W. L. & Lin, W. L. Quantitative evaluation of the use of microbubbles with transcranial focused ultrasound on blood–brain-barrier disruption. *Ultrason. Sonochem.* **15**, 636–643 (2008).
77. Treat, L. H. *et al.* Targeted delivery of doxorubicin to the rat brain at therapeutic levels using MRI-guided focused ultrasound. *Int. J. Cancer* **121**, 901–907 (2007).
78. Mullin, L. *et al.* Effect of anesthesia carrier gas on in-vivo circulation times of ultrasound microbubble contrast agents in rats. *Contrast Media Mol. Imaging* **6**, 126 (2011).
79. Itani, M. & Mattrey, R. F. The effect of inhaled gases on ultrasound contrast agent longevity in vivo. *Mol. Imaging Biol.* **14**, 40–46 (2012).
80. Weng, J. C., Wu, S. K., Lin, W. L. & Tseng, W. Y. I. Detecting blood–brain barrier disruption within minimal hemorrhage following transcranial focused ultrasound: A correlation study with contrast-enhanced MRI. *Magn. Reson. Med.* **65**, 802–811 (2011).

81. Kinoshita, M., McDannold, N., Jolesz, F. A., Hynynen, K. & Dunn, F. Noninvasive localized delivery of herceptin to the mouse brain by MRI-guided focused ultrasound-induced blood–brain barrier disruption. *Proc. Natl. Acad. Sci.* **103**, 11719–11723 (2006).
82. Kobus, T., Vykhodtseva, N., Pilatou, M., Zhang, Y. & McDannold, N. Safety validation of repeated blood–brain barrier disruption using focused ultrasound. *Ultrasound Med. Biol.* **42**, 492 (2016).
83. McDannold, N., Vykhodtseva, N., Raymond, S., Jolesz, F. A. & Hynynen, K. MRI-guided targeted blood-brain barrier disruption with focused ultrasound: Histological findings in rabbits. *Ultrasound Med. Biol.* **31**, 1527–1537 (2005).
84. Howles, G. P. *et al.* Contrast-enhanced in vivo magnetic resonance microscopy of the mouse brain enabled by noninvasive opening of the blood-brain barrier with ultrasound. *Magn. Reson. Med.* **64**, 995–1004 (2010).
85. Colen, R. R. & Jolesz, F. A. Future potential of MRI-guided focused ultrasound brain surgery. *Neuroimaging Clin. N. Am.* **20**, 355–366 (2010).
86. Lum, A. F. H. *et al.* Ultrasound radiation force enables targeted deposition of model drug carriers loaded on microbubbles. *J. Control. Release* **111**, 134 (2006).
87. Dayton, P., Klibanov, A., Brandenburger, G. & Ferrara, K. Acoustic radiation force in vivo: A mechanism to assist targeting of microbubbles. *Ultrasound Med. Biol.* **25**, 1195–1201 (1999).
88. Allen, J. S., May, D. J. & Ferrara, K. W. Dynamics of therapeutic ultrasound contrast agents. *Ultrasound Med. Biol.* **28**, 805–816 (2002).
89. Collis, J. *et al.* Cavitation microstreaming and stress fields created by microbubbles. *Ultrasonics* **50**, 273–279 (2010).
90. Dijkink, R. & Ohl, C. D. Measurement of cavitation induced wall shear stress. *Appl. Phys. Lett.* **93**, 254107 (2008).
91. Wiedemair, W., Tuković, Ž., Jasak, H., Poulikakos, D. & Kurtcuoglu, V. On ultrasound-induced microbubble oscillation in a capillary blood vessel and its implications for the blood–brain barrier. *Phys. Med. Biol.* **57**, 1019 (2012).
92. Yu, J. *et al.* Direct evidence for the role of caveolin-1 and caveolae in mechanotransduction and remodeling of blood vessels. *J. Clin. Invest.* **116**, 1284–1291 (2006).
93. Deng, J. *et al.* The role of caveolin-1 in blood-brain barrier disruption induced by focused ultrasound combined with microbubbles. *J. Mol. Neurosci.* **46**, 677–687 (2012).
94. Meijering, B. D. M. *et al.* Ultrasound and microbubble-targeted delivery of macromolecules is regulated by induction of endocytosis and pore formation. *Circ. Res.* **104**, 679–687 (2009).
95. Lionetti, V. *et al.* Enhanced caveolae-mediated endocytosis by diagnostic ultrasound in vitro. *Ultrasound Med. Biol.* **35**, 136–143 (2008).
96. Nag, S., Venugopalan, R. & Stewart, D. J. Increased caveolin-1 expression precedes decreased expression of occludin and claudin-5 during blood-brain barrier breakdown. *Acta Neuropathol.* **114**, 459–469 (2007).
97. Sharom, F. J. The P-glycoprotein efflux pump: How does it transport drugs? *J. Membr. Biol.* **160**, 161–175 (1997).
98. Zhang, Z. *et al.* Low intensity ultrasound promotes the sensitivity of rat brain glioma to doxorubicin by down-regulating the expressions of P-glucoprotein and multidrug resistance protein 1 in vitro and in vivo. *PLoS One* **8**, e70685 (2013).
99. Liu, H.-L. *et al.* Blood-brain barrier disruption with focused ultrasound enhances delivery of chemotherapeutic drugs for glioblastoma treatment. *Radiology* **255**, 415–425 (2010).
100. Aryal, M., Vykhodtseva, N., Zhang, Y.-Z., Park, J. & McDannold, N. Multiple treatments with liposomal doxorubicin and ultrasound-induced disruption of blood-tumor and blood-brain barriers improves outcomes in a rat glioma model. *J. Control. Release* **169**, 103–111 (2013).
101. Park, J., Aryal, M., Vykhodtseva, N., Zhang, Y.-Z. & McDannold, N. Evaluation of permeability, doxorubicin delivery, and drug retention in a rat brain tumor model after ultrasound-induced blood-tumor barrier disruption. *J. Control. Release* **250**, 77–85 (2017).
102. Kinoshita, M., McDannold, N., Jolesz, F. A. & Hynynen, K. Targeted delivery of antibodies through the blood-brain barrier by MRI-guided focused ultrasound. *Biochem. Biophys. Res. Commun.* **340**, 1085–1090 (2006).
103. Jordão, J. F. *et al.* Antibodies targeted to the brain with image-guided focused ultrasound reduces amyloid-β plaque load in the TgCRND8 mouse model of Alzheimer's disease. *PLoS One* **5**, e10549 (2010).

104. Kobus, T., Zervantonakis, I. K., Zhang, Y. & McDannold, N. J. Growth inhibition in a brain metastasis model by antibody delivery using focused ultrasound-mediated blood-brain barrier disruption. *J. Control. Release* **238**, 281–288 (2016).
105. Thévenot, E. *et al.* Targeted delivery of self-complementary adeno-associated virus serotype 9 to the brain, using magnetic resonance imaging-guided focused ultrasound. *Hum. Gene Ther.* **23**, 1144–1155 (2012).
106. Alonso, A. *et al.* Focal delivery of AAV2/1-transgenes into the rat brain by localized ultrasound-induced BBB opening. *Mol. Ther. Acids* **2**, e73 (2013).
107. Lin, C.-Y. *et al.* Non-invasive, neuron-specific gene therapy by focused ultrasound-induced blood-brain barrier opening in Parkinson's disease mouse model. *J. Control. Release* **235**, 72–81 (2016).
108. Burgess, A. *et al.* Targeted delivery of neural stem cells to the brain using MRI-guided focused ultrasound to disrupt the blood-brain barrier. *PLoS One* **6**, e27877 (2011).
109. Shen, W.-B. *et al.* Magnetic enhancement of stem cell-targeted delivery into the brain following MR-guided focused ultrasound for opening the blood-brain barrier. *Cell Transplant.* **26**, 1235–1246 (2017).
110. Xhima, K. *et al.* Ultrasound delivery of a TrkA agonist confers neuroprotection to Alzheimer-associated pathologies. *Brain* **145**, 2806–2822 (2022).
111. Kofoed, R. H. *et al.* Efficacy of gene delivery to the brain using AAV and ultrasound depends on serotypes and brain areas. *J. Control. Release* **351**, 667–680 (2022).
112. Aryal, M., Park, J., Vykhodtseva, N., Zhang, Y. Z. & McDannold, N. Enhancement in blood-tumor barrier permeability and delivery of liposomal doxorubicin using focused ultrasound and microbubbles: Evaluation during tumor progression in a rat glioma model. *Phys. Med. Biol.* **60**, 2527 (2015).
113. Park, J., Zhang, Y., Vykhodtseva, N., Jolesz, F. A. & McDannold, N. J. The kinetics of blood brain barrier permeability and targeted doxorubicin delivery into brain induced by focused ultrasound. *J. Control. Release* **162**, 134–142 (2012).
114. Aryal, M., Vykhodtseva, N., Zhang, Y. Z. & McDannold, N. Multiple sessions of liposomal doxorubicin delivery via focused ultrasound mediated blood–brain barrier disruption: A safety study. *J. Control. Release* **204**, 60–69 (2015).
115. Etame, A. B. *et al.* Enhanced delivery of gold nanoparticles with therapeutic potential into the brain using MRI-guided focused ultrasound. *Nanomedicine* **8**, 1142 (2012).
116. Diaz, R. J. *et al.* Focused ultrasound delivery of Raman nanoparticles across the blood-brain barrier: Potential for targeting experimental brain tumors. *Nanomedicine* **10**, 1087 (2014).
117. Liu, H. L. *et al.* Magnetic resonance monitoring of focused ultrasound/magnetic nanoparticle targeting delivery of therapeutic agents to the brain. *Proc. Natl. Acad. Sci. U. S. A.* **107**, 15205–15210 (2010).
118. Chen, P. Y. *et al.* Novel magnetic/ultrasound focusing system enhances nanoparticle drug delivery for glioma treatment. *Neuro. Oncol.* **12**, 1050–1060 (2010).
119. Alkins, R. *et al.* Focused ultrasound delivers targeted immune cells to metastatic brain tumors. *Cancer Res.* **73**, 1899 (2013).
120. Agliardi, G. *et al.* Intratumoral IL-12 delivery empowers CAR-T cell immunotherapy in a pre-clinical model of glioblastoma. *Nat. Commun.* **12**, 1–11 (2021).
121. Treat, L. H., McDannold, N., Zhang, Y., Vykhodtseva, N. & Hynynen, K. Improved anti-tumor effect of liposomal doxorubicin after targeted blood-brain barrier disruption by MRI-guided focused ultrasound in rat glioma. *Ultrasound Med. Biol.* **38**, 1725 (2012).
122. Jordão, J. F. *et al.* Amyloid-β plaque reduction, endogenous antibody delivery and glial activation by brain-targeted, transcranial focused ultrasound. *Exp. Neurol.* **248**, 29 (2013).
123. Wei, K. C. *et al.* Focused ultrasound-induced blood–brain barrier opening to enhance temozolomide delivery for glioblastoma treatment: A preclinical study. *PLoS One* **8**, e58995 (2013).
124. McDannold, N. *et al.* Acoustic feedback enables safe and reliable carboplatin delivery across the blood-brain barrier with a clinical focused ultrasound system and improves survival in a rat glioma model. *Theranostics* **9**, 6299 (2019).
125. Beccaria, K. *et al.* Ultrasound-induced blood-brain barrier disruption for the treatment of gliomas and other primary CNS tumors. *Cancer Lett.* **479**, 13–22 (2020).
126. Carpentier, A. *et al.* Clinical trial of blood-brain barrier disruption by pulsed ultrasound. **8** (2016).
127. Hynynen, K. *et al.* Pre-clinical testing of a phased array ultrasound system for MRI-guided noninvasive surgery of the brain—A primate study. *Eur. J. Radiol.* **59**, 149–156 (2006).

128. Jameel, A., Bain, P., Nandi, D., Jones, B. & Gedroyc, W. Device profile of exAblate Neuro 4000, the leading system for brain magnetic resonance guided focused ultrasound technology: An overview of its safety and efficacy in the treatment of medically refractory essential tremor. *Expert Rev. Med. Devices* **18**, 429–437 (2021).
129. Mainprize, T. *et al.* Blood-brain barrier opening in primary brain tumors with non-invasive MR-guided focused ultrasound: A clinical safety and feasibility study. *Sci. Rep.* **9**, 321 (2019).
130. Lipsman, N. *et al.* Blood-brain barrier opening in Alzheimer's disease using MR-guided focused ultrasound. *Nat. Commun.* **9**, 1–7 (2018).
131. Abrahao, A. *et al.* First-in-human trial of blood–brain barrier opening in amyotrophic lateral sclerosis using MR-guided focused ultrasound. *Nat. Commun.* **10**, 4373–4373 (2019).
132. Chen, K. T., Wei, K. C. & Liu, H. L. Theranostic strategy of focused ultrasound induced blood-brain barrier opening for CNS disease treatment. *Front. Pharmacol.* **10**, 86 (2019).
133. Ying Foo, C. *et al.* Medical device advances in the treatment of glioblastoma. *Cancers (Basel).* **14**, 5341 (2022).
134. Chen, K. T. *et al.* Neuronavigation-guided focused ultrasound for transcranial blood-brain barrier opening and immunostimulation in brain tumors. *Sci. Adv.* **7** (2021).
135. Pouliopoulos, A. N. *et al.* A clinical system for non-invasive blood-brain barrier opening using a neuronavigation-guided single-element focused ultrasound transducer. *Ultrasound Med. Biol.* **46**, 89 (2020).
136. Warton, K., Mahon, K. L. & Samimi, G. Methylated circulating tumor DNA in blood: Power in cancer prognosis and response. *Endocr. Relat. Cancer* **23**, R157–R171 (2016).
137. Westphal, M. & Lamszus, K. Circulating biomarkers for gliomas. *Nat. Rev. Neurol.* **11**, 556–566 (2015).
138. Malone, H. *et al.* Complications following stereotactic needle biopsy of intracranial tumors. *World Neurosurg.* **84**, 1084–1089 (2015).
139. Cohen, J. D. *et al.* Detection and localization of surgically resectable cancers with a multi-analyte blood test. *Science (80-.).* **359**, 926–930 (2018).
140. Touat, M. *et al.* Emerging circulating biomarkers in glioblastoma: Promises and challenges. *Expert Rev. Mol. Diagn.* **15**, 1311–1323 (2015).
141. Bettegowda, C. *et al.* Detection of circulating tumor DNA in early- and late-stage human malignancies. *Sci. Transl. Med.* **6** (2014).
142. D'Souza, A. L. *et al.* A strategy for blood biomarker amplification and localization using ultrasound. *Natl. Acad Sci.* **106**, 17152–17157 (2009).
143. D'Souza, A. L. *et al.* Tumor characterization by ultrasound-release of multiple protein and microRNA biomarkers, preclinical and clinical evidence. *PLoS One* **13** (2018).
144. Forbrich, A., Paproski, R., Hitt, M. & Zemp, R. Comparing efficiency of micro-RNA and mRNA biomarker liberation with microbubble-enhanced ultrasound exposure. *Ultrasound Med. Biol.* **40**, 2207–2216 (2014).
145. Peng, D., Xu, T., Mason, T. J. & Wu, W. A study of ovarian cancer biomarker amplification using ultrasound for early stage detection. *Ultrasonics* **54**, 451–454 (2014).
146. Chevillet, J. R. *et al.* Release of cell-free MicroRNA tumor biomarkers into the blood circulation with pulsed focused ultrasound: A noninvasive, anatomically localized, molecular liquid biopsy. *Radiology* **283**, 158–167 (2017).
147. Zhu, L. *et al.* Focused ultrasound-enabled brain tumor liquid biopsy. *Sci. Rep.* **8**, 1–9 (2018).
148. Zhu, L., Nazeri, A., Pacia, C. P., Yue, Y. & Chen, H. Focused ultrasound for safe and effective release of brain tumor biomarkers into the peripheral circulation. *PLoS One* **15** (2020).
149. Pacia, C. P. *et al.* Feasibility and safety of focused ultrasound-enabled liquid biopsy in the brain of a porcine model. *Sci. Rep.* **10**, 1–9 (2020).
150. Meng, Y. *et al.* MR-guided focused ultrasound liquid biopsy enriches circulating biomarkers in patients with brain tumors. *Neuro. Oncol.* **23**, 1789–1797 (2021).
151. Engelhardt, B. & Sorokin, L. The blood–brain and the blood–cerebrospinal fluid barriers: Function and dysfunction. *Semin. Immunopathol.* **31**, 497–511 (2009).
152. Abbott, N. J., Patabendige, A. A. K., Dolman, D. E. M., Yusof, S. R. & Begley, D. J. Structure and function of the blood-brain barrier. *Neurobiol. Dis.* **37**, 13–25 (2009).

153. Weerasuriya, A. & Mizisin, A. P. The blood-nerve barrier: Structure and functional significance. *Methods Mol. Biol.* **686**, 149–173 (2011).
154. Wachsmuth, J., Chopra, R. & Hynynen, K. Feasibility of transient image-guided blood-spinal cord barrier disruption. *AIP Conf. Proc.* **1113**, 256–259 (2009).
155. Payne, A. H. *et al.* Magnetic resonance imaging-guided focused ultrasound to increase localized blood-spinal cord barrier permeability. *Neural Regen. Res.* **12**, 2045–2049 (2017).
156. O'Reilly, M. A. *et al.* Preliminary investigation of focused ultrasound-facilitated drug delivery for the treatment of leptomeningeal metastases. *Sci. Rep.* **8**, 1–8 (2018).
157. Fletcher, S.-M. P., Ogrodnik, N. & O'Reilly, M. A. Enhanced detection of bubble emissions through the intact spine for monitoring ultrasound-mediated blood-spinal cord barrier opening. *IEEE Trans. Biomed. Eng.* **67**, 1387–1396 (2020).
158. Fletcher, S.-M. P., Choi, M., Ramesh, R. & O'Reilly, M. A. Focused ultrasound-induced blood-spinal cord barrier opening using short-burst phase-keying exposures in rats: A parameter study. *Ultrasound Med. Biol.* **47**, 1747–1760 (2021).
159. Montero, A.-S. *et al.* Ultrasound-induced blood-spinal cord barrier opening in rabbits. *Ultrasound Med. Biol.* **45**, 2417–2426 (2019).
160. Fletcher, S.-M. P., Choi, M., Ogrodnik, N. & O'Reilly, M. A. A porcine model of transvertebral ultrasound and microbubble-mediated blood-spinal cord barrier opening. *Theranostics* **10**, 7758–7774 (2020).
161. Weber-Adrian, D. *et al.* Gene delivery to the spinal cord using MRI-guided focused ultrasound. *Gene Ther.* **22**, 568–577 (2015).
162. Fletcher, S.-M. P. & O'Reilly, M. A. Analysis of multifrequency and phase keying strategies for focusing ultrasound to the human vertebral canal. *IEEE Trans. Ultrason. Ferroelectr. Freq. Control* **65**, 2322–2331 (2018).
163. Smith, P., Ogrodnik, N., Satkunarajah, J. & O'Reilly, M. A. Characterization of ultrasound-mediated delivery of trastuzumab to normal and pathologic spinal cord tissue. *Sci. Reports* **11**, 1–12 (2021).
164. Fletcher, S.-M. P. & O'Reilly, M. A. Analysis of a dual aperture approach and standing wave suppression pulse sequences for controlled transvertebral focused ultrasound delivery in ex vivo human thoracic vertebrae. *J. Acoust. Soc. Am.* **144**, 1925–1925 (2018).
165. Xu, R. & O'Reilly, M. A. A spine-specific phased array for transvertebral ultrasound therapy: Design and simulation. *IEEE Trans. Biomed. Eng.* **67**, 256–267 (2020).
166. Umansky, D. *et al.* Utilization of focused ultrasound for opening of the blood-nerve barrier. *Phys. Med. Biol.* **67**, 205003 (2022).

27

Histotripsy: Focused Ultrasound Therapy by Mechanical Tissue Fractionation

Zhen Xu, Timothy L. Hall, and Charles A. Cain

27.1 Introduction

Cavitation has often been thought of as a phenomenon to be avoided in both diagnostic and therapeutic ultrasound procedures, primarily because the temporal and spatial enucleation of tissue affecting bubbles has been remarkably unpredictable, and, once established, the bubbles were often sparsely distributed and difficult to control. Motivated by the physical limitations of ultrasound thermal therapies, our lab began a quest to make dense bubble clouds which could be generated predictably in time and space, and were sufficiently energetic and spatially dense to produce reliable and precise lesions with a minimum of deposited energy in the target volume. Progress in this direction led us to coin the term histotripsy in 2003.[1,2] A brief summary of what has been learned in the histotripsy project is presented in this chapter.

The key to predictability and controllability of the histotripsy cavitation process is the use of intense very short pulses, ideally a single quasi-monopolar negative pressure pulse.[3] Such a pulse, if its peak negative pressure (P-) exceeds an intrinsic threshold for water (or high water content tissue), generates a dense bubble cloud with 100% probability.[4] Because the pulse is so brief in duration, it propagates beyond the focus before the bubble cloud is large enough to interact chaotically with the expanding cloud it enucleates. Therefore, virtually every bubble cloud occupies the same predictable volume at its maximum expansion producing very precise and predictable lesions with a sufficient number of pulses (or histotripsy "dose").

Non-ideal histotripsy pulses are easy to generate where only a single half-cycle exceeds the intrinsic threshold.[4] Shorn of all non-essential elements, such as many positive half-cycles, often formed into thermally effective nonlinear shock fronts by nonlinear propagation, these pulses are minimally effective thermally, but generate reproducible dense bubble clouds.[5] Moreover, the pulse repetition frequency (PRF) can be adjusted, where necessary, to prevent unwanted thermal complications.[6]

Histotripsy fundamentally depends on a very nonlinear, exceedingly sharp, thresholding phenomenon which greatly increases the number of physical parameters to which the process is sensitive. The beginnings of an understanding of the underlying physics has made possible rational optimisation of histotripsy for many different applications.

Thus, histotripsy produces non-thermal lesions by generating dense energetic bubble clouds with very short intense acoustic pulses. Repeated expanding/contracting bubble clouds mechanically fractionate tissue in the focus until only small cellular fragments are left.[7] Because it is a highly nonlinear thresholding phenomenon, the non-migrating bubble clouds, and the subsequent lesions, are highly localised, with lesion boundaries often bisecting individual cells.[7]

27.2 Mechanisms

Dense bubble clouds are only initiated when some part of the negative pressure waveform(s) in the focus exceeds the intrinsic threshold. This is ~28 MPa for water and most soft tissues at physiological

DOI: 10.1201/9780429162671-27

temperature (Figure 27.1).[4] The intrinsic threshold is an interesting phenomenon in that it is independent of frequency and dissolved gas in the medium, and is 100% effective even for very short events. Moreover, the spatial extent of the resulting bubble cloud almost exactly corresponds to the volume of media exceeding this threshold. When the intensity is adjusted downwards until only the tip of the principal negative half-cycle exceeds the threshold, "bubble clouds" consisting of only a few bubbles (often only one) are generated, resulting in lesions which are much smaller than the diffraction limit at the frequency of the histotripsy pulse.[8] Since lesion size is spatially defined by the maximum extent of the generated bubble cloud, the end effector of histotripsy, very small lesions can be generated. Of course, by adjusting the intensity upwards, much larger lesions can be generated in the same focal volume by the same apparatus.

Pulses below the intrinsic threshold can generate sparsely distributed "incidental" bubbles which are often the unwanted "cavitation" reported in thermal therapies. These bubbles are not effective in generating useful lesions and are probabilistic in nature. However they can have a role in histotripsy.

The intrinsic threshold can be exceeded by two approaches, one direct (intrinsic threshold histotripsy)[4] and one indirect (shock scattering histotripsy).[5] Both methods have been successfully used in producing lesions in different tissues.[9–12]

If available transducer/driver systems are incapable of directly generating pulses with negative pressures exceeding the intrinsic threshold, a circumstance encountered all too often, there is an indirect method of generating dense bubble clouds called "shock scattering".[5] With histotripsy pulses exceeding about 3 cycles in length, but with P-values (from about 12 MPa to 25 MPa) lower than the intrinsic threshold, positive shock fronts with peak pressures greater than 50 MPa are easily formed by nonlinear propagation, particularly with lower f-number transducers. The lower pressure peak negative half-cycles cannot initiate dense bubble clouds directly, but do initiate the sparsely distributed aforementioned incidental bubbles in the focus. These bubbles invert the subsequent positive shock fronts at the pressure release bubble boundary. The scattered and inverted shock front, constructively interfering with the incoming negative pressure phase, can exceed the intrinsic threshold, inducing a dense bubble cloud. Subsequent shock fronts produce supra-intrinsic threshold regions by reflecting from the enlarging dense bubble cloud growing towards the transducer. Each inverted shock front can produce one layer of dense bubbles. After about 10–20 cycles, the bubble cloud exits the focus and longer excitations produce rapidly diminishing effects. Thus, shock scattering can be used when circumstances preclude higher peak negative pressures in a target volume. Shock scattering can be an effective approach for generating histotripsy lesions.[11–14]

If any part of the primary pulse exceeds the intrinsic threshold, a dense effective lesion producing bubble cloud is directly generated, even with a single negative half-cycle. These bubble clouds are more predictable and reproducible that those produced by shock scattering and the lesions are more precise. Moreover, the intrinsic threshold in different high water content tissue is essentially the same regardless of frequency or dissolved gas content.[4] It should be noted that enucleation of bubbles does not produce

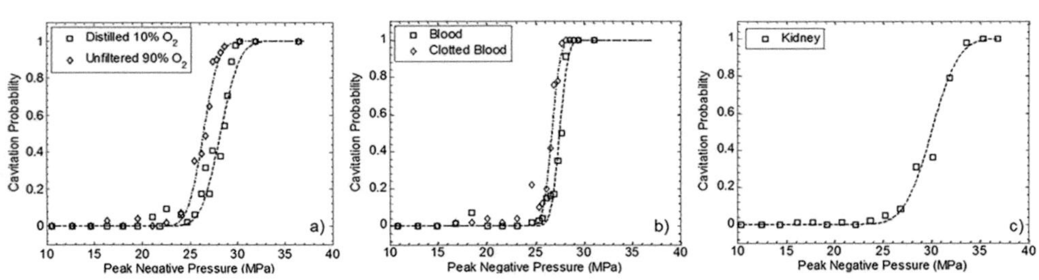

FIGURE 27.1 Cavitation probability as a function of peak negative pressure and fit curves for water of different gas concentrations, ex vivo porcine blood, clot, and kidney (after Maxwell et al.[4]). Each probability data point is the fraction of 100 pulses where cavitation was detected. Curves were fit by nonlinear least-squares regression to each data set. The peak negative pressure corresponding to cavitation probability of 0.5 was measured to be 26–28 MPa for all these water-based media.

effective lesions if the bubbles are constrained by very tough media from expanding.[15–17] Thus, tissues such as cartilage, tendon, and larger blood vessels are histotripsy resistant.[18]

The very sharp intrinsic threshold phenomenon has a number of very useful consequences. For short primary pulses fewer than 2 cycles long, a single principal negative cycle can exceed the intrinsic threshold directly, generating a dense lesion producing bubble cloud. Moreover, by changing the pressure, a variable fraction of the pulse can be made to exceed the threshold, resulting in very small to much larger bubble clouds and with no confounding shock scattering. If the bubble "cloud" is a single bubble, when only the tip of the waveform (P-) exceeds the intrinsic threshold, very small lesions, much less than the diffraction limit in size, can be generated. This is called microtripsy.[8]

Moreover, beam side lobes from distorting media aberrations can be "thresholded-out" if they do not change the shape of the main lobe of the intensity pattern and the main lobe still exceeds any side lobe (often the case even with severe aberrations). Thus, if the main lobe is still extant, and exceeds the intrinsic threshold, a clean bubble cloud and lesion is formed thus conferring significant immunity to aberrations. This allows clean lesions through ribs, skull, and other highly aberrating and attenuating structures without aberration correction.[13, 19, 20] This immunity to aberrations is enhanced by very short (less than about 3 cycles) histotripsy pulses and is optimised when the ideal histotripsy pulse is employed, namely, a single half cycle of negative pressure. Such pulses can be synthesised by the frequency compounding transducer which is described later.[8] Short pulses minimise unwanted and unpredicted foci produced by delay (sound speed) or multi-path interference patterns generated in some aberrating tissues (e.g., the ribs) for longer pulses.

If a high frequency probe waveform (possibly an imaging pulse) intersects a low frequency pump waveform in the focus, the compounded waveform negative pressure at the focus can momentarily exceed the intrinsic threshold, thus producing a lesion with the probe (imaging) transducer. Multi-beam histotripsy allows precise lesions with much smaller transducers, wherein the "heavy lifting" is accomplished with a much lower frequency pump (and larger) transducer.[21]

Negative pressure "monopolar" pulses, ideal for histotripsy, can be synthesised in a generalisation of the multi-beam histotripsy case, wherein very short pulses from transducer elements of many different frequencies are added at the focus of what is called a "frequency compounding" transducer. If the principal negative half-cycles of the waveforms produced by all transducer elements arrive at the focus at the same time, they add constructively, producing a very high negative pressure.[3] Since each element can emit a signal at a different frequency, the remaining cycles do not add constructively away from the focus, resulting in a diminution of the positive pressure part of the compounded waveform. Essentially, the frequency compounding transducer concentrates the negative half-cycles by appropriate delay time distributions ("phasing") while spreading out the positive half-cycles of all the elements in a quasi-random fashion. Such quasi-monopolar histotripsy pulses are shorn of all non-essential elements that could enhance unwanted thermal complications. Moreover, the very short high-bandwidth pulses minimise beam pattern distortions introduced by tissue aberrations.

There are opportunities to employ histotripsy and thermal approaches together to enhance therapeutic possibilities. Certainly, bubbles induced by histotripsy can increase ultrasound absorption in tissues, thus enhancing thermal therapies.[22–24] Also, the negative pressure intrinsic threshold (IT) for generating dense bubble clouds with 100% probability is a function of temperature. The IT in high water content tissue at 40 deg C is (20.4 MPa). At 80 deg C it is (13.7 MPa). The IT varies almost linearly between these temperature extremes. Therefore, reduction in the IT, to a point where special high intensity transducer/driver systems are not required, is possible. Moreover, if heating a volume with medium intensity thermal therapy continuous wave or long pulse waveforms, at some point the peak negative pressure IT will be reached, because of the rising temperature, with subsequent very rapid enucleation of a dense histotripsy bubble cloud. This bubble cloud, continuing to interact chaotically with the incident heating waveform, would rapidly increase in temperature until a boiling phenomenon ensues. Some form of such a complex process is likely to be a mechanism for producing "boiling histotripsy", a form of histotripsy employed in some applications.[25, 26] Boiling histotripsy is a complex phenomenon, initially described at the University of Washington (Seattle, USA), and is being studied extensively by several research groups.[27–31] Much of the complexity of boiling histotripsy is introduced by the chaotic interaction of the millisecond or longer pulses with the evolving bubble cloud once it is enucleated.

Histotripsy can perhaps be characterised by the specific mechanism of enucleation of the required energetically dense lesion forming bubble clouds. Certainly, sparsely distributed bubbles created at low pressures by long waveforms are not very useful for the mechanical fractionation necessary for effective lesion production. Three forms of histotripsy can be described, namely, intrinsic threshold histotripsy, shock-scattering histotripsy, and boiling histotripsy. These forms are different because of the way in which the threshold for dense bubble cloud formation is reached.

Intrinsic threshold histotripsy is the most straight-forward approach, only requiring a single negative half-cycle to generate the bubble cloud directly. Thus, it is characterised by very short pulses, 3 cycles or shorter, and very high intensities of around 30 MPa peak negative pressure (or higher).

Between about 10 MPa and 25 MPa peak negative pressure, shock scattering histotripsy is made possible by generating sparsely distributed incidental bubbles from which nonlinear propagation produced high positive pressure shock fronts are scattered from the pressure-release surface of the bubbles. The "phase reversal" this produces can easily result in peak negative pressures exceeding the intrinsic threshold. Since the incidental bubbles must be enucleated, and successive "shock scattering" events must occur (from successive negative half cycles scattering off the growing cloud) to generate a sufficiently large bubble cloud, 3–10 cycles are usually employed. After about 10 cycles, the shock-scattering bubble cloud grows sufficiently towards the transducer to exit the focal zone in which the intensities are insufficient to sustain the process.

Shock scattering as a useful form of histotripsy if transducer aperture sizes, and acoustic windows, are not large enough to allow the intrinsic threshold to be reached directly. Shock scattering, however, produces more chaotic and less reproducible bubble clouds, and so the lesions are less precise.

Boiling histotripsy generally uses apparatus designed for thermal therapies and must produce temperatures near the boiling point. Therefore the peak negative pressure may vary from 5 MPa up to around 20 MPa (if larger pressures are available, shock scattering histotripsy may be possible). Reaching focal temperatures near the boiling point at these intensities can take thousands of cycles and thus the pulse lengths are often measured in milliseconds.[31] The exact nature of the bubble cloud generation process in boiling histotripsy is complex and cannot be very exactly described. It is likely to involve both IT mechanisms, enabled by the higher temperatures, and true boiling phenomena. The characteristics of the three forms of histotripsy are summarised in Table 27.1.

27.3 Imaging Feedback

It would be difficult to overstate the importance of imaging feedback for histotripsy. Successful adoption of any non-invasive tissue ablation technique will require a high degree of confidence for the surgeon that only can be provided by effective imaging feedback. Therapy feedback is classified here into two broad categories: monitoring and evaluation. In the case of histotripsy, monitoring feedback refers to the detection and localisation of cavitation corresponding to the location of tissue ablation. Quantifying this information during the course of a treatment allows histotripsy doses (i.e., number of ultrasound pulses) to be assigned to targeted tissue volumes. For the second category, evaluation feedback refers to the ability to discern the specific locations where ablation has occurred as well as possibly the degree of ablation. At first glance, histotripsy damage to tissue would seem to be binary in nature, i.e. cells are either lysed, or unaffected, and the tissue matrix is either damaged or intact. However, in practice, some degree of heterogeneity in the distribution of tissue damage within a targeted volume is common, particularly for low cavitation doses. This heterogeneity may often be on a size scale smaller than the resolving power of the evaluation imaging feedback method. Thus, it can be useful to assign a "fractionation percentage" to describe tissue volumes containing both intact, and destroyed, cells and structures.

27.3.1 Treatment Monitoring

There are several possibilities that have been explored for detecting cavitation during histotripsy for monitoring feedback. One method would involve the detection of the rapid expansion of the bubble cloud stimulated by the passage of the negative pressure cycle(s) of the therapeutic sound wave. For

TABLE 27.1

Three Forms of Histotripsy

	Intrinsic Threshold Histotripsy	Shock Scattering Histotripsy	Boiling Histotripsy
Frequency	0.2–3 MHz	0.2–3 MHz	1–2 MHz
Pulse length	0.5–2 cycles 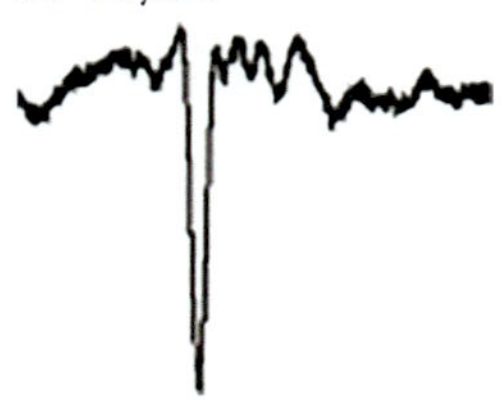 Frequency compounded (0.5–3 MHz) pulse with a dominate negative phase after Lin et al.[3]	3–20 cycles 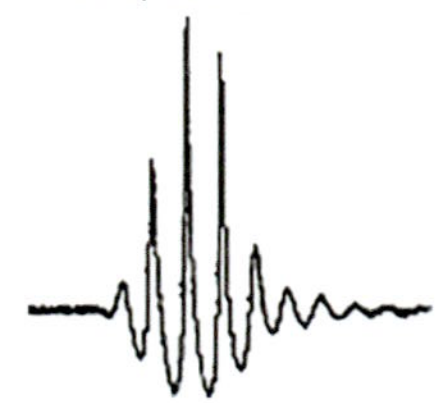 3-cycle pulse at 788 kHz after Xu et al.[2]	1–500 ms (>1k cycles) 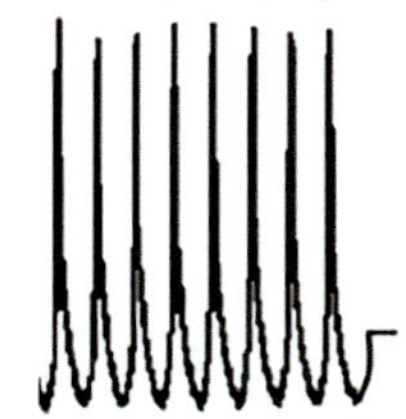 Millisecond long highly non-linear pulse at 1 MHz typically with >1 k cycles after Khokhlova et al.[26]
Pressure	P- >28 MPa	P- = 10–25 MPa P+ >50 MPa	P- = 5–20 MPa Shock > 70MPa
Time between pulses	1 ms – 5 s	1 ms – 5 s	1–5 s
Duty cycle	0.001%–1%	0.01%–5%	1–%
Image of bubble cloud in tissue phantom (bubbles are dark; ultrasound propagation from left to right)	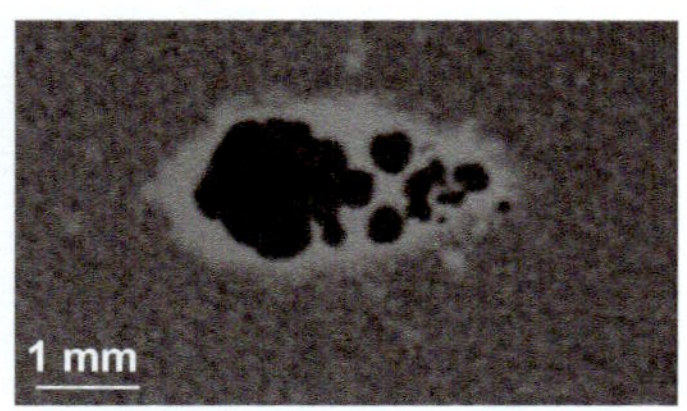 Tens to hundreds of cavitation microbubbles formed at the focus away from the transducer	 Hundreds of cavitation microbubbles formed at the focus back towards transducer by the scattered shockwave	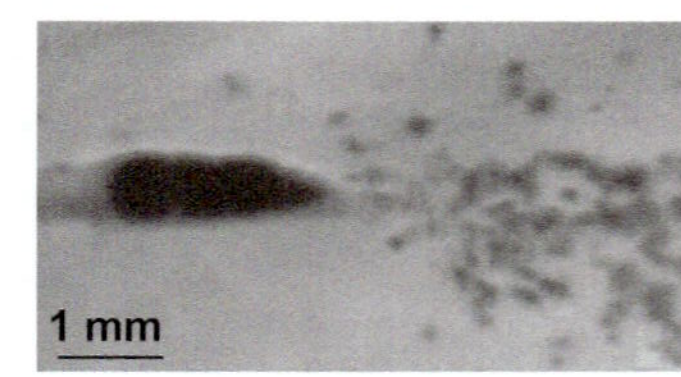 A millimeter boiling bubble explosively expand at the focus with cavitation microbubbles formed pre-focally (after Simon[32])
Lesion histology (H&E slides – all show complete cell disruption in the treatment area [left])	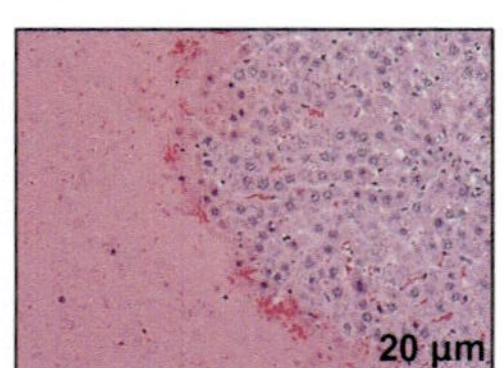	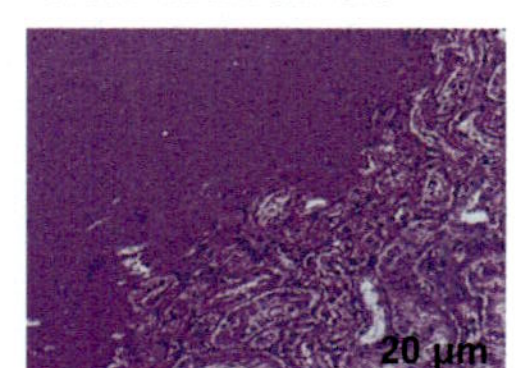	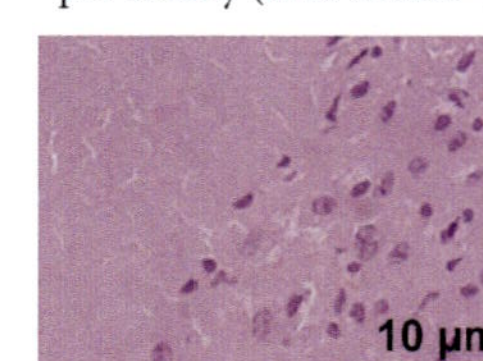 After Khokhlova et al.[26]

multi-cycle therapy pulses, succeeding cycles after the cloud has formed are backscattered from the cavitation bubbles, adding to the cloud expansion signal. This effect was noted during the first histotripsy studies by Tran and termed "therapy acoustic backscatter". Tran[33] showed a high correlation between variability in the backscatter signal received from a sequence of 10,000 bursts (suggestive of cavitation occurrence) and tissue damage, for a large set of therapeutic exposures just above and below threshold. Continuing this work, Xu showed a strong correlation between the received backscatter variability and the presence of cavitation bubbles imaged with a high-speed camera at a tissue fluid interface.[34]

A second method of histotripsy monitoring is to image the micrometer-sized remnant bubbles after the cavitation cloud collapses. These bubbles can persist up to a second or more before dissolving back into the tissue water[35, 36] and are an ideal size to act as strong scatterers of standard frequency diagnostic ultrasound imaging. The motion of these bubbles produces a dynamic, twinkling artifact (in the locations where cavitation has occurred) that is readily detected by standard B-mode imaging and further enhanced with harmonic imaging (Figure 27.2). Since the therapy acoustic bursts in histotripsy typically have very low duty cycles, interference with the ultrasound imaging is greatly reduced when compared with the long bursts used for thermal ablation. Imaging and therapy firings can be synchronised to entirely eliminate the interference. Virtually every in vivo histotripsy study has used B-mode ultrasound imaging guidance since first attempted for histotripsy type ultrasound exposures by Tran.[37] Most therapeutic targets suitable for histotripsy ablation are also good targets for ultrasound imaging, thus this remains the standard for monitoring.

Beyond acoustic detection of cavitation, Allen has developed an MRI-based method using a modified diffusion imaging sequence.[38, 39] Because the relaxation time constants in MRI are relatively very long, histotripsy cavitation can be modelled as a sudden random redistribution of water within the tissue. The MR signal is sensitised to this motion for only the brief period during which the histotripsy cavitation cloud expands and collapses. Because the motion of water during cavitation is orders of magnitude faster than typical diffusion and most blood flow, these effects are excluded. The result is an image displaying contrast where water molecules have been rapidly relocated through cavitation. By varying the size of the sensitising gradients, the spatial distance sensitivity can be adjusted as well, allowing for the detection of different spatial scales of cavitation. Indeed, Allen suggests this may be a more direct measure of the therapeutic action of histotripsy cavitation for appropriately chosen parameters. For

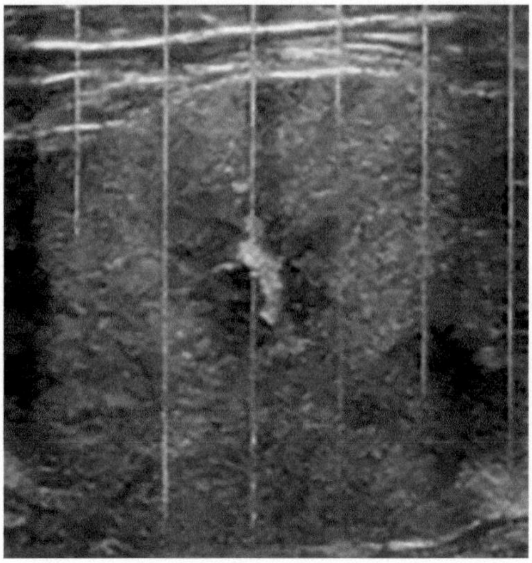

FIGURE 27.2 Standard B-mode trans-rectal ultrasound imaging of the canine prostate during histotripsy ablation (after Hempel et al.[14]). The bright elongated region in the centre (above arrow) is the cavitation cloud. In a live video, the cloud shows a dynamic, twinkling, "candle-flame" like appearance. Vertical streaks are caused by interference between the therapeutic ultrasound firings and the imaging system.

example, water molecules seen to have been displaced by 1 millimeter within 1 millisecond would probably only occur with the disruption of tissue boundaries and cell membranes.

27.3.2 Treatment Evaluation

In early histotripsy work, ultrasound imaging was found to be effective for evaluating lesions by detecting highly liquefied regions. As the tissue architecture is disrupted and mixed, a persistent change which can be detected, given sufficiently high resolving power, is produced. Hall showed a substantial reduction in the echogenicity of B-mode imaging for in vitro porcine liver tissue that had been thoroughly disrupted[40] (Figure 27.3). Wang explored the relationship between various histotripsy doses applied to porcine kidneys in vitro and the change in echogenicity, further correlating this with the density of intact cellular nuclei.[41] The echogenicity was found to decrease exponentially with increasing dose, and to vary linearly with the fraction of intact cellular nuclei. One of the general criticisms of B-mode echogenicity change for evaluating histotripsy ablation is that this change for increasing histotripsy doses appears to be significantly delayed with respect to the point at which a lethal dose is applied to target. The cell nuclei that correlate so well with echogenicity are amongst the last components of a targeted tissue to be fragmented with increasing dose, happening long after the cells are no longer viable. Thus, echogenicity change would be effective for detecting regions of complete tissue ablation, but not as useful for detecting partially damaged tissue.

Hypo-echogenicity has also been observed following histotripsy during in vivo treatments in the kidney,[43] liver,[12, 13] prostate,[14, 44–46] and an implanted prostate tumour model.[47] The effect was quite pronounced in the prostate where trans-rectal ultrasound imaging during therapy provided very high-quality images, although, in some circumstances, the hypo-echogenicity was observed to be transient.

Additional ultrasound imaging methods have been applied for evaluating histotripsy treatments. Wang showed that elasticity images of a targeted volume could be generated using shear waves produced by radiation force from the therapeutic transducer[42] (Figure 27.3). In applying various histotripsy doses, the Young's modulus was found to change more quickly with lower doses than echogenicity, suggesting that it could detect cavitation damage or partial treatments earlier. Intuitively, the Young's modulus could be expected to be a more direct measurement of tissue disruption, and perhaps provide a more accurate evaluation of treatments. Wang also looked at the frequency and decay rate of the shear waves and showed they could similarly be correlated with tissue disruption.[48]

To be successful, both B-mode echogenicity change and shear wave imaging are heavily reliant on high-quality ultrasound imaging. This can be challenging for deep tissue targets or for targets with low initial echogenicity. Miller[49] and Zhang[50] developed a method using Doppler ultrasound imaging to determine the state of tissue at the focal zone of the histotripsy ablation. Histotripsy-generated cavitation was found to induce a motion in the target tissue and this motion relaxation curve changed as

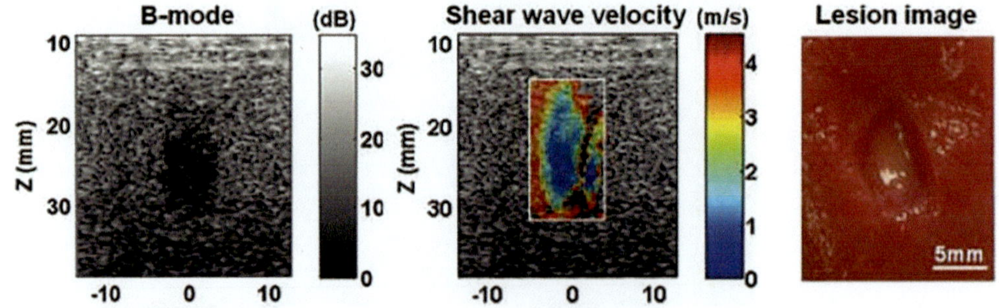

FIGURE 27.3 Standard B-mode ultrasound image of histotripsy lesion (left). Corresponding shear wave velocity map of the lesion (middle) produced by ARFI and plane wave imaging. Optical image of the lesion on gross dissection (right). This figure is cited from Wang et al.[42]

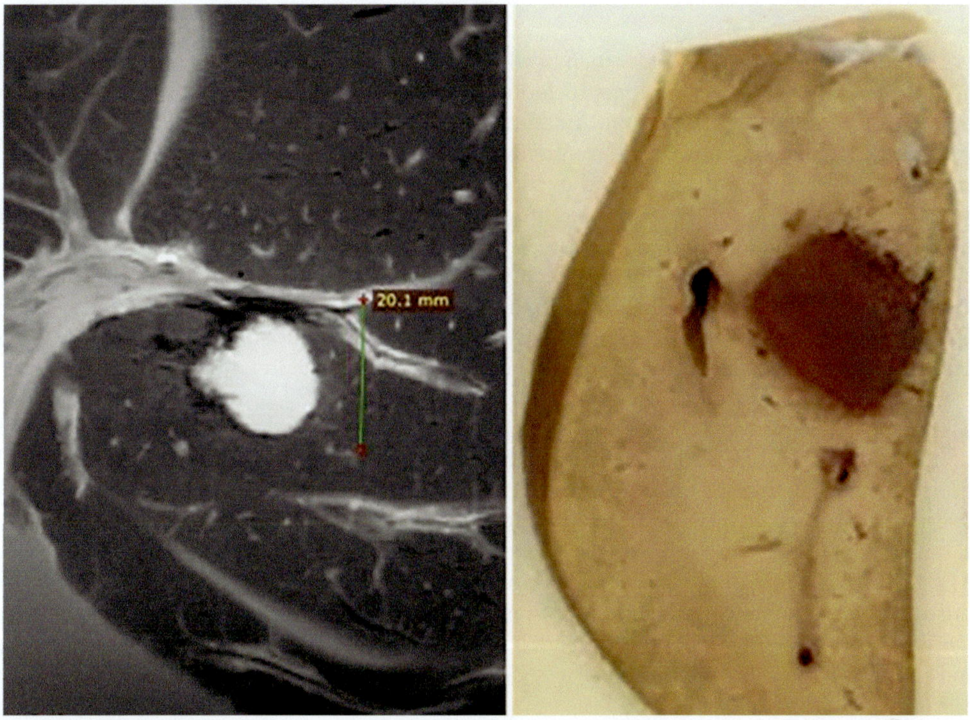

FIGURE 27.4 T2-weighted MR images and gross morphology pictures showing lesions generated by histotripsy in the in vivo porcine liver.

tissue was progressively fractionated. This bubble-induced motion could be readily detected with synchronised Doppler imaging at the appropriate time delay to give a real-time evaluation of the degree of tissue disruption at the focus. A related method based on 1-D spatial variability in the therapy acoustic backscatter that could distinguish between thermal coagulated lesions and more liquefied lesions has been reported by Parsons.[51]

With multiple contrast mechanisms available, MRI would seem to be a suitable method for evaluating histotripsy treatments. This work is still in its early stages. Preliminary studies have been reported in conference proceedings articles, showing contrast for the transverse relaxation process (R2) and the diffusion process (ADC) with sensitivity to histotripsy ablation.[52–54] Histotripsy lesions performed in vivo on liver and kidney have been imaged with MRI following organ dissection and showed a close correlation between R2 weighting and histology.[12, 13, 55] Many MR contrast parameters change substantially between in vivo and in vitro conditions, suggesting that further work will be needed to determine the ultimate effectiveness of MRI for histotripsy imaging feedback.

27.4 Pre-clinical and Clinical Results

Histotripsy has been investigated for a number of clinical applications where noninvasive tissue removal may be desired, including benign prostatic hyperplasia (BPH),[14, 44, 45, 46] congenital heart disease,[55–58] thrombosis,[11, 59] liver cancer,[12, 13, 60] renal cancer,[61, 62] prostate cancer,[46] and kidney stones.[63, 64] A histotripsy BPH human clinical trial is ongoing, whereas other applications are still at the stage of pre-clinical investigation using in vitro and in vivo animal models. In this section we summarise the pre-clinical and clinical results of using histotripsy and boiling histotripsy for prostate, congenital heart disease, thrombosis, and liver applications.

27.4.1 Prostate

BPH is a condition affecting many older men in whom enlargement of the prostate restricts the urethra, leading to lower urinary tract symptoms including increased voidance frequency, urinary hesitancy, incomplete emptying of the bladder, and nocturia.[65] While pharmaceuticals are effective at managing symptoms for some patients, many eventually seek surgical intervention for long-term relief. The standard treatment is to resect the central portion of the prostate, thus enlarging the urethral channel. Success rates are high, but the associated morbidity is significant, in part because of the advanced age and poor health of many subjects.[66] Minimally invasive thermal ablation techniques have not been effective because they fail to remove the obstructing tissue. Histotripsy was seen as a promising alternative because the liquefied tissue would be able to drain through the enlarged urethra providing immediate relief of symptoms. Trans-rectal ultrasound imaging is in common use for guiding prostate biopsies. The close access to the prostate from the rectum provides very high-quality ultrasound images that can aid in targeting, monitoring, and assessing histotripsy treatments.

Trans-perineal acoustic access to the prostate has been demonstrated for high intensity frequency ultrasound (HIFU) ablation[67] and modelled specifically for histotripsy,[68] suggesting that this could be a feasible approach for delivering acoustic energy. While trans-rectal insonation of the prostate for thermal ablation of prostate cancer has been in widespread clinical use, particularly outside the United States, trans-rectal insonation for histotripsy has not been attempted.

The first in vivo ablation of the prostate in a canine model using histotripsy was published by Lake.[43] After histotripsy, a retrograde urethrogram was performed on the subjects showing an enlarged channel in 4 of 6 subjects (Figure 27.5). Subsequent work looked at the acute and chronic responses of parenchymal and urethral tissues to varying histotripsy doses.[69] The mechanically tougher urethra was found

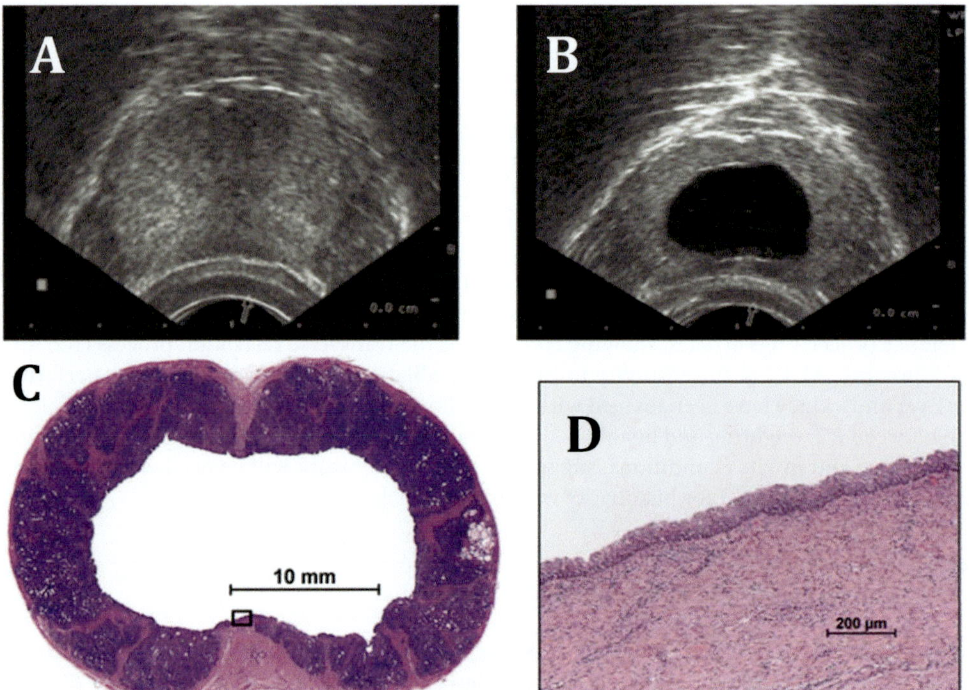

FIGURE 27.5 Histotripsy treatment of the canine prostate after Hempel et al.[14] (A) trans-rectal image of the prostate before treatment. (B) Trans-rectal image of the prostate 28 days post treatment displaying a large void. (C) Low-magnification H&E stain histology slide taken from the centre of the prostate. (D) High magnification image of the region marked on (C) by the small box showing regrowth of the urothelium lining on the enlarged channel.

to require a higher dose for irreversible tissue change. Additionally, the urothelial lining was seen to regrow and encapsulate the enlarged urethral channel in the prostate within 3 weeks. Histologic assessment showed limited inflammatory and fibrotic responses with the deposition of a narrow fibrotic band around the treatment cavity.[70] All prostate histotripsy studies were performed with a 750-kHz ultrasound transducer using bursts shorter than 10 μs duration, a PRF of 100–500 Hz, and a duty cycle of 0.05–0.5%. Peak negative pressures were extrapolated to be in the range of 30–50 MPa.

The general safety and tolerance of canine subjects to histotripsy therapy have been studied by Hempel.[14] Blood and urine parameters were collected along with daily veterinary pain scores up to 56 days post treatment. Results showed only transient laboratory value abnormalities and minimal hematuria. Pain scores indicated mild temporary discomfort. A significant safety concern to be noted for the development of a BPH intervention is that a majority of BPH patients are on anticoagulation therapy for cardiovascular diseases. This poses a severe complication risk from excessive bleeding for surgery. Wheat performed histotripsy on the prostate of canine subjects at varying levels of anticoagulation as measured by international normalisation ratio (INR) up to a supratherapeutic INR of 11.3.[44] Subjects survived 7–28 days following treatment and had no significant bleeding. Platelet activation, which could be the source of hemostasis, has been suggested as an effect of cavitation.[71, 72]

Additional studies were performed to assess the histotripsy sensitivity of certain periprostatic structures that are considered to be complication risks during traditional surgery, or could be at risk from mis-targeting during histotripsy prostate ablation. Stein targeted the urinary sphincter, neurovascular bundle, and rectum with various histotripsy doses and evaluated acute and chronic damage.[10] Only the rectum showed significant damage with doses typically used to ablate prostate tissue. Allam targeted the bladder trigone with large doses of histotripsy, and failed to produce any significant tissue damage or clinical complication.[73]

Schade undertook work to attempt to optimise histotripsy treatment parameters for prostate ablation, and, in particular the urethra for which there was concern that an impractically high dose might be required for sufficient ablation.[74] Higher PRFs (up to 2 kHz corresponding to duty cycle up to 2%) than in previous studies were tested. Interestingly, increasing the treatment PRF was found to improve ablation of the urethra, even when the total applied dose was kept constant and thus the treatment time was reduced. Acute disruption of the urethra was not always achieved with lower doses, but subsequently developed over the course of 2 weeks in many cases. A particular visual appearance of the urethra assessed by endoscopy immediately following treatment, was found to correlate with the 2-week outcome.[75] A further method of ablation was attempted in which the urethra was purposely spared, targeting only the adjacent, mostly glandular, tissue.[45] The disrupted tissue was found to be resorbed promptly, leaving a cavity adjacent to the urethra in most instances, and containing mostly fluid. Modest decreases in overall prostate volume were observed as well.

A clinical histotripsy prostate ablation system (Vortx R_X, Histosonics Inc., Ann Arbor, MI) has been approved for clinical trial (Clinicaltrials.gov identifier no: NCT01775488). This system has been tested on canine subjects and was effective at producing a reduction in prostate volume of 19%-53% at 28 day follow-up.[76]

27.4.2 Congenital Heart Disease

The congenital heart disease hypoplastic left heart syndrome (HLHS) is the clinical application that motivated the invention of histotripsy. This is a rare and complex congenital heart disease.[77] Infants born with HLHS have very small, or absent, left ventricles which are unable to pump enough blood to sustain life. If left untreated, all patients die within the first month of life.[78] The only successful treatment is a 3-stage reconstructive heart surgery performed over 3 years. To extend the patient's survival until the reconstructive surgery, and to optimise their physiological situation, a perforation must be created through the atrial septum (a membrane separating the left and right atria in the heart) to form a flow channel that allows the only functioning ventricle (right ventricle) to provide blood circulation for the entire body. The clinical approaches to creating this perforation (termed as the atrial septal defect [ASD]) are various forms of catheter-based septostomies, which are highly invasive and carry high morbidity and mortality rates. A clinical need for a less invasive ASD creation alternative motivated a paediatric cardiologist (Dr. Achi Ludomirsky) to approach Charles A. Cain at the University of Michigan in the late 1990s. As ASD creation requires tissue removal and cannot be achieved by the available thermal-based ablation methods, this motivated Cain's group to start investigating a mechanical tissue ablation method based on ultrasound-induced cavitation. In human neonates, a subcostal acoustic window which accesses the atrial septum, without bone and lung obstruction, exists.[56]

In 2004, Xu and Cain published the first paper demonstrating that in vitro porcine atrial wall and septum tissue was eroded layer by layer from the tissue-fluid interface using short, high-intensity ultrasound pulses, eventually resulting in sharply demarcated perforations[2] (Figure 27.6). This paper is the first journal publication in which the term histotripsy appeared. Pulse durations of 3–24 cycles at 788 kHz with duty cycle of 1–20% and peak negative pressures of 12 MPa were used. The erosion rate (defined in this paper as the thickness of tissue perforated/the time to produce the perforation) increased with shorter pulse duration. In fact, the erosion rate at 3-cycle pulse duration was almost 8-fold faster than that using 24 cycles. At a fixed pulse duration, there appeared to be a local peak with PRF or duty cycle with erosion rate, rather than increasing erosion rate with increasing duty cycle. The hypothesis was that each pulse produced a cavitation cloud at the tissue-fluid interface, and that the high strain and/or stress induced by the rapid expansion and collapse of the microbubbles at the tissue surface fractionated and removed tissue at the surface. Between 2005 and 2010, Xu and Cain published a number of papers correlating the erosion at a tissue-fluid interface to inertial cavitation, and further exploring the parameter regimen for tissue erosion.[34, 79, 80] To provide a rational explanation of why short pulses were more efficient, they studied the cavitation behaviour at the tissue-fluid interface using high-speed optical imaging.[81–83] The imaging results show that the rapid and violent collapse of the microbubbles occurred within the first few cycles of the pulses. In the following acoustic cycles, even though a larger cavitation cloud was formed, the growth of the microbubbles was less. More microbubbles were formed and collapsed more away from the interface, not effectively contributing to producing strain or stress to remove tissue. Additionally, as histotripsy fractionates tissue into small particles, there was a concern that the tissue debris particles from histotripsy ASD procedure may become hazardous emboli. To address this, the size distribution of tissue debris particles was measured, showing that there were no particles greater than 100 μm and >99% were smaller than 6 μm.[84] This particle size range is unlikely to form hazardous emboli, since 100 μm pore size filters have been used clinically to prevent embolisation during cardiovascular surgeries.

A series of follow-up in vivo studies were conducted to investigate the feasibility and safety of using histotripsy to produce intracardiac communications. In their first in vivo study,[85] histotripsy was tested in an open-chest adult canine model, where the therapy transducer was coupled to the outside of the heart through a water bag and ultrasound gel. Histotripsy treatment was delivered using 5 μs pulses at 1MHz frequency with 15 MPa peak negative pressure and 3.3 kHz PRF. The treatment was guided by ultrasound imaging using a 5-MHz phased array imaging probe inserted into the central hole of the therapy transducer. The ultrasound imaging was first used to place the therapy focus onto the target atrial septum. Prior to the procedure, histotripsy pulses were applied in a water bath, resulting in a

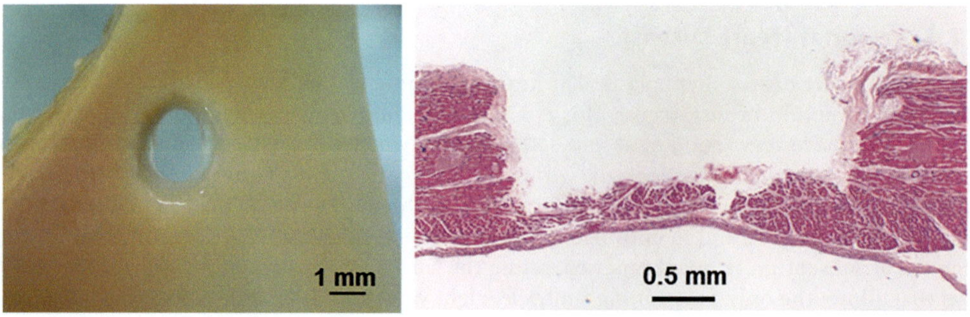

FIGURE 27.6 (a) Gross morphology of perforation generated in the in vitro atrial wall tissue. (2) H&E slide of the histology of tissue prior to perforation.

bright (hyperechoic) cavitation zone on a 2-dimensional ultrasound image and which was marked as the focal position. The therapeutic transducer was then moved using a 3-axis positioning system to align the focus marker on the atrial septum surface in the right atrium. During the treatment, the histotripsy-induced cavitation cloud appeared as a hyperechoic zone (Figure 27.7a), while erosion and perforation of the atrial septum showed as reduced speckle and a dark zone, allowing the monitoring of the treatment (Figure 27.7b). When the ASD was eventually generated, blood flow between the two atria through the ASD was detected using colour Doppler ultrasound. This was confirmation of treatment completion (Figure 27.7c). ASDs were generated in 9 of 10 animals in 6–16 minutes. The pathology of the ASD showed 3–5 mm perforation through the atrial septum with 1–3 mm hemorrhage surrounding the ASD and no damage to the heart wall.

In their subsequent in vivo studies,[57, 58] the feasibility of histotripsy for creating intracardiac communications noninvasively was investigated using an intact neonatal porcine model. The ultrasound transducer was coupled to the intact chest of the neonatal pigs submerged in the degassed water. In these neonatal pigs, the ventricular septum (the membrane separating the two ventricles in the heart) was targeted instead of the atrial septum, due to the difference in the heart orientation in humans versus quadruped animals. The acoustic window for histotripsy to target the ventricular septum in these animals included skin, muscle, some ribcage blockage and a small portion of the lung (<5%). The subcostal acoustic window expected in the human neonates is similar, but with no ribs and less lung coverage. Histotripsy treatment was delivered using 5 μs pulses at 1MHz frequency with 15 MPa peak negative pressure and 1 kHz PRF. The treatment was guided by ultrasound imaging similar to the canine study. A perforation through the ventricular septum (ventricular septal defect [VSD]) was created in 15 animals within 20 seconds to 13 minutes of therapy (3.1 ± 3.2 min). VSDs confirmed by Colour flow Doppler ranged in size from 2 to 6.5 mm (3.7 ± 1.6 mm). In all 15 neonatal pigs studied, gross morphology showed no damage to intervening tissues and the epicardial surfaces appeared intact. In acute animals (sacrificed within 2 hours) the VSD was filled with acellular debris and platelet/fibrin deposits with flanking Hemorrhage and myocyte injury spanning approximately 3.3 ± 1.1 mm from the VSD border. By 1 month the VSD was completely endothelialized, surrounded by fibroblastic scar tissue immediately adjacent to the defect, and flanked by normal myocardium. Brain MRI and lung pathology revealed no evidence of thromboembolic events.

Beyond the application in neonatal patients, the group at the University of Tokyo[86] and the histotripsy group at the University of Michigan[55] investigated the potential to create ASD or VSD in utero noninvasively, with the hope of establishing a flow channel in the fetal heart to prevent HLHS from developing, or to improve the patient's physiological condition in utero, in order to significantly improve their treatment outcome at birth. The University of Tokyo used an open-chest rabbit heart model, where a 3.3-MHz transducer was coupled to the outside of the heart wall. Much longer pulses (0.2–0.4 sec) were used at 10–20% duty cycle and I_{sa} of 6.5kWcm^{-2}.[86] These pulse durations and duty cycles are even higher than the typical boiling histotripsy parameters. An ASD was created in 8 of 9 rabbits, but Doppler flow

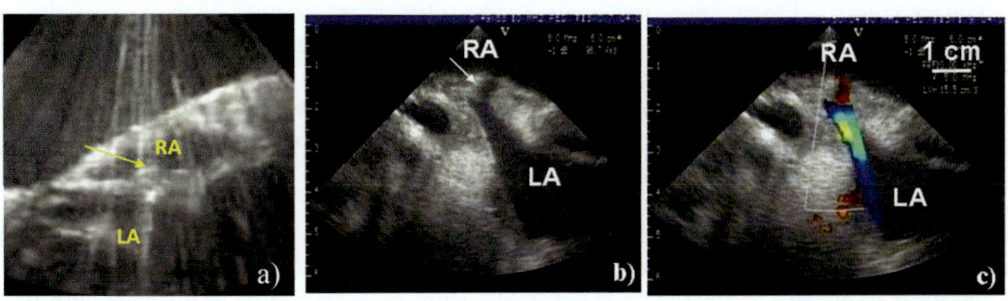

FIGURE 27.7 Ultrasound images of histotripsy ASD treatment in the open-chest canine heart model after Xu et al.[55] (a) The cavitation cloud shows as a hyperechoic zone (arrow) on the atrial septum above the "x" that marked the ultrasound therapy focus. (b) Ultrasound B-mode of the ASD (arrow) shown as a dark channel through the atrial septum created by histotripsy. (c) The blood flow through the ASD was viewed on colour Doppler. LA: left atrial; RA: right atrial.

was observed only in 2 of 9 treatments. The University of Michigan group used an intact pregnant sheep model.[55] The 1-MHz therapy transducer was coupled to the pregnant sheep's abdomen and targeted the ventricular septum of the fetal lamb through up to 8 cm of overlying maternal and fetal tissue. Fetal kidney and liver were also targeted to test application for fetal tumour treatment, and 5 μs pulses with 10–16 MPa peak negative pressure and 0.2–1 kHz PRF were used. Cavitation was generated in 19 of 31 treatment attempts in 27 organs. When cavitation was detected on ultrasound imaging, VSDs in the fetal heart and lesions in the fetal kidney and liver were created. No lesions were found when cavitation was absent. The inability to generate cavitation was primarily associated with the increased depth to target, and obstructing structures such as fetal limbs.

To summarise, histotripsy has been used to create intracardiac communications in the intact neonatal and fetal in vivo models under ultrasound imaging guidance, demonstrating its potential as a noninvasive treatment for HLHS. In addition to HLHS, histotripsy has been expanded to be investigated for various clinical applications where noninvasive perforations could be beneficial, including mitral chordal cutting,[87] ventriculostomy for hydrocephalus,[88] and ureterocele puncture.[89] In vitro and in vivo results have shown the potential of using histotripsy and boiling histotripsy to perforate tissue of various types from soft muscular tissue to tough fibrous tissue, including vascular, brain, and urologic tissue. Table 27.2 summarises the acoustic parameters used in all the studies to generate tissue perforation at a tissue-fluid interface for the various clinical applications mentioned in this section.

27.4.3 Liver Cancer

Every year >700,000 people are diagnosed with primary liver cancer or hepatocellular carcinoma (HCC). Liver is also a common site for metastasis originating from other organs such as the colon. Surgical resection remains the first line of treatment, but less than 25% of the liver cancer patients are candidates for surgical resection due to tumour burden, location, associated disease, and physiological condition.[90–92] Radiofrequency and microwave ablation have shown success in treating liver cancer. These required insertion of an electrode into the tumour to radiate heat, in order to thermally kill the tumour. As the blood flow dissipates heat (heat sink effect), they share three critical limitations: 1) the heating distribution is often inhomogeneous, leaving residual tumour[93–95]; 2) heating may be ineffective near major vessels[96]; and 3) they are ineffective for large (>3 cm diameter) and multiple (>3) tumours.[97] HIFU is an alternative liver ablation approach, delivered using an extracorporeal transducer,[98, 99] that can scan the focal zone to cover a large tumour. But the HIFU treatment is much slower than RFA, it is difficult to treat near major vessels and to achieve consistent thermal ablation in large tumours in the highly vascular liver.[98, 100] Further, skin burn and subcostal edema has been reported in clinical HIFU liver ablation cases[101, 102] due to the heating to the overlying tissue. There is a large unmet need for a new ablation method that can overcome the limitations of the current thermal therapies.

As histotripsy is not affected by the heat sink effect, it has the potential to overcome the limitations of thermal ablation. 1) Histotripsy can achieve homogeneous cell disruption even in highly vascular organs.[56–58] 2) As large vessels have greater mechanical strength[103–105] and higher resistance to histotripsy damage compared to surrounding tissue,[15, 18] histotripsy can completely fractionate the tissue near major vessels while preserving the vascular bundles.[106] 3) A large liver volume can be treated by histotripsy by mechanically or electronically moving the therapy focus to cover the target volume. 4) Histotripsy uses ultrasound imaging for real-time imaging feedback to guide and monitor the treatment. 5) Histotripsy can be applied noninvasively to the liver without overheating the overlying tissue, avoiding complications associated with device insertion in radiofrequency ablation (RFA) or microwave, including tumour cell seeding along the insertion pathway.[107, 108] Both histotripsy and boiling histotripsy have been investigated for liver ablation, and the studies are summarised in the following.

The in vivo feasibility of using histotripsy for noninvasive liver ablation was first investigated in an intact porcine liver model.[12] Histotripsy was generated using a 1-MHz focused transducer with 10 cycle pulses, 500 Hz PRF, and 0.5% duty cycle. A reported 30–50% of the transducer aperture was covered by the ribcage and the overlying tissue was 4–6 cm. The in situ peak negative pressure was estimated to be 14–17 MPa. Twelve lesions of ~1cm^3 were successfully created in the livers of 6 pigs (60–90 lb) by

TABLE 27.2

Summary of Research on Using Histotripsy to Generate Tissue Perforation

Clinical Area	Clinical Application	Papers	Experiments	Ultrasound Transducer Frequency	Pulse Sequence, PRF or Duty Cycle	Pressure/Intensity	Duration	Results
Cardiovascular	Intracardiac communication – HLHS neonatal	Xu et al. 2004, 2006	In vitro atrial wall or septum	788 kHz	3–24 cycle pulses; 2–20% duty cycle	p- = 8–12MPa I_{SPPA} = 3000–9000 W/cm^2	1–15 min/1mm thick tissue	232 1–4 mm perforations;
		Xu et al. 2010	In vivo canine extracardiac	1 MHz	5μs pulses; 3.3 kHz PRF	p- = 15MPa p+ = 61MPa	6–16 min	9 of 10–3–5 mm ASD; 9 of 10 Doppler flow
		Owens et al. 2011, 2013	In vivo porcine; noninvasive	1 MHz	5μs pulses; 1 kHz PRF	p- = 13MPa p+ = 32MPa	20 sec – 13 min	VSD with Doppler flow in all 15 pigs;
	Intracardiac communication – HLHS fetal	Fujisaki et al. 2010	In vivo rabbit; extracardiac	3.3 MHz	0.2–0.4 sec on; 2 sec off	Isa = 6500W/cm^2	10sec/appl; 3–4 appls.	8 of 9–1–3 mm ASD; 2 of 9 – Doppler flow
		Kim et al. 2011, 2013	In vivo sheep; noninvasive	1 MHz	5μs pulses; 0.2–1 kHz PRF	p- = 10–16MPa		VSD in fetal heart; lesions in fetal kidney, liver, and lung
	Mitralchordalcutting– Mitral regurgitation	Abe et al. 2008	In vitro calf mitral chordae	4.67 MHz	0.2–0.3 sec on; 2 sec off	I_{SPTA} = 26 kW/cm^2	Up to 120 pulses (4 min)	45%–67% completely cut; 0.6–0.7 mm average diameter
Brain	Third ventriculostomy for hydrocephalus	Alkins et al. 2013	In vivo porcine; Skull removed; w/o human skull	230 kHz 650 kHz	0.1–5 sec	p- > 8 MPa at 230kHz; p > 22 MPa at 650 kHz	1–3 pulses	Third ventriculostomy in 6 of 9 pigs; 2–9 mm diameter
Urology	Ureterocele puncture; ureterocele	Maxwell et al. 2014	In vitro bovine bladder	1 MHz	1–5000 cycle pulses; 0.5–0.6% duty cycle	p- = 17–20MPa p+ = 100–120 Mpa; I_{SPTA} = 145–190 W/cm^2	46–300 sec	0.8–2.8 puncture

mechanically scanning the therapy focus to follow a 5 × 5 × 5 mm cubic grid with 1-mm spacing at 8 seconds per location. The locations of these 12 lesions spanned the entire liver in the superior and inferior regions of the left, middle, and right lobes. For each treatment, a bubble cloud was clearly visualised on ultrasound imaging, providing real-time treatment monitoring. In addition, 2 larger lesioned volumes of 18 cm^3 (equivalent to 3.3-cm-diameter sphere) and 60 cm^3 (equivalent to 4.9-cm sphere) lesions were generated in 2 additional pigs in 26.7 minutes and 60 minutes by mechanical scanning the therapy focus to cover the treatment volume. The lesions formed appeared liquid. Histology shows homogeneous and complete cell fractionation within the treatment region with a sharply demarcated lesion boundary (<500 μm) (Figure 27.8a). The major hepatic vessels and bile ducts within the lesions remained intact (Figure 27.8b). In fact, an extensive network of intermediate and large vessels was observed throughout the completely fractionated liver volume. The number of vessels smaller than 300 μm was significantly reduced compared to that in the untreated region, whereas there was no statistically significant difference in vessel groups larger than 300 μm between the treated and untreated liver.

In order to investigate the ability of using histotripsy to treat through the ribs and the potential thermal effect on overlying tissue, a follow-up study was conducted using the same in vivo intact porcine liver model using pigs weighing 90–110 lb.[13] The ribs in the pathway cause periodic blockage of ultrasound, resulting in a decreased main lobe and increased grating lobes.[109–112] Due to the sharp cavitation threshold with histotripsy using microsecond pulses, a precise cavitation cloud can be generated through the ribs without aberration correction by using a pressure just above the cavitation threshold,

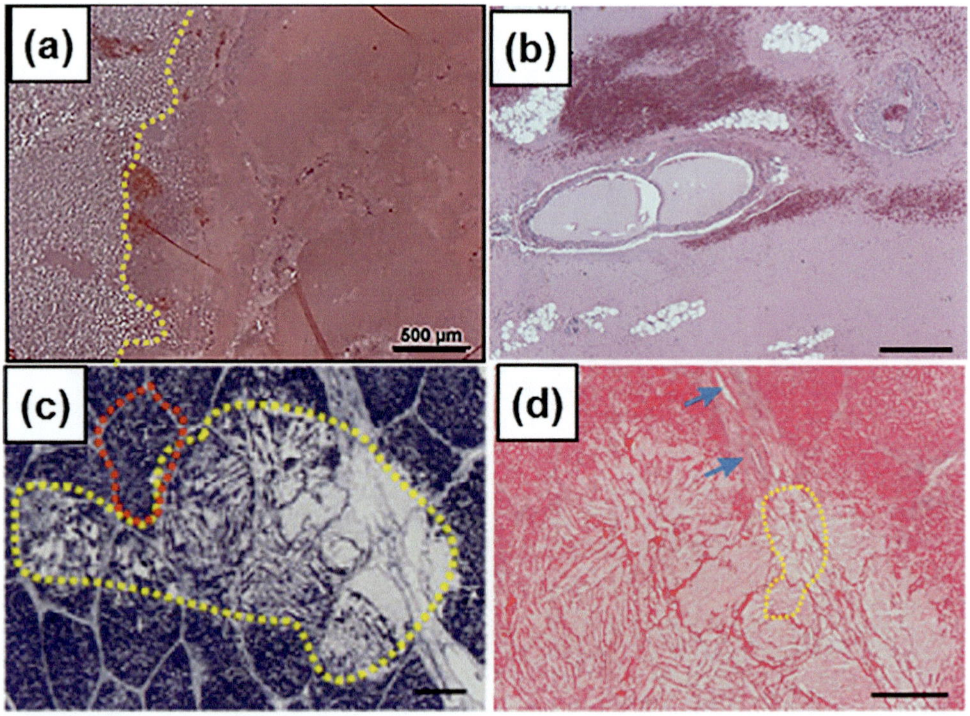

FIGURE 27.8 Representative histological sections of the in vivo porcine liver treated by histotripsy and boiling histotripsy. (a) H&E slide shows completely fractionated region in the liquid lesion generated by histotripsy with no cell structures in the treatment region (right of dotted line) and a sharply demarcated lesion boundary. (b) Intact vessels remain inside the completely fractionated histotripsy lesion on H&E slide. (c) Liquid lesion generated by boiling histotripsy using 10 ms pulses. The single lesion (outlined by yellow dotted line) contained no cellular structures with connective tissue with sharp margin. Red dotted line outlines a liver lobule surrounding by connective stroma tissue. NADH-d staining indicated no thermal damage. (d) A blood vessel (blue arrow) immediately adjacent to the boiling histotripsy lesion was not affected on H&E slide. The scale bar is 500 um. (a) and (b) are from paper by Vlaisavljevich et al.[12] (c) and (d) are from paper by Khokhlova et al.[25]

such that the main lobe peak is above, and the grating lobe peaks are below, the threshold.[19, 106] To apply the histotripsy treatment in vivo with various overlying tissue compositions and depths, the pressure was gradually increased until a cavitation bubble cloud was observed in the target region on ultrasound image. A pressure level right above the cavitation initiation threshold in situ was thus used for each treatment, in order to limit the cavitation within the main lobe. 5-cycle pulses at 750 kHz with 200Hz PRF and 0.13% duty cycle were used. The in situ peak negative pressure was estimated to be 13–17 MPa, corresponding to the pulse average acoustic power output of 5.1 ± 0.2 kW (6.6 ± 0.2 W time average,) through the rib coverage and 4.5 ± 0.8 kW (5.8 ± 1.1 W time average). Each lesion was generated by mechanically scanning the therapy focus to 125 (5 × 5 × 5) points separated by 1.25 mm and for 20 s per location. Lesions were created in the livers of 4 pigs through complete ribcage coverage and in the liver of another 4 pigs with abdominal soft tissue only (no ribcage coverage). The overlying tissue depth was 4–6 cm. No aberration correction was used. The lesions created through the complete ribcage coverage (3.6 ± 1.7 cm^3) and through abdominal tissue (4.5 ± 2.0 cm^3) had comparable dimensions, with no statistically significant difference, as measured on histology and MR images. All lesions generated had uniform cell fractionation with sharp margins, similar to the previous porcine study. The average of the highest temperature increase on the ribs with full ribcage covering the pathway was measured to be 4.1 ± 1.8 °C, which was not enough to cause any thermal damage to the ribs or surrounding tissue. The highest temperature increase recorded in abdominal tissue was 1.7 ± 1.3 °C.

Boiling histotripsy was also investigated for liver ablation and tested in the in vitro bovine liver[29] and in vivo externalised porcine liver model.[25] The treatment tissue effect of boiling histotripsy is determined by the ratio between the time to reach boiling in the target tissue and the pulse duration. The time to reach boiling is determined by the in situ shock amplitude, and is typically on the order of milliseconds. When using pulses not much longer than the time to reach boiling, the lesion generation is dominated by cavitation-induced mechanical effects, while longer pulses contribute to a thermal effect in its formation. In the in vitro study,[29] bovine liver was treated using 5–500ms pulses applied with a 2-MHz focused transducer with a duty cycle of 0.5–1%. The in situ peak negative pressure of 12 MPa, peak positive pressure of 67.5 MPa, shock amplitude of 73 MPa, and peak intensity of 20W/cm^2 were used. The calculated time to reach the boiling temperature using this shock amplitude in the liver was 4.5 ms. When using a pulse duration <10 ms, the lesion appeared visually as a liquid, with no thermal damage. Histological evaluation showed no recognizable cellular structures within the lesion and a sharply demarcated margin. The lesion size increased until reaching a plateau at 60 pulses. With pulses longer than 10 ms, the lesion contained thermal denaturation, with intact cell structures remaining and a less distinctive boundary. For the in vivo experiments,[25] the livers of 12 100–120 lb pigs were externalised prior to the treatment. Boiling histotripsy was applied using a 2MHz focused transducer. The transducer was attached to a sealed water cone, which was placed directly onto the liver. Ultrasound pulses of 1–500 ms in duration at 1% duty cycle with 87–102 MPa shock amplitude and acoustic output power of 240 W were used. Two to four single lesions were generated in each liver lobe, and the total treatment time for each single lesion was 50 s. The time to reach boiling was measured using ultrasound imaging, and varied within 0.9–1.5 ms depending on the depth of the focus from the front surface of the water cone, i.e. the depth of the overlying tissue (5–18 mm). For each pig, a liver lobe was also excised and treated, and the resulting lesions generated in the ex vivo liver were compared with the in vivo lesions. Pulses shorter than 20 ms produced liquefied lesions with only connective tissue remaining. No cell structures were observed within the lesion, while the margin was sharply demarcated between the fractionated and intact cells (<100 μm) (Figure 27.8c). Each single lesion was 3.8 ± 0.5 mm laterally by 6.1 ± 0.5 mm axially, as estimated from histology. Similar treatment results and lesion sizes were observed in the in vivo lesion. For pulses >20 ms, intact cell structures and thermal denaturation were observed inside the lesion, with a less distinctive boundary in both the ex vivo and in vivo samples. More thermal spread at the boundary was found in the in vivo lesions than the ex vivo lesions due to the heat perfusion by blood flow. It was also found that the large vessels remained intact in the treatment volumes (Figure 27.8d).

Overall, both histotripsy and boiling histotripsy studies have shown that homogenous cell fractionation was achieved in vivo in the highly vascular liver with vessel sparing ablation. Ultrasound imaging was used to visualise cavitation for real-time treatment monitoring. Histotripsy studies also demonstrated treatment of larger liver volumes and noninvasive ablation without thermal damage to the ribcage and other overlying tissue. These benefits suggest histotripsy and boiling histotripsy as new methods to overcome the limitations of the current liver tumour interventions. Technical advances can be made to further enhance the treatment precision and speed. For example, the lesion margin generated by histotripsy in the intact *in vivo* porcine liver was wider than the lesion margin generated by boiling histotripsy when it was externalised, probably because of the higher impact of the breathing motion in the intact model and the use of mechanical focus steering to generate a larger lesion. Breathing motion can be addressed by incorporating respiratory gating with the treatment. This should be straightforward to implement as histotripsy or boiling histotripsy uses short pulses and does not require a long time for temperature buildup. To improve the treatment speed, as histotripsy uses short pulses with long waiting time between pulses, the focus can be electrically steered using a phased array transducer to cover other locations in the treatment volume during the waiting time to significantly increase the treatment speed for volume ablation. For clinical translation, the treatment safety and efficacy will need to be studied in a liver tumour model. There are widely established rodent liver tumour models, but these will require miniaturised transducer setups for experimentation. Chronic studies will also be required to answer key questions regarding histotripsy and boiling histotripsy including the following: 1) What will happen to the liquid homogenate? 2) Are there intact cells in the liquid homogenate that can be released outside the treatment region to cause metastasis? 3) What is the local and systemic response to the treatment? Previous histotripsy studies in the kidney showed that the liquefied tissue homogenate was reabsorbed by the body in a month, with minimal fibrotic tissue left in situ, without changes in the kidney function.[113] Similar chronic studies in a liver tumour model are necessary.

27.4.4 Thrombosis

Thrombosis is the medical term for the process of pathologic blood clot formation, the key mechanism behind many cardiovascular diseases, including deep vein thrombosis (DVT), stroke, and myocardial infarction. Current treatment methods for thrombosis include thrombolytic drugs and catheter-based surgical procedures. Thrombolytic drugs (e.g., rt-PA) dissolve the blood clot by breaking down the cross-linked fibrin structures that solidify the clot.[114] As thrombolytic drugs are systemically administered and have a slow perfusion rate, this method has a low treatment efficacy, long treatment time, and can cause excessive bleeding.[115] Catheter-based devices are used for localised treatment of the target clot, including catheter-directed delivery of thrombolytic drugs[116] and thrombectomy for its mechanical removal.[117] Catheter-based procedures are invasive and associated with multiple complications.[118] There is an unmet clinical need to improve the therapeutic outcome and to increase the treatment efficacy and safety of thrombolysis.

Ultrasound can be combined with thrombolytic drugs and/or contrast agents to accelerate thrombolysis by enhancing the delivery of drugs into the clot, termed sonothrombolysis.[119–124] The effect of sonothrombolysis in enhancing clot lysis has been demonstrated in the in vitro model,[125–127] in vivo in animals,[128, 129] and in human clinical trials.[130–132] A strong correlation between cavitation and enhancement of clot lysis rate has established cavitation as the primary mechanism for sonothrombolysis,[127, 133] whereas its combination with radiation force and microstreaming can further enhance the effect.[134, 135] Typical sonothrombolysis pulses use continuous waves or pulses of various lengths at a low pressure (<2 MPa) with a wide range of frequencies (40 kHz – 3 MHz). These pulse sequences can be achieved even with diagnostic ultrasound.[136–139] Microbubbles help nucleate cavitation to enhance sonothrombolysis,[140, 141] and targeted microbubbles can further improve the therapeutic effect.[142, 143] There have been early signs of success in the clinical trials using sonothrombolysis for DVT (EKOS trial[144, 145]) and ischemic stroke (CLOTBUST trial[131, 132]). However, the treatment efficacy is still less than desired, and the treatment is operator-dependent. Sonothrombolysis also carries the adverse effects of thrombolytic drugs.

To further increase the treatment efficacy and speed, and to eliminate the risk associated with thrombolytic drugs, some researchers have studied thrombolysis via inertial cavitation using ultrasound alone.[146–148] In the late 1990s, Rosenschein et al. first reported using ultrasound alone to produce effective lysis in in vitro clots made with bovine blood inserted into the bovine femoral artery.[146, 147] Short pulses (200-µs at 2.5–10% duty cycle) at a higher intensity (I_{SPTA} >35 W/cm^2) were used. A cavitation cloud was clearly visualised in the clot using ultrasound imaging. Clot removal was seen on ultrasound imaging within 2 minutes of treatment. The clot debris from the treatment was measured, using serial filtration, with 93 ± 1% <8 μm. To examine the vessel damage for safety, in vivo porcine femoral arteries without clots were treated using 200-μs pulses at 4% duty cycle and 45 W/cm² for 5 minutes at one location. Arterial damage was observed, but the treatment duration was much longer than that used to remove clots at a single location.

Wright et al. (2012) and Burgess et al. (2012) from Sunnybrook Research Institute used pulse lengths of milliseconds (in the boiling histotripsy range) to investigate the use of ultrasound alone for thrombolysis in vitro and in vivo.[149–151] In Wright's study,[150] in vitro clots made with rabbit blood were treated with 0.1–10 ms pulses using a 1.5-MHz focused transducer at 0.1% duty cycle with acoustic power of 120–185 W and sonication duration of 5 and 20 seconds at each exposure location. Using 185 W and 1ms pulses, 99.2% of the clot was eroded. Whilst most of the clot debris was smaller than 60 μm, the filtered particle data indicated 1.1% above 0.5 mm in the in vitro flow bypass experiment. For Wright's in vivo experiments, the femoral artery of rabbits was exposed by surgical resection and a clot was formed by vessel occlusion using suture. The clot was treated with 1-ms and 10-ms pulses with power up to 300 W. Flow restoration was achieved in 6 of 10 clots using 1-ms pulses, with evidence of bleeding in 1 case. Treatments using 10-ms pulses were associated with substantial bleeding. Burgess used an intact rabbit embolic model of stroke,[151] where emboli were injected to the middle cerebral artery from the internal carotid artery. The transducer was acoustically coupled to the head using degassed water. Similar ultrasound parameters (1-ms pulse at 1 Hz and 20 s duration) were used but with higher power (415–550 W) to penetrate through the rabbit skull. The treatment was guided by MRI. At 550 W, reperfusion in 5 of 7 animals was achieved. Haemorrhage was detected outside the target vessel, probably because of the proximity of the vessel to the base of the rabbit skull.

Histotripsy using microsecond length pulses has also been investigated as an alternative for thrombolysis using ultrasound alone since 2007. Histotripsy thrombolysis has been demonstrated using in vitro clots[59] and an intact porcine in vivo DVT model.[11] For the in vitro study, clots made with canine blood were treated with histotripsy using a focused, 1 MHz transducer, with 5 cycle pulses at a PRF of 1 kHz.[59] At a peak negative pressure above 6 MPa (corresponding to 20 MPa peak positive pressure and I_{SPPA} of 2000 W/cm²), cavitation was detected using acoustic backscatter and ultrasound imaging, and clot lysis was observed. The thrombolysis rate increased with increasing pressure. At the peak negative pressure of 12 MPa (corresponding to 43 MPa peak positive pressure and I_{SPPA} of 7000 W/cm²), a 300-mg clot (4 mm diameter, 2 cm long) was completely lysed within 2 minutes. The clot debris was measured by serial filtration and Coulter Counter, showing >96% smaller than 5 μm diameter. There was no significant weight change for all 4 filters (5 μm, 20 μm, 100 μm, and 1 mm) used compared to the control. Histotripsy thrombolysis was also tested under pulsatile flow in vitro and remained effective.

The in vivo feasibility of using histotripsy for noninvasive thrombolysis was tested in an intact porcine DVT model.[11] Acute clots (20.1 ± 6mm length) were formed in the femoral vein (5.5 ± 1.0 mm diameter) of 30–40 kg pigs by balloon occlusion and thrombin injection. Histotripsy was applied using a 1-MHz focused transducer with 5 cycle pulses at 1 kHz PRF and peak negative pressure of 14–19 MPa (corresponding to I_{SPPA} = 9.8 k– 21 k W/cm² and I_{SPTA} = 49–105 W/cm²). A cavitation bubble cloud was produced in the femoral vein and visualised on ultrasound imaging as a hyperechoic zone (Figure 27.9a). The cavitation cloud was scanned along the long axis of the clot by moving the transducer, following a scan path determined by pre-treatment planning at a velocity of 0.1 mm/s. In 10 of 12 animals, the clot reduction was apparent on ultrasound imaging (Figure 27.9b), and flow restoration or improvement was observed on colour Doppler in 7 of 12 animals (Figure 27.9c and 27.9d). To evaluate the vessel damage without complication from the catheter-induced damage during clot formation, histotripsy was also applied to an empty femoral vein at 19 MPa for 300 seconds. Histology shows denudation of vascular endothelium and small pockets of hemorrhage in the vessel wall, but perforation of the vessel wall was never observed.

New techniques have been developed to further improve histotripsy thrombolysis treatment by reducing hazardous embolisation and avoiding vessel damage. First, the histotripsy-induced cavitation forms a vortex fluid flow in the vessel, which can capture, trap, and simultaneously erode clot fragments, functioning as a non-invasive emboli trap (NET). Shown by particle velocimetry imaging, cavitation in

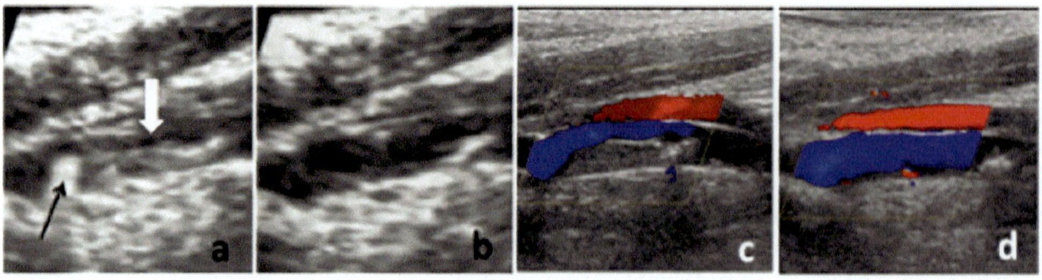

FIGURE 27.9 Ultrasound images of histotripsy thrombolysis in the in vivo porcine DVT model after Maxwell et al.[11] (a) During treatment, the bubble cloud (black arrow) was generated in the porcine femoral vein and appears as a bright zone on or in the thrombus (block arrow) on B-mode ultrasound imaging. (b) After the 300-s treatment using the bubble cloud to scan through the entire clot, the vessel lumen turned darker compared with (a), indicating clot removal. Correspondingly, pre-treatment colour Doppler (c) shows obstructed blood flow and post-treatment Doppler (d) shows flow restoration.

a vessel phantom enhanced streaming and generated fluid vortices adjacent to the focus with a negative pressure gradient, trapping the embolus near this location.[152] The NET was generated by a focused 1-MHz transducer at the peak negative pressure of 5–20 MPa, pulse length of 5–50 cycles, and PRF of 30–1 kHz.[153] The NET formed in a 6-mm vessel phantom was used to trap 1–4 mm emboli particles at flow rates up to 12 cm/s. Second, the histotripsy thrombolysis studies were conducted to initiate cavitation via the shock scattering mechanism, in which cavitation is generated from the weak cavitation nuclei on the vessel wall. To avoid damage to the vessel wall, the intrinsic threshold mechanism with 1-cycle pulses (microtripsy) was investigated for thrombolysis. Microtripsy was applied to in vitro clots in a vessel-mimicking phantom using a 1-MHz focused transducer at a PRF of 50 Hz with a peak negative pressure (P-) of 30–36 MPa.[154] The cavitation was generated entirely within the vessel lumen, resulting in a flow channel through the clot without contacting the vessel wall. Third, the clot composition plays an important role in the clot lytic rate, with retracted clot being more resistant to the treatment employing thrombolytic drugs.[155, 156] Histotripsy has also been shown to be effective for retracted clots, but the treatment efficacy is reduced. Histotripsy thrombolysis in combination with electronic focal steering using a phased array transducer has been used to significantly increase the treatment efficacy in treating retracted clots.

In summary, cavitation has been shown to enhance thrombolysis treatment in multiple facets. Sonothrombolysis enhances the delivery of thrombolytic drugs using low intensity ultrasound enhanced by contrast agents. Ultrasound alone can be used for thrombolysis treatment with high intensity ultrasound pulses. Histotripsy has been demonstrated in vitro and in vivo to be a noninvasive thrombolysis method without thrombolytic drugs or contrast agents. New techniques have been investigated to further improve the treatment efficacy and safety of histotripsy thrombolysis.

27.5 Expert Commentary

In order to understand the basic differences between thermal therapy (TT) and histotripsy (HT), it is useful to explore the concept of "dose" for each modality. In TT, the dose is a relatively complex spatial-temporal formulation of time and temperature. For longer treatment times, the temperature varies spatially and temporally and is a complex and not easily predicted function of energy deposition, perfusion, and thermal conductivity. Moreover, while the energy deposition is usually highest at the focus, energy is lost to absorption in intervening tissues. If the focus is scanned to treat larger volumes, intervening tissue temperature builds up quickly, often in ways not easy to predict, particularly at interfaces between different tissues. To get a precise dose distribution, the temperature should be measured (or imaged) throughout the target volume as well as in intervening tissues. This is difficult to accomplish with high spatial and temporal resolution, although MRI approaches have been employed usefully in the clinic.[157–161]

Several dose-related conundrums have persisted in TT. One is the problem of hot spots in intervening tissues when treating large volumes at depth. This can be alleviated somewhat by dose optimisation approaches[162] or by waiting until intervening tissues cool sufficiently. Cooling times add appreciably to overall treatment times and become prohibitive for larger volumes at depth, particularly when expensive MRI thermometry is being employed. Moreover, in cancer treatment, cooling around blood vessels can leave appreciable pockets of malignant cells receiving insufficient dose, a situation that cannot be predicted because of lack of sufficiently precise temperature monitoring and thermal deposition.

Another characteristic of TT is the difficulty in depositing an "optimal" dose. In cancer treatment, it is useful to treat with a safety margin because pockets of viable malignant cells can be the result of insufficient dose. However, the price paid for excess thermal dosing (safety margin) is hot spots in intervening tissues and unwanted (and unpredictable) local and systemic heating due to perfusion and heat conduction. This makes it very difficult to contour an optimal dose for larger volumes.

An additional complication is the difficulty in receiving immediate image feedback on the efficacy of a given delivered thermal dose. While MRI may provide useful feedback for small single-focus lesions, larger lesions produced by focal scanning are more difficult to monitor owing to the difficulties in controlling dose, and monitoring the results, as already discussed.

In HT, the dose is measured by the number of histotripsy pulses delivered to a focal volume. Since the end effectors are energetic bubble clouds (and rapidly expanding and contracting individual bubbles), and these bubbles last for short periods of time, they do not migrate. The lesions produced are almost exactly the spatial extent of the bubble clouds. Since every histotripsy bubble cloud, with the same acoustic pulse parameters, is remarkably similar, the lesion diameter is very precise and doesn't increase appreciably in diameter once the tissue has been highly fractionated. The process is self-limiting and excess dose for safety margins results in inconsequential increases in lesion diameters. As discussed elsewhere, fractionated tissues are easily seen with ultrasound (hypo-echogenicity owing to fractionated tissues having few particles large enough to scatter sound), or MRI (increased diffusion in liquefied tissues), or in ultrasound elasticity imaging (little or no shear wave propagation in homogenised volumes). Thus dose in HT is easily quantified and immediately observable by different image guidance modalities. Because it is non-thermal, the problem of "migrating" dose and intervening hot spots can be eliminated.

Because histotripsy is very nonlinear, it is sensitive to many acoustic parameters which have little effect on delivered dose in TT. For example, short pulses with variable but high peak intensities can result in large differences in HT efficacy while in TT it is only the time average intensity that really matters. HT offers a very rich parameter environment allowing many degrees of freedom in optimising HT for particular applications. HT phenomena are very sensitive to peak pulse intensities, small changes in pulse durations, changes in pulse repetition frequency, and many other parameters.

Many advantages accrue because HT depends fundamentally on sharp thresholding phenomena. Very short histotripsy pulses, often less than a full cycle in duration, makes HT relatively immune to tissue acoustic aberrations. Distortions in field patterns mostly increase field pattern side-lobes leaving the main lobe relatively unchanged in shape and spatial position. If the main lobe exceeds the intrinsic threshold for energetic bubble cloud production, but side-lobes remain below the threshold, clean bubble clouds and precise localised lesions can be generated without aberration correction, i.e., the side lobes are "thresholded out".

If the intrinsic threshold cannot be directly exceeded with the HT pulses, usually because of an insufficient acoustic window, nonlinear propagation can create large positive pressure shock fronts that can be inverted by sparse incidental bubbles created at acoustic intensities below the intrinsic threshold. These shock scattered pulses can exceed the intrinsic threshold allowing for dense lesion producing "shock-scattering" bubble clouds allowing tissue volumes with small acoustic access windows to be treated.

Thermal therapy techniques can be used to assist the creation of lesion, producing dense bubble clouds by the approach called "boiling histotripsy," a phenomenon occurring at elevated temperatures without the necessity for production of intense ultrasound pulses. The complex interaction of increasing temperatures on the intrinsic threshold, and the onset of true boiling phenomena, is a complex process increasing the range of application for histotripsy.

Histotripsy has many applications and can be seen as a platform technology for therapeutic ultrasound. It is a relatively new modality with many applications yet to be explored. Useful translation to the clinic is in progress but at a rate that can and should be increased. It is the hope that this chapter will stimulate an increase in interest in clinical application of this different therapeutic ultrasound modality.

27.6 Summary

A growing body of literature has demonstrated histotripsy and boiling histotripsy as promising image-guided noninvasive ultrasound ablation techniques for many clinical applications as described above. In the following text, histotripsy is used as a general term for both histotripsy and boiling histotripsy unless they are separately named. As a mechanical tissue fractionation technique, histotripsy has the following advantages compared to other thermal-based ablation techniques, such as radiofrequency ablation, microwave ablation, and HIFU ablation. 1) Histotripsy can mechanically remove tissue. This is required for some clinical applications and cannot be achieved via thermal means. 2) Histotripsy can completely fractionate tissue surrounding major vessels while preserving the vessels, whereas thermal therapy is often ineffective or inefficient near major vessels due to the heat sink effect. 3) Histotripsy can treat large volume tissue or multiple volumes quickly and homogeneously by mechanically or electrically steering the focus to cover the volume, as it is not impacted by the heat sink effect from variation of vasculatures in the target volume. 4) Histotripsy can treat through ribs and overlying tissue without aberration correction or overheating the overlying tissue, when an appropriate pressure level and a sufficiently low duty cycle are used. 5) Real-time imaging feedback is easily achievable with low-cost ultrasound imaging. 6) As the lesion zone is determined by the cavitation zone, this histotripsy-induced lesion boundary remains sharply demarcated, even when overdosed.

A 25-patient cohort of a BPH clinical safety trial of histotripsy has been completed by HistoSonics, Inc., demonstrating the safety of histotripsy in humans. Further clinical testing of BPH is underway, followed by clinical translation of other applications mentioned in this chapter. However, the clinical translation of histotripsy for different clinical applications is faced with multiple challenges. First, there are currently no established Food and Drug Administration (FDA) standards for histotripsy characterisation, as histotripsy uses significantly higher pressures than HIFU thermal therapy and cavitation as the effector. The lithotripsy standard is the closest alternative for histotripsy. The negative pressure used in the intrinsic threshold mechanism creates cavitation instantaneously and cannot be directly measured. The shock scattering approach and boiling histotripsy rely on the shock amplitude, which is difficult to measure accurately in situ in tissue. To provide accurate metrics for the acoustic parameters used in histotripsy, a combination of experimental calibration and sophisticated computational approach is necessary to characterise the ultrasound pressure waveform and beam profiles. Second, as histotripsy requires high pressure pulses, a sufficiently large acoustic window and a low f-number (often f# ≤1) transducer are essential. Such acoustic access may not exist for all clinical applications. Further investigation will be worth exploration to establish an upper limit on the f-number and the depth of the overlying tissue for histotripsy therapy. Third, there are clinical concerns or interesting questions to be addressed that are specially associated with this mechanical tissue fractionation modality. For example, for cancer treatment, are there fragments of intact cells within the treated liquefied volume that may be released into blood stream to increase the risk of metastasis? Or will the mechanical cell fractionation trigger local and systemic immune response to help fight cancer. Lastly, specialised equipment, especially driving electronics, is the key to generation of high-amplitude, short histotripsy pulses. This technical barrier has been the main hurdle that prevents widespread research on histotripsy. Boiling histotripsy can potentially be achieved using typical HIFU equipment. This has allowed additional researchers to step into this field. More researchers are needed to help characterise standards and to investigate more potential clinical applications to push forward this relatively new and growing area.

REFERENCES

1. Xu, Z., A. Ludomirsky, L. Y. Eun, T. L. Hall, B. C. Tran, J. B. Fowlkes, and C. A. Cain. 2003. "Controlled ultrasound tissue erosion." IEEE International Ultrasonics Symposium, Honolulu, HI, USA, October 5–8.
2. Xu, Z., A. Ludomirsky, L. Y. Eun, T. L. Hall, B. C. Tran, J. B. Fowlkes, and C. A. Cain. 2004. "Controlled ultrasound tissue erosion." *IEEE Transaction on Ultrasonics, Ferroelectrics, and Frequency Control* 51 (6):726–36.
3. Lin, K. W., T. L. Hall, R. J. McGough, Z. Xu, and C. A. Cain. 2014. "Synthesis of monopolar ultrasound pulses for therapy: The frequency-compounding transducer." *IEEE Transactions on Ultrasonics, Ferroelectrics, and Frequency Control* 61 (7):1123–36.
4. Maxwell, A. D., C. A. Cain, T. L. Hall, J. B. Fowlkes, and Z. Xu. 2013. "Probability of cavitation for single ultrasound pulses applied to tissues and tissue-mimicking materials." *Ultrasound in Medicine & Biology* 39 (3):449–65.
5. Maxwell, A. D., T. Y. Wang, C. A. Cain, J. B. Fowlkes, O. A. Sapozhnikov, M. R. Bailey, and Z. Xu. 2011. "Cavitation clouds created by shock scattering from bubbles during histotripsy." *The Journal of the Acoustical Society of America* 130 (4):1888–98.
6. Kieran, K., T. L. Hall, J. E. Parsons, J. S. Wolf, J. B. Fowlkes, C. A. Cain, and W. W. Roberts. 2007. "Refining histotripsy: Defining the parameter space for the creation of non-thermal lesions with high intensity, pulsed focused ultrasound of the in vitro kidney." *Journal of Urology* 178 (2):672–6.
7. Parsons, J. E., C. A. Cain, G. D. Abrams, and J. B. Fowlkes. 2006. "Pulsed cavitational ultrasound therapy for controlled tissue homogenization." *Ultrasound in Medicine & Biology* 32 (1):115–29.
8. Lin, K. W., Y. Kim, A. D. Maxwell, T. Y. Wang, T. L. Hall, Z. Xu, J. B. Fowlkes, and C. A. Cain. 2014. "Histotripsy beyond the intrinsic cavitation threshold using very short ultrasound pulses: Microtripsy." *IEEE Transactions on Ultrasonics, Ferroelectrics, and Frequency Control* 61 (2):251–65.
9. Roberts, William W., T. J. Hall, K. Ives, Jr. J. Stuart Wolf, J. B. Fowlkes, and C. A. Cain. 2006. "Pulsed cavitational ultrasound: A non-invasive technology for controlled tissue ablation (histotripsy) in the rabbit kidney." *Journal of Urology* 175 (2):734–8.
10. Styn, N., T. L. Hall, J. B. Fowlkes, C. A. Cain, and W. W. Roberts. 2011. "Histotripsy homogenization of the prostate: Thresholds for cavitation damage of periprostatic structures." *Journal of Endourology/ Endourological Society* 25 (9):1531–5.
11. Maxwell, A. D., G. Owens, H. S. Gurm, K. Ives, D. D. Myers, Jr., and Z. Xu. 2011. "Noninvasive treatment of deep venous thrombosis using pulsed ultrasound cavitation therapy (histotripsy) in a porcine model." *Journal of Vascular and Interventional Radiology* 22 (3):369–77.
12. Vlaisavljevich, E., Y. Kim, S. Allen, G. Owens, S. Pelletier, C. Cain, K. Ives, and Z. Xu. 2013. "Image-guided non-invasive ultrasound liver ablation using histotripsy: Feasibility study in an in vivo porcine model." *Ultrasound in Medicine & Biology* 39 (8):1398–409.
13. Kim, Y., E. Vlaisavljevich, G. E. Owens, S. P. Allen, C. A. Cain, and Z. Xu. 2014. "In vivo transcostal histotripsy therapy without aberration correction." *Physics in Medicine & Biology*59 (11):2553–68.
14. Hempel, C. R., T. L. Hall, C. A. Cain, J. B. Fowlkes, Z. Xu, and W. W. Roberts. 2011. "Histotripsy fractionation of prostate tissue: Local effects and systemic response in a canine model." *The Journal of Urology* 185 (4):1484–9.
15. Vlaisavljevich, E., A. Maxwell, M. Warnez, E. Johnsen, C. Cain, and Z. Xu. 2014. "Histotripsy-induced cavitation cloud initiation thresholds in tissues of different mechanical properties." *IEEE Transactions on Ultrasonics, Ferroelectrics, and Frequency Control* 61 (2):341–52.
16. Vlaisavljevich, E., K. W. Lin, A. Maxwell, M. T. Warnez, L. Mancia, R. Singh, A. J. Putnam, B. Fowlkes, E. Johnsen, C. Cain, and Z. Xu. 2015. "Effects of ultrasound frequency and tissue stiffness on the histotripsy intrinsic threshold for cavitation." *Ultrasound in Medicine & Biology* 41 (6):1651–67.
17. Xu, J., and T. A. Bigelow. 2011. "Experimental investigation of the effect of stiffness, exposure time and scan direction on the dimension of ultrasound histotripsy lesions." *Ultrasound in Medicine & Biology* 37 (11):1865–73.
18. Vlaisavljevich, E., Y. Kim, G. Owens, W. Roberts, C. Cain, and Z. Xu. 2014. "Effects of tissue mechanical properties on susceptibility to histotripsy-induced tissue damage." *Physics in Medicine and Biology* 59 (2):253–70.
19. Kim, Y., T-Y. Wang, Z. Xu, and C. A. Cain. 2011. "Lesion generation through ribs using histotripsy therapy without aberration correction." *IEEE Transactions on Ultrasonics, Ferroelectrics, and Frequency Control* 58 (11):2334–43.

20. Sukovich, J. R., Y. Kim, A. Pandey, H. Gurm, C. Cain, and Z. Xu. 2015. "Targeted lesion generation through the skull using histotripsy without aberration correction." International Society of Therapeutic Ultrasound Symposium, Uretcht, April 15–18.
21. Lin, K. W., A. P. Duryea, Y. Kim, T. L. Hall, Z. Xu, and C. A. Cain. 2014. "Dual-beam histotripsy: A low-frequency pump enabling a high-frequency probe for precise lesion formation." *IEEE Transactions on Ultrasonics, Ferroelectrics, and Frequency Control* 61 (2):325–40.
22. Coussios, C. C., C. H. Farny, G. T. Haar, and R. A. Roy. 2007. "Role of acoustic cavitation in the delivery and monitoring of cancer treatment by high-intensity focused ultrasound (HIFU)." *International Journal of Hyperthermia* 23 (2):105–20.
23. Liu, H. L., W. S. Chen, J. S. Chen, T. C. Shih, Y. Y. Chen, and W. L. Lin. 2006. "Cavitation-enhanced ultrasound thermal therapy by combined low- and high-frequency ultrasound exposure." *Ultrasound in Medicine & Biology* 32 (5):759–67.
24. Takagi, R., S. Yoshizawa, and S. I. Umemura. 2010. "Enhancement of ultrasonic heating by ultrasonically localized cavitation for high intensity focused ultrasound treatment." 2010 International Ultrasonics Symposium, Piscataway, NJ, USA, October 11–14.
25. Khokhlova, T. D., Y. N. Wang, J. C. Simon, B. W. Cunitz, F. Starr, M. Paun, L. A. Crum, M. R. Bailey, and V. A. Khokhlova. 2014. "Ultrasound-guided tissue fractionation by high intensity focused ultrasound in an in vivo porcine liver model." *Proceedings of the National Academy of Sciences of the United States of America* 111 (22):8161–6.
26. Khokhlova, V. A., J. B. Fowlkes, W. W. Roberts, G. R. Schade, Z. Xu, T. D. Khokhlova, T. L. Hall, A. D. Maxwell, Y. N. Wang, and C. A. Cain. 2015. "Histotripsy methods in mechanical disintegration of tissue: Towards clinical applications." *International Journal of Hyperthermia* 31 (2):145–62.
27. Simon, J. C., O. A. Sapozhnikov, V. A. Khokhlova, Y. N. Wang, L. A. Crum, and M. R. Bailey. 2012. "Ultrasonic atomization of tissue and its role in tissue fractionation by high intensity focused ultrasound." *Physics in Medicine & Biology*57 (23):8061–78.
28. Kreider, W., A. D. Maxwell, T. Khokhlova, J. C. Simon, V. A. Khokhlova, O. Sapozhnikov, and M. R. Bailey. 2013. "Rectified growth of histotripsy bubbles." *Proceedings of Meetings on Acoustics* 19 (1).
29. Wang, Y. N., T. Khokhlova, M. Bailey, J. H. Hwang, and V. Khokhlova. 2013. "Histological and biochemical analysis of mechanical and thermal bioeffects in boiling histotripsy lesions induced by high intensity focused ultrasound." *Ultrasound in Medicine & Biology* 39 (3):424–38.
30. Hoogenboom, M., D. Eikelenboom, M. H. den Brok, A. Heerschap, J. J. Futterer, and G. J. Adema. 2015. "Mechanical high-intensity focused ultrasound destruction of soft tissue: Working mechanisms and physiologic effects." *Ultrasound in Medicine & Biology* 41 (6):1500–17.
31. Khokhlova, T. D., M. S. Canney, V. A. Khokhlova, O. A. Sapozhnikov, L. A. Crum, and M. R. Bailey. 2011. "Controlled tissue emulsification produced by high intensity focused ultrasound shock waves and millisecond boiling." *The Journal of the Acoustical Society of America* 130 (5):3498–510.
32. Simon, J. C. 2013. *The thresholds and mechanisms of tissue injury by focused ultrasound*. Dissertation at Department of Bioengineering, University of Washington.
33. Tran, B. C., J. Brian Fowlkes, and C. Cain. 2004. "Correlation between acoustic backscatter variability and tissue damage prodcued by pulses cavitational ultrasound therapy." *Proceedings of the 2004 IEEE International Ultrasonics, Ferroelectric, and Frequency Control Joint 50th Anniversary Conference* 2:1461–4.
34. Xu, Z., J. B. Fowlkes, E. D. Rothman, A. M. Levin, and C. A. Cain. 2005. "Controlled ultrasound tissue erosion: The role of dynamic interaction between insonation and microbubble activity." *Journal of the Acoustical Society of America* 117 (1):424–35.
35. Wang, T-Y., Z. Xu, T. L. Hall, J. B. Fowlkes, and C. A. Cain. 2012. "An efficient treatment strategy for histotripsy by removing cavitation memory." *Ultrasound in Medicine and Biology* 38 (5):753–66.
36. Duryea, A. P., H. A. Tamaddoni, C. A. Cain, W. W. Roberts, and T. L. Hall. 2015. "Removal of residual nuclei following a cavitation event: A parametric study." *IEEE Transactions on Ultrasonics, Ferroelectrics, and Frequency Control* 62 (9):1605–14.
37. Tran, B. C., J. Seo, T. L. Hall, J. B. Fowlkes, and C. A. Cain. 2003. "Microbubble-enhanced cavitation for noninvasive ultrasound surgery." *IEEE Transactions on Ultrasonics, Ferroelectrics, and Frequency Control* 50 (10):1296–304.
38. Allen, S. P., L. Hernandez-Garcia, C. A. Cain, and T. L. Hall. 2015. "MR-based detection of individual histotripsy bubble clouds formed in tissues and phantoms." Magnetic resonance in medicine. 2016 Nov;76(5):1486–93.

39. Allen, S. P., T. L. Hall, C. A. Cain, and L. Hernandez-Garcia. 2015. "Controlling cavitation-based image contrast in focused ultrasound histotripsy surgery." *Magnetic Resonance in Medicine* 73 (1):204–13.
40. Hall, T. L., J. B. Fowlkes, and C. A. Cain. 2007. "A real-time measure of cavitation unduced tissue disruption by ultrasound imaging backscatter reduction." *IEEE Transactions on Ultrasonics, Ferroelectrics, and Frequency Control* 54 (3):569–75.
41. Wang, T. Y., Z. Xu, F. Winterroth, T. L. Hall, J. B. Fowlkes, E. D. Rothman, W. W. Roberts, and C. A. Cain. 2009. "Quantitative ultrasound backscatter for pulsed cavitational ultrasound therapy-histotripsy." *IEEE Transactions on Ultrasonics, Ferroelectrics, and Frequency Control* 56 (5):995–1005.
42. Wang, T. Y., T. L. Hall, Z. Xu, J. B. Fowlkes, and C. A. Cain. 2012. "Imaging feedback of histotripsy treatments using ultrasound shear wave elastography." *IEEE Transactions on Ultrasonics, Ferroelectrics, and Frequency Control* 59 (6):1167–81.
43. Kim, Y., C. G. Fifer, S. K. Gelehrter, G. E. Owens, D. R. Berman, E. Vlaisavljevich, S. P. Allen, M. F. Ladino-Torres, and Z. Xu. 2013. "Developmental impact and lesion maturation of histotripsy-mediated non-invasive tissue ablation in a fetal sheep model." *Ultrasound in Medicine & Biology* 39 (6):1047–55.
44. Lake, A. M., T. L. Hall, K. Kieran, J. B. Fowlkes, C. A. Cain, and W. W. Roberts. 2008. "Histotripsy: Minimally invasive technology for prostatic tissue ablation in an in vivo canine model." *Urology* 72 (3):682–6.
45. Wheat, J. C., T. L. Hall, C. R. Hempel, C. A. Cain, Z. Xu, and W. W. Roberts. 2010. "Prostate histotripsy in an anticoagulated model." *Urology* 75 (1):207–11.
46. Schade, G. R., T. L. Hall, and W. W. Roberts. 2012. "Urethral-sparing histotripsy of the prostate in a canine model." *Urology* 80 (3):730–5.
47. Schade, G. R., J. Keller, K. Ives, X. Cheng, T. J. Rosol, E. Keller, and W. W. Roberts. 2012. "Histotripsy focal ablation of implanted prostate tumour in an ACE-1 canine cancer model." *Journal of Urology* 188 (5):1957–64.
48. Wang, T. Y., T. L. Hall, Z. Xu, J. B. Fowlkes, and C. A. Cain. 2014. "Imaging feedback for histotripsy by characterizing dynamics of acoustic radiation force impulse (ARFI)-induced shear waves excited in a treated volume." *IEEE Transactions on Ultrasonics, Ferroelectrics, and Frequency Control* 61 (7): 1137–51.
49. Miller, R., X. Zhang, A. Maxwell, C. Cain, and Z. Xu. 2016. "Bubble-induced Colour Doppler Feedback for Histotripsy Tissue Fractionation." *IEEE Transactions on Ultrasonics, Ferroelectrics, and Frequency Control* 63 (3):408–19.
50. Zhang, X., R. M. Miller, A. D. Maxwell, C. A. Cain, and Z. Xu. 2014. "Real-time Feedback of Histotripsy Thrombolysis using Bubble-induced Colour Doppler." IEEE International Ultrasonics Symposium, Chicago, IL, USA, September 3–6.
51. Parsons, J. E., C. A. Cain, G. D. Abrams, and J. B. Fowlkes. 2007. "Spatial variability in acoustic backscatter as an indicator of tissue homogenate production in pulsed cavitational ultrasound therapy." *IEEE Transactions on Ultrasonics, Ferroelectrics, and Frequency Control* 54 (3):576–90.
52. Hall, T. L., G. R. Lee, L. Hernandez, and C. A. Cain. 2007. "Relaxation Properties of Cavitation Induced Tissue Lesions." Joint Annual Meeting ISMRM (International Society for Magnetic Resonance in Medcine)-ESMRMB (European Society for Magnetic Resonance in Medicine and Biology), May 19–25.
53. Allen, S. P., W. W. Roberts, T. L. Hall, C. A. Cain, and L. Hernandez. 2012. "Characterization of in vivo histotripsy lesions using high field MRI." The 20th Annual Meeting of ISMRM, Melbourne.
54. Partanen, A., N. Farr, W. Kreider, T. Khokhlova, A. Maxwell, Y-N. Wang, M. Bailey, and V. Khokhlova. 2014. "Use of MRI to visualize mechanically fractionated lesions generated by boiling histotripsy in tissue." 14th International Symposium for Therapeutic Ultrasound, Las Vegas.
55. Kim, Y., S. K. Gelehrter, C. G. Fifer, J. C. Lu, G. E. Owens, D. R. Berman, J. Williams, J. E. Wilkinson, K. A. Ives, and Z. Xu. 2011. "Non-invasive pulsed cavitational ultrasound for fetal tissue ablation: Feasibility study in a fetal sheep model." *Ultrasound in Obstetrics & Gynecology* 37 (4):450–7.
56. Xu, Z., G. Owens, D. Gordon, C. Cain, and A. Ludomirsky. 2010. "Noninvasive creation of an atrial septal defect by histotripsy in a canine model." *Circulation* 121 (6):742–9.
57. Owens, G. E., R. M. Miller, G. Ensing, K. Ives, D. Gordon, A. Ludomirsky, and Z. Xu. 2011. "Therapeutic ultrasound to non-invasively create intracardiac communications in an intact animal model." *Catheterization and Cardiovascular Interventions* 77 (4):580–8.
58. Owens, G. E., R. M. Miller, S. T. Owens, S. D. Swanson, K. Ives, G. Ensing, D. Gordon, and Z. Xu. 2012. "Intermediate-term effects of intracardiac communications created noninvasively by therapeutic ultrasound (histotripsy) in a porcine model." *Pediatric Cardiology* 33 (1):83–9.

59. Maxwell, A. D., C. A. Cain, A. P. Duryea, L. Yuan, H. S. Gurm, and Z. Xu. 2009. "Noninvasive thrombolysis using pulsed ultrasound cavitation therapy – histotripsy." *Ultrasound in Medicine & Biology* 35 (12):1982–94.
60. Khokhlova, T. D., Y. N. Wang, J. C. Simon, B. W. Cunitz, F. Starr, M. Paun, L. A. Crum, M. R. Bailey, and V. A. Khokhlova. 2014. "Ultrasound-guided tissue fractionation by high intensity focused ultrasound in an in vivo porcine liver model." *Proceedings of the National Academy of Sciences* 111 (22):8161–6.
61. Styn, N. R., J. C. Wheat, T. L. Hall, and W. W. Roberts. 2010. "Histotripsy of VX-2 tumour implanted in a renal rabbit model." *Journal of Endourology/Endourological Society* 24 (7):1145–50.
62. Wang, Y. N., T. Khokhlova, M. Bailey, J. H. Hwang, and V. Khokhlova. 2013. "Histological and biochemical analysis of mechanical and thermal bioeffects in boiling histotripsy lesions induced by high intensity focused ultrasound." *Ultrasound in Medicine & Biology* 39 (3):424–38.
63. Duryea, A. P., T. L. Hall, A. D. Maxwell, Z. Xu, C. A. Cain, and W. W. Roberts. 2011. "Histotripsy erosion of model urinary calculi." *Journal of Endourology/Endourological Society* 25 (2):341–4.
64. Duryea, A. P., A. D. Maxwell, W. W. Roberts, Z. Xu, T. L. Hall, and C. A. Cain. 2011. "In vitro comminution of model renal calculi using histotripsy." *IEEE Transactions on Ultrasonics, Ferroelectrics, and Frequency Control* 58 (5):971–80.
65. Barry, M. J., F. J. Fowler, Jr., M. P. O' Leary, R. C. Bruskewitz, H. L. Holtgrewe, W. K. Mebust, and A. T. Cockett. 1992. "The American Urological Association symptom index for benign prostatic hyperplasia. The Measurement Committee of the American Urological Association." *Journal of Urology* 148 (5):1549–57.
66. Roos, N. P., J. E. Wennberg, D. J. Malenka, E. S. Fisher, K. McPherson, T. F. Andersen, M. M. Cohen, and E. Ramsey. 1989. "Mortality and reoperation after open and transurethral resection of the prostate for benign prostatic hyperplasia." *New England Journal of Medicine* 320 (17):1120–4.
67. Hacker, A., K. U. Kohrmann, W. Back, O. Kraut, E. Marlinghaus, P. Alken, and M. S. Michel. 2005. "Extracorporeal application of high-intensity focused ultrasound for prostatic tissue ablation." *BJU International* 96 (1):71–6.
68. Hall, T. L., C. R. Hempel, B. J. Sabb, and W. W. Roberts. 2010. "Acoustic access to the prostate for extracorporeal ultrasound ablation." *Journal of Endourology* 24 (11):1875–81.
69. Hall, T. L., C. R. Hempel, K. Wojno, Z. Xu, C. A. Cain, and W. W. Roberts. 2009. "Histotripsy of the prostate: Dose effects in a chronic canine model." *Urology* 74 (4):932–7.
70. Darnell, S. E., T. L. Hall, S. A. Tomlins, X. Cheng, K. A. Ives, and W. W. Roberts. 2015. "Histotripsy of the Prostate in a Canine Model: Characterization of Post-Therapy Inflammation and Fibrosis." *Journal of Endourology* 29 (7):810–5.
71. Poliachik, S. L., W. L. Chandler, R. J. Ollos, M. R. Bailey, and L. A. Crum. 2004. "The relation between cavitation and platelet aggregation during exposure to high-intensity focused ultrasound." *Ultrasound in Medicine and Biology* 30 (2):261–9.
72. Devanagondi, R., X. Zhang, Z. Xu, K. Ives, A. Levin, H. Gurm, and G. E. Owens. 2015. "Hemodynamic and hematologic effects of histotripsy of free-flowing blood: Implications for ultrasound-mediated thrombolysis." *Journal of Vascular and Interventional Radiology* 26 (10):1559–65.
73. Allam, C. L., J. E. Wilkinson, X. Cheng, K. A. Ives, T. L. Hall, and W. W. Roberts. 2013. "Histotripsy effects on the bladder trigone: Functional and histologic consequences in the canine model." *Journal of Endourology* 27 (10):1267–71.
74. Schade, G. R., N. R. Styn, K. A. Ives, T. L. Hall, and W. W. Roberts. 2014. "Prostate histotripsy: Evaluation of prostatic urethral treatment parameters in a canine model." *BJU International* 113 (3):498–503.
75. Schade, G. R., N. R. Styn, T. L. Hall, and W. W. Roberts. 2012. "Endoscopic assessment and prediction of prostate urethral disintegration after histotripsy treatment in a canine model." *Journal of Endourology/Endourological Society* 26 (2):183–9.
76. Roberts, W. W., D. Teofilovic, R. C. Jahnke, J. Patri, J. M. Risdahl, and J. A. Bertolina. 2014. "Histotripsy of the prostate using a commercial system in a canine model." *Journal of Urology* 191 (3):860–5.
77. Abu-Harb, M., E. Hey, and C. Wren. 1994. "Death in infancy from unrecognised congenital heart disease." *Archives of Disease in Childhood Fetal & Neonatal Edition* 71:3–7.
78. Fyler, D C. 1980. "Report of the new England regional infant cardiac program." *Pediatrics* 65 (2 Pt 2):375–461.
79. Xu, Z., J. B. Fowlkes, and C. A. Cain. 2006. "A new strategy to enhance cavitational tissue erosion by using a high intensity initiating sequence." *IEEE Transactions on Ultrasonics, Ferroelectrics, and Frequency Control* 53 (8):1412–24.

80. Xu, Z., J. B. Fowlkes, A. Ludomirsky, and C. A. Cain. 2005. "Investigation of intensity threshold for ultrasound tissue erosion." *Ultrasound in Medicine & Biology* 31 (12):1673–82.
81. Wang, T-Y., A. D. Maxwell, S. Park, Zhen Xu, J. B. Fowlkes, and C. A. Cain. 2010. "Why are short pulses more efficient in tissue erosion using pulsed cavitational ultrasound therapy (histotripsy)?" 9th International Symposium on Therapeutic Ultrasound: ISTU – 2009, USA, September 24–26.
82. Xu, Z., M. Raghavan, T. L. Hall, C-W. Chang, M-A. Mycek, J. B. Fowlkes, and C. A. Cain. 2007. "High speed imaging of bubble clouds generated in pulsed ultrasound cavitational therapy-histotripsy." *IEEE Transactions on Ultrasonics, Ferroelectrics, and Frequency Control* 54 (10):2091–101.
83. Xu, Z., M. Raghavan, T. L. Hall, M. A. Mycek, and J. B. Fowlkes. 2008. "Evolution of bubble clouds induced by pulsed cavitational ultrasound therapy – histotripsy." *IEEE Transactions on Ultrasonics, Ferroelectrics, and Frequency Control* 55 (5):1122–32.
84. Xu, Z., Z. Fan, T. L. Hall, F. Winterroth, J. B. Fowlkes, and C. A. Cain. 2009. "Size measurement of tissue debris particles generated from pulsed ultrasound cavitational therapy-histotripsy." *Ultrasound in Medicine & Biology* 35 (2):245–55.
85. Leslie, T. A., J. E. Kennedy, R. O. Illing, G. R. ter Haar, F. Wu, R. R. Phillips, P. J. Friend, I. S. Roberts, D. W. Cranston, and M. R. Middleton. 2008. "High-intensity focused ultrasound ablation of liver tumours: Can radiological assessment predict the histological outcome?" *British Journal of Radiology* 81 (967):564–71.
86. Fujisaki, M., T. Chiba, S. Enosawa, T. Dohi, and S. Takamoto. 2010. "Cardiac intervention using high-intensity focused ultrasound: Creation of interatrial communication in beating heart of an anesthetized rabbit." *Ultrasound in Obstetrics and Gynecology* 36 (5):607–12.
87. Abe, Y., R. Otsuka, R. Muratore, K. Fujikura, K. Okajima, K. Suzuki, J. Wang, C. Marboe, A. Kalisz, J. A. Ketterling, F. L. Lizzi, and S. Homma. 2008. "In vitro mitral chordal cutting by high intensity focused ultrasound." *Ultrasound in Medicine and Biology* 34 (3):400–5.
88. Alkins, R., Y. Huang, D. Pajek, and K. Hynynen. 2013. "Cavitation-based third ventriculostomy using MRI-guided focused ultrasound: Laboratory investigation." *Journal of Neurosurgery* 119 (6):1520–29.
89. Maxwell, A. D., R. S. Hsi, M. R. Bailey, P. Casale, and T. S. Lendvay. 2014. "Noninvasive ureterocele puncture using pulsed focused ultrasound: An in vitro study." *Journal of Endourology* 28 (3):342–46.
90. Wu, F., Z. B. Wang, W. Z. Chen, J. Z. Zou, J. Bai, H. Zhu, K. Q. Li, C. B. Jin, F. L. Xie, and H. B. Su. 2005. "Advanced hepatocellular carcinoma: Treatment with high-intensity focused ultrasound ablation combined with transcatheter arterial embolization." *Radiology* 235 (2):659–67.
91. Parikh, S., and D. Hyman. 2007. "Hepatocellular cancer: A guide for the internist." *The American Journal of Medicine* 120 (3):194–202.
92. Jansen, M. C., R. van Hillegersberg, R. A. Chamuleau, O. M. van Delden, D. J. Gouma, and T. M. van Gulik. 2005. "Outcome of regional and local ablative therapies for hepatocellular carcinoma: A collective review." *European Journal of Surgical Oncology* 31 (4):331–47.
93. Nhan, T., A. Burgess, and K. Hynynen. 2013. "Transducer design and characterization for dorsal-based ultrasound exposure and two-photon imaging of in vivo blood-brain barrier disruption in a rat model." *IEEE Transactions on Ultrasonics, Ferroelectrics, and Frequency Control* 60 (7):1376–85.
94. Diaz, R. J., P. Z. McVeigh, M. A. O'Reilly, K. Burrell, M. Bebenek, C. Smith, A. B. Etame, G. Zadeh, K. Hynynen, B. C. Wilson, and J. T. Rutka. 2014. "Focused ultrasound delivery of Raman nanoparticles across the blood-brain barrier: Potential for targeting experimental brain tumours." *Nanomedicine: Nanotechnology, Biology, and Medicine* 10 (5):1075–87.
95. Goldberg, S. N., L. Solbiati, P. F. Hahn, E. Cosman, J. E. Conrad, R. Fogle, and G. S. Gazelle. 1998. "Large-volume tissue ablation with radio frequency by using a clustered, internally cooled electrode technique: Laboratory and clinical experience in liver metastases." *Radiology* 209 (2):371–9.
96. O'Reilly, M. A., and K. Hynynen. 2012. "Blood-brain barrier: Real-time feedback-controlled focused ultrasound disruption by using an acoustic emissions-based controller." *Radiology* 263 (1):96–106.
97. Etame, A. B., R. J. Diaz, C. A. Smith, T. G. Mainprize, K. Hynynen, and J. T. Rutka. 2012. "Focused ultrasound disruption of the blood-brain barrier: A new frontier for therapeutic delivery in molecular neurooncology." *Neurosurgical Focus* 32 (1):E3.
98. Okada A, Murakami T, Mikami K, Onishi H, Tanigawa N, Marukawa T, and Nakamura H. 2006. "A case of hepatocellular carcinoma treated by MR-guided focused ultrasound ablation with respiratory gating." *Magnetic Resonance in Medical Sciences* 5 (3):167–71.
99. Li, Y. Y., W. H. Sha, Y. J. Zhou, and Y. Q. Nie. 2007. "Short and long term efficacy of high intensity focused ultrasound therapy for advanced hepatocellular carcinoma." *Journal of Gastroenterology and Hepatology* 22 (12):2148–54.

100. Kopelman, D., Y. Inbar, A. Hanannel, G. Dank, D. Freundlich, A. Perel, D. Castel, A. Greenfeld, T. Salomon, M. Sareli, A. Valeanu, and M. Papa. 2006. "Magnetic resonance-guided focused ultrasound surgery (MRgFUS). Four ablation treatments of a single canine hepatocellular adenoma." *HPB (Oxford)* 8 (4):292–8.
101. Zhu, H., K. Zhou, L. Zhang, C. Jin, S. Peng, W. Yang, K. Li, H. Su, W. Chen, J. Bai, F. Wu, and Z. Wang. 2009. "High intensity focused ultrasound (HIFU) therapy for local treatment of hepatocellular carcinoma: Role of partial rib resection." *European Journal of Radiology* 72 (1):160–6. Epub 2008 Aug 15.
102. Illing, R. O., J. E. Kennedy, F. Wu, G. R. ter Haar, A. S. Protheroe, P. J. Friend, F. V. Gleeson, D. W. Cranston, R. R. Phillips, and M. R. Middleton. 2005. "The safety and feasibility of extracorporeal high-intensity focused ultrasound (HIFU) for the treatment of liver and kidney tumours in a Western population." *British Journal of Cancer* 93 (8):890–5.
103. Zhao, G., J. Cui, Q. Qin, J. Zhang, L. Liu, S. Deng, C. Wu, M. Yang, S. Li, and C. Wang. 2010. "Mechanical stiffness of liver tissues in relation to integrin beta1 expression may influence the development of hepatic cirrhosis and hepatocellular carcinoma." *Journal of Surgical Oncology* 102 (5):482–9.
104. Piana, G., L. Trinquart, N. Meskine, V. Barrau, B. V. Beers, and V. Vilgrain. 2010. "New MR imaging criteria with a diffusion-weighted sequence for the diagnosis of hepatocellular carcinoma in chronic liver diseases." *Journal of Hepatology* 23:23.
105. Umale, S., S. Chatelin, N. Bourdet, C. Deck, M. Diana, P. Dhumane, L. Soler, J. Marescaux, and R. Willinger. 2011. "Experimental in vitro mechanical characterization of porcine Glisson's capsule and hepatic veins." *Journal of Biomechanics* 44 (9):1678–83.
106. Vlaisavljevich, E., Y. Kim, S. Allen, G. Owens, S. Pelletier, C. Cain, K. Ives, and Z. Xu. 2013. "Image-guided non-invasive ultrasound liver ablation using histotripsy: Feasibility study in an in vivo porcine model." *Ultrasound in Medicine & Biology* 39 (8):1398–409.
107. O'Reilly, M. A., Y. Huang, and K. Hynynen. 2010. "The impact of standing wave effects on transcranial focused ultrasound disruption of the blood-brain barrier in a rat model." *Physics in Medicine and Biology* 55 (18):5251–67.
108. Chopra, R., N. Vykhodtseva, and K. Hynynen. 2010. "Influence of exposure time and pressure amplitude on blood-brain-barrier opening using transcranial ultrasound exposures." *ACS Chemical Neuroscience* 1 (5):391–98.
109. Kennedy, J. E., R. L. Clarke, and G. R. ter Haar. 2002. "The effects of absorbers such as ribs in the HIFU beam-path on the focal profile." *Proceedings of the Second International Symposium on Therapeutic Ultrasound*:185–92.
110. Wang, H., E. Ebbini, M. O'Donnell, and C. A. Cain. 1994. "Phase abberation correction and motion compensation for ultrasonic phased arrays: Experimental results." *IEEE Transactions on Ultrasonics, Ferroelectrics, and Frequency Control* 41 (1):34–43.
111. Khokhlova, V. A., S. M. Bobkova, and L. R. Gavrilov. 2010. "Focus splitting associated with propagation of focused ultrasound through the rib cage." *Acoustical Physics* 56 (Compendex):665–74.
112. Bobkova, S., L. Gavrilov, V. Khokhlova, A. Shaw, and J. Hand. 2010. "Focusing of high-intensity ultrasound through the rib cage using a therapeutic random phased array." *Ultrasound in Medicine and Biology* 36 (Copyright 2010, The Institution of Engineering and Technology):888–906.
113. Hall, T. L., K. Kieran, K. Ives, J. B. Fowlkes, C. A. Cain, and W. W. Roberts. 2007. "Histotripsy of rabbit renal tissue in vivo: Temporal histologic trends." *Journal of Endourology/Endourological Society* 21 (10):1159–66.
114. Collen, D., D. C. Stump, and H. K. Gold. 1988. "Thrombolytic therapy." *Annual Review of Medicine* 39:405–23.
115. Rogers, L. Q., and C. L. Lutcher. 1990. "Streptokinase therapy for deep vein thrombosis: A comprehensive review of the English literature." *The American Journal of Medicine* 88 (4):389–95.
116. Mewissen, M. W., G. R. Seabrook, M. H. Meissner, J. Cynamon, N. Labropoulos, and S. H Haughton. 1999. "Catheter-directed thrombolysis for lower extremity deep venous thrombosis: Report of a national multicenter registry." *Radiology* 211 (1):39–49.
117. Kim, H. S., A. Patra, B. E. Paxton, J. Khan, and M. B. Streiff. 2006. "Catheter-directed thrombolysis with percutaneous rheolytic thrombectomy versus thrombolysis alone in upper and lower extremity deep vein thrombosis." *Cardiovascular and Interventional Radiology* 29 (6):1003–7.
118. Sharafuddin, M. J., S. Sun, J. J. Hoballah, F. M. Youness, W. J. Sharp, and B. S. Roh. 2003. "Endovascular management of venous thrombotic and occlusive diseases of the lower extremities." *Journal of Vascular and Interventional Radiology* 14 (4):405–23.

119. Harpaz, D., X. Chen, C. W. Francis, V. J. Marder, and RS Meltzer. 1993. "Ultrasound enhancement of thrombolysis and reperfusion in vitro." *Journal of the American College of Cardiology* 21 (6):1507–11.
120. Luo, H., Y. Birnbaum, M. C. Fishbein, T. M. Peterson, T. Nagai, T. Nishioka, and R. J. Siegel. 1998. "Enhancement of thrombolysis in vivo without skin and soft tissue damage by transcutaneous ultrasound." *Thrombosis Research* 89 (4):171–7.
121. Siegel, R. J., S. Atar, M. C. Fishbein, A. V. Brasch, T. M. Peterson, T. Nagai, D. Pal, T. Nishioka, J. S. Chae, Y. Birnbaum, C. Zanelli, and H. Luo. 2000. "Noninvasive, transthoracic, low-frequency ultrasound augments thrombolysis in a canine model of acute myocardial infarction." *Circulation* 101 (17):2026–9.
122. Francis, C. W., and V. N. Suchkova. 2001. "Ultrasound and thrombolysis." *Vascular Medicine* 6 (3):181–7.
123. Frenkel, V., J. Oberoi, M. J. Stone, M. Park, C. Deng, B. J. Wood, Z. Neeman, M. Horne, and K. C. Li. 2006. "Pulsed high-intensity focused ultrasound enhances thrombolysis in an in vitro model." *Radiology* 239 (1):86–93.
124. Meunier, J. M., C. K. Holland, C. J. Lindsell, and G. J. Shaw. 2007. "Duty cycle dependence of ultrasound enhanced thrombolysis in a human clot model." *Ultrasound in Medicine & Biology* 33 (4):576–83.
125. Tachibana, K. 1992. "Enhancement of fibrinolysis with ultrasound energy." *Journal of Vascular and Interventional Radiology* 3 (2):299–303.
126. Francis, C. W., P. T. Onundarson, E. L. Carstensen, A. Blinc, R. S. Meltzer, K. Schwarz, and V. J. Marder. 1992. "Enhancement of fibrinolysis in vitro by ultrasound." *The Journal of Clinical Investigation* 90 (5):2063–8.
127. Datta, S., C. C. Coussios, L. E. McAdory, J. Tan, T. Porter, G. De Courten-Myers, and C. K. Holland. 2006. "Correlation of cavitation with ultrasound enhancement of thrombolysis." *Ultrasound in Medicine & Biology* 32 (8):1257–67.
128. Daffertshofer, M., Z. Huang, M. Fatar, M. Popolo, H. Schroeck, W. Kuschinsky, M. A. Moskowitz, and M. G. Hennerici. 2004. "Efficacy of sonothrombolysis in a rat model of embolic ischemic stroke." *Neuroscience Letters* 361 (1–3):115–9.
129. Hitchcock, K. E., N. M. Ivancevich, K. J. Haworth, D. N. Caudell Stamper, D. C. Vela, J. T. Sutton, G. J. Pyne-Geithman, and C. K. Holland. 2011. "Ultrasound-enhanced rt-PA thrombolysis in an ex vivo porcine carotid artery model." *Ultrasound in Medicine & Biology* 37 (8):1240–51.
130. Nacu, A., C. E. Kvistad, N. Logallo, H. Naess, U. Waje-Andreassen, A. H. Aamodt, R. Solhoff, C. Lund, H. Tobro, O. M. Ronning, R. Salvesen, T. T. Idicula, and L. Thomassen. 2015. "A pragmatic approach to sonothrombolysis in acute ischaemic stroke: The Norwegian randomised controlled sonothrombolysis in acute stroke study (NOR-SASS)." *BMC Neurology* 15:110.
131. Barlinn, K., G. Tsivgoulis, A. D. Barreto, J. Alleman, C. A. Molina, R. Mikulik, M. Saqqur, A. M. Demchuk, P. D. Schellinger, G. Howard, and A. V. Alexandrov. 2014. "Outcomes following sonothrombolysis in severe acute ischemic stroke: Subgroup analysis of the CLOTBUST trial." *International Journal of Stroke: Official Journal of the International Stroke Society* 9 (8):1006–10.
132. Eggers, J., I. R. Konig, B. Koch, G. Handler, and G. Seidel. 2008. "Sonothrombolysis with transcranial Colour-coded sonography and recombinant tissue-type plasminogen activator in acute middle cerebral artery main stem occlusion: Results from a randomized study." *Stroke; A Journal of Cerebral Circulation* 39 (5):1470–5.
133. Everbach, E. C., and C. W. Francis. 2000. "Cavitational mechanisms in ultrasound-accelerated thrombolysis at 1 MHz." *Ultrasound in Medicine and Biology* 26 (7):1153–60.
134. Chuang, Y. H., P. W. Cheng, and P. C. Li. 2013. "Combining radiation force with cavitation for enhanced sonothrombolysis." *IEEE Transactions on Ultrasonics, Ferroelectrics, and Frequency Control* 60 (1):97–104.
135. Bader, K. B., M. J. Gruber, and C. K. Holland. 2015. "Shaken and stirred: Mechanisms of ultrasound-enhanced thrombolysis." *Ultrasound in Medicine & Biology* 41 (1):187–96.
136. Kutty, S., J. Wu, J. M. Hammel, F. Xie, S. Gao, L. K. Drvol, J. Lof, S. J. Radio, S. L. Therrien, D. A. Danford, and T. R. Porter. 2012. "Microbubble mediated thrombus dissolution with diagnostic ultrasound for the treatment of chronic venous thrombi." *PloS One* 7 (12):e51453.
137. Barlinn, K., Z. Zivanovic, L. Zhao, M. Kesani, C. Balucani, G. Tsivgoulis, and A. V. Alexandrov. 2013. "Intracranial vessel localization with power motion Doppler (PMD-TCD) compared with CT angiography in patients with acute ischaemic stroke." *International Journal of Stroke: Official Journal of the International Stroke Society* 8 (6):398–402.
138. Holscher, T., R. Raman, K. Ernstrom, J. Parrish, D. T. Le, P. D. Lyden, and R. F. Mattrey. 2009. "In vitro sonothrombolysis with duplex ultrasound: First results using a simplified model." *Cerebrovascular Disease* 28 (4):365–70.

139. Eggers, J., S. Ossadnik, and G. Seidel. 2009. "Enhanced clot dissolution in vitro by 1.8-MHz pulsed ultrasound." *Ultrasound in Medicine & Biology* 35 (3):523–6.
140. Alexandrov, A. V., R. Mikulik, M. Ribo, V. K. Sharma, A. Y. Lao, G. Tsivgoulis, R. M. Sugg, A. Barreto, P. Sierzenski, M. D. Malkoff, and J. C. Grotta. 2008. "A pilot randomized clinical safety study of sonothrombolysis augmentation with ultrasound-activated perflutren-lipid microspheres for acute ischemic stroke." *Stroke; A Journal of Cerebral Circulation* 39 (5):1464–9.
141. Nedelmann, M., N. Ritschel, S. Doenges, A. C. Langheinrich, T. Acker, P. Reuter, M. Yeniguen, J. Pukropski, M. Kaps, C. Mueller, G. Bachmann, and T. Gerriets. 2010. "Combined contrast-enhanced ultrasound and rt-PA treatment is safe and improves impaired microcirculation after reperfusion of middle cerebral artery occlusion." *Journal of Cerebral Blood Flow and Metabolism: Official Journal of the International Society of Cerebral Blood Flow and Metabolism* 30 (10):1712–20.
142. Meairs, S., R. Kern, and A. Alonso. 2012. "Why and how do microbubbles enhance the effectiveness of diagnostic and therapeutic interventions in cerebrovascular disease?" *Current Pharmaceutical Design* 18 (15):2223–35.
143. Laing, S. T., M. R. Moody, H. Kim, B. Smulevitz, S. L. Huang, C. K. Holland, D. D. McPherson, and M. E. Klegerman. 2012. "Thrombolytic efficacy of tissue plasminogen activator-loaded echogenic liposomes in a rabbit thrombus model." *Thrombosis Research* 130 (4):629–35.
144. Parikh, S., A. Motarjeme, T. McNamara, R. Raabe, K. Hagspiel, J. F. Benenati, K. Sterling, and A. Comerota. 2008. "Ultrasound-accelerated thrombolysis for the treatment of deep vein thrombosis: Initial clinical experience." *Journal of Vascular and Interventional Radiology: JVIR* 19 (4):521–8.
145. Dumantepe, M., I. A. Tarhan, and A. Ozler. 2013. "Treatment of chronic deep vein thrombosis using ultrasound accelerated catheter-directed thrombolysis." *European Journal of Vascular and Endovascular Surgery* 46 (3): 366–71.
146. Rosenschein, U., A. Roth, T. Rassin, S. Basan, S. Laniado, and H. I. Miller. 1997. "Analysis of coronary ultrasound thrombolysis endpoints in acute myocardial." *Circulation* 95 (6):1411–6.
147. Rosenschein, U., V. Furman, E. Kerner, I. Fabian, J. Bernheim, and Y. Eshel. 2000. "Ultrasound imaging-guided noninvasive ultrasound thrombolysis: Preclinical results." *Circulation* 102 (2):238–45.
148. Schafer, S., S. Kliner, L. Klinghammer, H. Kaarmann, I. Lucic, U. Nixdorff, U. Rosenschein, W. G. Daniel, and F. A. Flachskampf. 2005. "Influence of ultrasound operating parameters on ultrasound-induced thrombolysis in vitro." *Ultrasound in Medicine & Biology* 31 (6):841–7.
149. Wright, C. C., K. Hynynen, and D. E. Goertz. 2012. "Pulsed focused ultrasound-induced displacements in confined in vitro blood clots." *IEEE Transactions on Bio-medical Engineering* 59 (3):842–51.
150. Wright, C., K. Hynynen, and D. Goertz. 2012. "In vitro and in vivo high-intensity focused ultrasound thrombolysis." *Investigative Radiology* 47 (4):217–25.
151. Burgess, A., Y. Huang, A. C. Waspe, M. Ganguly, D. E. Goertz, and K. Hynynen. 2012. "High-intensity focused ultrasound (HIFU) for dissolution of clots in a rabbit model of embolic stroke." *PloS One* 7 (8):e42311.
152. Maxwell, A. D., S. Park, B. L. Vaughan, C. A. Cain, J. B. Grotberg, and Z. Xu. 2014. "Trapping of embolic particles in a vessel phantom by cavitation-enhanced acoustic streaming." *Physics in Medicine and Biology* 59 (17):4927–43.
153. Park, S., A. D. Maxwell, G. E. Owens, H. S. Gurm, C. A. Cain, and Z. Xu. 2013. "Non-invasive embolus trap using histotripsy-an acoustic parameter study." *Ultrasound in Medicine & Biology* 39 (4):611–9.
154. Zhang, X., G. Owens, H. S. Gurm, Y. Ding, C. Cain, and Z. Xu. 2015. "Non-invasive thrombolysis using histotripsy beyond the 'intrinsic' threshold (microtripsy)." "International Society for Therapeutic Ultrasound Symposium, Utrecht, Netherlands, April 15–18.
155. Sutton, J. T., N. M. Ivancevich, S. R. Perrin, Jr., D. C. Vela, and C. K. Holland. 2013. "Clot retraction affects the extent of ultrasound-enhanced thrombolysis in an ex vivo porcine thrombosis model." *Ultrasound in Medicine & Biology* 39 (5):813–24.
156. Zhou, Y., S. K. Murugappan, and V. K. Sharma. 2014. "Effect of clot aging and cholesterol content on ultrasound-assisted thrombolysis." *Translational Stroke Research* 5 (5):627–34.
157. Cline, H. E., K. Hynynen, C. J. Hardy, R. D. Watkins, J. F. Schenck, and F. A. Jolesz. 1994. "MR temperature mapping of focused ultrasound surgery." *Magnetic Resonance in Medicine* 31 (6):628–36.

158. Elias, W. J., D. Huss, T. Voss, J. Loomba, M. Khaled, E. Zadicario, R. C. Frysinger, S. A. Sperling, S. Wylie, S. J. Monteith, J. Druzgal, B. B. Shah, M. Harrison, and M. Wintermark. 2013. "A pilot study of focused ultrasound thalamotomy for essential tremor." *The New England Journal of Medicine* 369 (7):640–8.
159. McDannold, N., C. Tempany, F. Jolesz, and K. Hynynen. 2008. "Evaluation of referenceless thermometry in MRI-guided focused ultrasound surgery of uterine fibroids." *Journal of Magnetic Resonance Imaging: JMRI* 28 (4):1026–32.
160. Quesson, B., C. Laurent, G. Maclair, B. D. de Senneville, C. Mougenot, M. Ries, T. Carteret, A. Rullier, and C. Moonen. 2011. "Real-time volumetric MRI thermometry of focused ultrasound ablation in vivo: A feasibility study in pig liver and kidney." *NMR in Biomedicine* 24 (2):145–53.
161. Jolesz, F., K. Hynynen, N. McDannold, and C. Tempany. 2005. "MR imaging-controlled focused ultrasound ablation: A noninvasive image-guided surgery." *Magnetic Resonance Imaging Clinics of North America* 13 (3):545–60.
162. Wan, H., J. Aarsvold, M. O'Donnell, and C. Cain. 1999. "Thermal dose optimization for ultrasound tissue ablation." *IEEE Transactions on Ultrasonics, Ferroelectrics, and Frequency Control* 46 (4):913–28.

28

Focused Ultrasound Ablation Enhancement of Specific Antitumour Immunity

Rodi Abdalkader and Mitsuru Hashida

28.1 Introduction

Cancer is considered to be a major health concern around the world. Malignant cells occupy specific tissues, leading to uncontrolled growth and to metastasis, formed when cancer cells migrate from the primary site to other, distant, organs.[1] When this occurs, treatment becomes difficult and patient survival is reduced.[2] To make things more complex, cancer cells can escape from the immune system's surveillance.[3] This is because these cells are derived originally from the body's own, normal, cells, and are therefore recognised as 'self'. The principle of immunotherapy is the activation of the immune system against these cancer cells. The immune system is divided into innate and adaptive cells. Cells of the innate system, such as natural killers (NKs), are non-antigen specific and can initiate fast reactions against cancer cells, causing cell lysis and the production of cytokines that inhibit tumour growth. The adaptive cells of the immune system include B and T lymphocytes, and these are antigen-specific cells. After being activated with antigens, B lymphocytes induce humoral immunity mediated by the production of antibodies, while T lymphocytes induce cellular immunity.[4, 5] To induce an immune response in cancer, tumour-associated antigens (TAAs) must be collected by dendritic cells (DCs). These are essential antigen-presenting cells (APCs). TAAs may exist in situ endogenously, or even, by administration exogenously. DCs then process the antigen to small pieces of peptides, which are presented on the major histocompatibility complex (MHC) class I and II. After receiving a maturation signal, dendritic cells can then migrate to the lymphoid tissues to elicit T-cell effectors (cytotoxic T cells $CD8^+$ and T helper $CD4^+$) that are important for the suppression of tumour progression.[6, 7] DCs will also induce a tolerance signal which leads to the depletion of T cells, and the activation of regulatory T cells (T_{reg}).[8, 9]

Ultrasound (US) is best known for its use in the medical field for diagnostic imaging.[10] In therapy, US can be used for various applications depending on the applied energy. High intensity focused ultrasound (HIFU) is mainly used for tumour ablation. This uses an external transducer that can generate a focal intensity of a few thousand W cm^{-2}. The ultrasound beam passes through the intact skin and is then concentrated in one region, which may be deep inside an organ, causing no damage to the surrounding tissues. The acoustic absorption in the focal volume leads to a temperature which can range from 60 to 95 °C. This temperature rise causes protein denaturation and coagulative necrosis in the tissue.[11, 12] However, cellular damage may also be caused by the mechanical effects of HIFU. In this case, pulsed ultrasound with low duty cycle (ranging from 1% to 5 %) is used. Unlike thermal HIFU, mechanical HIFU may not cause homogeneous cell lysis.[13] It has been suggested that mechanical HIFU mainly disrupts the cell membrane caused by effects that include acoustic cavitation, radiation force, shear stress, and acoustic streaming.[14] Early applications of HIFU included the targeted therapy of diseases of the central nervous system and some ophthalmic disorders.[15] HIFU tumour ablation therapy has recently become more common, as it has been recognised clinically for several tumour types, including those of the prostate, pancreas, liver, and breast.[16] All treatments are non-ionising and are carried out noninvasively, in contrast to other ablative therapies such as cryotherapy, radiofrequency, laser, and microwave.

DOI: 10.1201/9780429162671-28

In the drug delivery field, US has mainly been used in combination with gas-containing carriers such as micro- or nano-bubbles, usually filled with perfluorocarbons.[17, 18] Both focused and unfocused US can be used in these applications, with intensities of several W cm^{-2}. The combination with US has been found to improve the delivery of therapeutic compounds such as anticancer drugs and nucleic acids when combined or co-administered with these bubbles.[19–21] The effects are attributed to acoustic streaming effects and to cavitation forces that are associated with micro/nano bubbles during their interaction with an US wave.[22] Recently, it has been reported that US irradiation alone, or in combination with some micro/nano bubbles, could boost immunity against cancer.[23, 24] Therefore, in this chapter, we will discuss the role of US in harnessing cancer immunity. We will also focus on drug delivery system (DDS) aspects and discuss a new advanced material that has been found to be useful in enhancing immunity when combined with US irradiation.

28.2 Potential Mechanisms

In general, ablation therapy damages tumour tissue, leading to the formation of cellular debris. Tumour specific-antigens found in the debris can be collected by APCs such as DCs. For example, ablated tumour debris found in cryo-, laser, and radiofrequency ablation has been found to be a potent antigen source for DCs.[25] In principle, HIFU induces cell damage in the irradiated tumour in a way similar to that with other ablation therapies. Therefore, it may be expected that HIFU ablation therapy could elicit similar effects on tumour immunity. The theory of Matzinger suggests that cellular damage could initiate a danger response that, in return, can activate the immune system.[26, 27] HIFU, in both thermal and non-thermal (mechanical) modes, can cause cellular damage and thus it can provoke the release of danger signals which play a key role in activating APCs. Unlike thermal HIFU, mechanical HIFU causes cell membrane disruption with no protein denaturation. Endogenous danger signals can therefore be maintained, and this may explain the high efficacy in switching on APCs.[13, 24] In particular, a family of heat shock proteins (HSPs) are suspected to be behind the activation of tumour immunity post-HIFU ablation. In general, the expression of HSPs is increased when cells are exposed to heat or mechanical damage, oxidative stress, infection, or ischemia conditions. HSPs have been found to act as carriers of antigenic peptides derived from tumour or infectious cells.[28] It has also been reported that HSP–peptide complexes can be attached to MHC class I and then be internalised by receptor-mediated uptake on the surface of APCs. Consequently, APCs go through a maturation phase, and act later on the activation of T cytotoxic lymphocytes.[29, 30] The signal transducer and activator of transcription 3 (STAT3) was decreased after HIFU ablation. STAT3 is a critical factor in promoting tumourigenesis, in addition to its role in suppressing tumour immunity by inhibiting the expression of pro-inflammatory cytokines such as IL-12 and TNF-α, or by enhancing the expression of other immunosuppressive cytokines such as IL-10. More critically, STAT3 activation has a direct impact on DC differentiation and maturation which can lead to T cell tolerance.[31] However, the key molecules that moderate the delivery of tumour-specific peptides to APCs are still not well studied.

28.3 Pre-clinical Results

In one of the earliest reports, Yang et al. suggested that antitumour immunity could be enhanced after ablation with HIFU. In this study, a neuroblastoma tumour model was treated with HIFU. The treatment significantly prolonged survival. Tumour growth was also significantly inhibited after re-challenging the animals with a second inoculation of tumour cells.[32] In another study, HIFU ablation was performed in a murine model of H22 hepatocellular carcinoma.[33] After treatment, tumour debris from HIFU ablated animals was processed to generate a vaccine (HIFU vaccine). Interestingly, the HIFU vaccine induced significant and specific cytotoxic T-lymphocyte (CTL) cytotoxicity only in H22 cells. When vaccinated mice were challenged by H22 cell inoculation, tumour growth was significantly inhibited for 4 weeks using the HIFU vaccine compared to controls, or the ordinary tumour vaccine. Moreover, the incubation of immature DCs extracted from naïve mice with HIFU vaccine or with tumour vaccine increased the expression of MHC class II, CD80, and CD86, indicating the activation and maturation of DCs.

As mentioned earlier, HIFU can induce mechanical effects as well as thermal effects. Hu and co-workers investigated the effects of both mechanical and thermal HIFU on the activation of APCs in an in vitro setting using MC-38 tumour cells. Cells treated with mechanical HIFU had increased activation of APCs compared to thermal HIFU. Similarly to the study of Yang et al., the exposure of MC-38 tumour cell debris to DCs induced greater expression of CD80 and CD86. When exposed to mouse macrophages, the level of TNF-α was significantly increased compared to cells treated with 'thermal' HIFU. Based on these findings, it has been suggested that mechanical HIFU is more efficient at boosting immunity than thermal HIFU, presumably because of the widespread damage caused by thermal HIFU, that leads to the denaturation of some functional proteins such as HSPs.[13, 30] The findings discussed earlier were further investigated in an in vivo murine model of melanoma. Xing and colleagues evaluated the effects of both mechanical and thermal HIFU on increasing the risk of distant metastasis after excision of the primary tumour.[34] The extent of metastasis was significantly reduced in the group of animals having their tumour removed 2 days after HIFU ablation. CTL activity was also considerably increased when the splenocytes were exposed to B16 melanoma cells, implying that a specific immunity was formed against B16 melanoma cells. In addition, survival time was prolonged compared to the control groups. These results confirm that HIFU ablation, preferably mechanically produced, can provoke immunity against tumour progression, including distant metastasis. Huang et al. showed that mechanical HIFU could suppress STAT3 in a murine model of prostate tumour.[35] The decrease in the level of STAT3 was consistent with a significant increase in DC populations in mechanical HIFU-treated animals. A summary of these results and the US parameters used is shown in Table 28.1.

TABLE. 28.1

Overall summary of pre-clinical and clinical investigations related to the role of US ablation in harnessing tumour immunity

Tumour	Species	US parameters	Results	Ref.
1 Neuroblastoma (C1300)	Mice (Ajax)	4 MHz 550 W cm^{-2}	↓Tumour volume, ↑Survival	(32)
2 Hepatocellular carcinoma H22	Mice (C57BL/6J)	9.5 MHz 5W	↑CTL , ↑IL-12, ↑INF-γ, ↓Tumour volume, ↑Survival	(33)
3 Melanoma (B16F10)	Mice (C57BL/6J)	3.3 MHz	Mechanical HIFU: ↓ Metastasis, ↓CTL, ↑ Survival Thermal HIFU: ↓ Metastasis, ↓CTL, ↑ Survival	(34)
4 Murine prostate cancer (RM-9)	Mice (C57BL/6J)	3.3 MHz, 60 W	↓ STAT3, ↑CTL, ↑CD8+, ↑CD11c+ ↓Treg, ↓Tumour volume, ↑Survival	(35)
5 Osteosarcoma, Hepatocellular carcinoma, Renal cell carcinoma	Human	0.8 MHz (5000–20000) W cm^{-2}	↑ CD4+, ↑ CD4+/CD8+	(36)
6 Osteosarcoma, Hepatocellular carcinoma	Human	0.8 MHz (5000–20000) W cm^{-2}	↓ IL-6, ↓ VEGF, ↓ TGF-ß1, ↓ TGF-ß2 (In non metastatic patients)	(37)
7 Breast cancer	Human	1.6 MHz (5000–15000) W cm^{-2}	↑CD3+, ↑CD4+, ↑CD8+, ↑CD20+, ↑CD57+ ↑CTLs and NK, ↑Fas-ligand ↑Granzyme, ↑Perforin	(38)
8 Prostate cancer	Human	4 MHz (1260–2200) W cm-2	↑HSP72, ↑HSP73, ↑GRP75 ↑IL-2, ↑INF-γ, ↑TNF-α	(39)

28.4 Clinical Results

Wu and colleagues have investigated the possibility of immune activation after HIFU ablation in patients with different types of tumours. Among this patient population, some had metastasis prior to HIFU therapy. At 7 and 0 days post-treatment, peripheral blood was collected from patients, and T lymphocytes, B lymphocytes, and NK levels were measured. Significant increases in helper T cell $CD4^+$ and in the ratio of T helper/T suppressor ($CD4^+$/$CD8^+$) were observed post-treatment, indicating that an antitumour immunity had been activated.[36] In another study, patients with osteosarcoma and hepatocellular carcinoma were treated with HIFU, and several immunosuppressive cytokines such as VEGF, TGF-ß1, TGF-ß2, IL-6, and IL-10 in the serum were measured 1 week before and after HIFU ablation. The study also investigated metastasis among those patients who had already been diagnosed with distant metastasis. In nonmetastatic patients, a significant decrease in almost all immunosuppressive cytokines was noticed. However, metastatic patients had a higher level of immunosuppressive cytokines than nonmetastatic patients. These results could imply that provoking cancer immunity through HIFU ablation may not be sufficient in metastatic patients with aggressive tumours whose cytokine level is already high.[37] Lu and colleagues investigated the effects of HIFU ablation on activating tumour infiltrating lymphocytes (TILs) in patients with breast tumours. Mastectomy was performed 7–14 days post-HIFU ablation. TIL infiltration into tumour was increased in the HIFU treated group, with $CD3^+$ and helper $CD4^+$ being highest, followed by cytotoxic $CD8^+$. TILs were found to be located alongside the immune fibroblasts, new capillaries, and other inflammatory cells, thus confirming that infiltration of lymphocytes into the tumour from the periphery happened post-HIFU ablation.[38] In addition, Kramer and colleagues reported a significant increase in HSPs and glucose-regulated protein (GRP75) expression in patients with prostate cancer post-HIFU. Th1 cytokines (TNF-α, IL-2, and IFN-γ) were also significantly elevated.[39] For more experimental details, see Table 28.1.

28.5 Expert Commentary

28.5.1 Tumour Immunity Induction with US in Combination with Micro/Nano Bubbles

The co-treatment of gas bubbles with US accelerates the efficacy of US irradiation due to their strong cavitation capability.[40, 41] It has been reported that the co-treatment of HIFU with microbubbles (MBs) increases heat generation and thus the necrosis rate in ablated tissue compared to HIFU alone.[42, 43] Moreover, Farny et al. observed a correlation between cavitation power and heat generation. It was suggested that inertial cavitation could lead to temperature elevation.[44] In fact, the high intensities involved in HIFU may not always be beneficial for therapy, and in some cases such as in brain tumour treatments, HIFU may be of limited use. Low-intensity US in combination with MBs may be a useful alternative. Cavitation effects associated with MBs can disturb tumour vascularity without causing excessive heat.[45] For example, low-pressure amplitude focused US (FUS) in combination with conventional MBs such as Sonovue have induced antitumour immunity in mice. After treatment, tumour infiltrated $CD8^+$ and $CD4^+$ were significantly increased and an up-regulation in HSP expression levels in tumour was also noticed.[46] Suzuki et al. also reported that an intratumoural injection of NBs in combination with low-intensity US in colon 26 tumour-bearing mice led to a significant increase in the temperature in the tumour. Additionally, extensive necrosis was induced and tumour growth was inhibited. The in vivo depletion of $CD8^+$ cells completely blocked the effect of NBs with US on tumour suppression, indicating that $CD8^+$ cells are involved in the tumour inhibition mechanism after treatment involving NBs and US.[47]

28.5.2 Improving the Delivery of Immune Modulators by US Assisted by Targeted Nano Bubbles

DNA vaccine is considered to be a promising strategy for inducing specific tumour immunity. In this method, an exogenous gene that encodes specific cancer antigens can induce both humoral and cellular

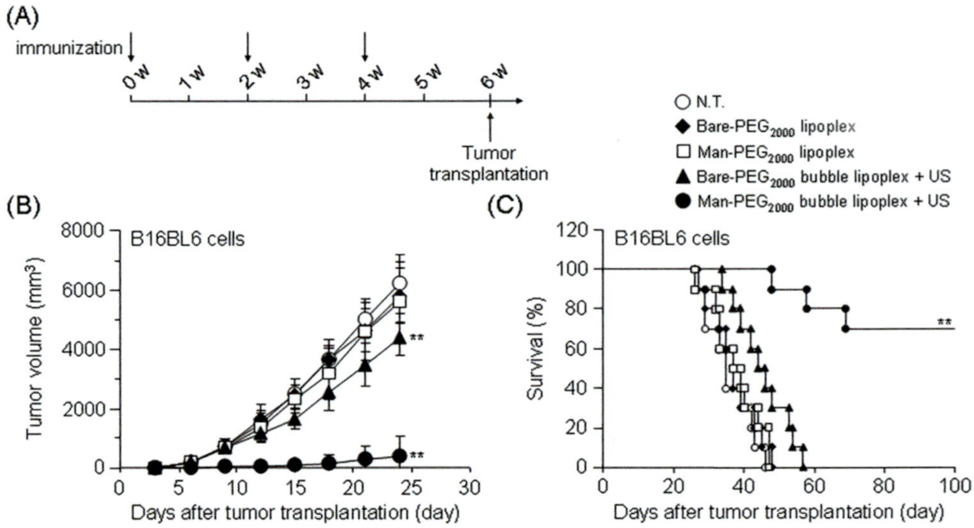

FIGURE 28.1 Cancer vaccine effects against solid tumours by DNA vaccination using Man-PEG2000 bubble lipoplexes and US exposure. (A) Schedule of therapeutic experiments in solid tumours. (B, C) The suppressing effects of tumour growth against solid tumours (B) and the prolongation of survival in tumour-transplanted mice (C) by DNA vaccination using Bare-PEG2000 lipoplexes, Man-PEG2000 lipoplexes, Bare-PEG2000 bubble lipoplexes with US exposure and Man-PEG2000 bubble lipoplexes with US exposure (50 μg of pDNA).

immunity.[48, 49] However, plasmid DNA is unstable in vivo and rapidly disappears from the circulation. Selective targeting and protection of pDNA is therefore critical for sufficient delivery into APCs. Cationic lipoplex modified with sugar ligand moieties, such as mannose, was found to be taken up selectively by APCs in the spleen due to the high levels of mannose receptor expression by the APCs there.[50–52] Here, a complex of DNA vaccine and mannose-modified lipoplex was reported to enhance cancer immunisation efficiency specifically in dendritic cells and macrophages with clear cytotoxic potential against melanoma.[53, 54]

Based on these findings, Un and colleagues developed a nano-sized US-responsive bubble lipoplex modified with mannose ligands. This formulation had 2 advantages: Firstly, selective targeting to APCs by mannose ligand recognition. Secondly, the direct internalisation of the DNA vaccine into the cytosol of APCs avoids the endocytotic pathway, and thus the immunisation yield was significantly improved. Specific Th1 cytokines such as IL-2 and IF-ɤ were significantly increased, and higher CTL activity was also noticed. Immunisation lasted 80 days after the first shot in mice treated with mannose bubble lipoplex with US irradiation.[55] Successful DNA vaccination was also achieved by delivering pDNA that encode genes of melanoma-specific antigens, such as gp100 and TRP-2, to dendritic cells specifically.[56] Potent DNA vaccination was obtained when mannose-modified bubble lipoplex was applied in combination with US, and immunisation was significant for at least 100 days post-immunisation against B16BL6 murine melanoma (see Figure 28.1).

28.5.3 Future Aspects of Some Advanced Materials

Novel formulations may also improve the ability of US to induce tumour immunity. For example, phase shift acoustic nanodroplets (PSANDs), which are emulsions that contain liquid perfluorocarbons, have recently been reported.[57, 58] PSANDs are characterised by their relatively small size (around 200 nm) compared to microbubbles. Under the effects of an ultrasound pressure wave, liquid perfluorocarbons shift from liquid to gas phase. This process leads to the formation of micron sized bubbles that can be clearly imaged by ultrasonography.[59–61] Interestingly, in an in vitro phantom, PSANDs in combination with HIFU were found to accelerate heat generation, due to bubble cavitation, and the energy needed for forming a lesion was significantly decreased.[41, 62]

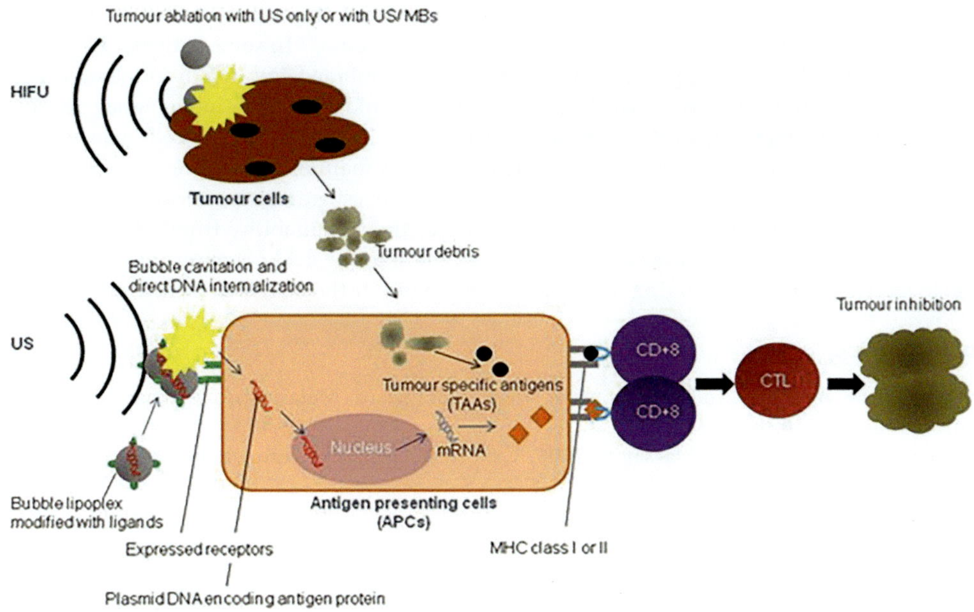

FIGURE 28.2 An illustration of the role of US in harnessing tumour immunity.

For example, lipid-based PSANDs can function as a theranostic dual modality where nanodroplets can emit heat upon exposure to US irradiation as well as the generation of a contrast signal that can be detected with ultrasonography. It has been shown that the intra-tumour injection of these PSANDs in combination with US irradiation can induce thermal emission in situ in B16BL6 melanoma tumour implanted into mice in areas that mostly covered the tumour site leading to the inhibition of the tumour growth as well as the significant upregulation of heat shock protein (HSP70).[63]

More recently, single-wall carbon nanotubes (SWCNTs) have shown great impact in tumour thermal ablation, when combined with near-infrared irradiation (NIR). The large area of these SWCNTs provides numerous possibilities for a variety of chemical modifications that may serve as a platform for drug and gene loading. SWCNTs in the tumour can absorb the energy received from NIR efficiently, leading to tissue necrosis and tumour suppression.[64] It was found also that heat shock proteins, such as HSP70, could be raised after tumour ablation in their presence with DNA having CpG motif.[65] Although there is still limited information about the possibility of the combination of these carriers with HIFU, the use of SWCNT as a US contrast agent further suggests the possibility of the combination of SWCNTs and US.[66] In terms of future potential, this method may provide a novel alternative in which SWCNTs could play the role of the thermal base to give sufficient coagulative necrosis with low US intensities as well as PSANDs.

28.6 Summary

US has shown great promise in harnessing cancer immunity, alone or in a combination with micro- or nano-sized bubbles. Tumour ablation with US has been the main interest in therapy. However, recently it has become clear that US could also function in many other ways in addition to causing thermal damage at the tumour site (see Figure 28.2). Preclinical studies in different murine tumour models strongly indicate that tumour immunity may be significantly stimulated after US ablation, compared with conventional cancer vaccines.[33] Two US interaction methods have been investigated: thermal and mechanical. The mechanical mode of US was found to be more effective in producing tumour immunity.[13]

Moreover, clinical studies have suggested an increase in cytotoxic T lymphocytes after US ablation in several patients, mostly those with breast cancer or hepatocarcinoma.[37] In some patients, T-lymphocyte infiltration into the tumour was significantly increased.[38] US combined with micro- or nano-sized bubbles also provides a new alternative in which low-intensity US could be used for inducing specific tumour immunity due to the cavitation effects. Moreover, specific targeting towards APCs cells may be achieved by modifying nano-sized bubbles with sugar moieties, such as mannose, for more efficient delivery of DNA vaccines to APCs.[55] This field is relatively new, and more investigations are needed, especially those related to determining the mechanisms involved and the clinical suitability from efficacy and safety viewpoints.[67] Collectively, US may make a useful contribution to the field of cancer immunotherapy, in addition to its critical role in providing novel delivery methods for the field of drug delivery.

REFERENCES

1. Brabletz, Thomas. 2012. 'To Differentiate or Not-Routes towards Metastasis.' *Nature Reviews Cancer* 12 (6): 425–436. doi:10.1038/nrc3265.
2. Gupta, Gaorav P., and Joan Massagué. 2006. 'Cancer Metastasis: Building a Framework.' *Cell* 127 (4): 679–695. doi:10.1016/j.cell.2006.11.001.
3. Cavallo, Federica, Carla De Giovanni, Patrizia Nanni, Guido Forni, and Pier Luigi Lollini. 2011. '2011: The Immune Hallmarks of Cancer.' *Cancer Immunology, Immunotherapy* 60 (3):319–326. doi:10.1007/s00262-010-0968-0.
4. Blattman, Joseph N., and Philip D. Greenberg. 2004. 'Cancer Immunotherapy: A Treatment for the Masses.' *Science (New York, N.Y.)* 305 (5681): 200–205. doi:10.1126/science.1100369.
5. Maruyama, Kouji, Zohair Selmani, Hidee Ishii, and Ken Yamaguchi. 2011. 'Innate Immunity and Cancer Therapy.' *International Immunopharmacology* 11 (3): 350–357. doi:10.1016/j.intimp.2010.09.012.
6. Mellman, Ira, and Ralph M. Steinman. 2001. 'Dendritic Cells.' *Cell* 106 (3) (August): 255–258. doi:10.1016/S0092-8674(01)00449-4.
7. Trombetta, E. Sergio, and Ira Mellman. 2005. 'Cell Biology of Antigen Processing in Vitro and in Vivo.' *Annual Review of Immunology* 23: 975–1028. doi:10.1146/annurev.immunol.22.012703.104538.
8. Steinman, Ralph M., Daniel Hawiger, and Michel C. Nussenzweig. 2003. 'Tolerogenic Dendritic Cells.' *Annual Review of Immunology* 21: 685–711. doi:10.1146/annurev.immunol.21.120601.141040
9. Darrasse-Jèze, Guillaume, Stephanie Deroubaix, Hugo Mouquet, Gabriel D Victora, Thomas Eisenreich, Kai-hui Yao, Revati F. Masilamani, et al. 2009. 'Feedback Control of Regulatory T Cell Homeostasis by Dendritic Cells in Vivo.' *The Journal of Experimental Medicine* 206 (9): 1853–1862. doi:10.1084/jem.20090746
10. Lencioni, Riccardo, Fabio Piscaglia, and Luigi Bolondi. 2008. 'Contrast-Enhanced Ultrasound in the Diagnosis of Hepatocellular Carcinoma.' *Journal of Hepatology* 48 (5): 848–857. doi:10.1016/j.jhep.2008.02.005.
11. ter Haar, Gail, and Constantin Coussios. 2007. 'High Intensity Focused Ultrasound: Physical Principles and Devices.' *International Journal of Hyperthermia : The Official Journal of European Society for Hyperthermic Oncology, North American Hyperthermia Group* 23 (2): 89–104. doi:10.1080/02656730601186138.
12. Al-Bataineh, Osama, Jürgen Jenne, and Peter Huber. 2012. 'Clinical and Future Applications of High Intensity Focused Ultrasound in Cancer.' *Cancer Treatment Reviews* 38 (5): 346–353. doi:10.1016/j.ctrv.2011.08.004.
13. Hu, Zhenlin, Yi Yang Xiao, Yunbo Liu, Michael A. Morse, H. Kim Lyerly, Timothy M. Clay, and Pei Zhong. 2005. 'Release of Endogenous Danger Signals from HIFU-Treated Tumour Cells and Their Stimulatory Effects on APCs.' *Biochemical and Biophysical Research Communications* 335 (1): 124–131. doi:10.1016/j.bbrc.2005.07.071.
14. Jang, H. J., J. Y. Lee, D. H. Lee, W. H. Kim, and J. H. Hwang. 2010. 'Current and Future Clinical Applications of High-Intensity Focused Ultrasound (HIFU) for Pancreatic Cancer.' *Gut Liver* 4 Suppl 1 (1976–2283 (Print)): S57–S61. doi:10.5009/gnl.2010.4.S1.S57.
15. Fry, W. J. 1954. 'Intense Ultrasound-A New Tool for Neurological Research.' *The British Journal of Psychiatry* 100 (418): 85–96. doi:10.1192/bjp.100.418.85.
16. Dogra, Vikram S., Man Zhang, and Shweta Bhatt. 2009. 'High-Intensity Focused Ultrasound (HIFU) Therapy Applications.' *Ultrasound Clinics* 4 (3): 307–321. doi:10.1016/j.cult.2009.10.005.

17. Suzuki, Ryo, Tomoko Takizawa, Yoichi Negishi, Naoki Utoguchi, and Kazuo Maruyama. 2008. 'Effective Gene Delivery with Novel Liposomal Bubbles and Ultrasonic Destruction Technology.' *International Journal of Pharmaceutics* 354: 49–55. doi:10.1016/j.ijpharm.2007.10.034.
18. Sirsi, Shashank R., and Mark A. Borden. 2012. 'Advances in Ultrasound Mediated Gene Therapy Using Microbubble Contrast Agents.' *Theranostics* 2 (12): 1208–1222. doi:10.7150/thno.4306.
19. Hernot, Sophie, and Alexander L. Klibanov. 2008. 'Microbubbles in Ultrasound-Triggered Drug and Gene Delivery.' *Advanced Drug Delivery Reviews* 60: 1153–1166. doi:10.1016/j.addr.2008.03.005.
20. Un, Keita, Shigeru Kawakami, Mitsuru Yoshida, Yuriko Higuchi, Ryo Suzuki, Kazuo Maruyama, Fumiyoshi Yamashita, and Mitsuru Hashida. 2011. 'The Elucidation of Gene Transferring Mechanism by Ultrasound-Responsive Unmodified and Mannose-Modified Lipoplexes.' *Biomaterials* 32 (20): 4659–4669. doi:10.1016/j.biomaterials.2011.03.013.
21. Abdalkader, Rodi, Shigeru Kawakami, Johan Unga, Ryo Suzuki, Kazuo Maruyama, Fumiyoshi Yamashita, and Mitsuru Hashida. 2015. 'Evaluation of the Potential of Doxorubicin Loaded Microbubbles as a Theranostic Modality Using a Murine Tumour Model.' *Acta Biomaterialia* 19: 112–118. doi:10.1016/j.actbio.2015.03.014.
22. Van Wamel, Annemieke, Klazina Kooiman, Miranda Harteveld, Marcia Emmer, Folkert J ten Cate, Michel Versluis, and Nico de Jong. 2006. 'Vibrating Microbubbles Poking Individual Cells: Drug Transfer into Cells via Sonoporation.' *Journal of Controlled Release* 112 (2): 149–155. doi:10.1016/j.jconrel.2006.02.007.
23. Wu, F. 2013. 'High Intensity Focused Ultrasound Ablation and Antitumour Immune Response.' *The Journal of the Acoustical Society of America* 134 (2): 1695–1701. doi:10.1121/1.4812893.
24. Unga, Johan, and Mitsuru Hashida. 2014. 'Ultrasound Induced Cancer Immunotherapy.' *Advanced Drug Delivery Reviews* 72: 144–153. doi:10.1016/j.addr.2014.03.004.
25. Den Brok, M. H. M. G. M., R. P. M. Sutmuller, S. Nierkens, E. J. Bennink, C. Frielink, L. W. J. Toonen, O. C. Boerman, C. G. Figdor, T. J. M. Ruers, and G. J. Adema. 2006. 'Efficient Loading of Dendritic Cells Following Cryo and Radiofrequency Ablation in Combination with Immune Modulation Induces Anti-Tumour Immunity.' *British Journal of Cancer* 95 (7): 896–905. doi:10.1038/sj.bjc.6603341.
26. Matzinger, Polly. 1994. 'Tolerance, Danger, and the Extended Family.' *Annual Review of Immunology* 12: 991–1045. doi:10.1146/annurev.iy.12.040194.005015.
27. Matzinger, Polly. 2002. 'The Danger Model: A Renewed Sense of Self.' *Science (New York, N.Y.)* 296 (5566): 301–305. doi:10.1126/science.1071059.
28. Wallin, R. P A, Andreas Lundqvist, Solveig H. Moré, Arne Von Bonin, Rolf Kiessling, and Hans Gustaf Ljunggren. 2002. 'Heat-Shock Proteins as Activators of the Innate Immune System.' *Trends in Immunology* 23 (3): 130–135. doi:10.1016/S1471-4906(01)02168-8.
29. Przepiorka, Donna, and Pramod K. Srivastava. 1998. 'Heat Shock Protein-Peptide Complexes as Immunotherapy for Human Cancer.' *Molecular Medicine Today* 4 (11): 478–484. doi:10.1016/S1357-4310(98)01345-8.
30. Chen, W., U. Syldath, K. Bellmann, V. Burkart, and H. Kolb. 1999. 'Human 60-kDa Heat-Shock Protein: A Danger Signal to the Innate Immune System.' *Journal of Immunology* 162 (6): 3212–3219.
31. Yu, Hua, and Richard Jove. 2004. 'The STATs of Cancer – New Molecular Targets Come of Age.' *Nature Reviews Cancer* 4 (2): 97–105. doi:10.1038/nrc1275.
32. Yang, Rong, Clarence R. Reilly, Frederick J. Rescorla, Narendra T. Sanghvi, Francis J. Fry, Thomas D. Franklin, and Jay L. Grosfeld. 1992. 'Effects of High-Intensity Focused Ultrasound in the Treatment of Experimental Neuroblastoma.' *Journal of Pediatric Surgery* 27 (2): 246–250. doi:10.1016/0022-3468(92)90321-W.
33. Zhang, Ying, Jian Deng, Jun Feng, and Feng Wu. 2010. 'Enhancement of Antitumour Vaccine in Ablated Hepatocellular Carcinoma by High-Intensity Focused Ultrasound.' *World Journal of Gastroenterology* 16 (28): 3584–3591. doi:10.3748/wjg.v16.i28.3584.
34. Xing, Yifei, Xiaochun Lu, Eric C. Pua, and Pei Zhong. 2008. 'The Effect of High Intensity Focused Ultrasound Treatment on Metastases in a Murine Melanoma Model.' *Biochemical and Biophysical Research Communications* 375 (4): 645–650. doi:10.1016/j.bbrc.2008.08.072.
35. Huang, Xiaoyi, Fang Yuan, Meihua Liang, Hui Wen Lo, Mari L. Shinohara, Cary Robertson, and Pei Zhong. 2012. 'M-HIFU Inhibits Tumour Growth, Suppresses STAT3 Activity and Enhances Tumour Specific Immunity in a Transplant Tumour Model of Prostate Cancer.' *PLoS ONE* 7 (7): e41632. doi:10.1371/journal.pone.0041632.

36. Wu, Feng, Zhi-Biao Wang, Pei Lu, Zhong-Li Xu, Wen-Zhi Chen, Hui Zhu, and Cheng-Bing Jin. 2004. 'Activated Anti-Tumour Immunity in Cancer Patients after High Intensity Focused Ultrasound Ablation.' *Ultrasound in Medicine & Biology* 30 (9): 1217–1222. doi:10.1016/j.ultrasmedbio.2004.08.003.
37. Zhou, Q., X. Q. Zhu, J. Zhang, Z. L. Xu, P. Lu, and F. Wu. 2008. 'Changes in Circulating Immunosuppressive Cytokine Levels of Cancer Patients after High Intensity Focused Ultrasound Treatment.' *Ultrasound in Medicine & Biology* 34 (1): 81–87. doi:10.1016/j.ultrasmedbio.2007.07.013.
38. Lu, Pei, Xue Qiang Zhu, Zhong Lin Xu, Qiang Zhou, Jun Zhang, and Feng Wu. 2009. 'Increased Infiltration of Activated Tumour-Infiltrating Lymphocytes after High Intensity Focused Ultrasound Ablation of Human Breast Cancer.' *Surgery* 145 (3): 286–293. doi:10.1016/j.surg.2008.10.010.
39. Kramer, Gero, Georg E. Steiner, Marion Gröbl, Kristian Hrachowitz, Franz Reithmayr, Ljubomir Paucz, Martin Newman, et al. 2004. 'Response to Sublethal Heat Treatment of Prostatic Tumour Cells and of Prostatic Tumour Infiltrating T-Cells.' *Prostate* 58 (2): 109–120. doi:10.1002/pros.10314.
40. Böhmer, M. R., C. H T Chlon, B. I. Raju, C. T. Chin, T. Shevchenko, and A. L. Klibanov. 2010. 'Focused Ultrasound and Microbubbles for Enhanced Extravasation.' *Journal of Controlled Release* 148: 18–24. doi:10.1016/j.jconrel.2010.06.012.
41. Umemura, Shin-ichiro, Shin Yoshizawa, Ryo Takagi, Yuta Inaba, and Jun Yasuda. 2013. 'Enhancement of Focused Ultrasound Treatment by Acoustically Generated Microbubbles.' *Japanese Journal of Applied Physics* 52 (7S): 07HA02. doi:10.7567/JJAP.52.07HA02. http://stacks.iop.org/1347-4065/52/07HA02.
42. Yu, Tinghe, Guoyun Wang, Kai Hu, Ping Ma, Jin Bai, and Zhibiao Wang. 2004. 'A Microbubble Agent Improves the Therapeutic Efficiency of High Intensity Focused Ultrasound: A Rabbit Kidney Study.' *Urological Research* 32 (1): 14–19. doi:10.1007/s00240-003-0362-x.
43. Kajiyama, K., K. Yoshinaka, S. Takagi, and Y. Matsumotod. 2010. 'Micro-Bubble Enhanced HIFU.' *Physics Procedia* 3 (1): 305–314. doi:10.1016/j.phpro.2010.01.041.
44. Farny, Caleb H., R. Glynn Holt, and Ronald A. Roy. 2010. 'The Correlation between Bubble-Enhanced HIFU Heating and Cavitation Power.' *IEEE Transactions on Biomedical Engineering* 57 (1): 175–184. doi:10.1109/TBME.2009.2028133.
45. Burke, Caitlin W., Alexander L. Klibanov, Jason P. Sheehan, and Richard J. Price. 2011. 'Inhibition of Glioma Growth by Microbubble Activation in a Subcutaneous Model Using Low Duty Cycle Ultrasound without Significant Heating.' *Journal of Neurosurgery* 114 (6): 1654–1661. doi:10.3171/2010.11.JNS101201.
46. Liu, Hao-Li, Han-Yi Hsieh, Li-An Lu, Chiao-Wen Kang, Ming-Fang Wu, and Chun-Yen Lin. 2012. 'Low-Pressure Pulsed Focused Ultrasound with Microbubbles Promotes an Anticancer Immunological Response.' *Journal of Translational Medicine* 10: 221. doi:10.1186/1479-5876-10-221.
47. Suzuki, Ryo, Yusuke Oda, Daiki Omata, Norihito Nishiie, Risa Koshima, Yasuyuki Shiono, Yoshikazu Sawaguchi, et al. 2015. 'Tumour Growth Suppression by the Combination of Nanobubbles and Ultrasound.' *Cancer Science*: n/a–n/a. doi:10.1111/cas.12867.
48. Condon, C., S. C. Watkins, C. M. Celluzzi, K. Thompson, and L. D. Falo. 1996. 'DNA-Based Immunization by in Vivo Transfection of Dendritic Cells.' *Nature Medicine* 2 (10): 1122–1128. doi:10.1038/nm1096-1122.
49. Rice, Jason, Christian H. Ottensmeier, and Freda K. Stevenson. 2008. 'DNA Vaccines: Precision Tools for Activating Effective Immunity against Cancer.' *Nature Reviews Cancer* 8 (2): 108–120. doi:10.1038/nrc2326.
50. Kawakami, S., A. Sato, M. Nishikawa, F. Yamashita, and M. Hashida. 2000. 'Mannose Receptor-Mediated Gene Transfer into Macrophages Using Novel Mannosylated Cationic Liposomes.' *Gene Therapy* 7 (4): 292–299. doi:10.1038/sj.gt.3301089.
51. Hattori, Yoshiyuki, Sachiko Suzuki, Shigeru Kawakami, Fumiyoshi Yamashita, and Mitsuru Hashida. 2005. 'The Role of Dioleoylphosphatidylethanolamine (DOPE) in Targeted Gene Delivery with Mannosylated Cationic Liposomes via Intravenous Route.' *Journal of Controlled Release* 108 (2–3): 484–495. doi:10.1016/j.jconrel.2005.08.012.
52. Ueki, Akiharu, Keita Un, Yuka Mino, Mitsuru Yoshida, Shigeru Kawakami, Hiromune Ando, Hideharu Ishida, Fumiyoshi Yamashita, Mitsuru Hashida, and Makoto Kiso. 2014. 'Synthesis and Evaluation of Glyco-Coated Liposomes as Drug Carriers for Active Targeting in Drug Delivery Systems.' *Carbohydrate Research* 405: 78–86. doi:10.1016/j.carres.2014.06.028.
53. Hattori, Yoshiyuki, Shigeru Kawakami, Yan Lu, Kazumi Nakamura, Fumiyoshi Yamashita, and Mitsuru Hashida. 2006. 'Enhanced DNA Vaccine Potency by Mannosylated Lipoplex after Intraperitoneal Administration.' *Journal of Gene Medicine* 8 (7): 824–834. doi:10.1002/jgm.910.

54. Lu, Yan, Shigeru Kawakami, Fumiyoshi Yamashita, and Mitsuru Hashida. 2007. 'Development of an Antigen-Presenting Cell-Targeted DNA Vaccine against Melanoma by Mannosylated Liposomes.' *Biomaterials* 28 (21): 3255–3262. doi:10.1016/j.biomaterials.2007.03.028.
55. Un, Keita, Shigeru Kawakami, Ryo Suzuki, Kazuo Maruyama, Fumiyoshi Yamashita, and Mitsuru Hashida. 2010. 'Development of an Ultrasound-Responsive and Mannose-Modified Gene Carrier for DNA Vaccine Therapy.' *Biomaterials* 31: 7813–7826. doi:10.1016/j.biomaterials.2010.06.058.
56. Un, Keita, Shigeru Kawakami, Ryo Suzuki, Kazuo Maruyama, Fumiyoshi Yamashita, and Mitsuru Hashida. 2011. 'Suppression of Melanoma Growth and Metastasis by DNA Vaccination Using an Ultrasound-Responsive and Mannose-Modified Gene Carrier.' *Molecular Pharmaceutics* 8 (2): 543–554. doi:10.1021/mp100369n.
57. Reznik, Nikita, Ross Williams, and Peter N. Burns. 2011. 'Investigation of Vaporized Submicron Perfluorocarbon Droplets as an Ultrasound Contrast Agent.' *Ultrasound in Medicine and Biology* 37 (8): 1271–1279. doi:10.1016/j.ultrasmedbio.2011.05.001.
58. Sheeran, Paul S., and Paul A. Dayton. 2014. 'Improving the Performance of Phase-Change Perfluorocarbon Droplets for Medical Ultrasonography: Current Progress, Challenges, and Prospects.' *Scientifica* 2014: 579684. doi:10.1155/2014/579684.
59. Williams, Ross, Cameron Wright, Emmanuel Cherin, Nikita Reznik, Mike Lee, Ivan Gorelikov, F. Stuart Foster, Naomi Matsuura, and Peter N. Burns. 2013. 'Characterization of Submicron Phase-Change Perfluorocarbon Droplets for Extravascular Ultrasound Imaging of Cancer.' *Ultrasound in Medicine and Biology* 39 (3): 475–489. doi:10.1016/j.ultrasmedbio.2012.10.004.
60. Sheeran, Paul S., Juan D. Rojas, Connor Puett, Jordan Hjelmquist, Christopher B. Arena, and Paul A. Dayton. 2015. 'Contrast-Enhanced Ultrasound Imaging and in Vivo Circulatory Kinetics with Low-Boiling-Point Nanoscale Phase-Change Perfluorocarbon Agents.' *Ultrasound in Medicine & Biology* 41 (3): 814–831. doi:10.1016/j.ultrasmedbio.2014.10.020.
61. Zhang, Peng, and Tyrone Porter. 2010. 'An in Vitro Study of a Phase-Shift Nanoemulsion: A Potential Nucleation Agent for Bubble-Enhanced HIFU Tumour Ablation.' *Ultrasound in Medicine and Biology* 36 (11): 1856–1866. doi:10.1016/j.ultrasmedbio.2010.07.001.
62. Abdalkader, Rodi, Johan Unga, Fumiyoshi Yamashita, Kazuo Maruyama, and Mitsuru Hashida. 2019. 'Evaluation of the Theranostic Potential of Perfluorohexane-Based Acoustic Nanodroplets.' *Biological and Pharmaceutical Bulletin* 42 (12): 2038–44. doi.org/10.1248/bpb.b19–00525.
63. Abdalkader, Rodi, Johan Unga, Kazuo Maruyama, Fumiyoshi Yamashita, and Mitsuru Hashida. 2020. 'The Application of the In-Situ Hyperthermia Emission from Acoustic Nanodroplets for Theranostic Dual-Imaging and Antitumor Modalities.' *Biological and Pharmaceutical Bulletin* 43 (7): 1141–5. doi:10.1248/bpb.b20–00171.
64. Hashida, Yasuhiko, Hironori Tanaka, Shuwen Zhou, Shigeru Kawakami, Fumiyoshi Yamashita, Tatsuya Murakami, Tomokazu Umeyama, Hiroshi Imahori, and Mitsuru Hashida. 2014. 'Photothermal Ablation of Tumour Cells Using a Single-Walled Carbon Nanotube-Peptide Composite.' *Journal of Controlled Release* 173: 59–66. doi:10.1016/j.jconrel.2013.10.039.
65. Zhou, Shuwen, Yasuhiko Hashida, Shigeru Kawakami, Junya Mihara, Tomokazu Umeyama, Hiroshi Imahori, Tatsuya Murakami, Fumiyoshi Yamashita, and Mitsuru Hashida. 2014. 'Preparation of Immunostimulatory Single-Walled Carbon nanotube/CpG DNA Complexes and Evaluation of Their Potential in Cancer Immunotherapy.' *International Journal of Pharmaceutics* 471 (1–2) 214–23. doi:10.1016/j.ijpharm.2014.05.037.
66. Delogu, Lucia Gemma, Gianpaolo Vidili, Enrica Venturelli, Cécilia Ménard-Moyon, Maria Antonietta Zoroddu, Giovannantonio Pilo, Paola Nicolussi, et al. 2012. 'Functionalized Multiwalled Carbon Nanotubes as Ultrasound Contrast Agents.' *Proceedings of the National Academy of Sciences of the United States of America* 109 (41): 16612–16617. doi:10.1073/pnas.1208312109.
67. Harris, Gerald R. 2009. 'FDA Regulation of Clinical High Intensity Focused Ultrasound (HIFU) Devices.' *Proceedings of the 31st Annual International Conference of the IEEE Engineering in Medicine and Biology Society: Engineering the Future of Biomedicine, EMBC 2009*, 145–148. doi:10.1109/IEMBS.2009.5332444.

29

Focused Ultrasound Therapy for Treatment of Pain

Matthew R.D. Brown, Paul Farquhar-Smith, and Nandita M. deSouza

29.1 Potential Mechanisms

The actual mechanism by which high intensity frequency ultrasound (HIFU) exerts its analgesic effects remains poorly understood. It is, however, likely that thermal effects result in localised denervation of the target, reducing the density of any nociceptive fibres present. This hypothesis is reinforced by evidence that unmyelinated nerve fibres are particularly vulnerable to (non-HIFU) thermal injury[1] and that direct sonication of neuronal structures in vivo results in demyelination and neural degeneration.[2] At lower temperatures, reversible blockade of nerve action potential conduction occurs,[3, 4] with unmyelinated fibres again proving to be the more susceptible to the effects of HIFU.

Transient neuromodulation has been shown to occur following the application of focused ultrasound to both the central nervous system[5] and peripheral nerves[6, 7] in animal and human subjects. The precise mechanism by which changes in neuronal excitation level are induced by HIFU has not been fully elucidated, but it is postulated that it causes temporary distortion of the cell membrane, thereby altering the function of stretch-activated ion channels present on the surface of neurons.[8] Acoustic pressure and cavitation changes caused by HIFU also result in ion flux both through existing ion channels and through a process termed sonoporation, whereby pores are formed in the neuronal membrane,[9] which has the effect of suppressing the transmission of action potentials.[10] Figure 29.1 summarises some of the multiple mechanisms by which HIFU is postulated to exert its effects.

29.2 Pre-clinical Studies

The ability of HIFU to induce a sensory nerve conduction block in a rat model of diabetic neuropathy has been investigated to determine its potential for pain relief. In vitro studies of compound muscle action potentials (CMAPs) and sensory action potentials (SAPs) in the sciatic and sural nerves, respectively, showed that HIFU temporarily inhibited mean $\pm$ (SD) SAPs of the control and diabetic rat nerves to 33.9 + 8.2 and 14.0 $\pm$ 10.7% of the baseline values, respectively, whereas the mean (SD) CMAPs were suppressed to 53.6 + 8.4 and 76.2 + 7.5% of baseline respectively. In vivo results showed that HIFU acutely blocked CMAPs to 32.9 + 12.6 and 19.9 + 10.9% of baseline in control and diabetic rat nerves, respectively, with a reversible blockade.[11] In another experiment the same authors showed that for nerves from controls and from a rat model of neuropathy, suppression of SAPs and CMAPs started 2 minutes post-HIFU treatment. Maximum suppression of SAPs was 34.4 ± 3.2% for the control rats and 11.6 ± 2.0% and 9.8 ± 3.0% for diabetic rats (4-week post-injection and 8-week post-injection of streptozotocin, respectively). Time to full recovery was 25 minutes in control rats, 70 minutes at week 4 and 80 minutes at week 8 post-sonication. Histological analysis revealed that the nerves in which SAPs and CMAPs did not fully recover were damaged thermally or mechanically by HIFU. Diabetic nerves were less suppressed by HIFU and were more vulnerable to permanent damage.[4]

These results are further supported by the demonstration of exposure-dependent effects of HIFU on nerve function.[3] In nerves treated with acoustic intensities of 390, 2,255, and 3,310 W/cm^2

 DOI: 10.1201/9780429162671-29

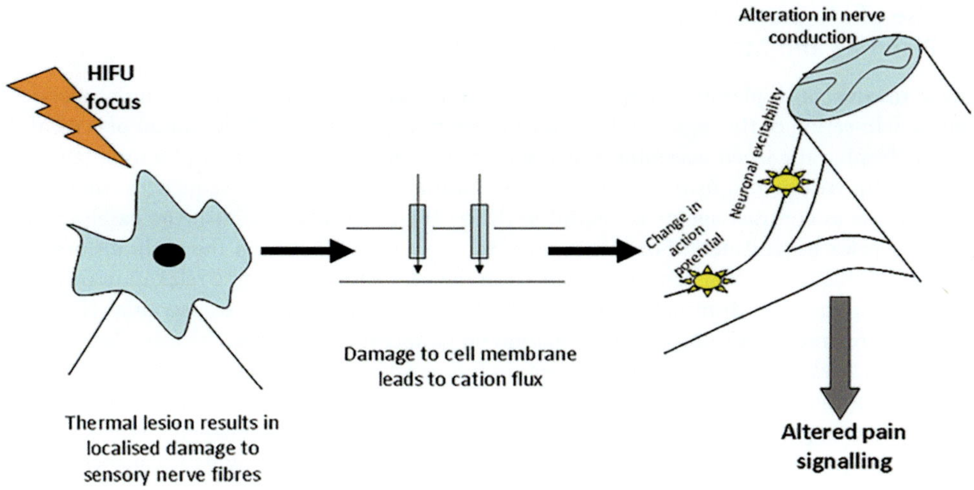

FIGURE 29.1 Schematic for a proposed mechanism of action of high-intensity focused ultrasound in alleviating pain.

CMAPs decreased initially within 4 hours or 7 days after HIFU treatment and then recovered to their baseline level at 28 days after treatment. For exposures of 7890W/cm^2, however, CMAPs remained absent even 28 days after treatment, consistent with irreversible damage. Experiments on rabbit sciatic nerve showed that acoustic intensities of 1480 to 1850 W/cm^2, applied using a scanning method, were effective in achieving complete conduction block in 100% of 22 nerve complexes with HIFU treatment times of 36 $\pm$ 14 seconds. Gross examination showed blanching of the nerve at the HIFU treatment site, and lesion volumes of 2.8 $\pm$ 1.4 cm^3 encompassing the nerve complex. Histologic examination indicated axonal demyelination and necrosis of Schwann cells as probable mechanisms of nerve block.[12] HIFU ablation of sciatic nerves done under MRI guidance in swine (n = 5) using a HIFU system integrated with a 3 T MRI scanner showed that acute lesions could be seen using T1-weighted contrast-enhanced (CE) MRI and histopathology using haematoxylin and eosin staining. There was macroscopic reddening, mild thickening of the nerve and pallor of the adjacent muscle in all animals. The HIFU-treated sections of the nerves displayed nuclear pyknosis of Schwann cells, vascular hyperaemia, perineural oedema, hyalinisation of the collagenous stroma of the nerve, myelin sheet swelling and loss of axons. The non-perfused volume of the lesions (5.8–64.6 cc) correlated linearly with estimated lethal thermal dose volume (4.7–34.2 cc),[13] indicating a direct thermal ablative effect.

Comparison of the effects of HIFU on neuronal tissue with other neurolytic techniques is variable; in a large animal model, intercostal nerve ablation in swine with HIFU showed evidence of well-demarcated, acute, focally extensive thermal necrosis. Similar results were obtained with a radiofrequency ablation technique, whereas the intercostal nerves appeared histologically intact with alcohol ablation.[14]

It has also been suggested that HIFU may have an additional role to play in the detection and diagnosis of neuropathic pain.[15] Recent studies have attempted to delineate its application in this field better. Paw withdrawal in response to focused ultrasound stimulation assessed in a rat tibial nerve neuroma model of neuropathic pain, demonstrated that focused ultrasound preferentially stimulated neuropathic tissue compared to normal tissue.[16] Results from similar work in a rat sciatic ligation model of neuropathic pain[17] mirrored these findings with a significantly lower paw withdrawal threshold for focused ultrasound stimulation in lesioned rats when compared to both a control group and a 'sham surgery' group. This work raises the possibility of HIFU being used in both the detection and treatment of neuropathic pain in the future.

29.2.1 Use of Magnetic Resonance Imaging Guidance for Planning and Monitoring Treatment

Imaging is invaluable in planning, delivering and monitoring HIFU. In the planning phase, detailed anatomical delineation of the region to be treated is essential, together with definition of critical structures in the beam path when accessing the lesion. It is essential to perform a planning study in the proposed patient treatment position to assess this. Standard T1 and T2-W sequences usually suffice, although the use of contrast agents is helpful to define the target and establish the baseline vascular enhancement prior to treatment. For treatment planning, where bone is in the path, ultrashort echo time (UTE) MR sequences that capture signals from the very short transverse relaxation time of bone have been explored.[18] This diminishes the need for CT-based planning for transcranial HIFU procedures. During treatment, MR provides information on temperatures achieved by using 'MR thermometry' sequences. These are usually proton resonance frequency shift (PRFS) sequences based on change in the proton resonance frequency with temperature.[19, 20] They are more robust than pure T1-based methods that interrogate T1 relaxation times as a function of temperature change.[21] During treatment delivery it is also possible to monitor acute tissue changes with diffusion-weighted sequences[22, 23] where an increase in the apparent diffusion coefficient indicates acute oedema within the area of tissue damage. Finally, post-treatment, both in the acute and more long-term follow-up, gadolinium enhanced T1-W sequences are recommended because the boundary between residual enhancing tumour and non-enhancing treated necrotic tissue is best appreciated after contrast enhancement.

29.3 Clinical Applications

29.3.1 Musculoskeletal Pain

29.3.1.1 Facet Joint Arthropathy

Back pain represents a significant societal burden both from a health an economic perspective, and the application of HIFU for the treatment of non-specific low back pain has been investigated. To date a single case series which investigates the use of MRgFUS in the treatment of low back pain caused by facet (zygapophyseal) joint arthropathy has been published.[24] A total of 18 patients were treated with sonications of multiple lumbar facet joints (mean number 5, range 2–8) with treatment on average lasting 188 minutes. Ten patients received sedation during the procedure and there were no reported adverse events. In 13 patients followed to 6 months, post-treatment reduction in average numerical rating scale (NRS) pain scores to 3.87 from a pre-treatment average of 6.42 (60.2% reduction) was observed. This was accompanied by a 45.8% improvement in Oswestry Disability Questionnaire score and a 61.9% reduction in the Brief Pain Inventory interference score. The results of this small series compare favourably with the outcomes observed with lumbar facet intra-articular injections for which there is only moderate (level III) evidence of long-term efficacy.[25] In a pilot study of 10 patients, a fluoroscopically guided HIFU treatment decreased the average numeric rating scale score for pain from 6.2 at baseline to 2.1 (n = 10) after 1 month, 4.9 (n = 9) after 3 months, 3.0 (n = 8) after 6 months and 3.0 (n = 6) after 12 months, indicating its potential in this clinical setting.[26]

29.3.1.2 Discogenic Back Pain

A modest amount of work has also been undertaken to explore the use of focused ultrasound in low back pain caused by intervertebral disc herniation. In vitro 'proof of concept' experiments have shown that HIFU is effective in producing localised heating, resulting in protein degradation and subsequent disc shrinkage.[27] However, the complex anatomy of the spine means that achieving uninterrupted sonication of intervertebral discs is difficult. To overcome this challenge, a minimally invasive approach, using a small probe inserted percutaneously to abut the disc has been proposed.[28] This study has progressed from in vitro proof-of-concept studies to in vivo animal work, with Forslund and colleagues successfully performing percutaneous sonication of porcine lumbar intervertebral discs.[29] Post-mortem histological analysis of tissues showed that disruption of collagen fibres occurred within the area of disc lesioning, and that importantly, no thermal damage to nerve roots was observed. Despite these promising findings from pre-clinical work, progression to trials in human subjects with discogenic pain has not been reported.

29.3.1.3 Joint Pain due to Osteoarthritis

Another common cause of pain in an ageing population, where the use of focused ultrasound has been examined is large joint osteoarthritis. To alleviate pain experienced by patients with advanced osteoarthritis of the knee joint, awaiting knee arthroplasty,[30] Izumi et al. describe the use of MRgHIFU to sonicate osteophytes inferior to the medial tibial plateau. The procedure was performed following infiltration of the periosteum with local anaesthetic. No intra-procedural complications were reported and cases took on average 74 minutes to complete. A post-treatment reduction in VAS scores on walking at 3, 10 and 28 days was recorded in 6 of 8 cases and 4 of these experienced a mean reduction in pain scores on a VAS of 72.6% at 6 months. Additionally a statistically significant increase in pressure pain thresholds (PPTs) at sites close to sonication was observed in responders, but not in non-responders, suggesting denervation of hypersensitive pressure-responsive nerve fibres in this group. No attempt was made to assess changes in functional level and quality of life scores in this small study.

Although there are no other published studies which describe the use of HIFU in osteoarthritis, its use in treating the pain caused by osteoid osteomas, a painful benign bone tumour, has received major attention. A small pilot study[31] in 6 patients demonstrated notable reductions in pain scores following sonication of the lesion from a pre-treatment average of 7.9 ± 1.4 to 0 ± 0 on an 11-point VAS at 1, 3 and 6 months, accompanied by a corresponding reduction in analgesic requirements. The same group of investigators reported a larger follow-on study of 29 patients which reinforced these findings, with similar marked reductions in pain scores on a VAS from a mean of 8 ± 1 pre-treatment to 1 ± 2 ($P < 0.001$) at 12 months.[32] There were no reported adverse events or complications in either study.

HIFU has also been trialled in patients with painful refractory osteoid osteomas where in small paediatric population, total pain resolution and cessation of analgesics were achieved in 88% of patients after 4 weeks.[33]

29.3.2 Cancer Pain

29.3.2.1 Pain from Bone Metastases

Approximately one third of patients with bone metastases experience pain,[34] which usually manifests itself as a background gnawing pain accompanied by severe episodic pain commonly triggered by weight-bearing or movement.[35] A variety of treatment options exist, including a variety of pharmacological approaches, radioisotopes and radiotherapy, but HIFU is not currently part of the treatment arsenal.[36] The relative safety and low toxicity of focused ultrasound when compared to the alternative, established, treatment (ionising radiation) for painful bone metastases has led to burgeoning interest in its use for treating these lesions. The pain from bone metastases arises due to a combination of factors including the release of chemical mediators, microfractures and increased pressure within the bone as a result of stretching of the periosteum.[37] The effect of these painful factors is amplified by the pathological sprouting of nociceptive nerve fibres in the periosteum associated with the metastases.[38, 39] It is thought that HIFU reduces pain by thermal denervation of the bone and periosteum, although debulking of the metastases may also contribute. The use of MR guidance to deliver HIFU allows sonication cells to be accurately placed to heat the cortical margin of the bone metastasis and provides near real-time monitoring of tissue temperature. The higher absorption of acoustic energy by bone than with soft tissue means that fewer sonications are required to achieve tissue heating thus permitting more rapid treatment of bone than soft tissue lesions.[40]

Initial pilot studies investigating the use of focused ultrasound in bone metastases demonstrated its efficacy and safety, albeit in small numbers of patients.[41–46] A recent placebo-controlled study demonstrated the efficacy of MRgFUS for relief of pain from bone metastases which had failed control by standard treatments in a larger cohort (n = 142).[47] A 3:1 randomisation of the 142 patients to either the intervention or placebo allowed subjects allocated to the placebo arm to crossover into the treatment arm of the study if they requested 'rescue treatment' within the 3-month follow-up period. Participants were deemed to be 'responders' if MRgFUS was found to be superior to placebo at 3 months, with 64.3% of participants in the intervention limb responding to treatment compared to 20.0% in the placebo limb (P <0.001, response being defined as a reduction in worst pain rating on NRS of 2 points or more from baseline and analgesic requirements assessed using the morphine equivalent daily dose [MEDD] not increasing by more than 25% from baseline). Interestingly, 17 patients crossed over from the placebo to the intervention limb during follow up and were treated with MRgFUS; 70.7% of these patients were deemed to be treatment responders, although this data was not included in the primary efficacy analysis. Statistically, significant differences were also observed at 3 months in worst pain on NRS and quality of life (QoL) (from brief pain inventory scores). This has subsequently been corroborated in other single-centre studies.[48–50] In a study of 21 patients, it was those with intraosseous rather than extraosseous metastases that experienced significant pain relief (Figure 29.2).[51] Local treatment of pain from bone metastases with MR-guided HIFU, even in the presence of disseminated malignancy, has a substantial positive effect on physical functioning, and improves other symptomatic QoL measures.[52] Investigation into the use of MRgFUS to treat painful bone metastases is ongoing with a large European Union (EU) consortium (FURTHER consortium) currently actively recruiting participants.

29.3.2.2 Pain from Extraosseous Primary and Metastatic Tumours

Advanced pancreatic cancer is characterised by debilitating, deep pain that substantially affects patient QoL. Therefore, in the treatment of cancer pain, this tumour has received disproportionately greater attention than others when considering potential applications of the use of HIFU for cancer pain treatment. There are at least a dozen reported single-centre pilot studies trialling the use of HIFU in pancreatic cancer. A study of 40 patients indicated pain relief in 87% of these cases for an average pain relief time of 10 weeks.[53] In the context of an overall survival of 6 months for stage 1V disease and 10 months for stage III disease, the procedure was of considerable benefit to patients. Another study undertaken in 25 patients showed a significant improvement in Karnofsky performance score in 23, with significant pain relief. A CT scan performed 1 month after HIFU showed tumour necrosis in 8 case.s[54] This was followed by a larger study in 32 patients which confirmed that there were no safety issues with the technique and a reduction in pain in 80% of cases.[55] Anzidei et al. reported successful ablation in 6 of 7 patients with advanced pancreatic cancer treated with MR-guided HIIFU. In one patient the treatment was suspended due to inadequate access to the lesion. Pain scores decreased from an average of 7 to 3 on the Visual Analogue Score (VAS).[56] In advanced pancreatic cancer, HIFU has been shown to improve QoL by improving a variety of factors, predominantly pain.[57]

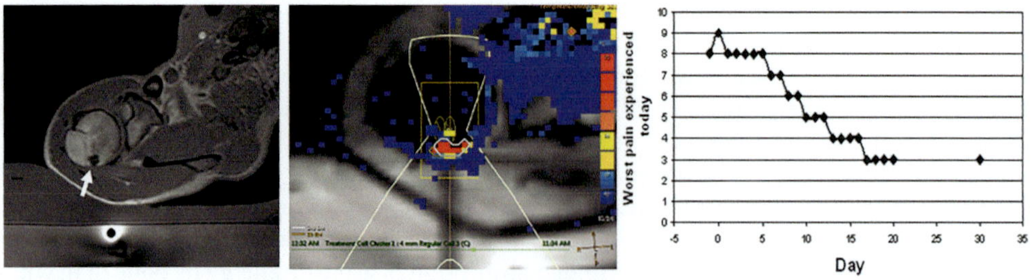

FIGURE 29.2 Axial T1-W image through the humeral head (left panel) in a patient with a painful bone metastasis (arrow) from breast cancer. The lesion was treated with HIFU under MR guidance and a temperature rise visualised at the precise location of the lesion (red pixels, middle panel). Worst pain monitored over 30 days showed a dramatic reduction in pain scores after a brief flare on Day 1 (right panel).

A systematic review by Keane and colleagues[58] comprehensively summarises the findings of 14 prospective studies, the bulk of which were undertaken in China. A total of 659 patients were treated with MRgFUS, and the majority included change in pain scores as an outcome measure. On average 86.4% of patients reported a reduction in pain scores following treatment, with minimal complications. However these favourable results are from studies which are predominantly unblinded and did not include placebo or sham treatments. A recently published meta-analysis of 19 articles including 939 patients indicated that patients treated with HIFU in conjunction with chemotherapy presented reduced levels of pain ($p < 0.05$) compared to the traditional treatment group of chemotherapy.[59]

A subsequent single-centre cohort study of 6 patients with unresectable pancreatic cancer also demonstrated notable reductions in pain scores from 7 to 3 one week after treatment ($P = 0.017$), and all but one patient completely stopped analgesic medication.[56] Interestingly tumour volumes remained stable post-treatment, with no regrowth in tumour in 5 of the 6 patients. HIFU has also been trialled in a combination schedule with gemcitabine chemotherapy to curtail tumour growth. The administration of both treatments concurrently was well tolerated and the overall survival in this phase 2 study was 12 months for patients with locally unresectable pancreatic adenocarcinoma.[60] Therefore, in addition to its role in pain palliation, HIFU is likely to demonstrate future utility in controlling tumour growth, not just in pancreatic cancer, but in a range of other tumour types where conventional treatments are no longer effective.

Liver cancer is another tumour type where HIFU has been trialled for pain relief with success. This is mainly in primary rather than metastatic tumour where 20% of 85 patients with primary disease compared to 1.6% of 190 patients with metastatic lesions experienced a 50% reduction in visual analogue pain score.[61] Several published case reports describe impressive reductions in pain emanating from other isolated primary malignancies including carcinoma of the cervix,[62] renal malignancies,[63] ovarian cancer[64] and metastatic gynaecological malignancies where extrapelvic tumours showed greater pain responses than intrapelvic ones.[65]

29.3.2.3 Neuropathic Pain

The use of HIFU in the treatment of neuropathic pain has also been investigated. Limited work has been conducted on the feasibility of sonicating peripheral nerves with MRgFUS systems. Staruch and colleagues published preliminary work which demonstrated the feasibility of inducing thermal lesions in the sciatic nerve of pigs.[66] However, despite the ability of HIFU to modulate peripheral neuronal excitability,[3] its clinical utility in neuropathic pain states remains to be established, and its exact effects on neuropathic conditions with both demonstrated central nervous system[67] and peripheral changes, is undetermined.

Transcranial MRgFUS is technically feasible and the ability to ablate cerebral structures safely and accurately has been demonstrated in the clinical environment.[68]

Martin and colleagues were the first to describe the MRgFUS treatment of both central and peripheral intractable neuropathic pain by ablating the medial thalamus of patients due to undergo central lateral thalamotomy.[69] A total of 9 patients were treated, and preliminary mean reductions in pain scores of 68% were demonstrated. This group then continued to treat a further 12 patients with chronic neuropathic pain caused by a range of conditions including post-herpetic neuralgia, avulsion of the brachial plexus and lumbar nerve root compression.[70] In those patients in whom an adequately sized lesion in the thalamus was judged to have been created ($n = 9$) a reduction from preoperative mean VAS scores of 59.5/100 to 34.3/100 at 3 months and 35.3/100 at 1 year ($n = 8$) occurred following treatment. Additionally the use of analgesic drugs in 5 of the 8 patients had ceased entirely at the 1-year time point, although the authors urge caution in drawing conclusions from this surrogate marker of pain levels. Adverse events were limited to one patient who developed an intracerebral haemorrhage at the target in the thalamus that resulted in persistent neurological impairment at 1 year.

The use of transcranial MRgFUS sonication for trigeminal neuralgia has been explored in a cadaveric feasibility study in which the root entry zone (REZ) and cisternal segments of 6 nerves were targeted.[71]

No evidence of aberrant heating of surrounding structures was demonstrated. Further clinical work which builds on these findings of transcranial MRgFUS is warranted.

29.4 Expert Commentary

Focused ultrasound is emerging as a viable treatment option in the therapeutic armamentarium available to clinicians. In particular, its use is being actively pursued in a range of painful conditions which differ both in aetiology and in underlying pathological process. The potential benefits of the use of MRgFUS in the targeting of specific pain generators, or structures involved in the transmission of pain signals, are apparent, because the use of MR guidance makes the safe generation of precise, well circumscribed thermal lesions possible. This precision and the quality of the monitoring of the lesion as it is generated is likely to improve as the image-based technology used in the treatment improves and operators gain experience and knowledge relating the intra-procedural imaging changes to subsequent outcome increases.[72]

HIFU is a safe treatment; adverse events, although possible, are uncommon. The vast majority of patients described in the various studies outlined earlier, experienced uncomplicated procedures. The bulk of adverse events reported have been localised minor burns arising at the site of the window through which the HIFU beam passes at the skin surface. These often arise due to the presence of air bubbles due to incomplete 'degassing' of the skin-transducer interface. Again it is conceivable that as HIFU technology improves, and as operator experience increases, that these skin burns will become even less common.

Another major beneficial feature of HIFU treatment for pain is the relative rapidity (within a day of sonication) of onset of the pain relief and its duration of effect, with many patients still experiencing benefit 1 year after treatment. Notably, these features appear to transcend the type of painful condition treated. Interestingly, many of the patients treated in preliminary studies had pain which had proved refractory to more traditional therapeutic approaches, thereby increasing the therapeutic value of MRgFUS as a 'rescue' or adjuvant therapy. In cancer patients (who make up a significant number of participants in clinical HIFU studies) marked reductions in opioid intake have been possible following sonication of painful lesions. This has major implications on quality of life, as opioids have a substantially negative effect on patient well-being. This opioid-sparing aspect of HIFU may be of further clinical relevance as there is some evidence that opioids may speed up rates of recurrence or metastasis formation,[73, 74] and therefore any opioid dose reduction achieved may be potentially additionally beneficial.

The limitations of HIFU as a treatment for pain revolve around its delivery in the clinical environment. Complex equipment and well trained staff are required to perform MRgFUS, and the positioning of patients within the MRI scanner to enable unobstructed passage of the HIFU beam to the target can sometimes prove challenging. Additionally the majority of patients treated for painful conditions require sedation, general anaesthesia or regional local anaesthetic blocks to tolerate the intraprocedural pain which may arise from the thermal effects. Moreover the fact that a patient often needs to lie with the painful site in contact with the equipment, increases the pressure and potentially the pain at this significant point. The relative advantages and disadvantages of MRgFUS when used to treat pain are remains incomplete, and a greater appreciation of what occurs to nociceptive pathways following sonication at the cellular level would be beneficial. Further basic science and clinical research regarding HIFU and pain is therefore warranted. An understanding of the exact mechanisms by which HIFU exerts its analgesic effects is listed in Table 29.1.

Although the effects of HIFU in pain have been encouraging, the majority of the results have come from small observational trials, often uncontrolled and the majority unblinded. In the future, larger studies with robust methodological design are indicated, not only to further delineate the analgesic efficacy of the treatment, but to enable the detection of rarer adverse events which smaller studies may not have been adequately powered to show.

TABLE 29.1

Current Advantages and Disadvantages of Using MRgHIFU for Managing Pain

	Disadvantages of MRgHIFU
PRECISION – Small, well-defined lesion produced	EQUIPMENT – Cost high and availability low
ACCURATE TARGETING – Under imaging guidance	TRAINING – Few centres able to do this
REAL-TIME TEMPERATURE MONITORING – MR thermometry	ANAESTHESTIC/SEDATION REQUIREMENT DURING PROCEDURE
NO IONISING RADIATION	MONITORING ANAESTHESIA IN MRI ENVIRONMENT
NON-INVASIVE – good safety profile	MECHANISM OF ACTION – poorly understood
EFFECTIVE – Increasing published literature	EVIDENCE FOR USE – Level 4

29.5 Summary

High intensity focused ultrasound is an emerging, novel and potentially effective treatment for certain painful conditions, with a good safety profile and, in the clinical literature published to date, encouraging efficacy. The ability to selectively and accurately lesion targets in both the peripheral and the central nervous system in a minimally invasive fashion, distinguishes it from existing treatments at the disposal of pain clinicians, which currently rely on the introduction of a needle, catheter or probe to close proximity of the target.

Ongoing developments in the technology used to deliver the treatment and an expansion in the clinical research supporting its adoption make it likely that HIFU will have a role in pain management in the future.

KEY POINTS

1. HIFU has a good safety profile in treatment of pain in a variety of benign and malignant conditions.
2. HIFU should be delivered under imaging guidance, preferably MRI, to accurately hit the target and to monitor intraprocedural temperature and tissue changes.
3. HIFU reduces pain through a variety of mechanisms including reduction in sensory action potentials as well as direct ablation of nerve endings.

REFERENCES

1. Xu D, Pollock M. Experimental nerve thermal injury. Brain. 1994 Apr;117:375–84.
2. Wang Q, Guo R, Rong S, Yang G, Zhu Q, Jiang Y, et al. Noninvasive renal sympathetic denervation by extracorporeal high-intensity focused ultrasound in a pre-clinical canine model. J Am Coll Cardiol. 2013 May 28;61(21):2185–92.
3. Foley JL, Little JW, Vaezy S. Effects of high-intensity focused ultrasound on nerve conduction. Muscle Nerve. 2008 Feb;37(2):241–50.
4. Lee Y-F, Lin C-C, Cheng J-S, Chen G-S. High-intensity focused ultrasound attenuates neural responses of sciatic nerves isolated from normal or neuropathic rats. Ultrasound Med Biol. 2015;41(1):132–42.
5. Tufail Y, Matyushov A, Baldwin N, Tauchmann ML, Georges J, Yoshihiro A, et al. Transcranial pulsed ultrasound stimulates intact brain circuits. Neuron. 2010 Jun 10;66(5):681–94.
6. Wahab RA, Choi M, Liu Y, Krauthamer V, Zderic V, Myers MR. Mechanical bioeffects of pulsed high intensity focused ultrasound on a simple neural model. Med Phys. 2012 Jul;39(7):4274–83.

7. Colucci V, Strichartz G, Jolesz F, Vykhodtseva N, Hynynen K. Focused ultrasound effects on nerve action potential in vitro. Ultrasound Med Biol. 2009 Oct;35(10):1737–47.
8. Kim H, Lee SD, Chiu A, Yoo S-S, Park S. Estimation of the spatial profile of neuromodulation and the temporal latency in motor responses induced by focused ultrasound brain stimulation. Neuroreport. 2014 May 7;25(7):475–9.
9. Tachibana K, Uchida T, Ogawa K, Yamashita N, Tamura K. Induction of cell-membrane porosity by ultrasound. Lancet. 1999;353(9162):1409.
10. Foley JL, Vaezy S, Crum LA. Applications of high-intensity focused ultrasound in medicine: Spotlight on neurological applications. Appl Acoust. 2007 Mar;68(3):245–59.
11. Lee Y-F, Lin C-C, Cheng J-S, Chen G-S. Nerve conduction block in diabetic rats using high-intensity focused ultrasound for analgesic applications. Br J Anaesth. 2015 May 1;114(5):840–6.
12. Foley JL, Little JW, Starr FL, Frantz C, Vaezy S. Image-guided HIFU neurolysis of peripheral nerves to treat spasticity and pain. Ultrasound Med Biol. 2004 Sep;30(9):1199–207.
13. Kaye EA, Gutta NB, Monette S, Gulati A, Loh J, Srimathveeravalli G, et al. Feasibility study on MR-guided high-intensity focused ultrasound ablation of sciatic nerve in a swine model: Preliminary results. Cardiovasc Intervent Radiol. 2015 Aug;38(4):985–92.
14. Gulati A, Loh J, Gutta NB, Ezell PC, Monette S, Erinjeri JP, et al. Novel use of noninvasive high-intensity focused ultrasonography for intercostal nerve neurolysis in a swine model. Reg Anesth Pain Med. 2014;39(1):26–30.
15. Davies IAI, Gavrilov LR, Tsirulnikov EM. Application of focused ultrasound for research on pain. Pain. 1996 Sep;67(1):17–27.
16. McClintic AM, Dickey TC, Gofeld M, Kliot M, Loeser JD, Richebe P, et al. Intense focused ultrasound preferentially stimulates subcutaneous and focal neuropathic tissue: Preliminary results. Pain Med. 2013 Jan;14(1):84–92.
17. Tych RE, Gofeld M, Jarvik JG, Kliot M, Loeser JD, McClintic AM, et al. Neuropathic tissue responds preferentially to stimulation by intense focused ultrasound. Ultrasound Med Biol. 2013 Jan;39(1):111–6.
18. Guo S, Zhuo J, Li G, Gandhi D, Dayan M, Fishman P, et al. Feasibility of ultrashort echo time images using full-wave acoustic and thermal modeling for transcranial MRI-guided focused ultrasound (tcMRgFUS) planning. Phys Med Biol. 2019 Apr 26;64(9):095008. doi: 10.1088/1361-6560/ab12f7. PMID: 30909173.
19. de Senneville BD, Mougenot C, Quesson B, Dragonu I, Grenier N, Moonen CTW. MR thermometry for monitoring tumor ablation. Eur Radiol. 2007 Sep;17(9):2401–10.
20. Gellermann J, Hildebrandt B, Issels R, Ganter H, Wlodarczyk W, Budach V, et al. Noninvasive magnetic resonance thermography of soft tissue sarcomas during regional hyperthermia: Correlation with response and direct thermometry. Cancer. 2006 Sep 15;107(6):1373–82.
21. Rieke V, Butts Pauly K. MR thermometry. J Magn Reson Imaging. 2008 Feb;27(2):376–90.
22. Giles S, Winfield J, Rivens I, Collins D, ter Haar G, DeSouza N. Investigating the utility of diffusion-weighted imaging (DWI) for monitoring treatment efficacy during MR guided high intensity focused ultrasound (MRgHIFU) therapy in bone applications. Proc Int Soc Magn Reonance Med. 2015;1:4047.
23. Giles SL, Winfield JM, Collins DJ, Rivens I, Civale J, ter Haar GR, et al. Value of diffusion-weighted imaging for monitoring tissue change during magnetic resonance-guided high-intensity focused ultrasound therapy in bone applications: An *ex-vivo* study. Eur Radiol Exp. 2018;2(1):10. doi: 10.1186/s41747-018-0041-x. Epub 2018 May 10. PMID: 29774894; PMCID: PMC5945713.
24. Weeks EM, Platt MW, Gedroyc W. MRI-guided focused ultrasound (MRgFUS) to treat facet joint osteoarthritis low back pain-case series of an innovative new technique. Eur Radiol. 2012 Dec;22(12):2822–35.
25. Boswell M V, Colson JD, Sehgal N, Dunbar EE, Epter R. A systematic review of therapeutic facet joint interventions in chronic spinal pain. Pain Physician. 2007 Jan;10(1):229–53.
26. Perez J, Gofeld M, Leblang S, Hananel A, Aginsky R, Chen J, et al. Fluoroscopy-guided high-intensity focused ultrasound neurotomy of the lumbar zygapophyseal joints: A clinical pilot study. Pain Med. 2022 Jan 3;23(1):67–75. doi: 10.1093/pm/pnab275. PMID: 34534337; PMCID: PMC8723143.
27. Persson J, Strömqvist B, Zanoli G, Mccarthy I, Lidgren L. Ultrasound nucleolysis: An in vitro study. Ultrasound Med Biol. 2002 Sep;28(9):1189–97.
28. Persson J, Hansen E, Lidgren L, McCarthy I. Modeling of the heat distribution in the intervertebral disk. Ultrasound Med Biol. 2005 May;31(5):709–17.

29. Forslund C, Persson J, Strömqvist B, Lidgren L, McCarthy ID. Effects of high-intensity focused ultrasound on the intervertebral disc: A potential therapy for disc herniations. J Clin Ultrasound. 2006 Sep;34(7):330–8.
30. Izumi M, Ikeuchi M, Kawasaki M, Ushida T, Morio K, Namba H, et al. MR-guided focused ultrasound for the novel and innovative management of osteoarthritic knee pain. BMC Musculoskelet Disord. 2013 Jan;14(1):267.
31. Napoli A, Mastantuono M, Cavallo Marincola B, Anzidei M, Zaccagna F, Moreschini O, et al. Osteoid osteoma: MR-guided focused ultrasound for entirely noninvasive treatment. Radiology. 2013 May;267(2):514–21.
32. Geiger D, Napoli A, Conchiglia A, Gregori LM, Arrigoni F, Bazzocchi A, et al. MR-guided Focused Ultrasound (MRgFUS) ablation for the treatment of nonspinal osteoid osteoma: A prospective multicenter evaluation. J Bone Joint Surg Am. 2014 May 7;96(9):743–51.
33. Sharma KV, Yarmolenko PS, Celik H, Eranki A, Partanen A, Smitthimedhin A, et al. Comparison of noninvasive high-intensity focused ultrasound with radiofrequency ablation of osteoid osteoma. J Pediatr. 2017 Nov;190:222–8.e1. doi: 10.1016/j.jpeds.2017.06.046. Epub 2017 Aug 17. PMID: 28823554.
34. Grond S, Zech D, Diefenbach C, Radbruch L, Lehmann KA. Assessment of cancer pain: A prospective evaluation in 2266 cancer patients referred to a pain service. Pain. 1996;64:107–14.
35. Falk S, Dickenson AH. Pain and nociception: Mechanisms of cancer-induced bone pain. J Clin Oncol. 2014 Jun 1;32(16):1647–54.
36. Kane CM, Hoskin P, Bennett M. Cancer induced bone pain. Br Med J. 2015;315:1–8.
37. Mercadante S. Malignant bone pain : Pathophysiology and treatment. Pain. 1997;69:1–18.
38. Jimenez-Andrade JM, Bloom AP, Stake JI, Mantyh WG, Taylor RN, Freeman KT, et al. Pathological sprouting of adult nociceptors in chronic prostate cancer-induced bone pain. J Neurosci. 2010 Nov 3;30(44):14649–56.
39. Jimenez-Andrade JM, Mantyh WG, Bloom AP, Xu H, Ferng AS, Dussor G, et al. A phenotypically restricted set of primary afferent nerve fibers innervate the bone versus skin: Therapeutic opportunity for treating skeletal pain. Bone. 2010 Feb;46(2):306–13.
40. Choi J, Raghavan M. Diagnostic imaging and image-guided therapy of skeletal metastases. Cancer Control. 2012;19(2):102–12.
41. Catane R, Beck A, Inbar Y, Rabin T, Shabshin N, Hengst S, et al. MR-guided focused ultrasound surgery (MRgFUS) for the palliation of pain in patients with bone metastases-preliminary clinical experience. Ann Oncol. 2007 Jan;18(1):163–7.
42. Gianfelice D, Gupta C, Kucharczyk W, Bret P, Havill D, Clemons M. Palliative treatment of painful bone metastases with MR imaging-guided focused ultrasound. Radiology. 2008 Oct;249(1):355–63.
43. Liberman B, Gianfelice D, Inbar Y, Beck A, Rabin T, Shabshin N, et al. Pain palliation in patients with bone metastases using MR-guided focused ultrasound surgery: A multicenter study. Ann Surg Oncol. 2009 Jan;16(1):140–6.
44. Mols F, Beijers T, Lemmens V, van den Hurk CJ, Vreugdenhil G, van de Poll-Franse L V. Chemotherapy-induced neuropathy and its association with quality of life among 2- to 11-year colorectal cancer survivors: Results from the population-based PROFILES registry. J Clin Oncol. 2013 Jul 20;31(21):2699–707.
45. Li C, Zhang W, Fan W, Huang J, Zhang F, Wu P. Noninvasive treatment of malignant bone tumors using high-intensity focused ultrasound. Cancer. 2010 Aug 15;116(16):3934–42.
46. Huisman M, Lam MK, Bartels LW, Nijenhuis RJ, Moonen CT, Knuttel FM, et al. Feasibility of volumetric MRI-guided high intensity focused ultrasound (MR-HIFU) for painful bone metastases. J Ther ultrasound. 2014;2(16):16.
47. Hurwitz MD, Ghanouni P, Kanaev S V, Iozeffi D, Gianfelice D, Fennessy FM, et al. Magnetic resonance-guided focused ultrasound for patients with painful bone metastases: Phase III trial results. J Natl Cancer Inst. 2014 Apr 23;106:1–9.
48. Bertrand AS, Iannessi A, Natale R, Beaumont H, Patriti S, Xiong-Ying J, et al. Focused ultrasound for the treatment of bone metastases: Effectiveness and feasibility. J Ther Ultrasound. 2018 Nov 30;6:8. doi: 10.1186/s40349-018-0117-3. PMID: 30519467; PMCID: PMC6267064.
49. Drost L, Hynynen K, Huang Y, Lucht B, Wong E, Czarnota G, et al. Ultrasound-guided focused ultrasound treatment for painful bone metastases: A pilot study. Ultrasound Med Biol. 2020 Jun;46(6):1455–63. doi: 10.1016/j.ultrasmedbio.2020.01.032. Epub 2020 Mar 4. PMID: 32146008.

50. Bongiovanni A, Foca F, Oboldi D, Diano D, Bazzocchi A, Fabbri L, et al. 3-T magnetic resonance-guided high-intensity focused ultrasound (3 T-MR-HIFU) for the treatment of pain from bone metastases of solid tumors. Support Care Cancer. 2022 Jul;30(7):5737–45. doi: 10.1007/s00520-022-06990-y. Epub 2022 Mar 24. PMID: 35332373.
51. Giles SL, Brown MRD, Rivens I, Deppe M, Huisman M, Kim YS, ter Haaret al. Comparison of imaging changes and pain responses in patients with intra- or extraosseous bone metastases treated palliatively with magnetic resonance-guided high-intensity-focused ultrasound. J Vasc Interv Radiol. 2019 Sep;30(9):1351–60.e1. doi: 10.1016/j.jvir.2019.02.019. Epub 2019 May 14. PMID: 31101417; PMCID: PMC6715806.
52. Harding D, Giles SL, Brown MRD, ter Haar GR, van den Bosch M, Bartels LW, et al. Evaluation of quality of life outcomes following palliative treatment of bone metastases with magnetic resonance-guided high intensity focused ultrasound: An international multicentre study. Clin Oncol (R Coll Radiol). 2018 Apr;30(4):233–42. doi: 10.1016/j.clon.2017.12.023. Epub 2018 Jan 6. PMID: 29317145; PMCID: PMC5842401.
53. Wang K, Chen Z, Meng Z, Lin J, Zhou Z, Wang P, et al. Analgesic effect of high intensity focused ultrasound therapy for unresectable pancreatic cancer. Int J Hyperth. 2011;27(2):101–7.
54. Li P-Z, Zhu S-H, He W, Zhu L-Y, Liu S-P, Liu Y, et al. High-intensity focused ultrasound treatment for patients with unresectable pancreatic cancer. Hepatobiliary Pancreat Dis Int. 2012 Dec;11(6):655–60.
55. Gao H-F, Wang K, Meng Z-Q, Chen Z, Lin J-H, Zhou Z-H, et al. High intensity focused ultrasound treatment for patients with local advanced pancreatic cancer. Hepatogastroenterology. 2013;60(128):1906–10.
56. Anzidei M, Marincola BC, Bezzi M, Brachetti G, Nudo F, Cortesi E, et al. Magnetic resonance-guided high-intensity focused ultrasound treatment of locally advanced pancreatic adenocarcinoma: Preliminary experience for pain palliation and local tumor control. Invest Radiol. 2014 Jun 13;49(12):759–65.
57. Marinova M, Feradova H, Gonzalez-Carmona MA, Conrad R, Tonguc T, Thudium M, Becher MU, et al. Improving quality of life in pancreatic cancer patients following high-intensity focused ultrasound (HIFU) in two European centers. Eur Radiol. 2021 Aug;31(8):5818–29. doi: 10.1007/s00330-020-07682-z. Epub 2021 Jan 23. PMID: 33486605.
58. Keane MG, Bramis K, Pereira SP, Fusai GK. Systematic review of novel ablative methods in locally advanced pancreatic cancer. World J Gastroenterol. 2014 Mar 7;20(9):2267–78.
59. Fergadi MP, Magouliotis DE, Rountas C, Vlychou M, Athanasiou T, Symeonidis D, et al. A meta-analysis evaluating the role of high-intensity focused ultrasound (HIFU) as a fourth treatment modality for patients with locally advanced pancreatic cancer. Abdom Radiol (NY). 2022 Jan;47(1):254–64. doi: 10.1007/s00261-021-03334-y. Epub 2021 Oct 31. PMID: 34718835.
60. Zhao H, Yang G, Wang D, Yu X, Zhang Y, Zhu J, et al. Concurrent gemcitabine and high-intensity focused ultrasound therapy in patients with locally advanced pancreatic cancer. Anticancer Drugs. 2010 Apr;21(4):447–52.
61. Ji Y, Zhu J, Zhu L, Zhu Y, Zhao H. High-intensity focused ultrasound ablation for unresectable primary and metastatic liver cancer: Real-world research in a Chinese tertiary center with 275 cases. Front Oncol. 2020 Oct 29;10:519164. doi: 10.3389/fonc.2020.519164. PMID: 33194582; PMCID: PMC7658544.
62. Machtinger R, Inbar Y, Ben-Baruch G, Korach J, Rabinovici J. MRgFUS for pain relief as palliative treatment in recurrent cervical carcinoma: A case report. Gynecol Oncol. 2008 Jan;108(1):241–3.
63. Wu F, Wang Z-B, Chen W-Z, Bai J, Zhu H, Qiao T-Y. Preliminary experience using high intensity focused ultrasound for the treatment of patients with advanced stage renal malignancy. J Urol. 2003 Dec;170(6 Pt 1):2237–40.
64. Lei T, Guo X, Gong C, Chen X, Ran F, He Y, et al. High-intensity focused ultrasound ablation in the treatment of recurrent ovary cancer and metastatic pelvic tumors: A feasibility study. Int J Hyperthermia. 2021;38(1):282–7. doi: 10.1080/02656736.2021.1889698. Erratum in: Int J Hyperthermia. 2021 Sep;38(2):103. PMID: 33612045.
65. Imseeh G, Giles SL, Taylor A, Brown MRD, Rivens I, Gordon-Williams R, ter Haar, et al. Feasibility of palliating recurrent gynecological tumors with MRGHIFU: Comparison of symptom, quality-of-life, and imaging response in intra and extra-pelvic disease. Int J Hyperthermia. 2021;38(1):623–32. doi: 10.1080/02656736.2021.1904154. PMID: 33882792.

66. Staruch R, Huisman M, Ladouceur-Wodzak M, Chhabra A, Chopra R. 3D MR neurography targeted peripheral nerve ablation with MR-guided high intensity focused ultrasound (MR-HIFU): Initial results of a feasibility study in a swine model. J Ther Ultrasound. 2015;3(Suppl 1):74–7.
67. Woolf CJ. Central sensitization: Implications for the diagnosis and treatment of pain. Pain. 2011 Mar;152(3 Suppl):S2–15.
68. McDannold N, Clement GT, Black P, Jolesz F, Hynynen K. Transcranial magnetic resonance imaging-guided focused ultrasound surgery of brain tumors: Initial findings in 3 patients. Neurosurgery. 2010 Feb;66(2):323–32.
69. Martin E, Jeanmonod D, Morel A, Zadicario E, Werner B. High-intensity focused ultrasound for noninvasive functional neurosurgery. Ann Neurol. 2009 Dec;66(6):858–61.
70. Jeanmonod D, Werner B, Morel A, Michels L, Zadicario E, Schiff G, et al. Transcranial magnetic resonance imaging-guided focused ultrasound: Noninvasive central lateral thalamotomy for chronic neuropathic pain. Neurosurg Focus. 2012 Jan;32(1):E1–11.
71. Monteith SJ, Medel R, Kassell NF, Wintermark M, Eames M, Snell J, et al. Transcranial magnetic resonance-guided focused ultrasound surgery for trigeminal neuralgia: A cadaveric and laboratory feasibility study. J Neurosurg. 2013 Mar;118(2):319–28.
72. Schlesinger D, Benedict S, Diederich C, Gedroyc W, Klibanov A, Larner J. MR-guided focused ultrasound surgery, present and future. Med Phys. 2013 Aug;40(8):080901.
73. Lee SK, Dawson J, Lee J a, Osman G, Levitin MO, Guzel RM, et al. Management of cancer pain: 1. Wider implications of orthodox analgesics. Int J Gen Med. 2014 Jan;7:49–58.
74. Afsharimani B, Cabot P, Parat M-O. Morphine and tumor growth and metastasis. Cancer Metastasis Rev. 2011 Jun;30(2):225–38.

Index

U

V

W

For Product Safety Concerns and Information please contact our
EU representative GPSR@taylorandfrancis.com Taylor & Francis
Verlag GmbH, Kaufingerstraße 24, 80331 München, Germany